Severe Stress and Mental Disturbance in Children

Severe Stress and Mental Disturbance in Children

Edited by

Cynthia R. Pfeffer, M.D.
Professor of Psychiatry
Cornell University Medical College
Chief, Child Psychiatry Inpatient Unit
The New York Hospital—Westchester Division
White Plains, New York

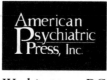

Washington, DC
London, England

Note: The authors have worked to ensure that all information in this book concerning drug dosages, schedules, and routes of administration is accurate as of the time of publication and consistent with standards set by the U.S. Food and Drug Administration and the general medical community. As medical research and practice advance, however, therapeutic standards may change. For this reason and because human and mechanical errors sometimes occur, we recommend that readers follow the advice of a physician who is directly involved in their care or the care of a member of their family.

Copyright © 1996 American Psychiatric Press, Inc.
ALL RIGHTS RESERVED
Manufactured in the United States of America on acid-free paper
99 98 97 96   4 3 2 1
First Edition

American Psychiatric Press, Inc.
1400 K Street, N.W., Washington, DC   20005

Library of Congress Cataloging-in-Publication Data
Severe stress and mental disturbance in children   /   edited by
   Cynthia R. Pfeffer.   —   1st ed.
       p.   cm.
   Includes bibliographical references and index.
   ISBN 0-88048-657-0
   1. Stress in children. 2. Psychic trauma in children.
I. Pfeffer, Cynthia R.
[DNLM: 1. Stress, Psychological—in infancy & childhood.
2. Mental Disorders—infancy and childhood. 3. Mental
Disorders—etiology. 4. Child Development. 5. Models,
Psychological. WS 350 S498 1996]
618.92′89—dc20   Library
DNLM/DLC
for Library of Congress   University of Texas   95-23086
                             at San Antonio   CIP
British Library Cataloguing in Publication Data
A CIP record is available from the British Library.

Contents

Section I

Neurodevelopmental and Neurobiological Models of Stress in Human and Nonhuman Subjects

Section II

Sudden Unexpected Trauma

Section III

Relationship Between Medical
Illness and Stress

Section IV

Suicide as Stressor and as Mediator of Stress

Section V

Abuse and Its Traumatic Impact

Section VI

Effects of Extreme Stress Factors on Developmental Processes

Contributors

Jack D. Barchas, M.D.
Barklie McKee Henry Professor and Chairman, Department of Psychiatry, Cornell University Medical College; Psychiatrist-in-Chief, The New York Hospital, New York, New York

Jacqueline A. Bartlett, M.D.
Associate Professor of Clinical Psychiatry and Director, Consultation/Liaison Service, University of Medicine and Dentistry of New Jersey, New Jersey Medical School, Newark, New Jersey

Seema Bhatnagar, M.Sc.
Doctoral Student, Developmental Neuroendocrinology Laboratory, Douglas Hospital Research Center, Department of Neurology and Neurosurgery, McGill University, Montreal, Quebec, Canada

Richard D. Bingham, M.D.
Assistant Professor of Psychiatry, University of Colorado School of Medicine; Medical Director, Day Treatment Program, The Children's Hospital, Denver, Colorado

David A. Brent, M.D.
Professor, Child Psychiatry, University of Pittsburgh; Chief, Division of Child and Adolescent Psychiatry, Western Psychiatric Institute and Clinic, Pittsburgh, Pennsylvania

Gene H. Brody, Ph.D.
Research Professor of Child and Family Development, The University of Georgia, Athens, Georgia

Dimitri A. Christakis, M.D.
Psychiatric Resident, Children's Hospital and Medical Center, University of Washington, Seattle, Washington

David C. Clark, Ph.D.
Professor of Psychiatry and Psychology, Director, Center for Suicide Research and Prevention, Rush Institute for Mental Well-Being, Rush-Presbyterian–St. Luke's Medical Center, Chicago, Illinois

Billie F. Corder, Ed.D.
Co-Director, Psychological Services, Dorothea Dix Hospital, Raleigh, North Carolina

Melissa K. Demetrikopoulos, M.S.
Department of Neurosciences, Graduate School of Biomedical Sciences, University of Medicine and Dentistry of New Jersey, Newark, New Jersey

Esther Elizur, Ph.D.
Family Therapist and Head of the Research Staff, Kibbutz Child and Family Clinic, Tel Aviv, Israel

Spencer Eth, M.D.
Assistant Professor of Psychiatry, University of California, Los Angeles, School of Medicine; Clinical Associate Professor of Psychiatry, University of Southern California School of Medicine; Associate Chief of Staff, VA Medical Center, Los Angeles, California

Victor Fornari, M.D.
Associate Professor of Clinical Psychiatry, Cornell University Medical College; Director of Training and Clinical Services, North Shore University Hospital–Cornell University Medical College, Manhasset, New York

Jared Fuss, M.D.
Instructor in Psychiatry, Cornell University Medical College; Physician-in-Charge, Child and Adolescent Psychiatry Consultation-Liaison Service, North Shore University Hospital–Cornell University Medical College, Manhasset, New York

William T. Garrison, Ph.D.
Associate Professor of Psychiatry, Behavioral Sciences and Pediatrics, The George Washington University; Chairperson, Department of Psychology, Children's National Medical Center, Washington, D.C.

Harris A. Gelbard, M.D., Ph.D.
Assistant Professor, Department of Neurology, University of Rochester School of Medicine, Rochester, New York

Carol A. Glod, Ph.D., R.N.
Clinical Director, Developmental Biopsychiatry Research Program, McLean Hospital, Belmont, Massachusetts

Ann E. Goebel, B.A.
Graduate Student, Department of Psychology, Boston University, Boston, Massachusetts

Thomas M. Haizlip, M.D.
Professor of Psychiatry, University of North Carolina School of Medicine, Chapel Hill; Associate Chair for Division of Child and Adolescent Psychiatry, Dorothea Dix Hospital, Raleigh, North Carolina

Fady Hajal, M.D.
Associate Professor of Clinical Psychiatry, Cornell University Medical College; Associate Director of Training Child and Adolescent Division, Chief, Adolescent Inpatient Service, The New York Hospital—Westchester Division, White Plains, New York

Robert J. Harmon, M.D.
Professor of Psychiatry and Pediatrics, Director, Division of Child and Adolescent Psychiatry, University of Colorado School of Medicine, Denver, Colorado

John K. Hickey, D.S.W.
Assistant Commissioner, Nassau County Department of Mental Health, Mental Retardation and Developmental Disabilities, Nassau, New York

J. Dee Higley, Ph.D.
Senior Staff Fellow, Laboratory of Clinical Studies, Primate Unit, National Institute on Alcohol Abuse and Alcoholism, National Institutes of Health, Bethesda, Maryland

Nancy L. Hornstein, M.D.
Assistant Clinical Professor, Department of Psychiatry and Behavioral Science, University of California, Los Angeles, California

Beth Houskamp, Ph.D.
Associate Professor, Marriage and Family Therapy, Azusa Pacific University, Azusa, California

Yutaka Ito, M.D.
Research Fellow in Child Psychiatry, Harvard Medical School and McLean Hospital; Clinical Assistant Professor, Department of Pediatrics, Tokyo Womans Medical College, Tokyo, Japan

Mordecai Kaffman, M.D.
Medical Director and Chief Psychiatrist, Kibbutz Child and Family Clinic, Tel Aviv, Israel

Sandra Kaplan, M.D.
Associate Professor of Clinical Psychiatry, Cornell University Medical College; Associate Chairman, Department of Psychiatry, Director, Child and Adolescent Psychiatry, North Shore University Hospital–Cornell University Medical College, Manhasset, New York

Anne E. Kazak, Ph.D.
Associate Professor, University of Pennsylvania School of Medicine; Director, Psychosocial Services, Division of Oncology, The Children's Hospital of Philadelphia, Philadelphia, Pennsylvania

Steven E. Keller, Ph.D.
Professor of Psychiatry, Associate Professor of Neurosciences, University of Medicine and Dentistry of New Jersey, New Jersey Medical School, Newark, New Jersey

Mary Klinnert, Ph.D.
Assistant Professor, Division of Pediatric Psychiatry, National Jewish Center for Immunology and Respiratory Medicine, Denver, Colorado

Richard P. Kluft, M.D.
Clinical Professor of Psychiatry, Temple University School of Medicine; Senior Attending Psychiatrist and Director, Dissociative Disorders Program, The Institute of Pennsylvania Hospital, Philadelphia, Pennsylvania

Sylvie Larocque, B.Sc.
Research Assistant, Developmental Neuroendocrinology Laboratory, Douglas Hospital Research Center, Montreal, Quebec, Canada

Laura Liotus, B.S.
Systems Analyst, University of Pittsburgh Medical Center, Western Psychiatric Institute and Clinic, Pittsburgh, Pennsylvania

Cheryl M. McCormick, Ph.D.
Post-Doctoral Fellow, Developmental Neuroendocrinology Laboratory, Douglas Hospital Research Center, Montreal, Quebec, Canada

Michael J. Meaney, Ph.D.
Associate Professor, Departments of Psychiatry and Neurology and Neurosurgery, McGill University; Director, Developmental Neuroendocrinology Laboratory, Douglas Hospital Research Center, Montreal, Quebec, Canada

Grace Moritz, A.C.S.W.
Project Coordinator, Peers of Adolescent Suicide Victims Study, University of Pittsburgh Medical Center, Western Psychiatric Institute and Clinic, Pittsburgh, Pennsylvania

David A. Mrazek, M.D., F.R.C.Psych.
Professor of Psychiatry and Pediatrics, George Washington University Medical Center; Chairman of Psychiatry, Children's National Medical Center, Washington, D.C.

Eileen Neubaum, M.S.
Research Coordinator, Department of Child and Family Development, The University of Georgia, Athens, Georgia

Linda Packman, C.S.W.
Psychiatric Social Worker, Division of Child and Adolescent Psychiatry, North Shore University Hospital–Cornell University Medical College, Manhasset, New York

Cynthia R. Pfeffer, M.D.
Professor of Psychiatry, Cornell University Medical College; Chief, Child Psychiatry Inpatient Unit, The New York Hospital—Westchester Division, White Plains, New York

Elizabeth T. Pinner, B.A.
Department of Psychology, New School for Social Research, New York, New York

Paul M. Plotsky, Ph.D.
Professor, Department of Psychiatry and Behavioral Sciences, Emory University, Atlanta, Georgia

Frank W. Putnam, M.D.
Senior Clinical Investigator, Laboratory of Developmental Psychology, National Institute of Mental Health, National Institutes of Health, Bethesda, Maryland

Robert S. Pynoos, M.D., M.P.H.
Associate Professor, Department of Psychiatry and Biobehavioral Sciences, University of California, Los Angeles; Director, University of California, Los Angeles, Program in Trauma, Violence, and Sudden Bereavement, Los Angeles, California

Fred Schiffer, M.D.
Clinical Instructor, Harvard Medical School; Attending Psychiatrist, McLean Hospital, Belmont, Massachusetts

Steven J. Schleifer, M.D.
Professor and Chairman of Psychiatry, University of Medicine and Dentistry of New Jersey, New Jersey Medical School, Newark, New Jersey

Nola Shanks, Ph.D.
Post-Doctoral Fellow, Developmental Neuroendocrinology Laboratory, Douglas Hospital Research Center, Montreal, Quebec, Canada

Shakti Sharma, B.Sc.
Research Assistant, Developmental Neuroendocrinology Laboratory, Douglas Hospital Research Center, Montreal, Quebec, Canada

James Smythe, Ph.D.
Post-Doctoral Fellow, Developmental Neuroendocrinology Laboratory, Douglas Hospital Research Center, Montreal, Quebec, Canada

Margaret L. Stuber, M.D.
Assistant Professor of Psychiatry and Behavioral Sciences, University of California, Los Angeles, California

Stephen J. Suomi, Ph.D.
Chief, Laboratory of Comparative Ethology, National Institute of Child
Health and Human Development, National Institutes of Health,
Bethesda, Maryland

Peter E. Tanguay, M.D.
Ackerly Professor of Child and Adolescent Psychiatry, Division of Child
and Adolescent Psychiatry, Department of Psychiatry and Behavioral
Sciences, University of Louisville, Louisville, Kentucky

Martin H. Teicher, M.D., Ph.D.
Associate Professor of Psychiatry, Harvard Medical School; Director,
Developmental Biopsychiatry Research Program, Hall Mercer Center
for Children and Adolescents, McLean Hospital, Belmont, Massachusetts

Victor Viau, M.Sc.
Doctoral Student, Developmental Neuroendocrinology Laboratory,
Douglas Hospital Research Center; Department of Neurology and
Neurosurgery, McGill University, Montreal, Quebec, Canada

Introduction

Cynthia R. Pfeffer, M.D.

In our current technological society, people experience intense and complex stressful events at all stages of the life cycle. There is a consensus that stress experienced early in life may have a profound impact on processes of development and social adaptation. Remarkably, the nature of stress and its immediate and long-term sequelae are not well understood or characterized. The major aim of this text is to describe features of stress as important etiologically relevant components of acute and chronic mental disturbance in children and adolescents.

Selye (1956) coined the term "disease of adaptation" to indicate the effects of stress on health. In the decades subsequent to his research, there have been major advances in the identification, classification, and methodology of study of psychiatric symptoms and disorders in children. For example, many clinical, research, and social policy issues have been discussed regarding childhood depression and suicidal behavior, posttraumatic stress disorder (PTSD), and dissociative disorders. This book integrates insights about how problems such as these are associated with events that were and continue to be experienced as stressful.

Knowledge has been rapidly acquired about the vast changes in epidemiological and sociocultural trends that are especially pertinent to youth. Illustrative of this rapid acquisition of knowledge is the attention that has been focused on accidents, homicide, and suicide, the three leading causes of death among youth (National Center for Health Statistics 1993). Together, they accounted for 77.5% of the 36,733 deaths in 1990 in the United States for youth of ages 15 to 24 years (National Center for Health Statistics 1993). The increased prevalence of suicide, violence, and depression, especially among youth born after World War II, appears to reflect cohort effects (Klerman 1989). Specific etiological factors for these birth cohort effects have not been identified. However, it is notable that these effects are not discernible from stressful period effects involving the changing sociocultural patterns of recent decades. In addition, the rise in tragic deaths among youth has been associated with sociocultural features such as increased availability of lethal agents such as firearms (Fingerhut and Kleinman 1989a) and motor vehicles (Fingerhut and Kleinman 1989b). Other social changes that appear to have adversely affected children and adolescents in the last several decades are increased divorce rate, heightened family mobility and disruption, and elevated prevalence in the abuse of illicit substances. Sophisticated technology applied in daily life to enhance travel or to provide complex medical procedures for assessment and treatment may be related to processes of stress that mediate the evolution of widespread increase in specific mental disturbances among youth.

Innovative, reliable psychiatric research methodologies in the study of correlates of normal and abnormal human development have burgeoned. Scientific inquiry and the use of advanced technology in the field of neuroscience foreshadow an explosion of knowledge about psychosocial, neuroanatomical, and neurophysiological development, and about etiological factors of psychopathology and neurobiological abnormalities. Applications of complex techniques for genetic research will make it possible to explore gene–environment interactions at a microscopic level involving cellular and intracellular mechanisms and to explore the macroscopic sphere regarding the longitudinal course of mental disturbance of children who have genetically based disorders. Given this immensely noteworthy progress, especially in areas related to child and adolescent psychiatry, it is timely to reevaluate what information exists about the impact of stress on children's development and abnormalities in these processes. This book offers a comprehensive view on topics important to those embarking on new phases of inquiry and clinical activities linking child development and mental disturbance in children who experience severe stress.

This book focuses on many of the concepts described above and has several major goals. Incorporating the insights of leading scholars on facets of stress pertinent to children and adolescents, this text attempts to synthesize clinical application involving psychiatric diagnostic nosology and treatment with an understanding of the definition, characterization, and sequelae of stress and the effects of these sequelae on the acute and long-term course of mental disturbance in children. Comprehensive clinical descriptions of PTSD, dissociative disorder, depression, and suicidal behavior as sequelae of severe stress are provided. This book presents theoretical models and empirically tested paradigms involving animal and human subjects and the use of neurobiological techniques that are important for an understanding of the developmental processes that are affected by stress. Stress-related aberrations of attachment and coping responses to stress that are determined, in part, by temperamental traits and social competence are explicitly detailed in the context of the rapid and extensive unfolding processes of development of human toddlers and nonhuman primates. The effects of stress on complex patterns of hormonal responses and the impact of hormonal variations on brain development, especially in the hippocampal neuronal region, are elucidated by descriptions of elegant neuroendocrine studies of stress-induced changes in hypothalamic-pituitary-adrenal axis hormones in young rodents. Innovative inquiry of brain electrophysiology (by use of electroencephalographic monitoring) in abused children highlights an important paradigm of how experiential factors contribute to limbic and cortical development of the brain.

This book describes situations that are considered to be stressful modifiers of the development of children. Among the more intense and universally stressful events are accidents, suicide, and violent and sexual abuse. In addition, new areas of research—for example, that of the stressful effects of sophisticated medical technology in the treatment of childhood life-threatening illnesses—are explored. The book illustrates genetic contributions to stress response patterns in discussions of chronic medical illnesses such as asthma, diabetes mellitus, and cancer. The book describes the immunological changes related to stress that are associated with depressive symptomatology. The book contains discussions of clinical approaches that are useful when one is attempting to understand and reduce the acute and prolonged sequelae of psychosocial stress in children, such as reactions to death, divorce, or adoption, and to cope with the complexities of organizing community resources when faced with the unexpected trauma of catastrophic violence, natural disasters, or airplane crashes.

A multitude of implications of the work discussed in this book—especially the importance of early identification of severely stressful states and the immense need for effective prevention techniques—are pertinent for the development of health care policy. Concepts that can guide national research priorities to support promising psychosocial and biological studies involving validating the relations between severe stress and mental disturbance in children can be gleaned from this book. Implicit in the emphasis in this book is the importance of integrating scientific inquiry with social policy planning. It is hoped that the knowledge gained from reading this book will stimulate innovative scientific research and foster effective clinical work that will be beneficial to children and their families.

Acknowledgments

Appreciation is extended to Hong Jiang, M.D., M.P.H., and Jerilyn H. Ferrante for excellent administrative assistance in preparation of this volume.

References

Fingerhut LA, Kleinman JC: Mortality among children and youth. Am J Public Health 79:899–901, 1989a

Fingerhut L, Kleinman JC: National Center for Health Statistics: trends and current status in childhood mortality, United States 1900–85. Vital and Health Statistics Ser 3, No 26. Washington, DC, U.S. Government Printing Office, 1989b

Klerman GL: Suicide, depression, and related problems among the baby boom cohort, in Suicide Among Youth: Perspectives on Risk and Prevention. Edited by Pfeffer CR. Washington, DC, American Psychiatric Press, 1989, pp 63–81

National Center for Health Statistics: Advance report of final mortality statistics, 1990. Monthly Vital Statistics Report, Vol 41, No 7, Suppl. Hyattsville, MD, National Center for Health Statistics, Public Health Service, 1993

Selye H: The Stress of Life. New York, McGraw-Hill, 1956

Prologue

Jack D. Barchas, M.D.

This volume is an important and valuable monograph that continues and expands a long-standing tradition in our field. The scientific study of the psychological impacts of severe stress has been a deep concern of American psychiatrists for half a century. The work of Erich Lindemann, based on his clinical experiences with survivors of a Boston fire, provided an early framework for the study of stress in adults (Lindemann 1979). The behavioral patterns of persons under stress were examined through time, and a new language dealing with the effects of stress was developed and has profoundly influenced our thinking and approach to patients.

Investigation of a variety of intense stressors was a major theme of the work of David and Beatrice Hamburg, who, in a pioneering set of studies, investigated environmental alterations ranging from leukemia to starting college. (This research provided the framework for the ideas and findings presented in Hamburg 1970.) The Hamburgs' particular focus was on coping styles and the ways in which individuals adapt and grow. Many of the persons studied established such adaptive patterns even in situations that the participants and others viewed as horrific. Common threads were seen through a diversity of stresses. This tradition of research has been continued by other scholars such as Ellen Frank in her consideration of the ways in which the psychological trauma of physical assault in women is handled and the processes that lead to better outcomes (Frank et al. 1988).

The issue of the effects of stress on children has received less satisfactory consideration despite the clear implications that stress is associated in some way with mental disorders and psychological suffering. The present volume performs a valuable service by bringing together literature on specific types of stress. Its emphasis on the *form* of stress is particularly interesting at this early phase of the enterprise. By emphasizing the form of stress and not prematurely committing to the implications of severity, the book encourages us to consider patterns of response. In addition, each stressor has its own set of clinical issues, and these are best addressed by a categorical approach. A future edition may therefore be organized around a quite different approach to the description of the stressors.

This volume highlights the broad range of scientific disciplines that are necessary for the study of stress and adaptation. We need knowledge in many areas and in the convergence of these areas, and this volume illuminates many aspects of such intersections. Biological and psychosocial research are important in this arena, and most critical is their interaction. In both the biological and the psychosocial disciplines we require more information about the cascade of effects of stress through time and development.

Although the biology of stress has been studied for decades, contemporary tools permit us to consider the patterns of change in ways that could only have been dreamed of by Selye and his colleagues (J. D. Barchas et al. 1978; Hyman and Nestler 1993). For example, from molecular neurobiology we are learning of changes in the expression of genes that respond within minutes to environmental perturbations. Stress activates the formation of the products of specific genes. These products in turn influence cellular processes at multiple levels. The complex set of steps in the cascade that leads to gene expression, protein formation, and alteration of eventual physiological and behavioral response will be continuing subjects for future investigation. We have just gained some of the necessary tools for studying the fundamental mechanisms—for example, the formation of messenger RNA can now be examined in single cells or a small group of cells. From such research it can be expected that we will find that the interaction of stress with developing systems is critical and influences the performance of organisms in the longer term. Such information is directly relevant to the study of stress in children and adolescents and to the study of severe mental disorders (J. D. Barchas et al. 1994a, 1994b).

Equally important are the detailed cascades of the psychosocial aspects of stress. Ultimately these will be linked to the cascades of biological events. Through time we can expect that one of the disciplines that will emerge is *sociophysiology,* the study of the interrelationships between social behavior and physiology (P. Barchas 1976, 1984; P. Barchas and Mendoza 1984). Many stressors arise in the context of social interactions. Social behavior, even that of daily life (e.g., establishment and maintenance of social hierarchies, alterations in roles, establishment of norms, conformity, and positive and negative evaluation and stigma), can be expected to exert an impact on physiology.

Although we tend to think of the interactions between social behavior and physiology as being led by physiology, in point of fact the converse may be equally important. Such investigation will require careful analysis of social behaviors and monitoring of endocrine, electrophysiological, brain metabolism, and other parameters. Through such investigations may come a clearer understanding of the ways in which social behavior and social stress have lasting effects. Social interaction may impact physiology and, in the process, alter future behavioral responses to stress. These malleable mechanisms, both behavioral and biological, will each be guided by the other.

It is also apparent that some forms of what we term "stress" may be highly adaptive and valuable for the developing organism. We live with considerable stress, but so too have generations far back; in fact, our evolution took place in the context of what we might consider to be extraordinary stress. Our knowledge base is too limited to formalize completely the relationships between severe stress, illness, and growth, but consideration of such issues will be a part of our developing perspective. From a clinical standpoint there are endless questions. We are all concerned with the issues as to how we can help individuals cope with what appears to be severe stress. Such questions require a wide range of investigation at a psychological level.

Many other types of studies will also be salient in the future for the study of severe stress in childhood. Substantial information on our current knowledge, as well as glimmerings of many future studies, is presented in this volume. The knowledge summarized in this book will be of enormous value to clinicians and will aid investigators as they develop a framework for the next generation of research.

References

Barchas JD, Akil H, Elliott GR, et al: Behavioral neurochemistry: neuroregulators and behavioral state. Science 20:964–973, 1978

Barchas JD, Faull KF, Quinn B, et al: Biochemical aspects of the psychotic disorders, in Basic Neurochemistry, 5th Edition. Edited by Siegel GJ, Agranoff BW, Albers RW, et al. New York, Raven, 1994a, pp 959–977

Barchas JD, Hamblin MW, Malenka RC: Biochemical hypothesis of mood and anxiety disorders, in Basic Neurochemistry, 5th Edition. Edited by Siegel GJ, Agranoff BW, Albers RW, et al. New York, Raven, 1994b, pp 979–1001

Barchas P: Physiological sociology: interface of sociological and biological processes. Annual Review of Sociology 2:299–333, 1976

Barchas P (ed): Social Hierarchies: Essays Toward a Sociophysiological Perspective. Westport, CT, Greenwood Press, 1984

Barchas P, Mendoza S: Social Cohesion. Westport, CT, Greenwood Press, 1984

Frank E, Anderson B, Stewart BD, et al: Efficacy of cognitive behavior therapy and systematic desensitization in the treatment of rape trauma. Behavior Therapy 19:403–420, 1988

Hamburg DA (ed) Psychiatry as a Behavioral Science. Englewood Cliffs, NJ, Prentice-Hall, 1970

Hyman SE, Nestler EJ: The Molecular Foundations of Psychiatry. Washington, DC, American Psychiatric Press, 1993

Lindemann E: Beyond Grief: Studies in Crisis Intervention. New York, Jason Aronson, 1979

Section I

Neurodevelopmental and Neurobiological Models of Stress in Human and Nonhuman Subjects

Chapter 1

Effect of Reactivity and Social Competence on Individual Responses to Severe Stress in Children: Investigations Using Nonhuman Primates

J. Dee Higley, Ph.D.
Stephen J. Suomi, Ph.D.

Study of Severe Stress in Human Children

Humans, like other animals, are highly adapted to respond to the day-to-day challenges and stress that they encounter. In response to such challenges, normally, individuals exhibit coping behaviors designed to marshal their psychological and emotional resources to eliminate or overcome the challenges that they face. Less frequently, stress is severe and at times threatens individual well-being. Traditionally, the initial response to severe stress has been called the "fight or flight response," a term that refers to the reaction of the central and peripheral nervous systems to stimuli that pose a danger to the individual. Typically, this response to threats or fear consists of internal changes that increase cardiovascular output, muscle tone, alertness, hormone output, and energy resources—changes that prepare an individual for swift actions to eliminate the present danger. This response is phylogenetically ancient, present in virtually all mammalian species, and is evident in small children and infants. Stressors, however, vary in intensity, and individuals vary in their capacity to cope with stressors. When stressors exceed the coping resources of an indi-

3

vidual or are prolonged, adverse health consequences and psycho-pathology may result. Understanding and predicting individual dif-ferences in the capacity to cope with stress could help produce treatment and prevention programs to ameliorate personal suffering and reduce the monetary cost to modern society.

The adverse consequences that result from stress are not limited to adults. Children are affected both emotionally and physically by stress. Researchers studying psychopathology and psychosomatic dis-orders have long recognized the roles that stress can play in producing behavior problems in children (Ainsworth et al. 1978; Biederman et al. 1990; Bowlby 1980; Kagan et al. 1991; Melamed and Siegel 1985; Trad 1987; Widom 1989), particularly when the stressors are severe or prolonged (Burt 1943; Dunsdon 1941; Freud and Dann 1951; Rut-ter 1979; Udwin 1993; Yule and Udwin 1991; Yule et al. 1990). Fur-thermore, it is also widely recognized that adult psychopathology frequently results from prolonged or severely stressful experiences that occurred earlier in life (Bifulco et al. 1991; Breier et al. 1988; Brown et al. 1986; Harris et al. 1986, 1987; Higley et al. 1992a, 1994; Hinde and Spencer-Booth 1971a, 1971b; Kraemer 1992; Suomi and Ripp 1983).

To reduce or eliminate distress in children, as well as prevent adult psychopathology, it is crucial that we understand how severe stress affects children and the developmental process. It is the thesis of this chapter that individual differences in the capacity to cope with stress are based, at least in part, on one's genetic background and prior ex-periences, particularly experiences that occur early in life, and that each of these factors affects or modifies the central nervous system (CNS) to change how the individual responds to future stressors. Us-ing findings from nonhuman primates, we will discuss three under-lying themes in this chapter that concern how infants and children respond to stress:

1. How the response to stress differs according to age and develop-mental status.
2. How same-aged individuals respond to identical stressors. It is our thesis that their response is based on two enduring tem-peramental traits. One, *individual reactivity,* affects the inten-sity of reactions to stress, and a second, parallel trait, *social competence,* affects coping styles. Social competence is based on the capacity to obtain and utilize social support. These two

traits affect how individuals approach and eliminate the stressors that they face.

3. How interindividual differences in both experiences and genetic background organize the CNS, which in turn affects and controls individuals' unique response at each step of development to the different stressors and challenges that they face.

For the purposes of this chapter, *stress* will be defined as the emotional response that results from an aversive event or stimulus. Stress, in this definition, is differentiated from a *stressor,* which is the stimulus that provokes the emotional response. The behaviors that are used as a method to eliminate the aversive emotional state are termed *coping responses.* Coping responses vary in their effectiveness—that is, some coping responses are less effective than others. Indeed, some coping responses may reduce emotional stress or anxiety but fail to effectively eliminate the stressor. For example, some young monkeys frequently suck their thumbs or toes under conditions of high stimulation or anxiety. This behavior has been shown to reduce tension and arousal in human infants (Rovee and Levin 1966). Although the immediate short-term effect of self-orality is a reduction of arousal and anxiety, if an infant has lost its mother, self-orality as a coping response will not elicit maternal return. This is an example of a less effective or even a maladaptive coping response. In contrast, an infant emitting high-pitched distress cries or using its limited motor skills to regain contact with its mother is less effective in the short-term at reducing arousal (indeed this coping response may even increase arousal), but these behaviors are clearly more effective coping behaviors than self-orality because they tend to elicit maternal solicitude and contact. It is also important to note that even when a stressor is equivalent for two individuals, differences in coping capacities are likely to produce differences in stress reduction.

Nonhuman Primates in the Study of Severe Stress

Because it is not possible to induce severe stress in children, systematic study of cause-and-effect relationships and developmental outcomes is difficult and frequently not possible. As a result of these methodological difficulties, many investigators have turned to animal models to assess and study how stress affects development, and the factors that place individuals at risk or protect them from developing psychopathology. Because their genetic backgrounds and early experiences can be closely controlled, nonhuman primates are ideal research subjects in the investigation of the effects of severe stress on adaptation in childhood and subsequent adult psychopathology. (For recent discussions of how primates have been used to study the effect of stress on development, cf. Higley 1985; Higley and Suomi 1989; McKinney 1988; Suomi 1991.) Indeed, some of the most important research findings in the study of how severe stress affects children and the long-term effect of such stress have come from longitudinal investigations of developing nonhuman primates.

Nonhuman primates are widely used as research subjects to study stress and development also because of their close genetic relationship with humans. For example, rhesus macaques, perhaps the most widely used nonhuman primate species in stress research, share between 92% and 94% of their genetic material with humans (Goodman and Lasker 1975; Kohne 1975; Koop et al. 1989; Sarich 1985; Sibley and Ahlquist 1987; Sibley et al. 1990). As a result of this close genetic relationship, rhesus macaques' CNS organization, function, and development closely parallel those of humans (Diamond and Goldman-Rakic 1989; Diamond et al. 1989; Gibson 1991; Goldman-Rakic 1987; Uylings and van Eden 1990). Such similarities to humans in complex CNS function enable nonhuman primates to live in large social groups (there may be over a hundred individuals in an typical rhesus monkey society) with highly evolved social networks and interchanges. As a result of the large social networks that infants are born into, nonhuman primates, particularly our closest phylogenetic relatives the Old World primates, are highly adapted to live in social groups.

Nevertheless, for a wide variety of primates, including humans, the greatest risk to physical well-being is typically from other conspecifics. Indeed, Cheney and colleagues (Cheney and Seyfarth 1990; Cheney et al. 1986) advance "competition between conspecifics" as the major factor influencing the evolution of primate intelligence and their advanced CNS. For example, with the exception of human encroachment, for a number of different primate species the most frequent cause of adolescent and adult wounding and even death is aggression by other troop members or intraspecies-related resource competition (Brain 1992; Dittus 1977a, 1977b, 1980; Hrdy 1977; Reynolds 1991; Southwick and Siddiqi 1977; Wheatley

1991). Moreover, as in humans, the risk is greater for males than for females (Brain 1992). For a few species high rates of infanticide are not unusual (Hrdy 1977). A consequence of this highly complex social life is that for most Old World primates, as for humans, under normal conditions, social stressors produce the greatest stress.

Although the day-to-day stressors that humans usually face in modern society vary in kind, most can be understood as pertaining to one of three general categories: loss of a loved one (either through death or divorce), a change in social relationships (including movement into new social settings or communities or the addition of a new family member), and interpersonal conflicts (including arguments, threats, or physical violence). Similarly, for most immature Old World nonhuman primates, loss or separation from family members, a change of social networks such as movement into a new social group or birth of an infant, and threats of or direct physical violence from other members of the nonhuman primate society constitute the three major stressors. In nonhuman primates, as in humans, how an immature individual faces and copes with these stressors can determine whether social adjustment and normative development will ensue. A crucial task of development is the acquisition of the behaviors and skills necessary to cope with social challenges and threats. These behaviors are controlled by the developing CNS, and normative early experiences stimulate normative CNS growth (Greenough 1987). Experientially based changes in the CNS are directly related to how individuals approach and cope with subsequent stressful challenges (Kraemer 1992). Moreover, these challenges vary with the developmental status of the young primate.

In Old World monkeys the primary caregiver is usually the mother, although, as in humans, males are also capable and in many species contribute, in some way, to the care of infants (Higley and Suomi 1986). The infant's mother is responsible for satisfaction of most of the infant's needs; as the infant matures, however, it becomes more and more self-reliant and, eventually, assumes responsibility for independently acquiring the resources and social support necessary for it to survive and to take its place in the social group. As the infant matures, the stressors it faces change and, accordingly, the behaviors it uses to cope with these changing stressful conditions develop and change. For example, the coping skills used in adolescence and adulthood are frequently seen in juvenile play bouts where they may be safely practiced under the mother's protection (Lindburg 1971;

Symons 1978). Whereas in infancy and childhood individuals seek their mothers, during adolescence they are more likely to attempt to cope with stress by active approach and problem solving, or avoidance and escape, or possibly, in the case of social stressors, by soliciting allies or responding with aggression (Higley 1985; Higley et al. 1994). As juveniles and young adolescents, monkeys are no longer able to use infantlike ventral clinging and maternal-directed orality as solutions to stressful stimuli and problems. Instead, these individuals must learn to seek social support and allies to defend their resources and alleviate anxiety. During late childhood and early adolescence, male and female roles diverge, producing somewhat different stressors and different methods of successfully coping with the stressors that the two sexes face. In most Old World primate species, males typically migrate from the family troop to a new and unfamiliar social setting. Females, on the other hand, typically remain in their family group and must integrate themselves into the adult social dominance hierarchy where they may face the prospect of diminished social ranking and preparation for child rearing.

Development of Coping Skills in Early Infancy

The normative sequence of development for rhesus monkeys follows a specific pattern of behavior change and developmental milestones. Initially, like most primates (including humans), infant rhesus monkeys are profoundly altricial; they are inextricably tied to their mother for their physical and psychological needs. As a result of these needs, the infants' first responses are social in nature. At birth, they exhibit reflexive clinging that is used to maintain contact with their mother as she provides physical warmth, nourishment, proprioceptive stimulation, and social interaction. Infants spend a large percentage of their early months clinging to their mother's ventrum (Berman 1980a, 1980b; Harlow and Harlow 1965; Hinde and Simpson 1967). When clinging, infants tightly clasp their mother with their hands, arms, and feet, and they typically place their mother's nipple in their mouth, behaviors that also allow the infants to meet their psychological needs for security and psychological warmth. This behavior profile declines across the early part of the first year, but the behaviors may be again activated even in older monkeys under conditions of fear or anxiety (Harlow 1969; Harlow and Harlow 1965; Harlow and Zimmerman 1959; Higley and Suomi 1989; Hinde and Simpson 1967; Hinde and Spencer-Booth 1971b). Ventral clinging to one' s mother is a primitive behavioral response seen across a wide number of Old World primate species, most likely reflecting the pressures that natural selection has imposed upon them as well as other adaptive functions (Higley and Suomi 1986).

At birth, the altricial neonate primate faces a number of physical challenges and potential stressors. The major developmental task of this period is to maintain homeostasis. The infant's first experience with stress typically occurs when its physical needs are not filled and a state of arousal occurs that motivates the infant to elicit care. Infants are preprogrammed with rather simple behaviors that allow them to cope with this state of arousal by eliciting care from their mothers. For example, when an infant loses contact with its mother's nipple, initially the rooting reflex allows it to cope with relocating the nipple, and the sucking reflex allows it to both fix and obtain nourishment (Harlow and Harlow 1965). When the infant is cold or uncomfortable, it both cries and performs a stereotyped jerking movement known as a "gecker" (Lindburg 1971). At this age, infants deprived of these basic needs for a prolonged period seldom survive. Mothers tenaciously defend and care for their infants, although other relatives (and in some species adult males) may provide social support. Mothers provide specific stimuli that serve to integrate their infant's preprogrammed behaviors in a coherent, organized response system, thus allowing the infant to maintain physiological and psychological homeostasis. In both human and nonhuman primates, maintaining arousal within an optimum range is believed to be crucial for normative emotional development and for a secure attachment to form (Mason 1978; Sroufe 1990). In the absence of the mother, the infant's capacity to maintain homeostasis is disturbed and the infant initiates a number of coping responses known as protest behaviors that are designed both to elicit maternal return and, in the interim, to maintain vigilance and preserve energy resources. These coping responses are organized into an orderly system of behaviors known as a *protest response* (Mineka and Suomi 1978), which includes increased distress vocals, locomotor activity, stress hormone output (e.g., adrenaline and cortisol), heart rate, and CNS monoamine activity (Boccia et al. 1992; Breese et al. 1973; Capitanio et al. 1986; Gunnar et al. 1980, 1981; Higley et al. 1992b; Kraemer et al. 1991; Rasmussen and Suomi

1989; Reite et al. 1978a, 1978b, 1981a; Scanlan 1988; Suomi et al. 1989; Wiener et al. 1990). Successful coping elicits the caregiver's return so that the infant can regain contact with the caregiver, resulting in a return to homeostasis.

Separation and Loss

Initially, infants are buffered from social stressors such as aggression and interpersonal conflict by their mothers (Berman 1980a, 1980b), although at times an infant may be injured when its mother is attacked by other group members. As infants develop and become more and more independent, mothers are quick to defend their infants when threatened. As a consequence of the buffering effects of maternal protection, infancy is perhaps the most stress-free period of life for most young primates. Perhaps the major, rare exception to this is when an infant is separated from its mother for a prolonged period or when its mother dies. When the initial protest response fails to elicit maternal return, a coping failure results and many of the homeostatic functions that mothers serve to organize break down. When the infant no longer has access to the caregiver, sleep patterns, thermoregulation, immune competence, and autonomic nervous system function become dysregulated (Boccia et al. 1989; Laudenslager et al. 1982, 1990; Reite and Short 1981, 1983; Reite et al. 1981a, 1981b).

Prolonged separation from or loss of the caregiver is one of the most potent stressors that a young infant may experience. If maternal death occurs prior to weaning, the infant usually dies, and even when an orphaned infant is old enough to obtain solid food and provide for its physical needs, stress-related deaths are not uncommon (Dolhinow and Murphy 1983). Studies investigating infants that survive such losses show that the development of the CNS is altered (Higley et al. 1991b, 1991c, 1992b; Kraemer and Clarke 1990; Kraemer et al. 1989), resulting in arrested behavioral development and pathological or diminished coping responses (Capitanio 1986; Capitanio and Reite 1984; Capitanio et al. 1986; Champoux et al. 1989; Higley and Suomi 1989; Higley et al. 1988; Hinde and Spencer-Booth 1971a; Kraemer and McKinney 1979; Suomi and Ripp 1983; Suomi et al. 1970). For example, infants reared with peers but without adult females typically show monoamine deficits, altered hypothalamic-pituitary-adrenal regulation, and autonomic nervous system dysregulation (Champoux 1988a, 1988b; Champoux et al. 1989; Higley and Suomi 1989; Higley et al. 1991c, 1992b) and increased predisposition for long-term psychopathology (Higley and Suomi 1989; Suomi et al. 1970). This condition is further aggravated for these infants because as orphans they fail to acquire the self-regulation and social skills with which to effectively cope with social challenges, resulting in increased frequency of childhood stress (Dolhinow and Murphy 1983; Higley and Suomi 1989; Stevenson-Hinde and Simpson 1980). Under normal conditions, the infant matures and develops the capacity to self-regulate such that subsequent short-term separations become less stressful; indeed, such separations are a normative part of developing independence and self-reliance.

As the infant develops self-reliance, short-term separation, both in feral and in laboratory environments, becomes increasingly frequent, and the infants become increasingly capable of coping with these brief separations. Nevertheless, the infants still perceive these separations as stressful. For example, while engaging in courtship behaviors during the breeding season, mothers leave their infants behind in trees or with the infants' older siblings while they consort with males, or, as another example, in the laboratory mothers and infants may be briefly separated for medical treatments. Indeed, in free-ranging troops of monkeys during the height of the breeding season (i.e., October and early November), the sounds of infants vocalizing to elicit maternal return are ubiquitous (J. D. Higley, personal observations, October 1991). Laboratory studies show that even when social separations occur after weaning, juvenile monkeys still respond intensely to the separation stressor exhibiting protest behaviors, hypothalamic-pituitary-adrenal activation, and CNS monoamine activation (Higley et al. 1991b, 1991c, 1992b). Studies have indicated that although prolonged social separation from an attachment source is highly stressful, one effective means of coping with social separation is to elicit social support from other monkeys. Infants that obtain social support from a familiar figure during separation are less likely to experience stress-related deaths (Dolhinow and Murphy 1983), distress cries (Coe et al. 1978; Gunnar et al. 1980; Higley et al. 1992a), behavioral depression (Boccia et al. 1991; Laudenslager et al. 1990; Rosenblum 1971; Rosenblum and Kaufman 1968), severe heart rate change (Caine and Reite 1981; Reite et al. 1989), and stress hormone elevations (Gunnar et al. 1980).

Attachment and Security

As the infant grows older, its motor skills improve rapidly and drastically, and it begins to leave its mother's ventrum to explore and investigate its surroundings. The infant's first exploration forays are brief, but with advancing age and increased motor skills, the time away from the mother increases. Mothers play a critical role during this period as the young primate learns to independently regulate its arousal and emotions. Self-regulation of arousal is a basic skill that the infant must learn during this period of development. As the infant leaves its mother's breast to explore its environment, the mother serves as a secure base from which the infant explores and returns, where the infant obtains psychological warmth and security. These "yo-yo–like" episodes function to teach the infant how to modulate its own internal arousal and anxiety. When the infant is overaroused, afraid, or threatened, it returns to its mother, where through physical contact its anxiety and arousal are reduced. Over repeated episodes, the infant learns to modulate its own emotional arousal, a fundamental coping skill that forms the basis of how to approach future challenges.

Research using nonhuman primates has played an important role in demonstrating the methods and mechanisms by which caregivers are able to reduce the infant's arousal and thus provide psychological warmth and security. Perhaps the most important among those mechanisms, particularly for young infants, is physical contact (Harlow 1958). Harlow referred to the reduction of arousal that resulted from physical contact and the resulting security "contact comfort." In his classic work with surrogate mothers, Harlow showed that physical contact is of central importance for the infant to acquire the capacity to regulate its emotions and exhibit emotional stability (Harlow 1958; Harlow and Harlow 1965). Studies using nonhuman primates were instrumental in demonstrating that physical contact reduces arousal and anxiety (Candland and Mason 1968; Harlow 1958). This reduction of stress through physical contact is phylogenetically old and is present in a wide variety of species, from rodents (Hofer 1987; Pauk et al. 1986; Schanberg and Field 1987) to higher primates (Candland and Mason 1968; Harlow 1958), including humans (Field 1986; Field et al. 1986; Schanberg and Field 1987). For example, premature human infants stimulated with tactile/kinesthetic contact such as stroking and passive arm movements by hospital personnel exhibit evidence of accelerated physical development, when compared with nonstimulated control infants. They also show evidence of facilitated CNS development—for example, increased activity and alertness during observations of behavior states; more mature habituation; orientation; and an increased range of state behaviors on the Brazelton scale (Field 1986; Field et al. 1986; Schanberg and Field 1987). Animal studies suggest that these more mature responses may be due to potentiated CNS development and increased secretion of growth hormone (Pauk et al. 1986; Schanberg and Field 1987).

The study of nonhuman primates has also aided in understanding the importance of other types of experience for normative CNS functioning and behavioral development. As mothers transport their infants they provide motion and vestibular stimulation. This variable appears to play an important role in proper development of the CNS and, as a consequence, affects the infant's capacity to cope with stress. Furthermore, this early stimulation appears to have long-term consequences on the adolescent and young adult's capacity to cope with stress. For example, Mason used inanimate surrogate mothers to control the types of experiences to which infants were exposed and to investigate the role that motion and vestibular stimulation play in developing emotional stability. He found that when other variables were held constant, infants reared on inanimate stationary surrogate mothers were less likely to explore and investigate their surroundings, exhibited more arousal and fearfulness, and exhibited more maladaptive methods to cope with their arousal than infants reared by surrogate mothers that moved (Eastman and Mason 1975; Mason and Berkson 1975). Infants reared on stationary surrogate mothers also appeared to be less capable of discriminating between differences in social cues and stimuli (Eastman and Mason 1975; Mason and Berkson 1975; Wood et al. 1979). As these infants—those reared on stationary surrogate mothers and those reared by surrogate mothers that moved—grew to adolescence and adulthood, Mason and colleagues paired them with opposite-sexed wild-born stimulus monkeys and observed their social behaviors (Anderson et al. 1977). Perhaps as a consequence of their failure to discriminate between social cues and between stimuli, males reared on stationary surrogate mothers were less likely to respond appropriately to wild-born females' social cues, resulting in increased aggression and attacks from the female stimulus animals; on the other hand, the young adult males reared by moving surrogate mothers were more likely to vary their behaviors according to the stimulus females' social cues and behaviors (Anderson et al. 1977). For both sexes, the stressor of the social tests produced more maladaptive coping responses, such as self-directed responses and stereotyped rocking behaviors, in the subjects reared on stationary surrogate mothers than in the subjects reared by moving surrogate mothers. When the young adult female subjects that had been reared on stationary surrogate mothers were paired with a wild-born stimulus male, they were less likely than females reared by moving surrogate mothers to initiate social contact, be approached, and engage in physical contact with the wild-born adult male with whom they were paired, and more likely to be threatened and attacked by the adult male (Anderson et al. 1977). These findings suggest that for the proper development of normative stress coping skills and arousal regulation, vestibular stimulation is of crucial importance. They also suggest that specific input during the formation of the CNS is integral for normative emotional regulation and that early experiences are crucial to long-term outcomes of adult coping skills and vulnerabilities.

These and similar findings from nonhuman primate studies were instrumental in the development of attachment theory (Bowlby 1969). Attachment behavior is markedly similar in developmental sequence and behavioral patterning across the primate order (Higley and Suomi 1986). Bowlby reviewed this and outlined in considerable detail the similarities between human and nonhuman primate attachment behavior (Bowlby 1969). Similarities in attachment are due at least in part to shared evolutionary ancestry and genetic material (Goodman and Lasker 1975; Kohne 1975; Koop et al. 1989; Sarich 1985; Sibley and Ahlquist 1987; Sibley et al. 1990). However, researchers have also found that the quality of mother-infant offspring relations shows consistent individual differences both within species and within specific rearing conditions (J. Altmann 1980; Higley and Danner 1988; Higley et al. 1992a; Lee 1986; Mason and Capitanio 1988; Nash and Wheeler 1982).

Attachment is a process by which an infant learns to use specific caregivers who possess stimulus features such as contact comfort, warmth, and motion as secure bases from which to obtain physical contact and contact comfort. This use of a secure base results in psychological security. As the infant's cognitive capabilities mature, it begins to respond selectively to one figure and organizes its behaviors according to its caregiver's responses. As the caregiver repeatedly responds to the infant's overarousal in a reliable and sensitive manner, a secure attachment results (Ainsworth et al. 1978; Bowlby 1969; Sroufe 1990). Mothers differ, however, in their response and sensitivity to their infants. Although all infants are innately predisposed to form an attachment bond with a mother or surrogate who provides contact comfort and other stimuli characteristic of adult females, the quality of that attachment bond varies according to the mother's treatment of the infant. There is evidence that among nonhuman primates, caregivers who respond inappropriately or insensitively produce anxious attachment relationships with their infants. For example, rhesus monkeys abused by their mothers are more likely to show anxious attachment-like social preferences. Sackett and colleagues (1967) found that in novel environments, infants who had been abused by their mother spent over twice as much time in close proximity to their abusive mother as normally reared infants did with their mother. In addition, when Mason and colleagues (1975, 1978, 1988) raised rhesus monkey infants either with an inanimate unresponsive surrogate mother or with surrogate mothers who provided contingent motion, or relatively more responsive canine surrogates, they found that the infants reared with responsive surrogates, of either type, were more likely to find comfort from their surrogate and explore both in novel environments and in the presence of strangers than were the infants raised with inanimate unresponsive surrogates.

Failure to reliably and sensitively respond to the infant's need for homeostasis results in a less secure attachment (Ainsworth et al. 1978; Bowlby 1969) and impairs the infant's capacity to respond to stress in the future (Bretherton and Waters 1985). This incapacity to respond to stress is believed to occur because the atachment bond becomes a prototype relationship that the infant uses to form future relationships with other individuals. Infants who fail to obtain secure attachment relationships with their caregivers have difficulties with future relationships (J. Altmann 1980; Higley et al. 1994), and experience additional stress through their relationships with other individuals (Sackett et al. 1967; Higley et al. 1994).

Some of the best indications of what happens to an infant when its caregiver fails to provide a consistently secure base for normative attachment development comes from studies of monkeys raised with mothers whose capacity to respond sensitively to their infant is circumscribed by experimental demands, or by rearing monkeys with caregivers who lack the social sophistication to respond contingently and sensitively to their infant's needs. To test the effect of maternal responsiveness on attachment sensitivity and infant development, Rosenblum and his colleagues (Andrews and Rosenblum 1991a; Rosenblum and Paully 1984), in an ingenious series of experiments, manipulated the daily foraging demands that mothers experienced. They placed mother-infant pairs in environments that forced the mothers to spend either prolonged or minimal portions of the day foraging for their daily food rations, hypothesizing that as each mother's available time was restricted by her need to obtain nourishment, her capacity to respond to her infant's needs would likewise be limited and less contingent on the infant's needs. To vary the predictability of the mother's response, a third experimental group was added for whom the environmental foraging demands varied in an unpredictable fashion (i.e., the foraging demands to find food were altered biweekly to force either high or low foraging demands on the mother). As predicted, when mothers were less accessible in the high foraging demand environment, infants made more efforts to obtain contact and increased the total amount of time that they spent in physical contact with their mother than did infants in the low foraging demand setting. Even more profound, however, was the behavior of the infants reared in the varied foraging demand setting. Relative to infants in both the low and the high foraging demand settings, these infants spent even more time in close contact with their mother, decreased their levels of social play, and exhibited behaviors characteristic of despair that are usually seen only in monkeys that are undergoing a prolonged social separation stressor. As predicted by attachment theory (Bowlby 1969), when these infants were provided with the challenge of exposure to a novel setting, they were less likely to leave their mother to explore the environment (Andrews and Rosenblum 1991a).

Other studies also have shown that the mother-infant attachment bond is less secure when an infant is reared by a mother that fails to respond to its needs in a sensitive fashion and to provide a secure base to reduce arousal. For example, Suomi and colleagues (1983) found that after infants underwent a series of separations from their mother, they were more likely to cling to and stay in close proximity to their mother than were a control group of infants that had been allowed to remain with their mother. Following the separations, both groups of infants were removed from their mothers and placed together as an all-peer group. Six months later, when both groups were given the opportunity to interact with their mothers in a social preference test, the infants who had been repeatedly separated from their mothers avoided close proximity to their mother, whereas the nonseparated control infants actively sought their mother and spent more time in close proximity. Other research has found also that social separation leads to more anxious-like mother-infant attachment bonds (Hinde and Spencer-Booth 1971a, 1971b). Similarly, infants with multiple mothers (i.e., infants who are rotated to a different mother-caregiver every 2 weeks) demonstrate little preference for their own mother (Sackett et al. 1967). On the other hand, as previously discussed and similarly to human infants (Schneider-Rosen et al. 1985), nonhuman primate infants that have been abused show excessive social preference and close proximity to their mother (Sackett et al. 1967). Both infants with multiple mothers and infants abused by their mothers are less interested in peer relations (Sackett et al. 1967) and show more inappropriate and less mature peer-related behavior (Arling and Harlow 1967; Sackett et al. 1967). It should also be noted that mothers that exhibit inappropriate maternal protectiveness, precluding infant investigation via restraint and retrieval during minimally challenging stimuli, produce infants that are less interested in the external environment, as measured by the percentage of time they spend orienting and visually investigating their surroundings (Fairbanks and McGuire 1988). As these restricted infants develop, they are more fearful and take longer to investigate novel environments than do juveniles who had less protective mothers (Fairbanks and McGuire 1988).

A second indication of the importance of a secure attachment for developing coping skills comes from studies of monkeys raised with other infants but without adults. Although these peer-only–reared monkeys form attachment bonds between themselves, infant agemates lack the psychological sophistication to respond sensitively to each other's needs and fears; thus, although these peer-only–reared infants are less fearful in their attachment figure's presence than in its absence, there is evidence that they are still more fearful than mother-reared infants under comparable conditions. For example, as predicted by some investigators (Sroufe 1979), peer-only–reared subjects are less likely to explore their environment and engage in social play even under conditions of minimal stress; instead, they are more likely to engage in high levels of infantlike ventral–ventral clinging, increased distress vocals, and closer proximity to the age-mate whom they have chosen as their attachment figure (Higley and Danner 1988; Higley et al. 1992a). When such intimate contact is provided, they are less able to find comfort and recover (Chamove et al. 1973; Harlow 1969). When these subjects are tested in a novel environment resembling that used in the Ainsworth Strange Situation procedure, they are less likely to explore the setting and interact with other adult monkeys, and more likely to exhibit distress cries, than are mother-reared infants (Higley and Danner 1988; Higley et al. 1992a). Compared with subjects reared by their mothers, peer-only–reared monkeys are highly fearful both as yearlings and as 2-year-olds in the absence of threatening stimuli, and in the face of a prolonged stressor such as social separation, they are more likely to exhibit behaviors characteristic of despair (Higley and Suomi 1989). There is evidence that these differences persist into early adulthood. Whereas mother-reared monkeys stop exhibiting infantlike clinging by late childhood and adolescence (Hinde and Simpson 1967), peer-reared monkeys continue to exhibit ventral clinging even as adolescents (Higley 1985). Furthermore, in a more recent study, 22 young adult rhesus monkeys (8 peer-reared and 14 mother-reared, 60 months of age), were tested prior to and after being removed from their social group. Removal occurred four times, with each separation lasting 4 days. Although there were fewer differences in behavior during the nonstressful baseline periods than when they were infants, during periods of the social separation stressor, the peer-reared monkeys were more likely to show regressive, infantlike behaviors such as self-orality and self-clasping (Higley et al. 1991c).

Studies of human infants have noted that insecure attachment bonds in infancy adversely affect early childhood development in numerous ways, including deficits in positive affect, emotional stability, self-reliance and resourcefulness, and future peer relations, and impaired cognition (e.g., see Bretherton and Waters 1985 for reviews of the effect of nonsecure attachment bonds). Bowlby (1973) and others (Sroufe 1983) have predicted that these deficits in early attachment relations portend subsequent risk for psychopathology, particularly depression and anxiety, not only in childhood but into adolescence and adulthood as well. Studies of human psychopathology have linked depression, as well as drug and alcohol problems, to dysfunctional parent–offspring relations (Brook et al. 1984; Hawkins et al. 1992; Holmes and Robins 1987, 1988). Similarly, in nonhuman primates, the severity of the despair response during separation is correlated with mother-infant relationship problems (Hinde and Spencer-Booth 1971a), and the risk for developing depression, as well as the risk for excessive alcohol consumption, is greater in peer-only–reared monkeys than in mother-reared monkeys (Higley and Suomi 1989; Higley et al. 1991a, 1992a; Kraemer and McKinney 1979; Kraemer et al. 1991). Attachment bonds play a crucial role in the development of the skills to cope with stress. From this attachment bond, the infant primate learns self-regulation and how to form other relationships that it can use as a buffer to ameliorate the effects of future stressful experiences and challenges.

Deficits in coping responses and increased fear in peer-reared monkeys may be a result not only of insecure attachment bonds. Adults also serve a crucial function by acting as social references for infants and children so that the latter can gauge the potential risk from novel and uncertain social stimuli. Studies with humans indicate that in infants and toddlers, a primary response to unfamiliar or uncertain stimuli is the use of the emotional expression of another individual to interpret the safety or danger of the situation. This is called *social referencing* (Feinman 1985; Klinnert et al. 1983). Perhaps because of their familiarity to the infants and their capacity to reduce other fears, caregivers are most often used by human infants as social referents (Zarbatany and Lamb 1985). Because of their experiences and knowledge, adults are capable of providing clear cues as to the degree of danger (and potential pleasure) or safety of individuals who are strangers to infants and young children. Nonhuman primate infants and juveniles are also capable of using the emotional cues that adults provide to process new and novel stimuli (Andrews and Rosenblum 1991b; Feinman 1985; Mineka et al. 1984; Plimpton et al. 1981). However, when peer-only–reared monkeys use other infants to interpret the safeness of a novel environment, the response of their infant age-mate social referent is most likely similar to their own—that is, uncertainty or fear; hence, unlike the adult referent who can reduce the infant's arousal and provide security to the infant in uncertain situations, the immature infant referent is unlikely to reduce fear and may, in fact, increase the infant's anxiety. A vicious cycle may, in fact, ensue, with one infant providing fearful signals for a second infant, and the second infant, now more fearful because of the first, as a social referent, increasing the anxiety of the first infant, and so forth. Novak (1973) found evidence for this effect in peer-reared infants. She exposed juvenile monkeys who had been reared with either an inanimate surrogate, their mother, or only peers to an uncertain, potentially fearful stimulus. The infants were accompanied by their respective attachment source (surrogate, mother, or age-mate) during the stimulus. Inanimate surrogates are unable to exhibit fearful expression, and hence, as might be expected, surrogate-reared juveniles exhibited minimal fear; the mother-reared juveniles exhibited intermediate fear, and the peer-only–reared subjects exhibited the greatest amount of fear. (Similarly, in another study, vervet monkeys whose mothers spent excessive amounts of time directing "worried" visual glances at their infants exhibited increased anxiety and arousal [Fairbanks and McGuire 1988].) Thus the differences between the groups may also lie in a fundamental difference in adults' and immature attachment figures' capacity to provide emotional signals to indicate safety in the face of uncertainty.

Other variables may affect the developing infant's capacity to cope with stressors in its environment. As with studies of rats reared in enriched environments (Greenough 1987), monkeys reared in environments that are physically enriched show less fear and increased problem solving in the face of stressful challenges (Champoux et al. 1990). This increased adaptiveness in the face of stressful challenges may be in part because the infant learns about cause-and-effect relationships. Such experiences are postulated to affect the infant's expectations concerning its capacity to solve future challenges as they arise. In human terms, they may learn "If first I don't succeed, try again." In a test of this hypothesis, infants were reared in one of two conditions: they either had controlled access to rewards such as food and sweet treats or received the same number and type of treats, but on a noncontingent basis. When the two groups were subsequently tested in a number of stressful challenges, the infants reared with the capacity to maintain control over their environment exhibited less fearful behavior and were more likely to explore and actively manipulate their environment than were the monkeys reared without control over their environment (Mineka et al. 1986). Interestingly, however, when the stressful challenge was severe (as during a social separation), the group differences disappeared (Mineka et al. 1986).

Effect of Early Experiences on the Central Nervous System and Their Role in Determining Subsequent Responses to Stress

Caregivers play an important role in organizing and facilitating CNS growth and development. It is probably no accident that many of the milestones in myelination and neuronal connections correspond to developmental milestones in the mother-infant relationship (e.g., weaning, independence, stranger fear, etc.) (Gibson 1991; Goldman-Rakic 1987; Lawrence and Hopkins 1976). More recently, Kraemer (1992) discussed the importance of the attachment bond for normative CNS development and for adaptive strategies for responding to stress. He outlined how normative attachment organizes an infant's CNS, particularly the noradrenergic system. Within Kraemer's model, attachment failures become more than behavior difficulties; attachment failures result in diminished CNS norepinephrine function and result in a diminished CNS capacity to cope with stress.

Consistent with this model, subjects with attachment failures are more likely to have low levels of cerebrospinal fluid (CSF) norepinephrine and to exhibit depression and helplessness (Kraemer 1986; Kraemer and Clarke 1990; Kraemer and McKinney 1979; Kraemer et al. 1989, 1991). In addition to the evidence that nonhuman primates reared in impoverished environments possess diminished concentrations of CSF norepinephrine, there is also some evidence that nonhuman primates that exhibit excessive behavioral responses to stress and increased anxiety possess excessive norepinephrine activity; high concentrations of the norepinephrine end-product 3-methoxy-4-hydroxyphenylglycol (MHPG) are found in individuals who are more likely to exhibit high levels of behavioral withdrawal (Higley et al. 1990, 1991a, 1991b, 1991c; Kraemer and McKinney 1979; Redmond et al. 1986). Similarly, Redmond and colleagues (Redmond 1987; Redmond et al. 1976) found that stimulating the major noradrenergic cell bodies in the locus coeruleus of stumptail macaques resulted in behaviors characteristic of fear and behavior withdrawal. Other studies by his group demonstrated that pharmacologically increasing or decreasing norepinephrine concentrations resulted in parallel increased or decreased displays of behavioral withdrawal (Redmond 1987). Thus, while the direction and nature of the relationship is less well understood, it appears that the noradrenergic system is involved in stress coping and that early mothering experiences that affect self-regulation of arousal and stress coping behaviors diminish the noradrenergic system's capacity to respond to future stressors.

The organization of the stress hormones is also altered by early experiences that reduce a monkey's capacity to cope with stress. Peer-reared monkeys exhibit increased plasma concentrations of the stress hormone cortisol and the peptide that stimulates its release, ACTH (adrenocorticotropin). Even when infants who had been removed from their mothers at birth were reared in the nursery by surrogate mothers that provided nourishment, motion, heat, and contact comfort, at 30 days of age these infants' plasma cortisol concentrations were elevated and plasma growth hormone concentrations were diminished relative to those of mother-reared control infants (Champoux et al. 1989). Cortisol concentrations remained elevated at 6 and 18 months of age both during baseline and during stressful conditions (Higley et al. 1992b). Two years later, as young adults, when faced with stressful conditions, these same peer-reared monkeys exhibited higher plasma concentrations of ACTH and cortisol (Higley et al. 1991c). It is noteworthy that the young adult peer-reared monkeys were also more likely to abuse alcohol than were the mother-reared monkeys (Higley et al. 1991a).

From Attachment to Independence: Social Cognition, Social Inhibition, and Social Dominance

As the young primate continues to develop, its mother begins to play a less central role in its development, and peers become a major force in organizing behavior and social development. Nevertheless, mothers are still quick to respond to threats to their offspring and are the primary individual to protect their juvenile offspring (Berman 1980b; Bernstein and Ehardt 1985; Cheney 1977; Netto and van Hooff 1986). Developing independence from one's mother is a major task of this developmental period. Achieving independence from the mother occurs primarily because of the infant's increased motor capabilities and its motivation to explore the environment and interact with age-mates through play. The mother, however, takes an active role in promoting independence by leaving her infant while it plays and punishing and rejecting the infant's attempts to obtain ventral contact (Higley and Suomi 1986). Without the mother's active involvement in promoting independence and self-reliance, prolonged dependency and infantlike clinging may continue into adolescence (Higley 1985; Higley and Suomi 1989). The process of weaning is challenging, but the stress the infant experiences during this period is a normal part of development; the infant learns to cope with anxiety and arousal in a relatively safe setting in which social support from other family and group members is readily available.

The next major developmental milestone that a maturing primate undertakes involves the process of adopting adult roles and forming social bonds with the individuals with whom it will live. Two of the primary methods juveniles use to form these bonds are *social grooming* and *social play*. Although social grooming clearly serves hygienic purposes (it cleans the coat and fur), a number of studies have shown that its major function is to promote social interaction. It is clear that nonhuman primates relish being groomed (Goosen 1981). Social grooming, particularly among adults, is the most frequent and widespread behavior that most nonhuman primates use to express affection and social attraction. In infancy, reciprocal grooming is infrequent, although mothers may at times groom infants. However, as infants become juveniles and young adolescents, social grooming begins to form a more central aspect of social life, particularly for females. Social play, particularly in young males, is one of the most frequent juvenile social behaviors among some species. Play increases young primates' capacity to cope with stress by allowing immature individuals to practice skills requisite to their future adult roles and to increase their social sophistication in a safe setting, while at the same time allowing them to develop social bonds with other individuals whom they may call upon for aid or support in future stressful challenges (Janus 1992; Lee 1983). Both kinship and same-sex social bonds formed during juvenile grooming and play interactions are long-lasting and form the basis of subsequent preferred social interactions (Abegglen 1984; Bernstein et al. 1974; Chism 1978; Erwin and Flett 1974; Erwin et al. 1975; Fedigan 1982; Hansen et al. 1966; Janus 1992; Noë 1986; Owens 1975). As in humans, social support functions as an important force for ameliorating stress both in infants and in juveniles (Berman 1980a; Bernstein and Ehardt 1986; Caine and Reite 1981; Cheney 1977; Chism 1978; Noë 1986; Rosenblum and Kaufman 1967).

Although play undoubtedly serves a wide variety of purposes (Smith 1982), a number of researchers have suggested that the most important function that play serves is in the development of appropriate use and inhibition of aggression (Higley et al. 1994; Ruppenthal et al. 1974; Suomi 1979). For example, as adolescents and young adults, monkeys who were deprived or limited in their opportunities to play are likely to exhibit excessive aggression in situations that call for a mild response (Alexander 1966; Alexander and Harlow 1965;

Kondo et al. 1981) or to exhibit inappropriate submissive communication signals when they are threatened by a more dominant or dangerous animal (Kondo et al. 1981; Møller et al. 1968). Subjects deprived of opportunities to play also demonstrate deficits in perceiving social cues. They may, for example, miss important social signals and emotional expressions that indicate a specific response is required (Møller et al. 1968). As a result of these deficits, these individuals as adolescents and young adults ultimately exhibit less competent social skills, thus adding to the potential for increased stressful episodes in the future (Alexander 1966; Alexander and Harlow 1965; Kondo et al. 1981). It is also noteworthy that peer relations have therapeutic effects on nonhuman primates reared in impoverished environments and can be used to reverse most of the deficits that resulted from such rearing (Novak 1979; Novak and Harlow 1975; Suomi 1972; Suomi et al. 1974).

Stressful experiences may also inhibit the acquisition of socially competent behaviors by limiting the levels of play to which a juvenile primate is exposed and the potential partners with whom the individual can form a relationship. For example, a number of studies have shown that in individuals who have been separated from their mothers or in orphans, play decreases considerably in the short term (Dolhinow 1981; Dolhinow and Murphy 1983; Mineka and Suomi 1978; Mineka et al. 1981; Suomi et al. 1970, 1976) and remains attenuated in the long term, when compared with play in nonseparated control subjects (Capitanio and Reite 1984; Hinde and Spencer-Booth 1971a). During periods of stress due to limited food, threats from other hostile troops, inclement weather, or intragroup tension, play is limited and may even stop entirely (Baldwin and Baldwin 1973, 1976; Lee 1983; Loy 1970; Oliver and Lee 1978; Richard 1974; Zimmerman et al. 1975). Prolonged exposure to these and other stressful experiences may prevent or limit both play opportunities and the range of partners with whom individuals can form playful relations and form social bonds. Juveniles reared by low-ranking mothers are kept in close physical contact, resulting in limited social interactions (Tartabini et al. 1980). A direct consequence is that low-ranking monkeys initiate and participate in play bouts less frequently, and with fewer partners, than juveniles reared by higher-ranking mothers (J. Altmann 1980; Cheney 1978a, 1978b; Tartabini and Dienske 1991), whereas high-ranking juveniles are preferred and sought more frequently as play partners (J. Altmann 1980; Cheney 1978a, 1978b; Gouzoules 1975).

Having a low-ranking mother may also contribute to other forms of stress for developing individuals because low-ranking juveniles are more likely to be attacked by other monkeys and are less likely to receive aid from other troop members (J. Altmann 1980; Berman 1980a; Cheney 1977; Datta 1986; Janus 1991; Netto and van Hooff 1986). On the other hand, even when high-ranking infants are not aided by other associates, they are less likely to exhibit fear when they are threatened by other individuals (Berman 1980a).

Sex-role differences in how males and females approach stressful events and stimuli begin to emerge following infancy. For juvenile males, the bonds that are formed during play episodes are of crucial import later in life when they are forced to move into new societies. Whereas juvenile females direct most of their social play and grooming behaviors to a small nucleus of troop members, juvenile males play with a larger network of individuals, including unrelated age-mates and age-mates from other troops (Hausfater 1972; Symons 1978; Vessey 1968). In many ways these sex differences portend future differences in social roles. For many Old World primate species, the society is formed around matrilineal families headed by a grandmother, her daughters, and her daughters' offspring. As discussed previously, whereas females remain with their natal group to form these matrilines, for most Old World species, males leave their natal troop to join a new troop at puberty (Pusey and Packer 1987).

The capacity to cope with these gender-related role differences is based at least in part on these early interactions. In what appears to have some function in building relationships with males with whom they will interact later in life, among species in which males migrate to new troops, males are more likely than females to play and interact with numerous different individuals, both within and outside of their natal troop (Owens 1975; Packer 1979; Symons 1978; Vessey 1968), and are more likely than females to play with older monkeys (Abegglen 1984; Caine 1979; Cheney 1978a; Fedigan 1972; Hayaki 1985; Lindburg 1971; Owens 1975; Symons 1978). Females, on the other hand, play with fewer partners (Bramblett and Coelho 1987; Cheney 1978b), seldom play with individuals in other troops (Cheney 1978b; Ehardt and Bernstein 1987; Symons 1978; Vessey 1968), and exhibit less aggressive play (S. A. Altmann 1968; Harlow 1969; Janus 1991; Lindburg 1971; Symons 1978). Instead, juvenile females groom more often and exhibit more of their social behaviors to their own family with whom they spend their life (S. A. Altmann 1968; Berman 1982; Capitanio and Reite 1984; Cheney 1977; Ehardt and Bernstein 1987) and, perhaps in preparation of their future role as mothers, are intrinsically more interested in (Chamove et al. 1967) and spend more time interacting with infants (Cheney 1978a, 1978b; Higley and Suomi 1986; Lancaster 1971; Lindburg 1971) than do males. In addition, when female juveniles are threatened by other conspecifics, they are more likely to form defensive coalitions with other females within their group than are males (Cheney 1977; Lindburg 1971). Also, when females form long-lasting relationships with other, unrelated females, it is virtually always within their own troop (Ehardt and Bernstein 1987; Sade 1966). In addition, among females, social grooming is more often directed at female infants and juveniles both by kin and by unrelated individuals within a female's social troop (Loy and Loy 1987).

Migration to a new troop is a dangerous and highly stressful event for young males. Wounding and death are not uncommon (J. Altmann 1980; Dittus 1977a, 1977b; Gartlan 1975; Henzi and Lucas 1980; Ohsawa 1991; Packer 1979; Pusey and Packer 1987; van Noordwijk and van Schaik 1985). With the exception of human encroachment, for a number of different primates the most frequent cause of adolescent and young adult male death is aggression by other monkeys or intraspecies-related resource competition (Brain 1992; Dittus 1977a, 1977b, 1980; Southwick and Siddiqi 1977). Even before young males leave their natal troop, maternal rates of protective intervention may decrease and the rates of aggression the males receive from other natal troop members may increase (Cheney 1978a; Itoigawa 1975). Indeed, Cheney and colleagues (1986), arguing from an evolutionary perspective, assert that the major selective pressure on nonhuman primates is the challenge of competing and interacting with conspecifics.

There is evidence that when males leave their natal troop, they may attempt to cope with the increased stress by utilizing the social bonds that they formed during play and other interactions. When males leave their natal social group to join a new troop, they often leave in the company of friends with whom they have had long-standing relationships (Cheney and Seyfarth 1977; Drickamer and Vessey 1973; Itoigawa 1975; Sugiyama and Ohsawa 1975), and even when they leave by themselves, frequently they emigrate to a troop that friends or older brothers have already joined (Boelkins and Wilson 1972; Colvin 1983a, 1983b, 1986; Itoigawa 1975; Matsumura 1991; Packer 1979). Indeed, just before leaving its natal troop, an adolescent male may increase play relations with individuals in the troop that it will join (Cheney 1981; Matsumura 1991). In one study of male emigration, researchers found that 93% of the male migrants moved into troops to which partners from their previous natal troop had already immigrated (Cheney 1983). After immigrating into these new troops, males spend significantly more time interacting with males from their previous natal troop than with males whom they did not know previous to entering the new troop (Boelkins and Wilson 1972; Packer 1979). Newly immigrated males also use the skills that they have acquired to integrate themselves into the new troop. They may groom the offspring of females or the females themselves; in fact, it is the only time in their adult life when they groom females as often as they are groomed by females (Kaufman 1967). When young migrating males are threatened by conspecifics in a new troop, they form coalitions with their familiar partners to solve aggressive disputes, and as a result they are able to facilitate their integration into the new troop and to obtain high social ranks in a relatively rapid fashion (Meikle and Vessey 1981). Males may also decrease the levels of stress that they experience and increase the probability of remaining in new troops by caring for and forming bonds with male infants born into the new troop into which they immigrate (Breuggeman 1973). For example, the most frequent infant care and affiliative social behaviors shown by adult males are directed at younger males (Breuggeman 1973; Kaufman 1967), and infant care is more likely to be shown to male infants than to female infants (Breuggeman 1973).

Interindividual Differences

In her study of baboons, Smuts (1985) gives examples of two types of young adolescent males who migrate into new troops: one, socially clever and sophisticated, and a second, socially incompetent and oblivious to social cues. In the first case, the young male's interactions with the females in the troop led to his eventual integration and prolonged tenure in the new troop. Smuts describes how this competent male, as he interacted with the females, maintained a constant awareness of the females' state and the social signals indicating their emotions. If any female appeared nervous, he responded with behaviors designed to alleviate her fears and to elicit social reciprocation. Because of his social adeptness and finesse, within a short time he reversed the social initiation process and the females were actively seeking his company. A male representative of the second, less competent type, on the other hand, seemed somewhat unaware of the social cues that the females exhibited. When the females failed to respond to the male's cues or when they exhibited fearfulness and anxiety, the male chased the females and used aggression to force proximity. Within a relatively short time, the less socially adroit male was expelled from the new troop into which he was attempting to immigrate (Smuts 1985). On the other hand, when Sapolsky (1983) studied this same group of baboons 5 years later, one of these same socially incompetent males was still present in the troop and had gone on to become the male with whom the females were most likely to consort during their period of sexual receptivity.

In still another study of males immigrating into new troops, van Noordwijk (van Noordwijk and van Schaik 1985) found that males that tried to force themselves into new monkeys troops using aggression were more likely to receive wounds and high rates of aggression and, in larger social groups, were less likely to remain in the troop. Similarly, in vervets, Raleigh and colleagues (Raleigh and McGuire 1989) found that males who were approached by and formed coalitions with females were more likely to obtain high standing in their social group and spend time in close social proximity, and less likely to receive aggression from the females.

Individual differences are also present in how young monkeys react to a major stressor such as social separation, with responses ranging from minimal protest to profound depression, illness, and at times even death when intervention is not forthcoming (Dolhinow 1981; Dolhinow and Murphy 1983; Kaufman and Stynes 1978; van Lawick-Goodall 1971). Furthermore, these individual differences in the severity of the response that infant primates exhibit during social separation appear to have traitlike interindividual qualities that exhibit long-term stability. For example, when we investigated individual differences in the response to social separation in peer-reared monkeys, we found that a severe response to separation in infancy was predictive of a severe response in childhood and in early adolescence 3 years later (Higley 1985). A number of other studies have found similar continuity of individual differences in the response to a severe stressor such as social separation (Capitanio et al. 1986; Suomi 1981). These examples of individual differences in both stress-related social behavior and social separation illustrate two important variables: first, there are traitlike individual differences in how individuals approach and attempt to cope with a severe stressor such as migration to a new troop or response to separation from one's attachment source, and, second, these differences can be maintained across major stages of development.

As discussed earlier in this chapter, individual differences in temperament or personality appear to affect how individuals approach and attempt to cope with stress. One personality trait receiving much attention across a wide variety of species is behavioral reactivity (also known as timidity, fearfulness, or behavioral inhibition) (Blizard 1989; Higley and Suomi 1989; Kagan et al. 1989). Reactivity is characterized by prolonged latencies to approach novel objects, excessive fearfulness in new social settings, and behavioral withdrawal to challenging stimuli. In one study of reactivity using rhesus monkeys, two researchers, each blind to the other's methodology and ratings, rated temperament in the same neonatal rhesus monkeys. The correlation between their two ratings was greater than .90 (Higley and Suomi 1989). Four months later, when these same subjects were exposed to a novel environment, the subjects rated as highly reactive took longer to approach and explore a novel but interesting environment and spent more time in close proximity to their surrogate mothers (Higley and Suomi 1989). Neonatal ratings of reactivity were also predictive of the severity of depression in 6-month-old rhesus monkeys undergoing a social separation (Becker et al. 1984), with higher ratings for reactivity correlating positively with the severity of depression seen in the monkeys during the separation. Other researchers have also rated different traits that are related to how nonhuman primates respond to physical and social stress (Raleigh et al. 1989; Stevenson-Hinde and Simpson 1980; Stevenson-Hinde and Zunz 1978) and have shown that these traits are predictive of the response to subsequent stressors.

As the above findings suggest, interindividual differences in temperamental traits related to stress appear to be stable over time and across situations. Indeed, Stephenson-Hinde rated confidence (a trait that, by the definition used in this study, included fearfulness) in juvenile monkeys and found that individual differences exhibited a strong positive correlation over a 4-year period (Stevenson-Hinde and Simpson 1980). Furthermore, these ratings predicted the response to a novel environment, with highly confident juvenile males spending more time exploring and investigating a novel environment than did less confident males (Stevenson-Hinde and Simpson 1980), and highly confident females exhibiting fewer distress cries than did less confident females (Stevenson-Hinde et al. 1980). Higley (1985) found that measures of play and distress during baseline home-cage day-to-day interactions were predictive of the intensity of social separation distress, with low levels of play and high levels of distress correlating with increased behavioral withdrawal and measures of depression during a social separation. Similarly, Reite and colleagues (1981b) found that levels of self-directed disturbance during home-cage nonstressful interactions were predictive of self-directed disturbance behavior during social separation. The converse also appears to be true: Individual differences in the severity of a behavioral response and heart rate levels during a social separation 2 to 5 years earlier are predictive of increased fear and reactivity during future stressors such as exposure to novel environments and new social partners (Capitanio et al. 1986).

Direct behavioral measures of traits related to how one responds to stress also exhibit continuity over time. For example, individual differences in a behavioral measure of sociality, the time that a monkey spends in close proximity to other animals, are strongly correlated between the 6th and 18th month of life, a period roughly corresponding to infancy and childhood in rhesus monkeys (Higley 1985). In addition, individual differences in the time spent in social play are correlated from the 18th to the 30th month of life (early adolescence) in rhesus monkeys (Higley 1985). The time spent in social interactions and close social proximity is strongly correlated with the acquisition of social dominance, a measure of social competence in rhesus monkeys (Higley et al. 1994), suggesting that the capacity to elicit social support is traitlike and exhibits long-term interindividual stability. In a similar fashion, interindividual differences in the response to the stress of social separation show long-term interindividual stability, with the levels of distress and depression during separations in infancy predictive of individual differences during the juvenile years and even into adolescence and early adulthood 3 to 5 years later (Capitanio et al. 1986; Higley 1985). This traitlike response to social separation is also predictive of other psychopathological behavior later in life, such as excessive alcohol consumption (Higley et al. 1991a).

A reoccurring theme in this chapter is that interindividual differences in the CNS underlie the stress-related behavioral differences. Interindividual differences in CNS norepinephrine, dopamine, and serotonin activity have been measured by assaying concentrations of the final product of each neurotransmitter in the CSF obtained from the base of the brain. These differences in neurotransmitter metabolite concentrations, particularly norepinephrine and its end-product MHPG, are correlated with the behavioral response to separation (Higley and Suomi 1989; Higley et al. 1988; Kraemer 1992; Kraemer and McKinney 1979; Kraemer et al. 1983, 1989, 1991). Concentrations of the major serotonin end product, 5-hydroxyindoleacetic acid (5-HIAA), are correlated positively with levels of social behavior and social dominance rankings (Higley et al. 1994; Raleigh et al. 1986, 1989). The correlation between neurotransmitters and behavior appears to be, at least in part, an indication of a cause-and-effect relationship. For example, pharmacological modifications that increase CNS norepinephrine decrease measures of behavioral depression, and, conversely, pharmacological modifications that decrease norepinephrine increase measures of behavioral depression, during social separation (Kraemer 1992; Kraemer and Clarke 1990; Kraemer and McKinney 1979; Suomi et al. 1978). Likewise, treatments that increase serotonin increase the frequency of and competence shown in social behavior, whereas treatments that decrease serotonin decrease the frequency of and competence shown in social behavior (Raleigh 1987; Raleigh et al. 1980, 1986, 1991). As with the behavior and personality traits reactivity and social competence, interindividual differences in the concentrations of the end-products of norepinephrine and serotonin (MHPG and 5-HIAA, respectively) are strongly correlated from infancy through the second and third years of life (Higley et al. 1992b).

Two of the most frequently used biological measures of stress and sympathetic nervous system activation are heart rate and pituitary-adrenal activation. Both the sympathetic nervous system and the hypothalamic-pituitary-adrenal system are controlled, at least in part, by central norepinephrine and serotonin stimulation (Angelucci and Montez 1988; Bennett 1990; Feldman and Quenzer 1984). A number of studies have investigated the relationship between sympathetic nervous system activity and levels of anxiety and distress during a social separation. Reite and colleagues (1981a, 1981b) found that individual differences in heart rate during home-cage nonstressful baseline periods were positively correlated with individual differences in the same measures during a social separation. Other measures of sympathetic nervous system arousal, such as body temperature, alpha waves, and sleep states, also exhibited daily interindividual stability (Reite et al. 1981a, 1981b). In a series of studies investigating heart rate changes and anxiety (Higley and Suomi 1989; Suomi 1981, 1983), neonatal heat rate reactivity was strongly predictive of distress during social separation, during a highly stressful medical procedure, and during exposure to a novel environment.

Perhaps the most traditional measure of stress is hypothalamic-pituitary-adrenal output, as measured by assessment of plasma concentrations of the peripheral stress hormones ACTH and cortisol. A number of studies have shown that interindividual differences in cortisol are positively correlated with interindividual differences in distress and despair levels exhibited during a social separation (e.g., see Higley and Suomi 1989). Moreover, individual differences in both heart rate and cortisol stabilize early in life and, like behavioral measures of stress, exhibit long-term interindividual stability (Champoux 1988a, 1988b; Higley and Suomi 1989; Higley et al. 1992b; Suomi 1981, 1983). These and the aforementioned findings on heart rate are particularly noteworthy because they suggest a possible biological substrate underlying how individuals respond to stress. They also suggest that individuals that are at risk for stress anxiety problems could be identified early in life.

Given this possibility of early identification, we have developed a series of early neonatal tests and biological measurements in non-human primates that are used to identify and follow individuals at risk for future problems. In one early study that assessed the relationship of early temperament ratings and future reactivity, Suomi (1983) found that heart rate and cortisol levels obtained during the first 30 days of life were predictive of levels of distress during a brief social separation 18 months later. Higley, Scanlan, and Thompson (Higley and Suomi 1989) found that early neonatal temperament ratings of high irritability were correlated with heart rate levels during exposure to a novel environment 4 months later. In two independent replications, one early neonatal measure that has demonstrated substantial predictive capacity is neonatal state patterning. When neonates that exhibited increased time in a restless state were compared with neonates that showed early self-regulation with increased episodes of deep sleep that were punctuated with episodes of alert directed activity, the latter group of infants exhibited significantly less distress than during a social separation 6 months later (Champoux 1988a, 1988b; Scanlan 1988).

Etiology of Interindividual Differences

We discussed earlier the role that early experiences play in the individual's acquisition of coping skills and the response to stress. Clearly, early experiences affect how individuals approach future stressors. One of the most profound early experiences that affect the future response to a wide variety of challenges is early attachment loss or prolonged social separation. Among human children, early loss of a parent can modify the underlying biological substrate in such a manner that as adults these individuals exhibit chronically higher levels of cortisol, particularly if the home life for the child is less supportive and more chaotic (Breier et al. 1988). In nonhuman primates, Hinde and Spencer-Booth (1971a, 1971b) found that infants who had undergone a 6-day forced separation from mother when they were approximately 6 months of age, when compared with infants who had been treated identically except that they had not been separated from mother, still exhibited less frequent social play and longer latencies to approach novel objects and explore new environments up to 2 years later. Similar findings were obtained by Capitanio (1984) using a different species of nonhuman primate over even a longer period of time between testings. Thus early, severely stressful experiences, such as loss or prolonged separation, may have long-term consequences in the coping capacities that individuals develop, and differences in early stress experiences also offer a potential explanation for the sources of variation seen between individuals.

However, even in homogenous rearing and separation environments, some juvenile and adolescent monkeys seem to cope better with stressful experiences, such as social separation, than others. An illustration of this comes from observations of young adult female monkeys. One of the primary stresses that most adolescent or young adult females face is the birth of their first infant. Females that are peer-reared are more likely to exhibit aggression to a new born infant (Higley et al. 1994; Suomi and Ripp 1983), and when they do care for an infant, they are more likely to exhibit slight deficiencies in otherwise adequate maternal behavior. For example, in the case of our laboratory-born females, all of the mothers who carried their first infant inappropriately (e.g., upside down) had been peer-reared (four cases). Thus, early experiences can influence the response to the birth of a first infant. However, not all peer-reared females exhibit such behavior. In an assessment of maternal competence of females with identical peer-rearing backgrounds, the probability of a given female's reject-ing her firstborn infant was directly related to the levels of depression that she had exhibited as an infant during a social separation. None of the females who as infants had exhibited a mild response to social sepa-ration rejected their infant, but seven of the nine females that had exhib-ited severe depression during a social separation rejected their firstborn infant (Suomi and Ripp 1983). These findings suggest that early experi-ence can affect how an individual responds to a severe stressor such as social separation and that differences in an early reaction to stress tend to show long-term stability. Because these females had been reared in identical environments, but differed both in their response to separation and in their treatment of their infant, these findings also suggest that individual differences in the reaction to a severe stressor have other un-derlying causes than just early experience.

Recently, studies have turned to examining genetic factors as one possible explanation for the source of variance seen between individu-als. These genetic influences in reactivity and their underlying biologi-cal substrates are present both between species and within species. For example, between-species comparisons have shown that among the closely related macaque species, cynomologus macaques (*Macaca fascicularis*) exhibit more fearfulness and behavioral reactivity when compared with rhesus macaques, with higher concentrations of plasma cortisol when exposed to a wide variety of stressors and chal-lenges (Clarke and Mason 1988; Clarke et al. 1988a, 1988b). Simi-larly, cynomologus macaques are more fearful than liontail macaques (Clarke and Lindburg 1993).

Genetic contributions to individual differences in reactivity have also been demonstrated within species. In the series of studies by Suomi in which heart rate was correlated with behaviors characteris-tic of anxiety (Suomi 1983; Suomi et al. 1981), subjects were statisti-cally compared using sibling relationships as an independent variable; a significant portion of the variance in heart rate was accounted for by genetic contributions. Similar genetic effects have been shown for individual differences in plasma ACTH and cortisol concentrations (Scanlan 1988; Scanlan et al. 1982). There are also clear genetic con-tributions to the behavioral response to novelty and challenges (Champoux and Suomi 1986; Suomi 1983, 1991; Suomi et al. 1981). It should be emphasized that the expression of these genetic effects on reactivity varies according to the environmental setting. For exam-ple, in the above genetic study of the behavioral reaction to stress

(Champoux and Suomi 1986; Suomi 1991), rhesus macaques were selectively bred to be reactive or relatively nonreactive. At birth they were taken from their biological mother and placed with one of two different types of mothers, a nurturing-solicitous, or a rejecting-punitive mother, resulting in four different conditions: 1) reactive infant-nurturing mother, 2) reactive infant-punitive mother, 3) nonreactive infant-nurturing mother, and 4) nonreactive infant-punitive mother. During home-cage mother-infant interactions there were few differences between the selectively bred infants other than the expected differences in the response to mothers' maternal styles (i.e., there was no effect of genetic background; both types of infants responded similarly to punitive mothers or to nurturing mothers). However, under the challenge of a greater stressor (i.e., the stress of a social separation), regardless of rearing experience, the infants who had been selectively bred to be reactive exhibited more distress than the infants who had been bred to be nonreactive. After the infants were permanently removed from their mothers and placed together as a social group, the reactive infants, when compared with the nonreactive infants, were more likely to spend time in infantlike ventral-clinging to the other infants. (Clinging to age-mates is not typically seen in mother-reared monkeys.) They were also more likely to initiate aggression toward the other members of their social group. Interestingly, despite the more fearful and anxiouslike behavior seen in the monkeys who had been bred to be reactive, one of the most reactive monkeys was able to become the dominant member of its group by eliciting social support and care from an adult female member who had been placed with the group to maintain order, again showing that the expression of genetic influences can be understood only when the environmental setting and rearing history are taken into account. This finding also illustrates that, contrary to popular notions, a genetic risk does not inevitably produce an unalterable fixed outcome.

Summary and Conclusions

Although it has long been argued that severely stressful experiences early in life may produce long-lasting outcomes, it has only recently been recognized that early traumatic experiences in children can produce long-lasting psychological outcomes similar to the posttraumatic stress syndrome seen in adults (Udwin 1993). One intriguing study, however, investigated the role of subsequent family life and so-cial support in children who experienced early parental loss, finding that social support and the quality of home life following the early parental loss were strongly predictive of adult psychopathology and problems (Breier et al. 1988). However, to date there are virtually no studies that have investigated the roles that interindividual differ-ences prior to the traumatic experience play in coping with and over-coming these potentially long-lasting effects. Data presented and reviewed in this chapter suggest that one's temperament affects the recovery and long-term outcome of early trauma and that the inter-actions between social support and reactivity seem to be crucial in-dependent variables to consider when predicting developmental outcomes and long-term adjustment. The data presented here also indicate that the age at which children are exposed to specific trau-matic and severely stressful events must be taken into account, be-cause the cognitive and emotional readiness for certain experiences will dictate the short and long-term response to these stressors.

Another issue involves the somewhat independent roles that the two individual traits—reactivity and social competence—play in an individ-ual's coping with stress. Although one might predict some overlap be-tween the two traits, large factor analysis studies consistently have demonstrated that these traits are independent entities (Eysenck et al. 1988; Olweus et al. 1980), and other studies have proposed different underlying CNS substrates (Cloninger 1988; Olweus et al. 1980) and different environmental and genetic influences (Pedersen et al. 1988). Numerous studies have investigated each as a separate, enduring trait that predicts behavior across both time and situations; however, few, if any, studies have assessed in long-term longitudinal investigation the in-teractive role that both traits play in stress responsiveness. Indeed, it may be that simultaneous consideration of these two traits and of their inter-action is crucial in understanding how individuals approach and elimi-nate the stressors that they face. These types of studies may add considerably to our understanding of how children, and ultimately adults, respond to stress across the life-span.

References

Abegglen J: On Socialization in Hamadryas Baboons: A Field Study. Lewisburg, PA, Bucknell University Press, 1984

Ainsworth MDS, Blehar MC, Waters E, et al: Patterns of Attachment: A Psychological Study of the Strange Situation. Hillsdale, NJ, Lawrence Erlbaum, 1978

Alexander BK: The effects of early peer deprivation on the juvenile behavior of rhesus monkeys. Unpublished doctoral dissertation, University of Wisconsin, Madison, 1966

Alexander BK, Harlow HF: Social behavior of juvenile rhesus monkeys subjected to different rearing conditions during the first six months of life. Zoologische Jahrbüucher Physiologie 71:489–508, 1965

Altmann J: Baboon Mothers and Infants. Cambridge, MA, Harvard University Press, 1980

Altmann SA: Sociobiology of rhesus monkeys, IV: testing Mason's hypothesis of sex differences in affective behavior. Behaviour 32:49–69, 1968

Anderson CO, Kenney AM, Mason WA: Effects of maternal mobility, partner, and endocrine state on social responsiveness of adolescent rhesus monkeys. Dev Psychobiol 10:421–434, 1977

Andrews MW, Rosenblum LA: Attachment in monkey infants raised in variable- and low-demand environments Child Dev 62:686–693, 1991

Andrews MW, Rosenblum LA: Dominance and social competence in differentially reared bonnet macaques, in Primatology Today. Edited by Ehara A, Kimura T, Takenaka O, et al. New York, Elsevier, 1991, pp 347–350

Angelucci L, Montez R: Order and disorder in the hypothalamo-pituitary-adrenocortical stress activation, in Psychobiology of Stress. Edited by Puglisi-Allegra S, Oliverio A. Boston, MA, Kluwer Academic, 1988, pp 73–80

Arling GL, Harlow HF: Effects of social deprivation on maternal behavior of rhesus monkeys. Journal of Comparative and Physiological Psychology 64:361–377, 1967

Baldwin JD, Baldwin JI: The role of play in social organization: comparative observations on squirrel monkeys (*Saimiri*). Primates 14:369–381, 1973

Baldwin JD, Baldwin JI: Effects of food ecology on social play: a laboratory simulation. Zeitschrift für Tierpsychologie 40:1–14, 1976

Becker MS, Suomi SJ, Marra L, et al: Developmental data as predictors of depression in infant rhesus monkeys (abstract). Infant Behavior and Development 7:26, 1984

Bennett GW: Functional interactions between neuropeptides and noradrenaline in the brain and spinal cord, in The Pharmacology of Noradrenaline in the Central Nervous System. Edited by Heal DJ, Marsden CA. New York, Oxford University Press, 1990, pp 454–494

Berman CM: Early agonistic experience and rank acquisition among free-ranging infant rhesus monkeys. International Journal of Primatology 1:153–170, 1980a

Berman CM: Mother-infant relationships among free-ranging rhesus monkeys on Cayo Santiago: a comparison with captive pairs. Animal Behaviour 28:860–873, 1980b

Berman CM: Ontogeny of social relationships with group companions among free-ranging companies among free-ranging infant rhesus monkeys, I: social networks and differentiation. Animal Behaviour 30:149–162, 1982

Bernstein IS, Ehardt CL: Agonistic aiding: kinship, rank, age, and sex influences. American Journal of Primatology 8:37–52, 1985

Bernstein IS, Ehardt CL: Selective interference in rhesus monkey (*Macaca mulatta*) intragroup agonistic episodes by age-sex class. J Comp Psychol 100:380–384, 1986

Bernstein IS, Gordon TP, Rose RM: Aggression and social controls in rhesus monkey (*Macaca mulatta*) groups revealed in group formation studies. Folia Primatol (Basel) 21:81–107, 1974

Biederman J, Rosenbaum JF, Hirshfeld DR, et al: Psychiatric correlates of behavioral inhibition in young children of parents with and without psychiatric disorders. Arch Gen Psychiatry 47:21–26, 1990

Bifulco A, Brown GW, Adler Z: Early sexual abuse and clinical depression in adult life. Br J Psychiatry 159:115–122, 1991

Blizard DA: Analysis of stress susceptibility using the Maudsley reactive and non-reactive strains, in Coping With Uncertainty: Behavioral and Developmental Perspectives. Edited by Palermo DS. Hillsdale, NJ, Lawrence Erlbaum, 1989, pp 75–99

Boccia ML, Reite M, Kaemingk K, et al: Behavioral and autonomic responses to peer separation in pigtail macaque monkey infants. Dev Psychobiol 22:447–461, 1989

Boccia ML, Reite M, Laudenslager M: Early social environment may alter the development of attachment and social support: two case reports. Infant Behavior and Development 14:253–260, 1991

Boccia ML, Laudenslager ML, Broussard CL, et al: Immune responses following competitive water tests in two species of macaques. Brain Behav Immun 6:201–213, 1992

Boelkins RC, Wilson AP: Intergroup social dynamics of the Cayo Santiago rhesus with special reference to changes in group membership by males. Primates 13:125–140, 1972

Bowlby J: Attachment and Loss, Vol 1: Attachment. New York, Basic Books, 1969

Bowlby J: Attachment and Loss, Vol 2: Separation: Anxiety and Anger. New York, Basic Books, 1973

Bowlby J: Attachment and Loss, Vol 3: Loss: Sadness and Depression. New York, Basic Books, 1980

Brain C: Deaths in a desert baboon troop. International Journal of Primatology 13:593–599, 1992

Bramblett CA, Coelho AM: Development of social behavior in vervet monkeys, Syke's monkeys, and baboons, in Comparative Behavior of African Monkeys. Edited by Zucker EL. New York, AR Liss, 1987, pp 67–79

Breese GR, Smith RD, Mueller RA, et al: Induction of adrenal catecholamine synthesizing enzymes following mother-infant separations. Nature New Biology 246:94–96, 1973

Breier A, Kelsoe JRJ, Kirwin PD, et al: Early parental loss and development of adult psychopathology. Arch Gen Psychiatry 45:987–993, 1988

Bretherton I, Waters E: Growing points in attachment theory and research. Monogr Soc Res Child Dev 50 (1–2, Ser No 209), 1985

Breuggeman JA: Parental care in a group of free-ranging rhesus monkeys Macaca mulatta). Folia Primatol (Basel) 20:178–210, 1973

Brook JS, Whiteman M, Gordon AS, et al: Identification with paternal attributes and its relationship to the son's personality and drug use. Developmental Psychology 20:1111–1119, 1984

Brown GW, Bifulco A, Harris T, et al: Life stress, chronic subclinical symptoms and vulnerability to clinical depression. J Affect Disord 11:1–19, 1986

Burt C: War neuroses in British children. Nervous Child 2:324–327, 1943

Caine NG: The relationship between maternal rank and companion choice in immature macaques (*Macaca mulatta* and *M. radiata*). Primates 20:583–590, 1979

Caine N, Reite M: The effect of peer contact upon physiological response to maternal separation. American Journal of Primatology 1:271–276, 1981

Candland DK, Mason WA: Infant monkey heart rate: habituation and effects of social substitutes. Dev Psychobiol 1:254–256, 1968

Capitanio JP: Early experience and social processes in rhesus macaques (*Macaca mulatta*), I: dyadic social interaction. J Comp Psychol 98:35–44, 1984

Capitanio JP: Behavioral pathology, in Comparative Primate Biology: Behavior, Conservation and Ecology. Edited by Mitchell G, Erwin J. New York, AR Liss, 1986, pp 411–454

Capitanio JP, Reite M: The roles of early separation experience and prior familiarity in the social relations of pigtail macaques: a descriptive multivariate study. Primates 25:475–484, 1984

Capitanio JP, Rasmussen KL, Snyder DS, et al: Long-term follow-up of previously separated pigtail macaques: group and individual differences in response to novel situations. J Child Psychol Psychiatry 27:531–538, 1986

Chamove AS, Harlow HF, Mitchell GD: Sex differences in the infant-directed behavior of preadolescent rhesus monkeys. Child Dev 38:329–335, 1967

Chamove AS, Rosenblum LA, Harlow HF: Monkeys (*Macaca mulatta*) raised with only peers: a pilot study. Animal Behaviour 21:316–325, 1973

Champoux M: Behavioral development of nursery-reared rhesus monkeys (*Macaca mulatta*) neonates. Infant Behavior and Development 11:367–371, 1988a

Champoux M: Behavioral development and temporal stability of reactivity to stressors in mother-reared and nursery/peer–reared rhesus macaques. Unpublished doctoral dissertation, University of Wisconsin, Madison, 1988b

Champoux M, Suomi SJ: Adaptation to a social group by rhesus monkey juveniles differing in infant temperament. Paper presented at the International Society for Developmental Psychobiology, Annapolis, MD, November 1986

Champoux M, Coe CL, Schanberg S, et al: Hormonal effects of early rearing conditions in the infant rhesus monkey. American Journal of Primatology 19:111–117, 1989

Champoux M, DiGregorio G, Schneider ML, et al: Inanimate environmental enrichment for group-housed rhesus macaque infants. American Journal of Primatology 22:61–67, 1990

Cheney DL: The acquisition of rank and the development of reciprocal alliances among free-ranging immature baboons. Behavioral Ecology and Sociobiology 2:303–318, 1977

Cheney DL: Interactions of immature male and female baboons with adult females. Animal Behaviour 26:389–408, 1978a

Cheney DL: The play partners of immature baboons. Animal Behaviour 26:1038–1050, 1978b

Cheney DL: Intergroup encounters among free-ranging vervet monkeys. Folia Primatol (Basel) 35:124–146, 1981

Cheney DL: Proximate and ultimate factors related to the distribution of male migration, in Primate Social Relationships: An Integrated Approach. Edited by Hinde RA. Sunderland, MA, Sinauer Associates, 1983, pp 241–249

Cheney DL, Seyfarth RM: Behaviour of adult and immature male baboons during intergroup encounters. Nature 269:404–406, 1977

Cheney DL, Seyfarth RM: The representation of social relations by monkeys. Cognition 37:167–196, 1990

Cheney DL, Seyfarth R, Smuts B: Social relationships and social cognition in nonhuman primates. Science 234:1361–1366, 1986

Chism J: Relationships between patas infants and group members other than the mother, in Recent Advances in Primatology. Edited by Chivers DJ, Herbert J. London, Academic, 1978, pp 173–176

Clarke AS, Lindburg DG: Behavioral contrasts between male cynomologus and lion-tailed macaques. American Journal of Primatology 29:49–59, 1993

Clarke AS, Mason WA: Differences among three macaque species in responsiveness to an observer. International Journal of Primatology 9:347–364, 1988

Clarke AS, Mason WA, Moberg GP: Differential behavioral and adrenocortical responses to stress among three macaque species. American Journal of Primatology 14:37–52, 1988a

Clarke AS, Mason WA, Moberg GP: Interspecific contrasts in responses of macaques to transport cage training. Lab Anim Sci 38:305–309, 1988b

Cloninger CR: A unified biosocial theory of personality and its role in the development of anxiety states: a reply to commentaries. Psychiatric Developments 6:83–120, 1988

Coe CL, Mendoza SP, Smotherman WP, et al: Mother-infant attachment in the squirrel monkey: adrenal response to separation. Behavioral Biology 22:256–263, 1978

Colvin JD: Familiarity, rank, and the structure of rhesus male peer networks, in Primate Social Relationships: An Integrated Approach. Edited by Hinde RA. Sunderland, MA, Sinauer Associates, 1983a, pp 190–200

Colvin JD: Influences of the social situation on male emigration, in Primate Social Relationships: An Integrated Approach. Edited by Hinde RA. Sunderland, MA, Sinauer Associates, 1983b, pp 160–171

Colvin JD: Proximate causes of male emigration at puberty in rhesus monkeys, in The Cayo Santiago Macaques. Edited by Rawlins RG, Kessler JJ. Albany, State University of New York Press, 1986, pp 131–157

Datta SB: The role of alliances in the acquisition of rank, in Primate Ontogeny, Cognition, and Social Behaviour. Edited by Else JG, Lee PC. New York, Cambridge University Press, 1986, pp 219–225

Diamond A, Goldman-Rakic PS: Comparison of human infants and rhesus monkeys on Piaget's AB task: evidence for dependence on dorsolateral prefrontal cortex. Exp Brain Res 74:24–40, 1989

Diamond A, Zola-Morgan S, Squire LR: Successful performance by monkeys with lesions of the hippocampal formation on AB and object retrieval, two tasks that mark developmental changes in human infants. Behav Neurosci 103:526–537, 1989

Dittus WPJ: The social regulation of population density and age-sex distribution in the toque monkey. Behaviour 63:281–322, 1977a

Dittus WPJ: The socioecological basis for the conservation of the toque monkey (*Macaca sinica*) of Sri Lanka (Ceylon), in Primate Conservation. Edited by Prince Rainier III of Monaco, Bourne GH. New York, Academic, 1977b, pp 238–265

Dittus WPJ: The social regulation of primate populations, in The Macaques: Studies in Ecology, Behavior and Evolution. Edited by Lindburg D. New York, Van Nostrand Reinhold, 1980, pp 131–157

Dolhinow P: An experimental study of mother loss in the Indian Langur monkey (*Presbytis entellus*). Folia Primatol (Basel) 33:77–128, 1981

Dolhinow P, Murphy G: Langur monkey mother loss: profile analysis with multivariate analysis of variance for separation subjects and controls. Folia Primatol (Basel) 40:181–196, 1983

Drickamer LC, Vessey SH: Group changing in free-ranging male rhesus monkeys. Primates 14:249–254, 1973

Dunsdon MI: A psychologist's contribution to air raid problems. Mental Health 2:37–41, 1941

Eastman RF, Mason WA: Looking behavior in monkeys raised with mobile and stationary artificial mothers. Dev Psychobiol 8:213–221, 1975

Ehardt CL, Bernstein IS: Patterns of affiliation among immature rhesus monkeys (*Macaca mulatta*). American Journal of Primatology 13:255–269, 1987

Erwin J, Flett M: Responses of rhesus monkeys to reunion after long-term separation. Psychol Rep 35:171–174, 1974

Erwin J, Maple T, Welles JF: Responses of rhesus monkeys to reunion, in Contemporary Primatology: Fifth International Congress of Primatology. Edited by Kondo S, Kawai M, Ehara A. New York, S Karger, 1975, pp 254–262

Eysenck SB, von Knorring AL, von Knorring L: A cross-cultural study of personality: Swedish and English children. Scand J Psychol 29:152–161, 1988

Fairbanks LA, McGuire MT: Long-term effects of early mothering behavior on responsiveness to the environment in vervet monkeys. Dev Psychobiol 21:711–724, 1988

Fedigan LM: Social and solitary play in a colony of vervet monkeys. Primates 13:347–364, 1972

Fedigan LM: Primate Paradigms: Sex Roles and Social Bonds. Montreal, Eden Press, 1982

Feinman S: Emotional expression, social referencing, and preparedness for learning in infancy—mother knows best, but sometimes I know better, in The Development of Expressive Behavior: Biology-Environment Interactions. Edited by Zivin G. New York, Academic, 1985, pp 291–318

Feldman RS, Quenzer LF: Fundamentals of Neuropsychopharmacology. Sunderland, MA, Sinauer Associates, 1984

Field TM: Interventions for premature infants. J Pediatr 109:183–191, 1986

Field TM, Schanberg SM, Scafidi F, et al: Tactile/kinesthetic stimulation effects on preterm neonates. Pediatrics 77:654–658, 1986

Freud A, Dann S: An experiment in group upbringing. Psychoanal Study Child 6:127–168, 1951

Gartlan JS: Adaptive aspects of social structure in *Erythrocebus patas*, in Proceedings From the Symposia of the Fifth Congress of the International Primatological Society. Edited by Kondo S, Kawai M, Ehara A. Tokyo, Japan Science Press, 1975, pp 161–171

Gibson KR: Myelination and behavioral development: a comparative perspective on questions of neoteny, altriciality and intelligence, in Brain Maturation and Cognitive Development. Edited by Gibson KR, Peterson AC. New York, Walter DeGruyter, 1991, pp 29–63

Goldman-Rakic PS: Development of cortical circuitry and cognitive function. Child Dev 58:601–622, 1987

Goodman M, Lasker GW: Molecular evidence as to man's place in nature, in Primate Functional Morphology and Evolution. Edited by Tuttle RH. Chicago, IL, Aldine, 1975, pp 71–101

Goosen C: On the function of allogrooming in Old World monkeys, in Primate Behavior and Sociobiology. Edited by Chiarelli AB, Corruccini RS. New York, Springer-Verlag, 1981, pp 110–120

Gouzoules H: Maternal rank and early social interaction of infant stumptail macaques, *Macaca arctoides*. Primates 16:405–418, 1975

Greenough WT: Experience and brain development. Child Dev 58:539–559, 1987

Gunnar MR, González CA, Levine S: The role of peers in modifying behavioral distress and pituitary-adrenal response to a novel environment in year-old rhesus monkeys. Physiol Behav 25:795–758, 1980

Gunnar MR, González CA, Goodlin BL, et al: Behavioral and pituitary-adrenal responses during a prolonged separation period in infant rhesus macaques. Psychoneuroendocrinology 6:65–75, 1981

Hansen EW, Harlow HF, Dodsworth RO: Reactions of rhesus monkeys to familiar and unfamiliar peers. Journal of Comparative and Physiological Psychology 61:274–279, 1966

Harlow HF: The nature of love. Am Psychol 13:673–685, 1958

Harlow HF: Age-mate or peer affectional system. Advances in the Study of Behavior 2:333–383, 1969

Harlow HF, Harlow MK: The affectional systems, in Behavior of Nonhuman Primates. Edited by Schrier AM, Harlow HF, Stollinitz F. New York, Academic, 1965, pp 287–334

Harlow HF, Zimmerman RR: Affectional responses in the infant monkey. Science 130:421–432, 1959

Harris T, Brown GW, Bifulco A: Loss of parent in childhood and adult psychiatric disorder: the role of lack of adequate parental care. Psychol Med 16:641–659, 1986

Harris T, Brown GW, Bifulco A: Loss of parent in childhood and adult psychiatric disorder: the role of social class position and premarital pregnancy. Psychol Med 17:163–183, 1987

Hausfater G: Intergroup behavior of free-ranging rhesus monkeys (*Macaca mulatta*). Folia Primatol (Basel) 18:78–107, 1972

Hawkins JD, Catalano RF, Miller JY: Risk and protective factors for alcohol and other drug problems in adolescence and early adulthood: Implications for substance abuse prevention. Psychol Bull 112:64–105, 1992

Hayaki H: The social interactions of juvenile Japanese monkeys on Koshima Islet. Primates 24:139–153, 1985

Henzi SP, Lucas JW: Observations on the inter-troop movement of adult vervet monkeys (*Cercopithecus aethiops*). Folia Primatol (Basel) 33:220–235, 1980

Higley JD: Continuity of social separation behaviors in rhesus monkeys from infancy to adolescence. Unpublished doctoral dissertation, University of Wisconsin, Madison, 1985

Higley JD, Danner GR: Attachment in rhesus monkeys reared either with only peers or with their mothers as assessed by the Ainsworth Strange Situation procedure (abstract). Infant Behavior and Development 11:139, 1988

Higley JD, Suomi SJ: Parental behavior in non-human primates, in Parental Behavior in Animals and Humans. Edited by Sluckin W. Oxford, UK, Blackwell Scientific, 1986, pp 152–207

Higley JD, Suomi SJ: Temperamental reactivity in non-human primates, in Temperament in Childhood. Edited by Kohnstamm GA, Bates JE, Rothbart MK. New York, Wiley, 1989, pp 153–167

Higley JD, Suomi SJ, Linnoila M: Central amine correlates of timidity and affective disturbances in rhesus monkeys (abstract). American Journal of Primatology 14:425, 1988

Higley JD, Suomi SJ, Linnoila M: Parallels in aggression and serotonin: consideration of development, rearing history, and sex differences, in Violence and Suicidality: Perspectives in Clinical and Psychobiological Research. Edited by van Praag HM, Plutchik R, Apter A. New York, Brunner/Mazel, 1990, pp 245–256

Higley JD, Hasert MF, Suomi SJ, et al: Nonhuman primate model of alcohol abuse: effects of early experience, personality, and stress on alcohol consumption. Proc Natl Acad Sci U S A 88:7261–7265, 1991a

Higley JD, Mehlman P, Taub D, et al: CSF monoamine metabolite and adrenal correlates of aggression in free-ranging rhesus monkeys (abstract). American Journal of Primatology 24:108, 1991b

Higley JD, Suomi SJ, Linnoila M: CSF monoamine metabolite concentrations vary according to age, rearing, and sex, and are influenced by the stressor of social separation in rhesus monkeys. Psychopharmacology (Berl) 103:551–556, 1991c

Higley JD, Hopkins WD, Thompson WW, et al: Peers as primary attachment sources in yearling rhesus monkeys (*Macaca mulatta*). Developmental Psychology 28:1163–1171, 1992a

Higley JD, Suomi SJ, Linnoila M: A longitudinal study of CSF monoamine metabolite and plasma cortisol concentrations in young rhesus monkeys: effects of early experience, age, sex and stress on continuity of interindividual differences. Biol Psychiatry 32:127–145, 1992b

Higley JD, Linnoila M, Suomi SJ: Developing social competence: experiential and genetic contributions to the expression and inhibition of aggression in primates, in Handbook of Aggressive and Destructive Behavior in Psychiatric Patients. Edited by Ammerman RT, Hersen M, Sisson L. New York, Plenum, 1994, pp 17–32

Hinde RA, Simpson MJA: Qualities of mother-infant relationships in monkeys. Ciba Found Symp 33:39–68, 1967

Hinde RA, Spencer-Booth Y: Effects of brief separation from mother on rhesus monkeys. Science 173:111–118, 1971a

Hinde RA, Spencer-Booth Y: Toward understanding individual differences in rhesus mother-infant interaction. Animal Behaviour 19:165–173, 1971b

Hofer MA: Shaping forces within early social relationships, in Perinatal Development: A Psychobiological Perspective. Edited by Krasnegor NA, Blass EM, Hofer MA, et al. New York, Academic, 1987, pp 251–274

Holmes SJ, Robins LN: The influence of childhood disciplinary experience on the development of alcoholism and depression. J Child Psychol Psychiatry 28:399–415, 1987

Holmes SJ, Robins LN: The role of parental disciplinary practices in the development of depression and alcoholism. Psychiatry 51:24–35, 1988

Hrdy SB: The Langurs of Abu. Cambridge, MA, Harvard University Press, 1977

Itoigawa N: Variables in male leaving a group of Japanese macaques, in Proceedings From the Symposia of the Fifth Congress of the International Primatological Society. Edited by Kondo S, Kawai M, Ehara A. Tokyo, Japan Science Press, 1975, pp 330–334

Janus M: Aggression in interactions of immature rhesus monkeys: components, context and relation to affiliation levels. Animal Behaviour 41:121–134, 1991

Janus M: Interplay between various aspects in social relationships of young rhesus monkeys: dominance, agonistic help, and affiliation. American Journal of Primatology 26:291–308, 1992

Kagan J, Reznick JS, Gibbons J: Inhibited and uninhibited types of children. Child Dev 60:838–845, 1989

Kagan J, Snidman N, Julia-Sellers M, et al: Temperament and allergic symptoms. Psychosom Med 53:332–340, 1991

Kaufman JH: Social relations of adult males in a free-ranging band of rhesus monkeys, in Social Communication Among Primates. Edited by Altmann SA. Chicago, IL, University of Chicago Press, 1967, pp 73–98

Kaufman JH, Stynes AJ: Depression and conservation-withdrawal in bonnet macaque infants. Psychosom Med 40:71–75, 1978

Klinnert MD, Campos JJ, Sorce JF, et al: Emotions as behavior regulators: social referencing in infancy, in Emotion: Theory, Research, and Experience. Edited by Plutchik R, Kellerman H. New York, Academic, 1983, pp 57–86

Kohne DE: DNA evolution data and its relevance to mammalian phylogeny, in Phylogeny of the Primates: A Multidisciplinary Approach. Edited by Luckett WP, Szalay FS. New York, Plenum, 1975, pp 249–261

Kondo K, Minami T, Itoigawa N: Behavioral differences between feral group-reared and mother-reared young Japanese monkeys, in Primate Behavior and Sociobiology. Edited by Chiarelli AB, Corruccini RS. New York, Springer-Verlag, 1981, pp 64–71

Koop BF, Tagle DA, Goodman M, et al: A molecular view of primate phylogeny and important systematic and evolutionary questions. Mol Biol Evol 6:580–612, 1989

Kraemer GW: Causes of changes in brain noradrenaline systems and later effects on responses to social stressors in rhesus monkeys: the cascade hypothesis. Ciba Found Symp 123:216–233, 1986

Kraemer GW: A psychobiological theory of attachment. Behavioral and Brain Sciences 15:493–541, 1992

Kraemer GW, Clarke AS: The behavioral neurobiology of self-injurious behavior in rhesus monkeys. Prog Neuropsychopharmacol Biol Psychiatry 14(suppl):S141–S168, 1990

Kraemer GW, McKinney WT: Interactions of pharmacological agents which alter biogenic amine metabolism and depression—an analysis of contributing factors within a primate model of depression. J Affect Disord 1:33–54, 1979

Kraemer GW, Ebert MH, Lake R, et al: Neurobiological measures in rhesus monkeys: correlates of the behavioral response to social separation and alcohol, in Stress and Alcohol Use. Edited by Pohorecky LA, Brick J. New York, Elsevier, 1983, pp 171–184

Kraemer GW, Ebert MH, Schmidt DE, et al: A longitudinal study of the effect of different social rearing conditions on cerebrospinal fluid norepinephrine and biogenic amine metabolites in rhesus monkeys. Neuropsychopharmacology 2:175–189, 1989

Kraemer GW, Ebert MH, Schmidt DE, et al: Strangers in a strange land: a psychobiological study of infant monkeys before and after separation from real or inanimate mothers. Child Dev 62:548–566, 1991

Lancaster JB: Play-mothering: the relations between juvenile females and young infants among free ranging vervet monkeys. Folia Primatol (Basel) 15:161–182, 1971

Laudenslager ML, Reite M, Harbeck RJ: Suppressed immune response in infant monkeys associated with maternal separation. Behav Neural Biol 36:40–48, 1982

Laudenslager ML, Held PE, Boccia ML, et al: Behavioral and immunological consequences of brief mother-infant separation: a species comparison. Dev Psychobiol 23:247–264, 1990

Lawrence DG, Hopkins DA: The development of motor control in the rhesus monkey: evidence concerning the role of corticomotoneuronal connections. Brain 99:235–254, 1976

Lee PC: Play as a means for developing relationships, in Primate Social Relationships: An Integrated Approach. Edited by Hinde RA. Sunderland, MA, Sinauer Associates, 1983, pp 82–89

Lee PC: Environmental influences on development: play, weaning and social structure, in Primate Ontogeny, Cognition and Social Behaviour. Edited by Else JG, Lee PC. Cambridge, UK, Cambridge University Press, 1986, pp 227–237

Lindburg DG: The rhesus monkey in North India: an ecological and behavioral study, in Primate Behavior: Developments in Field and Laboratory Research. Edited by Rosenblum LA. New York, Academic, 1971, pp 1–106

Loy J: Behavioral responses of free-ranging rhesus monkeys to food shortage. Am J Phys Anthropol 33:263–272, 1970

Loy KM, Loy J: Sexual differences in early social development among captive patas monkeys, in Comparative Behavior of African Monkeys. Edited by Zucker EL. New York, AR Liss, 1987, pp 23–37

Mason WA: Social experience and primate cognitive development, in The Development of Behavior: Comparative and Evolutionary Aspects. Edited by Burghardt GM, Bekoff M. New York, Garland STPM Press, 1978, pp 233–251

Mason WA, Berkson G: Effects of maternal mobility on the development of rocking and other behaviors in rhesus monkeys: a study with artificial mothers. Dev Psychobiol 8:197–211, 1975

Mason WA, Capitanio JP: Formation and expression of filial attachment in rhesus monkeys raised with living and inanimate mother substitutes. Dev Psychobiol 21:401–430, 1988

Matsumura S: Social interactions of young male Japanese monkeys during inter-troop transfer, in Primatology Today. Edited by Ehara A, Kimura T, Takenaka O, et al. New York, Elsevier, 1991, pp 163–166

McKinney WT: Models of Mental Disorders: A New Comparative Psychiatry. New York, Plenum, 1988

Meikle DB, Vessey SH: Nepotism among rhesus monkey brothers. Nature 294:160–161, 1981

Melamed BG, Siegel LJ: Children's reactions to medical stressors: an ecological approach to the study of anxiety, in Anxiety and the Anxiety Disorders. Edited by Tuma AH, Maser J. Hillsdale, NJ, Lawrence Erlbaum, 1985, pp 369–386

Mineka S, Suomi SJ: Social separation in monkeys. Psychol Bull 85:1376–1400, 1978

Mineka S, Suomi SJ, DeLizio R: Multiple separations in adolescent monkeys: an opponent-process interpretation. J Exp Psychol Gen 110:56–85, 1981

Mineka S, Davidson M, Cook M, et al: Observational conditioning of snake fear in rhesus monkeys. J Abnorm Psychol 93:355–372, 1984

Mineka S, Gunnar M, Champoux M: Control and early socioemotional development: infant rhesus monkeys reared in controllable versus uncontrollable environments. Child Dev 57:1241–1256, 1986

Møller GW, Harlow HF, Mitchell GD: Factors affecting agonistic communication in rhesus monkeys *Macaca mulatta*. Behaviour 31:336–357, 1968

Nash LT, Wheeler RL: Mother-infant relationships in nonhuman primates, in Child Nurturance: Studies of Development in Nonhuman Primates. Edited by Fitzgerald HE, Mullins JA, Gage P. New York, Plenum, 1982, pp 27–51

Netto WJ, van Hooff JARAM: Conflict interference and the development of dominance relationships in immature *Macaca fascicularis*, in Primate Ontogeny, Cognition and Social Behaviour. Edited by Else JG, Lee PC. New York, Cambridge University Press, 1986, pp 291–300

Noë R: Lasting alliances among adult male savannah baboons, in Primate Ontogeny, Cognition and Social Behaviour. Edited by Else JG, Lee PC. New York, Cambridge University Press, 1986, pp 381–392

Novak MA: Fear-attachment relationships in infant and juvenile rhesus monkeys. Unpublished doctoral dissertation, University of Wisconsin, Madison, 1973

Novak MA: Social recovery of monkeys isolated for the first year of life, II: long-term assessment. Developmental Psychology 15:50–61, 1979

Novak MA, Harlow HF: Social recovery of monkeys isolated for the first year of life, I: rehabilitation and therapy. Developmental Psychology 11:453–465, 1975

Ohsawa H: Take-over of a harem and the subsequent promiscuity in patas monkeys, in Primatology Today. Edited by Ehara A, Kimura T, Takenaka O, et al. New York, Elsevier, 1991, pp 221–224

Oliver JI, Lee PC: Comparative aspects of the behavior of juveniles in two species of baboon in Tanzania, in Recent Advances in Primatology: Behaviour. Edited by Chivers DJ, Herbert J. New York, Academic, 1978, pp 104–109

Olweus D, Mattsson A, Schalling D, et al: Testosterone, aggression, physical, and personality dimensions in normal adolescent males. Psychosom Med 42:253–269, 1980

Owens NW: Social play behaviour in free-living baboons, *Papio anubis*. Animal Behaviour 23:387–408, 1975

Packer C: Inter-troop transfer and inbreeding avoidance in *Papio anubis*. Animal Behaviour 27:1–36, 1979

Pauk J, Kuhn CM, Field TM, et al: Positive effects of tactile versus kinesthetic or vestibular stimulation on neuroendocrine and ODC activity in maternally-deprived rat pups. Life Sci 39:2081–2087, 1986

Pedersen NL, Plomin R, McClearn GE, et al: Neuroticism, extraversion, and related traits in adult twins reared apart and reared together. J Pers Soc Psychol 55:950–957, 1988

Plimpton EH, Swartz KB, Rosenblum LA: Responses of juvenile bonnet macaques to social stimuli presented through color videotapes. Dev Psychobiol 14:109–115, 1981

Pusey AE, Packer C: Dispersal and philopatry, in Primate Societies. Edited by Smuts BB, Cheney DL, Seyfarth RM, et al. Chicago, IL, University of Chicago Press, 1987, pp 250–266

Raleigh MJ: Differential behavioral effects of tryptophan and 5-hydroxytryptophan in vervet monkeys: influence of catecholaminergic systems. Psychopharmacology (Berl) 93:44–50, 1987

Raleigh MJ, McGuire MT: Female influences on male dominance acquisition in captive vervet monkeys, *Cercopithecus aethiops sabaeus*. Animal Behaviour 38:59–67, 1989

Raleigh MJ, Brammer GL, Yuwiler A, et al: Serotonergic influences on the social behavior of vervet monkeys (*Cercopithecus aethiops sabaeus*). Exp Neurol 68:322–334, 1980

Raleigh MJ, Brammer GL, Ritvo ER, et al: Effects of chronic fenfluramine on blood serotonin, cerebrospinal fluid metabolites, and behavior in monkeys. Psychopharmacology (Berl) 90:503–508, 1986

Raleigh MJ, McGuire MT, Brammer GL: Subjective assessment of behavioral style: links to overt behavior and physiology in vervet monkeys. American Journal of Primatology 18:161–162, 1989

Raleigh MJ, McGuire MT, Brammer GL, et al: Serotonergic mechanisms promote dominance acquisition in adult male vervet monkeys. Brain Res 559:181–190, 1991

Rasmussen KLR, Suomi SJ: Heart rate and endocrine responses to stress in adolescent male rhesus monkeys on Cayo Santiago. P R Health Sci J 8:65–71, 1989

Redmond DEJ: Studies of the nucleus locus coeruleus in monkeys and hypotheses for neuropsychopharmacology, in Psychopharmacology: The Third Generation of Progress. Edited by Meltzer HY. New York, Raven, 1987, pp 967–975

Redmond DEJ, Huang YH, Snyder DR, et al: Behavioral effects of stimulation of the nucleus locus coeruleus in the stump-tailed monkey *Macaca arctoides*. Brain Res 116:502–510, 1976

Redmond DEJ, Katz MM, Maas JW, et al: Cerebrospinal fluid amine metabolites: relationships with behavioral measurements in depressed, manic, and healthy control subjects. Arch Gen Psychiatry 43:938–947, 1986

Reite M, Short R: Circadian rhythms in monkeys: variability and behavioral correlations. Physiol Behav 27:663–671, 1981

Reite M, Short R: Maternal separation studies: rationale and methodological considerations. Prog Clin Biol Res 131:219–253, 1983

Reite M, Short R, Kaufman IC, et al: Heart rate and body temperature in separated monkey infants. Biol Psychiatry 13:91–105, 1978a

Reite M, Short R, Seiler C: Loss of your mother is more than loss of a mother. Am J Psychiatry 135:370–371, 1978b

Reite M, Harbeck R, Hoffman A: Altered cellular immune response following peer separation. Life Sci 29:1133–1136, 1981a

Reite M, Short R, Seiler C, et al: Attachment, loss, and depression. J Child Psychol Psychiatry 22:141–169, 1981b

Reite M, Kaemingk K, Boccia ML: Maternal separation in bonnet monkey infants: altered attachment and social support. Child Dev 60:473–480, 1989

Reynolds V: Social incompetence in a rhesus monkey (*Macaca mulatta*), in Primatology Today. Edited by Ehara A, Kimura T, Takenaka O, et al. New York, Elsevier, 1991, pp 151–154

Richard A: Intra-specific variation in the social organization and ecology of *Propithecus verreauxi*. Folia Primatol (Basel) 22:178–207, 1974

Rosenblum LA: The ontogeny of mother-infant relations in macaques, in Ontogeny of Vertebrate Behavior. Edited by Moltz H. New York, Academic, 1971, pp 315–367

Rosenblum LA, Kaufman IC: Laboratory observations of early mother-infant relations in pigtail and bonnet macaques, in Social Communication Among Primates. Edited by Altmann SA. Chicago, IL, University of Chicago Press, 1967, pp 33–41

Rosenblum LA, Kaufman IC: Variations in infant development and response to maternal loss in monkeys. Am J Orthopsychiatry 38:418–426, 1968

Rosenblum LA, Paully GS: The effects of varying environmental demands on maternal and infant behavior. Child Dev 55:305–314, 1984

Rovee CK, Levin GR: Oral "pacification" and arousal in the human newborn. J Exp Child Psychol 3:1–17, 1966

Ruppenthal GC, Harlow MK, Eisele CD, et al: Development of peer interactions of monkeys reared in a nuclear-family environment. Child Dev 45:670–682, 1974

Rutter M: Maternal deprivation, 1972–1978: new findings, new concepts, new approaches. Child Dev 50:283–305, 1979

Sackett GP, Griffin GA, Pratt CL, et al: Mother-infant and adult female choice behavior in rhesus monkeys after various rearing experiences. Journal of Comparative and Physiological Psychology 63:376–381, 1967

Sade DS: Ontogeny of social relations in a group of free-ranging rhesus monkeys. Unpublished doctoral dissertation, University of California, Berkeley, 1966

Sapolsky RM: Endocrine aspects of social instability in the olive baboon (*Papio anubis*). American Journal of Primatology 5:365–379, 1983

Sarich V: A molecular approach to the question of human origins, in Primate Evolution and Human Origins. Edited by Ciochon RL, Fleagle JG. Menlo Park, CA, The Benjamin/Cummings Publishing Company, 1985, pp 314–322

Scanlan JM: Continuity of stress responsivity in infant rhesus monkeys (*Macaca mulatta*): state, hormonal, dominance, and genetic influences. Unpublished doctoral dissertation, University of Wisconsin, Madison, 1988

Scanlan JM, Suomi SJ, Higley JD, et al: Stress and heredity in adrenocortical response in rhesus monkeys. Paper presented at the annual meeting of the Society for Neuroscience, Minneapolis, MN, November 1982

Schanberg SM, Field TM: Sensory deprivation stress and supplemental stimulation in the rat pup and preterm human neonate. Child Dev 58:1431–1447, 1987

Schneider-Rosen K, Braunwald KG, Carlson V, et al: Current perspectives in attachment theory: illustration from the study of maltreated infants. Monogr Soc Res Child Dev 50(1–2, Ser No 209): 194–210, 1985

Sibley CG, Ahlquist JE: DNA hybridization evidence of hominoid phylogeny: results from an expanded data set. J Mol Evol 26:99–121, 1987

Sibley CG, Comstock JA, Ahlquist JE: DNA hybridization evidence of hominoid phylogeny: a reanalysis of the data. J Mol Evol 30:202–236, 1990

Smith PK: Does play matter? Functional and evolutionary aspects of animal and human play. Behavioral and Brain Sciences 5:139–184, 1982

Smuts BB: Sex & Friendship in Baboons. New York, Aldine, 1985

Southwick CH, Siddiqi MF: Population dynamics of rhesus monkeys in Northern India, in Primate Conservation. Edited by Prince Rainier III of Monaco, Bourne GH. New York, Academic, 1977, pp 339–362

Sroufe LA: The coherence of individual development: early care, attachment, and subsequent developmental issues. Am Psychol 34:834–841, 1979

Sroufe LA: Infant-caregiver attachment and patterns of adaptation in preschool: the roots of maladaptation and competence. Minnesota Symposia on Child Psychology 16:41–81, 1983

Sroufe LA: Considering normal and abnormal together: the essence of developmental psychopathology. Development and Psychopathology 2:335–347, 1990

Stevenson-Hinde J, Simpson MJA: Subjective assessment of rhesus monkeys over four successive years. Primates 21:66–82, 1980

Stevenson-Hinde J, Zunz M: Subjective assessment of individual rhesus monkeys. Primates 19:473–482, 1978

Stevenson-Hinde J, Zunz M, Stillwell-Barnes R: Behaviour of one-year-old rhesus monkeys in a strange situation. Animal Behaviour 28:266–277, 1980

Sugiyama Y, Ohsawa H: Life history of male Japanese macaques at Ryozenyama, in Contemporary Primatology: Fifth International Congress of Primatology. Edited by Kondo S, Kawai M, Ehara A. New York, S Karger, 1975, pp 407–410

Suomi SJ: Social rehabilitation of isolate-reared monkeys. Developmental Psychology 6:487–496, 1972

Suomi SJ: Peers, play and primary prevention in primates, in Primary Prevention of Psychopathology: Social Competence in Children. Edited by Kent M, Rolf J. Hanover, NH, University Press of New England, 1979, pp 127–149

Suomi SJ: Genetic, maternal, and environmental influences on social development in rhesus monkeys, in Primate Behavior and Sociobiology. Edited by Chiarelli AB, Corruccini RS. New York, Springer-Verlag, 1981, pp 81–87

Suomi SJ: Social development in rhesus monkeys: consideration of individual differences, in The Behavior of Human Infants. Edited by Oliverio A, Zappella M. New York, Plenum, 1983, pp 193–202

Suomi SJ: Early stress and adult emotional reactivity in rhesus monkeys. Ciba Found Symp 156:171–183, 1991

Suomi SJ, Ripp C: A history of mother-less mother monkey mothering at the University of Wisconsin Primate Laboratory, in Child Abuse: The Nonhuman Primate Data. Edited by Reite M, Caine N. New York, AR Liss, 1983, pp 50–78

Suomi SJ, Harlow HF, Domek CJ: Effect of repetitive infant-infant separation of young monkeys. J Abnorm Psychol 76:161–172, 1970

Suomi SJ, Harlow HF, Novak MA: Reversal of social deficits produced by isolation rearing in monkeys. Journal of Human Evolution 3:527–534, 1974

Suomi SJ, Collins ML, Harlow HF, et al: Effects of maternal and peer separations on young monkeys. J Child Psychol Psychiatry 17:101–112, 1976

Suomi SJ, Seaman SF, Lewis JK, et al: Effects of imipramine treatment of separation-induced social disorders in rhesus monkeys. Arch Gen Psychiatry 35:321–325, 1978

Suomi SJ, Kraemer GW, Baysinger CM, et al: Inherited and experiential factors associated with individual differences in anxious behavior displayed by rhesus monkeys, in Anxiety: New Research and Changing Concepts. Edited by Klein DF, Rabkin J. New York, Raven, 1981, pp 179–199

Suomi SJ, Mineka S, DeLizio RD: Short- and long-term effects of repetitive mother-infant separations on social development in rhesus monkeys. Developmental Psychology 19:770–786, 1983

Suomi SJ, Scanlan JM, Rasmussen KLR, et al: Pituitary-adrenal response to capture in Cayo Santiago–derived group M rhesus monkeys. P R Health Sci J 8:171–176, 1989

Symons D: Play and Aggression: A Study of Rhesus Monkeys. New York, Columbia University Press, 1978

Tartabini A, Dienske H: Social play and rank order in rhesus monkeys *Macaca mulatta*. Behavioural Processes 4:375–383, 1991

Tartabini A, Genta ML, Bertacchini PA: Mother-infant interaction and rank order in rhesus monkeys *Macaca mulatta*. Journal of Human Evolution 9:139–146, 1980

Trad PV (ed): Infant and Childhood Depression: Developmental Factors. New York, Wiley, 1987

Udwin O: Children's reactions to traumatic events. J Child Psychol Psychiatry 34:115–127, 1993

Uylings HB, van Eden CG: Qualitative and quantitative comparison of the prefrontal cortex in rat and in primates, including humans. Prog Brain Res 85:31–62, 1990

van Lawick-Goodall J: In the Shadow of Man. Boston, MA, Houghton-Mifflin, 1971

van Noordwijk MA, van Schaik CP: Male migration and rank acquisition in wild long-tailed macaques (*Macaca fascicularis*). Animal Behaviour 33:849–861, 1985

Vessey SH: Interactions between free-ranging groups of rhesus monkeys. Folia Primatol (Basel) 8:228–239, 1968

Wheatley BP: The role of females in inter-troop encounters and infanticide among Balinese *Macaca fascicularis,* in Primatology Today. Edited by Ehara A, Kimura T, Takenaka O, et al. New York, Elsevier, 1991, pp 169–172

Widom CS: Child abuse, neglect, and adult behavior: research design and findings on criminality, violence, and child abuse. Am J Orthopsychiatry 59:355–367, 1989

Wiener SG, Bayart F, Faull KF, et al: Behavioral and physiological responses to maternal separation in squirrel monkeys (*Saimiri sciureus*). Behav Neurosci 104:108–115, 1990

Wood BS, Mason WA, Kenney MD: Contrasts in visual responsiveness and emotional arousal between rhesus monkeys raised with living and those raised with inanimate substitute mothers. Journal of Comparative and Physiological Psychology 93:368–377, 1979

Yule W, Udwin O: Screening child survivors for post-traumatic stress disorders: experiences from the 'Jupiter' sinking. Br J Psychiatry 30:131–138, 1991

Yule W, Udwin O, Murdoch K: The 'Jupiter' sinking: effects on children's fears, depression and anxiety. J Child Psychol Psychiatry 31:1051–1061, 1990

Zarbatany L, Lamb M: Social referencing as a function of information source: mothers versus strangers. Infant Behavior and Development 8:25–33, 1985

Zimmerman RR, Strobe DA, Steere P, et al: Behaviour and malnutrition in the rhesus monkey, in Primate Behavior. Edited by Rosenblum LA. New York, Academic, 1975, pp 241–265

Chapter 2

Neurophysiological Mechanisms of Stress Response in Children

Martin H. Teicher, M.D., Ph.D.
Yutaka Ito, M.D.
Carol A. Glod, Ph.D., R.N.
Fred Schiffer, M.D.
Harris A. Gelbard, M.D., Ph.D.

During the last decade an intellectual evolution has taken place in psychiatry, with the gradual recognition that many psychiatric patients have been victims of early childhood trauma. Many scholars who endeavor to understand the effects of early abuse neglect to consider that this intense trauma occurs during a time in which the brain is growing at an astounding rate. Although the development of the brain is strongly guided by genetic factors, the final product is largely sculpted through experience. In this chapter we propose a model through which we can perhaps more completely understand the sequelae of childhood abuse, by considering the possible effects of abuse on brain development. Preliminary data are provided that offer some support for this model. We believe that this framework provides an important bridge between psychological and biological theories of psychopathology and may have important implications for the treatment of patients who have experienced intense childhood stress.

Psychological Effects of Early Abuse

Physical and sexual traumatization in childhood may lead to the development of psychiatric difficulties in both children and adults

(Brown and Anderson 1991; Bryer et al. 1987). The initial sequelae of abuse may manifest through an array of internalizing symptoms such as depression, anxiety, suicidal ideation, and posttraumatic stress (Famularo et al. 1988; Finkelhor 1986; Kashani and Carlson 1987) or through externalizing signs such as aggressive-impulsivity, delinquency, and substance abuse (Burgess et al. 1987; Finkelhor 1986). Childhood trauma may be a factor in the development of somatoform disorder (Krystal 1978), panic disorder with agoraphobia (Faravelli et al. 1985), borderline personality disorder (BPD) (Herman 1986; Herman et al. 1989; Stone 1981; Westen et al. 1990; Zanarini et al. 1989), severe, intractable psychosis (Beck and van der Kolk 1987), and multiple personality disorder (MPD) (Bliss 1980; Horevitz and Braun 1984; Putnam et al. 1986). Thus, persistent childhood abuse may produce a spectrum of psychiatric disorders. The consequences may range from extreme adaptive reactions, as seen in MPD and refractory psychosis; to intermediate adaptive reactions, as present in BPD; to more delimited reactions, as manifest in somatoform disorders and panic disorder (Herman et al. 1989). We suggest that this spectrum of psychopathology may be related to different types and degrees of limbic system or cortical dysfunction.

Limbic and Cortical Regulation of Human Affect and Emotion

The limbic system is a somewhat ill-defined collection of neuroanatomical regions linked by common phylogeny, cytoarchitecture, membrane proteins, and neural connections (Levitt 1984; Lopes da Silva et al. 1990; Reep 1984). This complex system consists of the subcallosal, cingulate, and parahippocampal gyri and the underlying hippocampal formation, dentate gyrus, and amygdaloid complex in the temporal lobe; portions of the frontal cortex; septal nuclei; the hypothalamus; anterior thalamic nuclei; olfactory bulbs and tracts; and parts of the basal ganglia (limbic striatum) (Figure 2–1). Together these regions influence memory, learning, emotional states and responses, and behavior, particularly aggressive, oral, and sexual activity (Pinchus and Tucker 1978).

Hippocampus.   The hippocampus has long been known to play a critical role in memory storage and retrieval (Pinchus and Tucker 1978) and is postulated to be a critical locus for the generation of dissociative states (Mesulam 1981). The hippocampus and parahippocampal gyrus may also play a dominant role in the pathophysiology of generalized anxiety and panic disorders (Gray et al. 1983; Reiman et al. 1984; Teicher 1988). These disorders possibly arise from excess noradrenergic influences on the hippocampus that ascend from the locus coeruleus (Gorman et al. 1989). Recent research also suggests that the septal area and hippocampus are crucial components of the behavioral inhibitory system, which acts to arrest ongoing behavior when it is environmentally inappropriate (Depue and Spoont 1986).

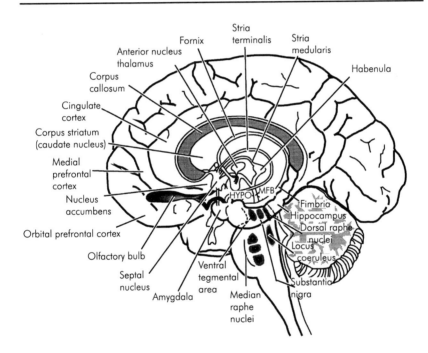

Figure 2–1.   Schematic illustration of the brain, sliced down the middle (midsagittal section), showing the major regions of the limbic system and related brain nuclei. Note that the hippocampus and amygdala are part of the overlying temporal lobe that has been removed for illustrative purposes. *Abbreviations:* HYPO = hypothalamus; MFB = medial forebrain bundle. Aspects of this figure are based on previous illustrations published by Pinchus and Tucker (1978), Goodwin and Jamison (1990), and Hyman and Nestler (1993).

Serotonergic projections from the median raphe nuclei to the hippocampus presumably play an important role in establishing an individual's overall level of behavioral inhibition (Depue and Spoont 1986). Thus, the hippocampal area may subserve the anxiogenic, dissociative, amnestic, and disinhibitory aspects of posttraumatic stress disorder (PTSD).

Amygdala. The interconnecting amygdaloid nuclei have been strongly implicated in the control of aggressive, oral, and sexual behaviors (Pinchus and Tucker 1978). Episodic dyscontrol and impulsive violence in humans may be due to irritable foci in the amygdaloid nuclei (Pinchus and Tucker 1978). It is also likely that the amygdala is involved in the formation and recollection of emotional memory and in the learning of nonverbal motor patterns. The amygdaloid nuclei are some of the most sensitive structures in the brain for the emergence of *kindling,* an important phenomenon in which repeated intermittent stimulation produces greater and greater alteration in neuronal excitability that may eventually result in seizures (Goddard et al. 1969; Post et al. 1984). However, the emergence of seizure activity is not critical; kindling results in long-term alterations in neuronal excitability that can have major impact on behavioral control (Post et al. 1984). van der Kolk and Greenberg (1987) have proposed that repeated traumatization, particularly child abuse, may lead to limbic kindling and to the emergence of neurological abnormalities, which can then lead to inappropriate aggression and sexual activity.

Limbic striatum. The limbic striatum, another key component of the limbic system, consists of the nucleus accumbens and associated portions of the caudate nucleus (Domesick 1988). It receives overlapping projections from the hippocampal formation, the basolateral nucleus of the amygdala, and the cingulate and prefrontal cortex. The limbic striatum is densely innervated by serotonergic projections from the dorsal raphe nuclei, by dopamine projections from the ventral tegmental area, and it is also well innervated by enkephalin projections. The limbic striatum provides a major gateway through which behavioral action can be inhibited or disinhibited (Depue and Spoont 1986). In adults the prefrontal cortex plays a decisive role in controlling activity within this circuit. Damage to the prefrontal cortex, particularly irritative lesions, can produce marked changes in personality with emergence of impulsive behavior, "emotional incontinence," poor self-control, and dulled awareness of the consequences of one's actions (Pinchus and Tucker 1978). van der Kolk and Greenberg (1987) have postulated that enkephalin projections within this region play a role in the addictive repetition of traumatic experience.

Temporolimbic seizures.   Seizure foci producing partial complex seizures are often localized to limbic structures in the temporal lobe, or to the frontal cortex. As indicated below, a number of studies suggest that there may be an increased incidence of electroencephalogram (EEG) abnormalities, and seizure foci, in patients with a history of early abuse. There is considerable controversy regarding the possible behavioral consequences of partial complex seizures. One consequence may be a tendency toward aggressive behavior. Though the relationship is controversial, some studies suggest that EEG abnormalities are frequently present in patients with episodic violence. For instance, in a study of 130 violent patients with substantial histories of childhood deprivation, parental psychiatric illness, and family violence, Bach-Y-Rita and co-workers (1971) found that one-half of all patients for whom EEGs were obtained showed abnormalities, particularly temporal spikes, on the EEGs.

Electroencephalogram abnormalities have also been reported to be a significant risk factor for suicidal ideation or attempts. One of the earliest pioneering studies on the physiological determinants of suicide reported a strong positive association between paroxysmal disturbances on the EEG and suicidal ideation, attempts, and assaultive-destructive behavior (Struve et al. 1972). It has also been reported, in the neurological literature, that the risk of completed suicide is four to five times greater in patients with epilepsy than in nonepileptic patients, and that this risk may be 25-fold greater in patients with temporal lobe epilepsy (Barraclough 1981; W. S. Matthews and Barabas 1981). As many as one-third of all epileptic patients have attempted suicide at some point in their life (Delay et al. 1957; Jensen 1975). The risk of attempted suicide is far greater for epileptic patients than for patients with other medical disorders that produce a comparable degree of handicap or disability (Mendez et al. 1986). More recently, Mendez and co-workers (1989) provided data suggesting that this risk may be related to interictal psychopathological changes, particularly BPD, which is highly prevalent in this population.

Previous research has suggested a possible relationship between BPD and temporal lobe–limbic system dysfunction (Andrulonis et al.

1981; Cowdry et al. 1985; Snyder and Pitts 1984). Snyder and Pitts (1984) reported that unmedicated patients with BPD had a higher incidence of sleep or wake EEG abnormalities (38% abnormal) than a contrast group of dysthymic patients (13% abnormal). Similarly, Cowdry and co-workers (1985) found that 41% of BPD patients (41% of whom were on medication) had a definite sharp wave abnormality on sleep-deprived EEG, compared with only 5% of patients with unipolar depression (75% of whom were on medication) ($P < .005$). On the other hand, Cornelius and co-workers (1986) reported that conventional EEG abnormalities did not occur statistically more frequently in unmedicated patients with BPD (18.8%) than in a comparison group consisting of patients with other personality disorders (9.1%). This finding is complicated, because more than half of the comparison group had either antisocial personality disorder (which shares important clinical features with BPD) or a mixed personality disorder (which may have included borderline traits). In short, EEG abnormalities may represent a significant risk factor for personality disturbance in some patients.

The relationship between abnormal EEG activity, temporal lobe epilepsy, dissociative phenomena, and the emergence of MPD is also complex and unresolved. Both Mesulam (1981) and Schenk and Baer (1981) have suggested that there is a strong association between temporal lobe epilepsy, dissociation, and MPD. However, Coons and co-workers (1988) reported that significant neurological and EEG abnormalities were "infrequently observed in patients with MPD." However, 23% of their population had grossly abnormal EEGs with paroxysmal spike and sharp waves—between 5 and 10 times the reported incidence of paroxysmal EEG events observed in other studies of psychiatric patients (Goodin and Aminoff 1984). Given that one would expect to observe interictal EEG abnormalities in no more than 40% of patients with actual partial complex seizures, this may indeed be a very high incidence.

Right-hemisphere function.   The right hemisphere appears to play a pivotal role in the perception and expression of emotion. Some authors have theorized that the right hemisphere is specialized for emotional processing in a fashion analogous to left-hemispheric specialization for language (e.g., Ross 1980). Most studies that focus on the perception or expression of human emotion (through vocal tone or facial expression) suggest that the right hemisphere is particularly specialized for the perception and expression of negative emotion

(Silberman and Weingartner 1986; Tomarken et al. 1992). Others suggest that the right hemisphere may be specialized for perception of all emotion, as well as for the expression of negative affect (Borod 1992; Hirschman and Safer 1982). Under normal circumstances, our capacity to appropriately identify and evaluate the affect of others, and in turn to appropriately communicate affect, depends on a healthy interaction between right-hemisphere emotional perception, and left-hemisphere linguistic processing and reason.

Summary

Evidence suggests that the anxiogenic, amnestic, somatic, and dissociative effects of trauma may be mediated via hippocampal projections in the limbic system and controlled by norepinephrine. The inappropriate release of aggressive and sexual behaviors that often occurs in traumatized individuals may be related to the development of irritative kindled foci in the amygdala or prefrontal cortex, or to deficient serotonergic modulation of the septo-hippocampal behavioral inhibitory system. The emergence of EEG abnormalities and possible epileptogenic foci may also enhance an individual's risk for both aggressive and self-destructive behavior. Damage to the right hemisphere can produce an array of affective disturbances, including indifference, depression, hysteria, gross social–emotional disinhibition, florid manic excitement, childishness, euphoria, impulsivity, and abnormal sexual behavior (Joseph 1988). Contemporary understanding of right-hemisphere function suggests that the right hemisphere can maintain a highly developed social–emotional mental system that can independently perceive, recall, and act on certain memories and experiences without the active participation of the left hemisphere (Joseph 1988). Deficient integration of the right and left hemispheres could result in the misperception of affect and foster a situation in which the right and left cerebral cortex may act at least partially independent of each other, giving rise to intrapsychic conflict and splitting (Joseph 1988; Muller 1992).

Possible Role of Early Experience on the Development of Limbic and Cortical Circuits

The prefrontal cortex, hippocampus, and amygdala are among the most plastic brain regions. The prefrontal cortex has the most delayed ontogeny of any brain region. Major projections to the prefrontal cortex scarcely begin to myelinate until adolescence, and this process continues into the third decade (Alexander and Goldman 1978; Fuster 1980; Goldman 1971; Weinberger 1987). Dopamine projections to the prefrontal cortex are specifically activated by stress (Deutch et al. 1985; Knorr et al. 1989; Reinhard et al. 1982). Thus, it is conceivable that stress activates the developing prefrontal cortex and alters its development. We theorize that stress may produce precocial maturation of the prefrontal cortex, leading to signs of early maturation ("parentified child"), but may arrest the development of this region, preventing it from reaching full adult capacity.

The hippocampus is a region in which neurogenesis continues into postnatal life, and the cellular organization of the hippocampus can be markedly affected by levels of corticosteroids, which can produce cell death (Sapolsky et al. 1990). Indeed, in a carefully controlled study on the effects of adult posttraumatic stress on regional brain anatomy, Bremner and co-workers (1995) reported that the most significant finding was a 12% reduction in hippocampal volume. The amygdala is a major site where overstimulation at any age can result in persistent kindled changes in neuronal excitability and behavior (Post et al. 1984).

Cynader and co-workers (1981) have shown, in kittens, that the normal bidirectional flow of information from the right and left hemispheres through the corpus callosum can be affected by early experience. In extreme circumstances the corpus callosum can be so affected that communication becomes entirely unidirectional. In such a situation a portion of one hemisphere becomes capable of transmitting information to the corresponding region of the other hemisphere and can affect its activity. However, this portion of the receiving hemisphere is unable to exert any influence on the transmitting hemisphere. Such unidirectionality could lead to an extreme instance of hemispheric dominance. Human research suggests that lateralized differences in frontal cortical activity may be established very early in life and play a decisive role in temperamental reactions (Fox and Davidson 1986). Evidence suggests that the degree and direction of lateralized function are controlled by genetic, hormonal, and experiential factors (Denenberg 1983; Galin 1977; Joseph 1988; Muller 1992). We believe that these anatomical structures may be particularly vulnerable to the effects of early abuse and trauma, which in turn may result in persistent neuropsychiatric disturbances that affect mood, cognition, and behavior.

Effects of Early Abuse on
Human Brain Development and Function

Researchers have long believed, based on animal studies, that early deprivation or abuse may result in neurobiological abnormalities (Hofer 1975; Hubel 1978; Teicher 1989); however, there has been little evidence for this in humans (van der Kolk and Greenberg 1987). Green and co-workers (1981) suggested that many abused children show evidence of neurological damage, even in the absence of apparent or reported head injury. These authors found that soft neurological signs and nonspecific EEG abnormalities were more common in abused children, and considered this to be an additional source of trauma, amplifying the pathological impact of the abusive environment (Green 1983). Childhood incest has been associated with reports of abnormal EEG activity. Davies (1979) reported that in a sample of 22 patients who had been involved, as a child or as the younger member, in an incestuous relationship, 77% had abnormal EEGs, and 36% had clinical seizures. These patients also experienced impulsivity and depersonalization. Davies suggested that these individuals were more at risk for being sexually abused by family members because of this neurological handicap. We wonder if the trauma of the abuse, and the need to repress memories of the abuse, may have overwhelmed the developing limbic system, to help bring about these abnormalities.

Association Between Early Abuse and
Ratings of Limbic Dysfunction in Adulthood

To better study the potential relationship between early abuse and limbic system dysfunction, we devised a self-report questionnaire, the Limbic System Checklist–33 (LSCL-33), to evaluate the frequency with which patients experienced 33 symptoms often encountered as ictal temporal lobe epilepsy phenomena (Teicher et al. 1993). The items, which were taken from the work of Spiers and co-workers (1985), consisted of paroxysmal somatic disturbances, brief hallucinatory events, visual phenomena, automatisms, and dissociative experiences. Subjects rated the lifetime frequency with which they experienced these disturbances using the predefined descriptors of "never," "rarely," "sometimes," and "often." From these descriptors, a total score was derived, as well as factor scores for somatic, sensory, behavioral, and mnemonic disturbances.

Psychometric evaluation indicated that LSCL-33 scores were low in healthy control subjects (<10) and elevated in patients with documented temporal lobe epilepsy (>23). LSCL-33 scores correlated well with scores on the Dissociative Experiences Scale (Bernstein and Putnam 1986) ($r = .81$, $n = 16$). They also significantly correlated with scores on the somatization ($r = .65$) and psychoticism ($r = .57$) subscales of the Hopkins Symptom Checklist–90 (SCL-90; Derogatis et al. 1974). However, none of the other SCL-90 subscales (e.g., depression, anxiety, paranoid ideation) added to the overall correlation. Test-retest reliability was found to be very high for total scores on the LSCL-33 ($r = .92$; $n = 16$; 1- to 2-week intertest interval) and for scores on each of the subscales. Thus, the LSCL-33 appears to have promise as a test instrument.

To ascertain whether there was an association between early abuse and limbic system dysfunction, we evaluated 253 adult outpatients who presented for assessment at an adult outpatient clinic. Mean age of the sample was 34 years (range 17–69), and 58% were female. The Life Experience Questionnaire (LEQ; Bryer et al. 1987) was used to ascertain abuse history. Each subject reported the type of abuse experienced (physical, sexual), age at onset, duration, and perpetrator of the abuse. Approximately 56% of patients reported a history of abuse during their lifetime. Of these, 16% reported a history of both physical and sexual abuse, 30% reported a history of physical abuse without sexual abuse, and 10% reported a history of sexual abuse without physical abuse.

Overall, abuse had a prominent effect on limbic system functioning, as reflected by total LSCL-33 scores ($P < .0001$). Subjects who indicated that they had never been abused ($n = 109$) had mean LSCL-33 scores of 13.6 (±11.3). Total LSCL-33 scores were 38% greater in patients who indicated a history of physical abuse and no sexual abuse ($P < .01$, $n = 77$) and were 49% greater in patients who indicated a history of sexual abuse but no physical abuse ($P < .02$, $n = 26$) than in patients who indicated that they had never been abused. Patients who indicated a history of both physical and sexual abuse ($n = 41$) had scores that were 113% greater than those of patients who indicated that they had never been abused ($P < .0001$). Both males and females who had indicated a history of abuse showed comparably increased LSCL-33 scores compared with patients who did not indicate having been abused, although among the latter, males had insignificantly lower LSCL-33 scores than females.

As expected, abuse before the age of 18 had a greater impact on limbic system functioning than abuse after age 18. Patients who were sexually abused before the age of 18 (but not physically abused) had scores that were 66% higher than those of patients who had never been abused ($P < .003$). In contrast, patients who had been sexually abused after age 18 (but not physically abused) had scores that were no different from those of patients who had never been abused. Similarly, patients who had been physically abused before age 18 (but not sexually abused) had scores that were 52% higher than those of patients who had never been abused ($P < .004$), whereas patients who had been physically abused after age 18 (but not sexually abused) had scores that were not significantly greater than those of patients who had not been abused. Although age at the time of first abuse was a significant factor for those patients subjected to either physical or sexual abuse, patients who had been abused both physically and sexually were strongly affected regardless of the age at first abuse. Hence, patients with combined abuse prior to age 18 had scores that were 147% greater than those of patients who had not been abused ($P < .0001$), whereas patients who had been abused both physically and sexually for the first time after age 18 had scores 127% greater ($P < .0002$).

As with total LSCL-33 scores, abuse was associated with elevated scores on each of the subscales of the LSCL-33. Each subscale was most markedly elevated in patients with a history of combined physical and sexual abuse, whereas a history of either physical or sexual abuse alone was associated with intermediate scores. Gender differences were present only on the somatic subscale, with females having overall somatic scores 39% greater than those in males ($P < .01$). There were no significant gender by abuse category interactions.

Overall, these findings are consistent with our hypothesis that early childhood abuse may lead to limbic system dysfunction. However, despite the high association between abuse and LSCL-33 scores, a number of serious limitations exist in the present study. First, the LSCL-33 is a new instrument, and further analysis of the validity and reliability of this scale is necessary. Confirmation of limbic system dysfunction through more direct assessment of brain function or anatomy is crucial. Second, the present study is purely correlational. It identifies a strong statistical association, but no claims regarding a cause-and-effect relationship can be established. It may be true, as

Davies (1979) proposed, that limbic dysfunction may increase the risk for early abuse. It is also possible that limbic dysfunction may be a hereditary disturbance, passed from generation to generation, and associated with a greater likelihood of abusive behavior on the part of parents, siblings, or relatives.

Association Between Early Abuse and Electroencephalogram Abnormalities in Childhood

In another study we attempted to ascertain whether childhood physical, sexual, or psychological abuse was associated with direct evidence of neurobiological abnormalities. A chart review was conducted to blindly examine the association between different categories of abuse and evidence for abnormalities on electroencephalography, brain electrical activity mapping (BEAM), computed tomography (CT), magnetic resonance imaging (MRI), neurological examination, and neuropsychological testing (Ito et al. 1993). We hypothesized that early abuse would be associated with an increased incidence of abnormalities on some of these tests. Furthermore, we suspected that abuse may be associated with a relatively circumscribed constellation of abnormalities in abused children.

Medical records were reviewed on 115 consecutive admissions to a child and adolescent psychiatric hospital. The admissions occurred between June 1988 and May 1989. Eleven patients were eliminated from consideration for inclusion in the study because of possible preexisting (i.e., prior to the onset of the abuse) neurological abnormalities or traumatic brain injuries. The mean age of the remaining 104 patients was 13 years. Sixty percent were adolescents (13 years or older), and 51% were male. Most of the subjects were Caucasian (86%). IQ test scores were above 85 in 84% of the patients, and 7% of the patients were mildly or moderately retarded (IQ below 71). Pharmacological treatment was not assessed or controlled.

Medical records were transcribed by research assistants, who prepared separate sheets for abuse history and neurological results on each subject. These sheets were separated and coded for independent blind scoring by two experienced clinicians. Any discrepant item was reviewed by a third blind clinician. Final scores required identical assessment by two of three raters. Neurological evaluations and tests were ordered based on clinical need, and the specialists who conducted these tests were unaware of our research interest or hypotheses.

Four broad categories of childhood trauma were evaluated: physical abuse, sexual abuse, psychological abuse (e.g., witnessing domestic violence, verbal abuse), and neglect. Each category was classified on a three-point scale: 0 = no known abuse or neglect; 1 = possible history of serious abuse or neglect, or known incidence of abuse of moderate severity; 2 = documented history of serious abuse or neglect. Physical abuse included physical assault or provoked injury other than ordinary physical punishment, such as rare slaps. Sexual abuse referred to sexual intrusion, penetration, molestation with genital contact or fondling by others. Exposure was not considered sexual abuse. Rare episodes of fondling were rated 1; digital penetration was rated 2. Neglect was defined as failure or refusal to provide necessary care and adequate supervision. Frequent witnessing of verbal fights between parents, or of verbal threats toward siblings by parents, was rated 1. Neurological assessments were divided into four categories: imaging studies (CT or MRI scans), electrophysiological studies (EEG or BEAM), neurological examination, and neuropsychological testing. Each category was rated as normal or abnormal. Neurological examinations were performed on 96% of the subjects. Ninety percent received electrophysiological assessment, 86% underwent neuropsychological testing, and 67% had neuroimaging studies. Overall, 98% of the neurological assessment categories, and 80% of the abuse categories, were scored identically by the two assigned clinician raters. All discrepancies were satisfactorily resolved by the blind third rater, who agreed with one of the two discrepant scores.

Four groups were established based on the abuse category scores:

1. *The nonabused group.* Patients in this group had no evidence of abuse in any of the four categories.
2. *The psychological abuse group.* Patients in this group had scores of 1 or 2 for psychological abuse or neglect, but scores of 0 for physical and sexual abuse.
3. *The overall physical/sexual abuse group.* Patients in this group had either physical or sexual abuse scores of 1 or 2, regardless of scores on the other categories.
4. *The severe physical/sexual abuse group.* Patients in this group had physical or sexual abuse scores of 2, indicating a documented history of severe abuse.

Altogether, 27 patients were assigned to the nonabused group, 22 patients to the psychological abuse group, and 55 patients to the overall physical/sexual abuse group. Thirty-eight patients in the physical/sexual abuse group had documented histories of unequivocal serious physical or sexual abuse.

There were no differences between patients with a history of abuse and patients with no history of abuse in the prevalence of abnormal neurological exams or abnormal neuropsychological tests. Abnormal imaging studies were found in 15.0% of the nonabused patients and in 26.0% of the abused patients, although this difference was not statistically significant. Abnormal electrophysiological studies were found in 26.9% of the nonabused patients but in 54.4% of the patients with a history of early trauma ($P = .021$). Abnormal electrophysiological studies were observed in 42.9% of the patients with psychological abuse, 59.6% of the total sample of patients with physical/sexual abuse ($P = .014$), and 71.9% of the subsample of patients with serious physical/sexual abuse ($P = .0013$). The overall prevalence of abnormal electrophysiological studies in patients with a significant history of abuse or neglect was about the same (53.3%–57.1%), regardless of age or gender (Table 2–1). Both the psychological abuse group and the physical/sexual abuse group had a statistically comparable prevalence of abnormal electrophysiological results (42.9% vs. 59.6%, respectively).

The majority of abnormal electrophysiological results occurred in frontotemporal or anterior regions (Figure 2–2). In the nonabused group, 19.2% of the patients had abnormalities within this area. In contrast, 47.1% of patients with a history of abuse had electrophysiological abnormalities in this region ($P = .018$). Patients with a history of physical/sexual abuse had a three- to fourfold greater prevalence of EEG abnormalities localized to the frontotemporal and anterior regions than patients who had not been abused.

Abused and nonabused patients differed most clearly in the prevalence of left-sided frontotemporal abnormalities ($P = .036$) (Figure 2–3). They did not differ either in the prevalence of abnormalities that were localized in the right side ($P > .8$) or in the prevalence of abnormalities that were seen bilaterally or that were not specifically localized ($P > .5$). In the group of patients who had not experienced abuse, left-sided electrophysiological abnormalities were rare, whereas in the group of patients who had experienced some kind of abuse, left-sided abnormalities were 2.5-fold more prevalent than right-sided abnormalities. This difference was particularly evident in the psychological abuse group, in which left-sided electrophysiological abnormalities were present in five cases, and right-sided abnormalities were present in none. Furthermore, all of the left-sided abnormalities in the psychological abuse group were restricted to the temporal lobes. It thus appears that although the overall incidence of electrophysiological abnormalities was numerically, but not statistically, increased in the psychological abuse group, there was a trend for a specific increase in the prevalence of left-sided temporal abnormalities. In the physical/sexual abuse group there was an overall increase in the prevalence of frontotemporal abnormalities, with less evidence for left-sided localization, particularly in the subgroup with a history of unequivocal serious abuse.

To further explore the possibility that psychological abuse may affect the development of the left hemisphere, the results of neuropsychological testing were reviewed for evidence of right–left hemispheric asymmetries (i.e., substantially better visuospatial ability than verbal performance). Overall, in patients with no history of abuse, left-hemisphere deficits were 2.25-fold more prevalent than right-hemisphere deficits. In patients with a history of abuse (any type), left-sided deficits were 6.67-fold more prevalent than right-sided deficits; left-sided deficits were 8-fold more prevalent than right-sided deficits in patients with a history of psychological abuse. Thus, abuse appears to be associated with an

Table 2–1. Prevalence of abnormal electrophysiological studies by age group and gender in study of association between abuse and neurobiological abnormalities in 104 patients admitted to a child and adolescent psychiatric hospital

Group	Prevalence	
Nonabused	26.9%	(7/26)
Any abuse		
Males	55.6%	(15/27)
Children	56.3%	(9/16)
Adolescents	54.5%	(6/11)
Females	53.7%	(22/41)
Children	53.3%	(8/15)
Adolescents	53.8%	(14/26)

increased prevalence of left-sided EEG abnormalities and an increased prevalence of right–left hemispheric asymmetries.

As in the previous study, there are a number of different ways to interpret a positive association between abuse history and electrophysiological abnormalities. Davies (1979) postulated that EEG abnormalities may be a risk factor for being abused, leading to a higher rate of victimization. It is also conceivable that EEG abnormalities may be inherited, and present in parents or siblings, and associated with a greater incidence of abusive behavior on their part. We propose that these EEG abnormalities may be a consequence of early abuse in at least some, and possibly many, of these patients. It will, however, be necessary to conduct a prospective, longitudinal assessment study with unmedicated subjects to test this hypothesis.

It is also worth pondering what it may mean that psychological abuse seemed to be most strongly associated with left-hemisphere abnormalities. The research reviewed above suggests that the right hemisphere may be specialized for the processing of emotion, particularly negative emotions (see also Ahern and Schwartz 1985; Schwartz et al. 1975). Galin (1974) and Joseph (1988) further speculated that painful childhood memories may be preferentially stored in the right hemisphere, outside of consciousness, but capable of influencing conscious behavior and affect. The present findings suggest that childhood abuse may be associated with greater left-sided dysfunction,

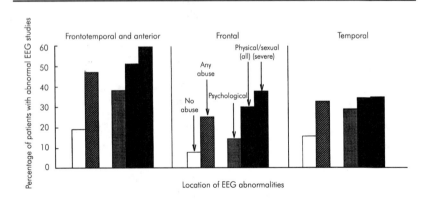

Figure 2–2.   Incidence of electroencephalogram (EEG) abnormalities associated with abuse history based on the regional localization of the EEG abnormality.

which may lead to greater dependence on the right hemisphere. Increased right frontal function, in turn, may lead to enhanced perception and reaction to negative affect (Tomarken et al. 1992) and may facilitate unconscious storage of painful childhood memories (Joseph 1988). Although purely hypothetical, such speculation is consistent with clinical observation that traumatized individuals are often hypersensitive to perception of negative affect and that memories of early abuse may be fully repressed, but eventually retrievable. Muller (1992), in a provocative article, has argued that early difficulties in maternal-child interaction may foster poor integration in right–left hemispheric function and produce a necessary or sufficient neural substrate for borderline splitting.

Right–Left Evoked Response Asymmetry During Recall of Unpleasant Early Memories in Psychologically Traumatized Subjects

Schiffer and colleagues (1995) have used probe auditory evoked potential (AEP) attenuation as a measure of hemispheric activity to further study the effects of early trauma on cerebral laterality. We were

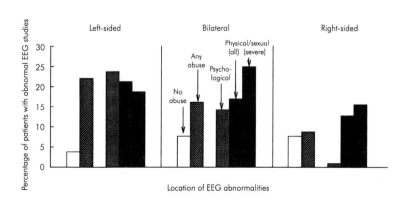

Figure 2–3.   Incidence of electroencephalogram (EEG) abnormalities associated with abuse history based on the left- and right-hemispheric localization of the EEG abnormality.

particularly interested in exploring Galin's (1974) and Joseph's (1988) hypothesis that painful childhood memories might be preferentially stored, outside of awareness, in the right hemisphere. To evaluate this hypothesis, hemispheric brain activity was measured in adult subjects under two conditions: first, during recall of a neutral memory and, then, during recall of an unpleasant affectively laden early experience. Probe AEPs were used as an index of hemispheric activity. Subjects were exposed to repeated auditory clicks, during which the amplitude of the average evoked potential EEG response was measured. While exposed to the clicks, the subjects were asked to engage in a mental activity. When one hemisphere is more actively involved than the other, the AEP response is attenuated in that hemisphere (Papanicolaou and Johnstone 1984; Papanicolaou et al. 1983a, 1983b). AEPs were studied in 10 right-handed adult subjects who all were psychotropic-free. Each subject was first asked to remember and reflect on an ordinary work or school situation. AEPs were recorded after the subject indicated that he or she was actively remembering the situation. Following the recording, the subject was asked a number of questions taken from the Profile of Mood States (POMS; Lorr et al. 1971). Each subject was then engaged in an empathic psychiatric interview, lasting about 15 minutes. The psychiatrist tried to affectively engage the subject and to get him or her to share, with emotion, a painful childhood memory. When the psychiatrist felt that the subject was affectively reexperiencing the memory, he asked the subject to try to continue to maintain the memory, without speech or motion, so that AEPs could be measured. Following recording of the AEPs, the POMS was used again to measure the subject's emotional state. All results from the AEP recordings were scored blindly by a research electrophysiologist.

Of the 10 subjects studied, 5 had experienced extreme psychological trauma during childhood, 2 severe trauma, 2 moderate trauma, and 1 no significant trauma. Overall, the neutral memory task produced a low mood score, which was increased by about eightfold during recall of the early abusive memory. Specifically, recall of this early memory resulted in substantially increased levels of tension, anger, sadness, hopelessness, nervousness, and panic. During the neutral task, 8 subjects had higher amplitudes over the right auditory cortex than over the left, implying greater relative left-sided cortical activity (left-sided attenuation). During recall of the unpleasant memory, 7 subjects had lower amplitudes over the right auditory cortex than over the left, implying greater relative right-sided cortical activity (right-sided attenuation; $P < .02$). Moreover, there was a significant correlation between ratings of severity of early psychiatric trauma and blind assessment of the degree of shift in the asymmetry index between tasks (Spearman's $\rho = .586, P < .05$).

These findings are consistent with findings from a large number of studies demonstrating increased right-hemisphere involvement with a number of affective tasks. Of particular interest was the observation that the degree of left–right shift correlated with estimates of the severity of the subject's early abuse. This observation suggests that early traumatic experience may play a role in fostering the specialization of the right hemisphere or in preventing the development of greater hemispheric interconnectivity. Unfortunately, it is not possible to distinguish between the possibility that the right hemisphere is merely specialized to handle emotions and the intriguing possibility that early abusive memories may be stored in the right hemisphere outside of conscious awareness. In any case, these findings are consistent with a hypothesis that childhood trauma influences hemispheric laterality. One could speculate that increased right-hemispheric dominance may contribute to a more affectively laden, negative perception of the world (Tomarken et al. 1992), which may be part of the problem in certain abused individuals.

Conclusions

Overall, findings from the studies discussed in this chapter support our initial hypothesis that early abuse may be associated with features of limbic system dysfunction, EEG abnormalities, and measures of hemispheric asymmetry. However, these studies do not provide strong proof, which would require prospective demonstration of the emergence of electrophysiological abnormalities or hemispheric asymmetries in previously healthy children after the occurrence of early abuse. Obviously, such a study would be logistically and ethically difficult. The present studies lend additional support to previous observations that there is a significant association between childhood abuse and evidence of neurobiological abnormalities. We cannot, however, disentangle the hypothesis that early abuse may lead to neurobiological abnormalities, from the equally plausible hypothesis that neurobiological abnormalities may increase the risk of childhood abuse. Regardless of the direction, the nature of the association indicates that in order to obtain a complete understanding of the causes and consequences, and therefore the treatment and prevention, of childhood abuse, an integrated biopsychosocial model is necessary.

We specifically hypothesize that early abuse can lead to a variety of neurodevelopmental abnormalities with different behavioral sequelae. When noradrenergic inputs to the hippocampus are affected, as has been implicated to happen following abuse, anxiogenic, amnestic, somatic, and dissociative effects may result. Kindled foci in the amygdala, or serotonin deficiencies in the septo-hippocampal behavioral inhibitory system, can lead to the inappropriate release of aggressive and sexual behavior, as can irritability in the prefrontal cortex. Deficient integration of left- and right-hemisphere function may result in the misperception of affect and may foster a situation in which the right and left halves of the brain act uncooperatively. Lack of appropriate hemispheric interdependence may give rise to intrapsychic conflict or may create affective instability if the right hemisphere floods the left with emotions and moods that do not make logical sense. If this model is valid, then the consequences of abuse would depend on the age at which the trauma occurs and the duration and severity of the trauma, as different regions would have different windows, and thresholds, of vulnerability. This model also suggests that psychotherapy, in adulthood, may be insufficient to correct the effects of early abuse, if abuse results in irreversible neurological alterations. Indeed, it is even conceivable that attempting to recall the abuse and "work through the trauma" may lead to temporary, or even persistent, worsening, if such a process further exacerbates kindling or neuronal irritability. Although this last point is highly speculative, what is not speculative is that prevention of abuse, or early corrective intervention in those cases in which prevention was not possible, is the ultimate goal. Certainly, additional research is necessary. We hope that this hypothesis helps foster the development of a more comprehensive understanding of the mechanisms through which early severe stress may produce pervasive psychiatric difficulties.

References

Ahern GL, Schwartz GE: Differential lateralization for positive and negative emotion in the human brain: EEG spectral analysis. Neuropsychologia 23:745–756, 1985

Alexander GE, Goldman PS: Functional development of the dorsolateral prefrontal cortex: an analysis utilizing reversible cryogenic depression. Brain Res 143:233–249, 1978

Andrulonis PA, Glueck BC, Stroebel CF, et al: Organic brain dysfunction and the borderline syndrome. Psychiatr Clin North Am 4:47–66, 1981

Bach-Y-Rita G, Lion JR, Climent CE, et al: Episodic dyscontrol: a study of 130 violent patients. Am J Psychiatry 127:1473–1478, 1971

Barraclough B: Suicide and epilepsy, in Epilepsy and Psychiatry. Edited by Reynolds E, Trimble MR. New York, Churchill Livingstone, 1981, pp 72–76

Beck JC, van der Kolk BA: Reports of childhood incest and current behavior of chronically hospitalized psychotic women. Am J Psychiatry 144:1474–1476, 1987

Bernstein EM, Putnam FW: Development, reliability and validity of a dissociation scale. J Nerv Ment Dis 174:727–735, 1986

Bliss EL: Multiple personalities: a report of 14 cases with implications for schizophrenia and hysteria. Arch Gen Psychiatry 37:1388–1397, 1980

Borod JC: Interhemispheric and intrahemispheric control of emotion: a focus on unilateral brain damage. J Consult Clin Psychol 60:339–348, 1992

Bremner JD, Randall P, Scott TM, et al: MRI-based measurement of hippocampal volume in patients with combat-related posttraumatic stress disorder. Am J Psychiatry 152:973–981, 1995

Brown GR, Anderson B: Psychiatric morbidity in adult inpatients with childhood histories of sexual and physical abuse. Am J Psychiatry 148:55–61, 1991

Bryer JB, Nelson BA, Miller JB, et al: Childhood sexual and physical abuse as factors in adult psychiatric illness. Am J Psychiatry 144:1426–1430, 1987

Burgess AW, Hartmann CR, McCormack A: Abused to abuser: antecedents of socially deviant behavior. Am J Psychiatry 144:1431–1436, 1987

Coons PM, Bowman ES, Milstein V: Multiple personality disorder: a clinical investigation of 50 cases. J Nerv Ment Dis 176:519–527, 1988

Cornelius JR, Brenner RP, Soloff PH, et al: EEG abnormalities in borderline personality disorder: specific or nonspecific. Biol Psychiatry 21:977–980, 1986

Cowdry RW, Pickar D, Davies R: Symptoms and EEG findings in the borderline syndrome. Int J Psychiatry Med 15:201–211, 1985

Cynader M, Lepore F, Guillemot JP: Inter-hemispheric competition during postnatal development. Nature 290:139–140, 1981

Davies RK: Incest: some neuropsychiatric findings. Int J Psychiatry Med 9:117–121, 1979

Delay J, Deniker P, Barande R: Le suicide des épileptiques. Encephale 46:401–436, 1957

Denenberg VH: Lateralization of function in rats. Am J Physiol 245:R505–R509, 1983

Depue RA, Spoont MR: Conceptualizing a serotonin trait: a behavioral dimension of constraint. Ann N Y Acad Sci 487:47–62, 1986

Derogatis LR, Lipman RS, Rickels K, et al: The Hopkins Symptom Checklist (HSCL): a self-report symptom inventory. Behav Sci 19:1–15, 1974

Deutch AY, Tam S-Y, Roth RH: Footshock and conditioned stress increase 3,4-dihydroxyphenylacetic acid (DOPAC) in the ventral tegmental area but not in the substantia nigra. Brain Res 333:143–146, 1985

Domesick VB: Neuroanatomical organization of the dopamine neurons in the ventral tegmental area. Ann N Y Acad Sci 537:10–26, 1988

Famularo R, Kinscherff R, Fenton T: Propranolol treatment for childhood posttraumatic stress disorder, acute type: a pilot study. Am J Dis Child 142:1244–1247, 1988

Faravelli C, Webb T, Ambonetti A: Prevalence of traumatic early life events in 31 agoraphobic patients with panic attacks. Am J Psychiatry 142:1493–1494, 1985

Finkelhor D: A Sourcebook on Child Sexual Abuse. Beverly Hills, CA, Sage, 1986

Fox NA, Davidson RJ: Taste-elicited changes in facial signs of emotion and the asymmetry of brain electrical activity in human newborns. Neuropsychologia 24:417–422, 1986

Fuster JM: The Prefrontal Cortex: Anatomy, Physiology, and Neuropsychology of the Frontal Lobe. New York, Raven, 1980

Galin D: Implications for psychiatry of left and right cerebral specialization. Arch Gen Psychiatry 31:572–583, 1974

Galin D: Lateral specialization and psychiatric issues: speculations on development and the evolution of consciousness. Ann N Y Acad Sci 299:397–411, 1977

Goddard CV, McIntrye DC, Leech CK: A permanent change in brain functioning resulting from daily electrical stimulation. Exp Neurol 25:295–330, 1969

Goldman PS: Functional development of the prefrontal cortex in early life and the problem of neuronal plasticity. Exp Neurol 32:366–387, 1971

Goodin DS, Aminoff MJ: Does the interictal EEG have a role in the diagnosis of epilepsy? Lancet ii:837–839, 1984

Goodwin FK, Jamison KR: Manic-Depressive Illness. New York, Oxford University Press, 1990

Gorman JM, Liebowitz MR, Fryer AJ, et al: A neuroanatomical hypothesis for panic disorder. Am J Psychiatry 146:148–161, 1989

Gray JA, Holt L, McNaughton N: Clinical implications of the experimental pharmacology of the benzodiazepines, in The Benzodiazepines: From Molecular Biology to Clinical Practice. Edited by Costa E. New York, Raven, 1983, pp 147–171

Green AH: Dimensions of psychological trauma in abused children. Journal of the American Academy of Child Psychiatry 22:231–237, 1983

Green AH, Voeller K, Gaines R, et al: Neurological impairment in maltreated children. Child Abuse Negl 5:129–134, 1981

Herman JL: Histories of violence in an outpatient population. Am J Orthopsychiatry 56:137–141, 1986

Herman JL, Perry JC, van der Kolk BA: Childhood trauma in borderline personality disorder. Am J Psychiatry 146:490–495, 1989

Hirschman RS, Safer MA: Hemispheric differences in perceiving positive and negative emotions. Cortex 18:569–580, 1982

Hofer MA: Studies on how early maternal deprivation produces behavioral change in young rats. Psychosom Med 37:245–264, 1975

Horevitz RP, Braun BR: Are multiple personalities borderlines? Psychiatr Clin North Am 7:69–87, 1984

Hubel DH: Effects of deprivation on the visual cortex of cat and monkey. Harvey Lect 72:1–51, 1978

Hyman SE, Nestler EJ: The Molecular Foundations of Psychiatry. Washington, DC, American Psychiatric Press, 1993

Ito Y, Teicher MH, Glod CA, et al: Increased prevalence of electrophysiological abnormalities in children with psychological, physical and sexual abuse. J Neuropsychiatry Clin Neurosci 5:401–408, 1993

Jensen I: Temporal lobe epilepsy: late mortality in patients treated with unilateral temporal lobe resections. Acta Neurol Scand 52:374–380, 1975

Joseph R: The right cerebral hemisphere: emotion, music, visual-spatial skills, body-image, dreams, and awareness. J Clin Psychol 44:630–673, 1988

Kashani JH, Carlson GA: Seriously depressed preschoolers. Am J Psychiatry 144:348–350, 1987

Knorr AM, Deutch AY, Roth RH: The anxiogenic carboline FG-7142 increases in vivo and in vitro tyrosine hydroxylation in the prefrontal cortex. Brain Res 495:335–361, 1989

Krystal H: Trauma and affects. Psychoanal Study Child 33:81–116, 1978

Levitt P: A monoclonal antibody to limbic system neurons. Science 223:299–301, 1984

Lopes da Silva FH, Witter MP, Boeijinga PH, et al: Anatomic organization and physiology of the limbic cortex. Physiol Rev 70:453–511, 1990

Lorr M, McNair DM, Droppleman LF: Profile of Mood States Manual. San Diego, CA, Educational and Industrial Testing Service, 1971

Matthews WS, Barabas G: Suicide and epilepsy: a review of the literature. Psychosomatics 22:515–524, 1981

Mendez MF, Cummings JL, Benson DF: Depression in epilepsy: significance and phenomenology. Arch Neurol 43:766–770, 1986

Mendez MF, Lanska DJ, Manon-Espaillat R, et al: Causative factors for suicide attempts by overdose in epileptics. Arch Neurol 46:1065–1068, 1989

Mesulam M-M: Dissociative states with abnormal temporal lobe EEG: multiple personality and the illusion of possession. Arch Neurol 38:176–181, 1981

Muller RJ: Is there a neural basis for borderline splitting? Compr Psychiatry 33:92–104, 1992

Papanicolaou AC, Johnstone J: Probe evoked potentials: theory, method and applications. Int J Neurosci 24:107–131, 1984

Papanicolaou AC, Levin HS, Eisenberg HM, et al: Evoked potential indices of selective hemispheric engagement in affective and phonetic tasks. Neuropsychologia 21:401–405, 1983a

Papanicolaou AC, Schmidt AL, Moore BD, et al: Cerebral activation patterns in an arithmetic and a visuospatial processing task. Int J Neurosci 20:289–294, 1983b

Pinchus JH, Tucker GJ: Behavioral Neurology, New York, Oxford University Press, 1978

Post RM, Rubinow DR, Ballenger JC: Conditioning, sensitization and kindling: implications for the course of affective illness, in Neurobiology of Mood Disorders. Edited by Post RM, Ballenger JC. Baltimore, MD, Williams & Wilkins, 1984, pp 432–466

Putnam FW, Post RM, Guroff JJ, et al: One hundred cases of multiple personality disorder. J Clin Psychiatry 47:285–293, 1986

Reep R: Relationship between prefrontal and limbic cortex: a comparative anatomical review. Brain Behav Evol 25:5–80, 1984

Reiman EM, Raicle ME, Butler FK, et al: A focal brain abnormality in panic disorder, a severe form of anxiety. Nature 310:683–685, 1984

Reinhard JF Jr, Bannon MJ, Roth RH: Acceleration by stress of dopamine synthesis and metabolism in prefrontal cortex: antagonism by diazepam. Naunyn-Schmiedebergs Arch Pharmacol 318:374–377, 1982

Ross ED: The aprosodias: functional-anatomic organization of the affective components of language in the right hemisphere. Arch Neurol 38:561–569, 1980

Sapolsky RM, Uno H, Rebert CS, et al: Hippocampal damage associated with prolonged glucocorticoid exposure in primates. J Neurosci 10:2897–2902, 1990

Schiffer F, Teicher MH, Papanicolaou AC: Evoked potential evidence for right brain activity during recall of traumatic memories. J Neuropsychiatry Clin Neurosci 7:169–175, 1995

Schenk L, Baer D: Multiple personality and related dissociative phenomena in patients with temporal lobe epilepsy. Am J Psychiatry 138:1311–1316, 1981

Schwartz GE, Davidson RJ, Maer F: Right hemisphere lateralization for emotion in the human brain: interaction wih cognition. Science 190:286–288, 1975

Silberman EK, Weingartner H: Hemispheric lateralization of functions related to emotion. Brain Cogn 5:322–353, 1986

Snyder S, Pitts WM Jr: Electroencephalograph of DSM-III borderline personality disorder. Acta Psychiatr Scand 69:129–134, 1984

Spiers PA, Schomer DL, Blume HW, et al: Temporolimbic epilepsy and behavior, in Principles of Behavioral Neurology. Edited by Mesulam M-M. Philadelphia, PA, FA Davis, 1985, pp 289–326

Stone MH: Borderline syndromes: a consideration of subtypes and an overview, directions for research. Psychiatr Clin North Am 4:3–13, 1981

Struve FA, Klein DF, Saraf KR: Electroencephalographic correlates of suicide ideation and attempts. Arch Gen Psychiatry 27:363–365, 1972

Teicher MH: Biology of anxiety. Med Clin North Am 72:791–814, 1988

Teicher MH: Psychological factors in neurological development, in Neurobiological Development (Nestle Nutrition Workshop Series, Vol 12). Edited by Evrard P, Minkowski A. New York, Raven, 1989, pp 243–258

Teicher MH, Glod CA, Surrey J, et al: Early childhood abuse and limbic system ratings in adult psychiatric outpatients. J Neuropsychiatry Clin Neurosci 5:301–306, 1993

Tomarken AJ, Davidson RJ, Wheeler RE, et al: Individual differences in anterior brain asymmetry and fundamental dimensions of emotion. J Pers Soc Psychol 64:676–687, 1992

van der Kolk BA, Greenberg MS: The psychobiology of the trauma response: hyperarousal, constriction, and addiction to traumatic reexposure, in Psychological Trauma. Edited by van der Kolk BA. Washington, DC, American Psychiatric Press, 1987, pp 63–87

Weinberger DR: Implications of normal brain development for the pathogenesis of schizophrenia. Arch Gen Psychiatry 44:660–669, 1987

Westen D, Ludolph P, Misle B, et al: Physical and sexual abuse in adolescent girls with borderline personality disorder. Am J Orthopsychiatry 60:55–66, 1990

Zanarini MC, Gunderson JG, Marino MF, et al: Childhood experiences of borderline patients. Compr Psychiatry 30:18–25, 1989

Chapter 3

Early Environment and the Development of Individual Differences in the Hypothalamic-Pituitary-Adrenal Stress Response

Michael J. Meaney, Ph.D.
Seema Bhatnagar, M.Sc.
Sylvie Larocque, B.Sc.
Cheryl M. McCormick, Ph.D.
Nola Shanks, Ph.D.
Shakti Sharma, B.Sc.
James Smythe, Ph.D.
Victor Viau, M.Sc.
Paul M. Plotsky, Ph.D.

The adrenal glucocorticoids and catecholamines constitute a frontline of defense for mammalian species under conditions that threaten homeostasis. (The conditions are commonly referred to as "stress" and

The research described in this chapter was supported by grants from the Medical Research Council of Canada (MRCC) to MJM and from the National Institute of Mental Health to PMP. MJM is the recipient of an MRCC Scientist Career Award. NS, JS, and CMM were supported by postdoctoral fellowships from the Natural Sciences and Engineering Research Council of Canada. SB is a graduate fellow of the Canadian Heart Foundation and the MRCC. CMM is currently Assistant Professor of Psychology in the Department of Psychology, Bates College, Lewiston, Maine.

the provocative stimuli as "stressors.") These hormones serve as major regulators of carbohydrate and lipid metabolism, cardiovascular tone, muscle function, immunocompetence, and behavior. The adrenal glucocorticoids represent the end product of the hypothalamic-pituitary-adrenal (HPA) axis. Under most conditions, this axis lies under the dominion of specific peptides secreted by neurons located in the paraventricular nuclei (PVN) of the hypothalamus. Most notable among these peptides are corticotropin-releasing factor (CRF) and arginine vasopressin (AVP). The neurons of the PVN are thus the major target for both the activational effects of the neural signals associated with stress and the inhibitory effects associated with glucocorticoid negative feedback. The nature of the HPA response to stress is a function of the integration of these signals at the level of the CRF/AVP neurons in the hypothalamus.

The ability of the organism to rapidly mount an endocrine response to stress is imperative. Under stressful conditions, adrenalectomized animals are unable to sustain the necessary cardiovascular tone and blood glucose levels and thus perish. However, inappropriate or exaggerated HPA activity is also threatening to the health of the organism. Prolonged exposure to elevated glucocorticoid levels results in a general suppression of anabolic processes, muscle atrophy, decreased sensitivity to insulin and a risk of steroid-induced diabetes, hypertension, hyperlipidemia, hypercholesterolemia, arterial disease, amenorrhea, impotency, and the impairment of growth and tissue repair, as well as immunosuppression (Brindley and Rolland 1989; Munck et al. 1984). In addition, elevated glucocorticoid levels are also associated with psychopathology. Hence, an efficient response to stress is one that is rapidly mobilized in the presence of a threat and then effectively "turned off" once the threatening condition is no longer present.

The development of the HPA response is shaped by events occurring early in life. These effects are surprisingly robust and account, in part at least, for the individual differences that occur in neuroendocrine responses to stress. There is now considerable evidence for the idea that these early environmental factors ultimately influence activity at the level of the hypothalamic CRF/AVP neurons, either directly or indirectly via their effects on systems that mediate the inhibitory signals associated with glucocorticoid negative feedback. These changes persist throughout the life of the animal and are accompanied by altered endocrine responses to stress. Such developmental effects likely represent one way in which early life events can predispose an individual to pathology in later life. Thus, early environment can determine vulnerability to pathology in later life by determining the efficiency with which the animal responds to stress.

The Adrenocortical Response to Stress

The HPA axis, as described by Selye (1950), is highly responsive to stress. Neural signals associated with the stressor are transduced into endocrine responses via their effects at the level of the hypothalamus (Figure 3–1). Thus, the secretion of CRF and AVP from PVN neurons into the portal system of the anterior pituitary during stress causes an increase in the release of adrenocorticotropin (ACTH) from pituitary corticotrophes into circulation (see, e.g., Antoni 1986; Gibbs 1986; Linton et al. 1985; Nakane et al. 1985; Plotsky 1987; Rivier and Vale 1983; Rivier et al. 1982). The elevated ACTH levels, in turn, stimulate an increase in the synthesis and release of adrenal glucocorticoids. The highly catabolic glucocorticoids produce lipolysis, increasing the level of free fatty acids; glycogenolysis, increasing blood glucose levels; and protein catabolism, increasing availability of amino acids as substrates for gluconeogenesis, which further increases blood glucose levels (Brindley and Rolland 1989; Munck et al. 1984). Together, these actions assist the organism under stressful conditions, in part at least, by increasing the availability of energy substrates. The glucocorticoids also suppress immunological responses (Munck et al. 1984), protecting against the occurrence of inflammation at a time when mobility may be important to the animal.

However, for the reasons stated above, once the stressor is terminated, it is very clearly in the animal's best interest to terminate the HPA stress response. The efficacy of this process is determined by the ability of the glucocorticoids to inhibit subsequent ACTH release (i.e., glucocorticoid negative feedback; see Figure 3–1). The HPA axis is a classical closed-loop feedback system in which the end product of the axis, the adrenal glucocorticoids, feed back onto higher structures in the axis to inhibit activity. Thus, circulating glucocorticoids feed back onto the pituitary and specific brain regions to inhibit the release of ACTH from the anterior pituitary cells (Dallman et al. 1987a; Jones et al. 1982; Keller-Wood and Dallman 1984; Plotsky and Vale

1984; Plotsky et al. 1987; Van Loon and DeSouza 1987). The focus for glucocorticoid negative-feedback inhibition is the population of CRF and CRF/AVP neurons in the parvocellular region of the PVN. Thus, glucocorticoids serve to decrease mRNA levels (e.g., Beyer et al. 1988;

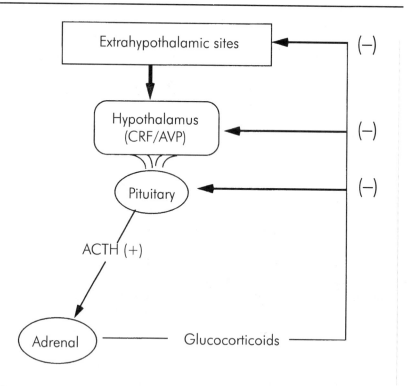

Figure 3–1. A schema describing the hypothalamic-pituitary-adrenal (HPA) response to stress. Neural signals associated with the stressor impinge upon hypothalamic (and extrahypothalamic) sites to stimulate the release of corticotropin-releasing factor (CRF) and/or arginine vasopressin (AVP) stores from hypothalamic neurons into the hypophysial portal system of the anterior pituitary. These peptides stimulate the release of adrenocorticotropin (ACTH) from corticotrophes into circulation, and ACTH, in turn, stimulates the release of adrenal glucocorticoids (primarily cortisol in primates and corticosterone in rodents). Activity within the HPA axis is regulated by a negative-feedback loop whereby the end products of the axis, the adrenal glucocorticoids, act at various levels to inhibit CRF/AVP synthesis and release.

Lightman and Young 1988; Swanson and Simmons 1989; Wolfson et al. 1985; Young et al. 1987), content (e.g., Kiss et al. 1984; Merchenthaler et al. 1983; Swanson et al. 1983), and release (Plotsky and Sawchenko 1987) of both CRF and AVP. In producing these effects, glucocorticoids act either directly on CRF and CRF/AVP neurons or indirectly via other brain regions that, in turn, regulate activity within the PVN neurons. Thus, the pituitary and the hypothalamus are not the only relevant brain sites for glucocorticoid feedback effects.

There is now considerable evidence for the importance of extrahypothalamic regions in the inhibition of CRF synthesis and HPA activity. Most notable among these regions is the hippocampus (Jacobson and Sapolsky 1991). In the rat, hippocampal lesions or ablations are associated with elevated corticosterone (the principal glucocorticoid in rodents) levels under basal, stress, and poststress conditions (e.g., Feldman and Conforti 1976, 1980; Fischette et al. 1980; Sapolsky et al. 1984a; Wilson et al. 1980). Moreover, hippocampectomized animals show reduced suppression of ACTH following exogenous glucocorticoid administration (Feldman and Conforti 1976, 1980) and increased CRH and AVP mRNA levels in the PVN of the hypothalamus (Herman et al. 1989), and fornix lesions were shown to decrease glucocorticoid inhibition of CRF and AVP release in the portal system (Sapolsky et al. 1990). These findings, together with the fact that the hippocampus is rich in corticosteroid receptors (McEwen et al. 1986), suggest that this structure is involved in the inhibitory influence of glucocorticoids over adrenocortical activity. (See Jacobson and Sapolsky 1991 and McEwen et al. 1986 for reviews of the issues and controversies on this topic.)

Corticosteroid Receptors and Their Action

Corticosteroids exert their intracellular effects via soluble, high-affinity corticosteroid receptors. As will be discussed later in this chapter, there are at least two corticosteroid receptor subtypes, the mineralocorticoid and glucocorticoid receptors (also referred to as type I and type II corticosteroid receptors, respectively). The importance of corticosteroid action is reflected by the presence of corticosteroid receptors in virtually every cell type in the body (see Burnstein and

Cidlowski 1989). The recent cloning of the human (Hollenberg et al. 1985), rat (Meisfeld et al. 1984), and mouse (Danielson et al. 1986) glucocorticoid receptor, as well as the human mineralocorticoid receptor (Arriza et al. 1988), has marked a period of tremendous progress in our knowledge of steroid receptor action. The basic features of the prevailing understanding of steroid receptor action are summarized schematically in Figure 3–2 (see Carson-Jurica et al. 1990; Evans and Arriza 1989).

These receptors belong to a family of ligand-dependent transcription factors. Briefly, the steroid diffuses across the cell membrane and then binds to soluble, unoccupied receptor sites. The receptor is then "activated," a process that corresponds to the dissociation of a 90-kDa heat-shock protein into a form that is then capable of binding to specific DNA sequences referred to as *hormone regulatory (or responsive) elements* (Pratt et al. 1989). Receptors complexed with a heat-shock protein are unable to bind DNA. Corticoid effects on the transcription of target genes are then mediated by an interaction between the hormone-receptor complex and specific DNA sequences. The results of this interaction are then reflected in changes in mRNA transcription and protein synthesis. It should be noted that this summary does not include any reference to the effects of various intracellular factors such as protein kinases and the early gene products cFOS/JUN that can regulate glucocorticoid receptor function. Indeed, there are a number of potential sites for the regulation of corticosteroid receptor action (see Burnstein and Cidlowski 1989).

An essential feature of this model is that it predicts that receptor density (or binding capacity) is a major determinant of target cell sensitivity to glucocorticoids. This appears to be true in many, but not all, cases (see Burnstein and Cidlowski 1989; Ringold 1985). The presence of corticosteroid receptors in a cell is a prerequisite for a glucocorticoid response. Moreover, variations in corticosteroid receptor levels have often been found to predict the magnitude of cellular responses to glucocorticoids (e.g., as we shall see, changes in receptor density in certain brain structures can alter glucocorticoid negative-feedback efficacy). These conclusions are also supported by studies indentifying glucocorticoid receptor anomalies as a major source of naturally occurring syndromes of glucocorticoid resistance.

The uptake of corticosterone in rat brain, as alluded to earlier, is associated with at least two distinct corticosteroid receptor subtypes (see, e.g., Beaumont and Fanestil 1983; Emadian et al. 1986; Funder and Sheppard 1987; McEwen et al. 1986; Reul and De Kloet 1985, 1986; Reul et al. 1987; Sheppard and Funder 1987). The *mineralocor-*

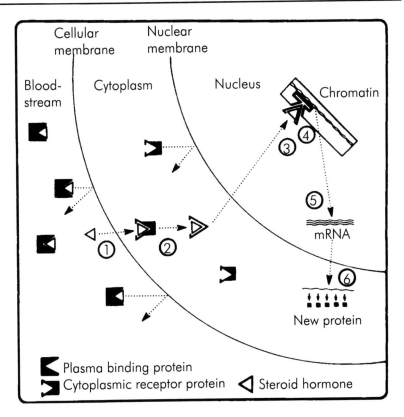

Figure 3–2. A summary of current models of steroid receptor action. *(1)* The free steroid (i.e., steroid that is not bound to plasma binding proteins, such as corticosteroid-binding globulin [CBG]) diffuses across the cell membrane *(2)* to where it binds to an unoccupied intracellular receptor (which can be located in either the cytoplasmic or nuclear compartments), forming an activated hormone-receptor complex. *(3–4)* The complex then binds to specific sites on the DNA *(5)*, resulting in the regulation of mRNA transcription and *(6)* protein synthesis. According to this model the sensitivity of the cell to circulating steroid is determined, in part, by the number of intracellular receptors.

ticoid (or type I) receptor binds in vitro to both corticosterone and the mineralocorticoids aldosterone, spironolactone, and RU 26752 with high affinity and binds the synthetic glucocorticoid RU 28362 with very low affinity. In the brain, mineralocorticoid receptor density is highest in the septo-hippocampal system. The *glucocorticoid (or type II) receptor,* which is far more diffusely distributed throughout the brain, binds corticosterone, dexamethasone, and RU 28362 with high affinity and binds RU 26752 and aldosterone with lower affinity. Although both receptors bind corticosterone with high affinity, the K_d of the mineralocorticoid receptor for corticosterone (~0.5 nM) is lower than that of the glucocorticoid receptor (~2.0–5.0 nM) (e.g., Reul and De Kloet 1985).

A physiological consequence of this difference in affinity for corticosterone is the fact that these receptors then show different rates of ligand occupancy under basal corticosterone levels. About 50% to 90% of the mineralocorticoid sites are occupied under basal corticosterone levels (~5 µg/dl) (Reul and De Kloet 1985; Reul et al. 1987). Because of this high occupancy rate, the hippocampal mineralocorticoid receptor is relatively insensitive to dynamic variations in corticosterone levels above those seen in the resting state. In contrast, the glucocorticoid receptor is highly responsive to dynamic changes in corticosterone titers, such as those occurring during the circadian peak or during stress (Meaney et al. 1988a; Reul and De Kloet 1985; Reul et al. 1987). Under conditions of basal circulating corticosterone only about 10% to 15% of the glucocorticoid receptors are occupied. Stress results in a dramatic increase in the hormone receptor signal, such that immediately following a 20-minute period of restraint, about 75% of glucocorticoid receptors are occupied. Corticosterone injections that mimic the steroid levels seen during stress (~30 µg/dl) also result in about 75% occupancy of glucocorticoid receptors. These findings, together with the known negative-feedback efficacy of the synthetic corticoids such as dexamethasone, once thought to selectively bind to the glucocorticoid receptor, suggested that it was this site, and not the mineralocorticoid-like receptor, that underlies the negative-feedback actions of glucocorticoids.

However, Dallman and her colleagues have recently provided evidence for the involvement of both hippocampal mineralocorticoid and glucocorticoid receptors in the regulation of ACTH levels in rats. In these studies, hippocampal implants of the glucocorticoid receptor antagonist RU 38486 and implants of the mineralocorticoid receptor antagonist RU 26752 both resulted in elevated levels of plasma ACTH (Bradbury and Dallman 1991; also see Dallman et al. 1991). Moreover, Ratka and co-workers (1989) have found that systemic injections of either antagonist resulted in elevated poststress corticosterone levels in intact rats. These findings suggest that glucocorticoid negative feedback may involve both mineralocorticoid and glucocorticoid receptor sites. In addition, it should also be noted that although there is presently considerable emphasis on the role of the hippocampus and hippocampal corticosteroid receptors in glucocorticoid negative-feedback regulation of HPA function, several other corticolimbic sites are likely to be relevant. Kovacs and Makara (1988) reported that glucocorticoid implants into the septum attenuated adrenalectomy-induced increases in plasma ACTH. Moreover, Diorio and co-workers (1993) have found that corticoid implants into the frontal cortex–cingulate gyrus dampen plasma ACTH responses to restraint stress. Interestingly, these regions contain both mineralocorticoid and glucocorticoid receptor sites (Diorio et al. 1993; Meaney and Aitken 1985; Meaney et al. 1985a, 1985b).

Probably the strongest support for the importance of the hippocampus in the regulation of HPA activity comes from studies on the role of hippocampal corticosteroid receptor systems. Evidence from a number of models (see Goldman et al. 1978; Jacobson and Sapolsky 1991; McEwen et al. 1986; Meaney et al. 1993; Sapolsky and Meaney 1986) suggests that a decrease in hippocampal corticosteroid receptor density is associated with a hypersecretion of corticosterone both under basal conditions and following the termination of stress (i.e., less effective negative feedback). There are decreased levels of hippocampal corticosteroid receptor binding in the aged rat, lactating rats, and immature rats, and these animals also hypersecrete corticosterone under basal and/or stressful conditions. Perhaps the most impressive evidence comes from studies with the vasopressin-deficient Brattleboro rat (Sapolsky et al. 1984a). These animals show a deficit in corticosteroid receptors in the hippocampus and pituitary, and hypersecrete corticosterone following stress. The hippocampal receptor deficit is reversed with vasopressin treatment, and so long as the treatment is continued, receptor levels remain elevated and the animals exhibit normal corticosterone secretion following subsequent stress (Sapolsky et al. 1984a).

Effects of Postnatal Handling on Hypothalamic-Pituitary-Adrenal Responses to Stress

During the late 1960s, Levine, Denenberg, Ader, and others (Ader and Grota 1969; Hess et al. 1969; Levine 1957, 1962; Levine et al. 1967) described the effects of postnatal "handling" (outlined below) on the development of behavioral and endocrine responses to stress. As adults, handled rats exhibited attenuated fearfulness in novel environments and a less pronounced increase in the secretion of the adrenal glucocorticoids in response to a variety of stressors. These findings clearly demonstrated that the development of rudimentary, adaptive responses to stress could be modified by environmental events. In addition, the handling paradigm provides a marvelous opportunity to examine how subtle variations in the early environment alter the development of specific neurochemical systems, leading to stable individual differences in biological responses to stimuli that threaten homeostasis.

The studies to be described in this section have been performed using laboratory rats. The following description of developmental landmarks is provided to give the reader an impression of the maturational process and its timing in this rodent species. Rat pups are born following a 21- to 22-day period of gestation. The animals remain highly dependent upon the mother for the first 2 weeks of life. During the third week of life the weaning process begins and the animals begin to regulate their own body temperature. Rat pups are weaned at 22 days of age, and puberty begins over the next few weeks of life (generally during days 35 to 40 in females and 40 to 50 in males, depending upon the measures used to indicate the onset of sexual maturity). By 70 days of life the animals have reached maturity. In each case, the postnatal manipulations described below are most effective during the first week of life.

The handling procedure usually involves removing rat pups from their cage, placing the animals together in small containers, and, 15 to 20 minutes later, returning the animals to their cage and their mothers. The manipulation is generally performed daily for the first 21 days of life, and the animals are tested as fully mature adults.

In response to a wide variety of stimuli, handled (H) rats secrete less corticosterone and show a faster return of corticosterone to basal levels following the termination of stress than do nonhandled (NH) animals (Ader and Grota 1969; Hess et al. 1969; Levine 1957, 1962; Levine et al. 1967; Meaney et al. 1988b, 1989). Another way to evaluate hormone data is to calculate the integrated response, which is a measure of hormone secretion over time (i.e., [area under the curve]/[time]). This procedure reflects the integrated hormonal signal and for certain hormones, such as ACTH, is physiologically very relevant. The integrated plasma corticosterone response to stress (calculated from the prestress to 120 minutes poststress time points) is usually 75% to 100% higher in the NH rats. These endocrine differences are apparent as late as 24 to 26 months of age (Meaney et al. 1988b), indicating that the handling effect persists over the entire life of the animal. The differences in HPA function are not due to changes in adrenal sensitivity to ACTH or in pituitary sensitivity to CRF (Grota 1975; Meaney et al. 1989). Moreover, there are no differences between H and NH animals in the metabolic clearance rate for ACTH or corticosterone (Grota 1975; Meaney et al. 1989). Rather, the difference lies in the fact that the NH animals show increased hormone secretion both during and following stress.

Young adult H and NH animals do not differ in levels of corticosteroid-binding globulin (CBG), the principal plasma binder for corticosterone (Meaney et al. 1989, 1992), or in free corticosterone levels (Meaney et al. 1992). These findings are of considerable importance because brain uptake of corticosterone appears to approximate the non-CBG-bound (free + albumin-bound) portion of the steroid (Partridge et al. 1983). Thus, differences in total corticosterone are likely predictive of differences in brain uptake of the steroid. Interestingly, the handling effects on HPA function are specific to conditions of stress. Young adult H and NH animals do not differ in basal corticosterone levels at any time point over the diurnal cycle (Meaney et al. 1989, 1992), which also indicates that differences in HPA activity observed during stress cannot be accounted for by differences in prestress, basal glucocorticoid levels.

Handled and nonhandled animals also differ in plasma ACTH responses to stress. As with levels of corticosterone, plasma ACTH levels are higher both during and following stress in NH compared with H animals (Meaney et al. 1989; Viau et al. 1993). Generally, the integrated plasma ACTH response (prestress to 60 minutes poststress) is about 50% to 100% higher in the NH rats. These findings, along with findings from an earlier report (Zarrow et al. 1972) on differences in

CRF-like bioactivity between H and NH animals, suggest that the mechanism(s) underlying differences in CRF-like bioactivity between H and NH animals is located above the level of the pituitary and may be related to differential sensitivity of central nervous system negative-feedback processes.

Effects of Postnatal Handling on Hypothalamic-Pituitary-Adrenal Negative-Feedback Processes

Taking into account the findings in the previous section, we examined whether the relative hypersecretion of ACTH and corticosterone by NH animals might be related to differences in negative-feedback sensitivity to circulating glucocorticoids between H and NH animals. We (Meaney et al. 1989) used a classical negative-feedback paradigm based on the finding that high levels of circulating glucorticoids feed back onto the brain and/or pituitary to inhibit subsequent HPA activity (see Jones et al. 1982; Keller-Wood and Dallman 1984). Such delayed, negative feedback persists for hours following the animal's exposure to elevated glucocorticoid levels. H and NH animals were injected with one of five doses of either corticosterone or dexamethasone 3 hours prior to a 20-minute period of restraint. Both glucocorticoids were more effective in suppressing stress-induced HPA responses in the H animals (i.e., the ID_{50} for both corticosterone and dexamethasone was 5 to 10 times lower in the H animals). These data suggest that H animals are indeed more sensitive to the negative-feedback effects of circulating glucocorticoids on HPA activity.

Because this delayed form of negative feedback is mediated by the binding of corticosterone to soluble intracellular receptors, we measured both mineralocorticoid and glucocorticoid receptor sites in selected brain regions and the pituitary of young adult H and NH animals (Meaney and Aitken 1985; Meaney et al. 1985a, 1985b, 1987, 1988b, 1989, 1992; Sarrieau et al. 1988). The results of these studies demonstrated significant and tissue-specific differences in glucocorticoid receptor binding capacity as a function of handling. H animals showed increased glucocorticoid receptor binding capacity in the hippocampus, but not in the septum, amygdala, hypothalamus, or pituitary. The difference in the receptor binding capacity was clearly related to the number of receptor sites and not to the affinity of the receptor for a ^{3}H-labeled radioligand, RU 28362. Moreover, the difference occurred in glucocorticoid receptors, but not in mineralocorticoid receptors. Finally, using in situ hybridization with probes selective for either glucocorticoid or mineralocorticoid receptor mRNA, we (O'Donnell et al. 1994) compared levels of glucocorticoid and mineralocorticoid receptor mRNA expression in H and NH animals. We found that, compared with NH animals, H animals had higher glucocorticoid receptor mRNA expression (grains/cell) throughout the hippocampus. There were no differences in mineralocorticoid receptor mRNA expression between the H and NH animals. These data indicate that postnatal handling permanently increases glucocorticoid receptor biosynthesis (perhaps by increasing basal transcription rates of the glucocorticoid receptor gene).

The difference in hippocampal glucocorticoid receptor density appears to be related to the more efficient suppression of poststress HPA activity in the H animals. Chronic administration of corticosterone results in a 30% to 45% down-regulation of hippocampal glucocorticoid receptor binding sites that persists for about 7 days following the cessation of treatment (Sapolsky et al. 1984b; Tornello et al. 1982). The effect is highly specific to the hippocampus, such that receptor binding capacity in the hypothalamus and pituitary is unaffected. This somewhat peculiar effect provided us with an opportunity to examine the importance of differences in hippocampal glucocorticoid receptor density between H and NH animals for HPA responses to stress. Thus, in one experiment H animals were treated for 5 days with corticosterone and then allowed 2 days for steroid clearance (Meaney et al. 1989). Hippocampal glucocorticoid receptor density was down-regulated in the H + corticosterone animals to levels that were indistinguishable from those of the NH animals, and significantly less than those of the H + vehicle animals. There were no differences in glucocorticoid receptor density in the hypothalamus or pituitary among these three groups. When the animals in these groups were exposed to a 20-minute period of restraint, we found that the H + corticosterone animals, like the NH animals, hypersecreted corticosterone 60 and 120 minutes poststress in comparison to the H + vehicle control animals. These data suggest that the differences in negative-feedback efficiency and in HPA responses to stress between H and NH animals are related to the differences in hippocampal glucocorticoid receptor density. Thus, the chronic corticosterone treatment reversed both the handling-induced increase in hippocampal glucocorticoid receptor binding capacity and the difference in poststress HPA activity.

It appears that the increase in glucocorticoid receptor sites in the hippocampus is a critical feature for the handling effect on HPA function. The increase in receptor density appears to increase the sensitivity of the hippocampus to circulating glucocorticoids, enhancing the efficacy of negative-feedback inhibition over HPA activity, and serving to reduce poststress secretion of ACTH and corticosterone in H animals.

The effect of postnatal handling on HPA negative feedback likely involves glucocorticoid receptor differences in at least one other region. Handling also increases glucocorticoid receptor density in the frontal cortex (Meaney et al. 1985a). We have recently provided evidence for the role of the prefrontal cortex in the regulation of stress-induced HPA activity (Diorio et al. 1993). Medial prefrontal cortex lesions produced increased levels of ACTH and corticosterone both during and following the termination of stress. Corticosterone implants directly into this region produced a 40% to 50% decrease in stress-induced ACTH and corticosterone levels. Interestingly, these effects were apparent only with more moderate stimuli, in this case restraint. Neither the medial prefrontal cortex lesions nor corticosterone implants into this region had any effect on ACTH or corticosterone levels observed during stress induced by ether (a more severe stressor associated with two to three times higher levels of ACTH). Moreover, these effects were observed only during or following stress; neither treatment altered basal ACTH or corticosterone levels at any point over the diurnal cycle. These findings suggest that the handling effect on HPA function may involve altered glucocorticoid receptor density in the frontal cortex.

The Nature of the Glucocorticoid Negative-Feedback Signal

In recent studies we have provided a more detailed description of plasma ACTH responses to ether and restraint stress in H and NH animals (Viau et al. 1993). The results of these studies have shown that very shortly following the onset of stress, plasma ACTH levels are higher in the NH rats. Although ACTH levels rise in both groups, this increase is greater in the NH animals. Thus, the integrated ([hormone levels] × [time]) plasma ACTH response in the NH rats is generally about twofold greater than that in the H animals. At this point it is important to note that H and NH animals do not differ in gluco-corticoid fast-feedback sensitivity (the inhibitory signal associated with the rapidly increasing levels of plasma corticosterone that occur during the first few minutes of stress) (Viau et al. 1993).

These data raise an interesting set of problems. First, assuming that differences in fast feedback are not relevant here, the other important negative-feedback signal in determining the magnitude of the plasma ACTH response to stress is that associated with basal gluco-corticoid levels. Moreover, although we have previously shown that basal corticosterone levels do not differ in H vs. NH rats, there are differences in glucocorticoid receptor levels in brain regions known to regulate HPA activity. Because the increased receptor density confers a greater sensitivity to corticosterone, it remains possible that the basal glucocorticoid feedback signal might be stronger in the H rats despite the fact that basal hormone levels are comparable in H and NH rats.

The second problem concerns the differences in poststress levels of HPA activity. H and NH rats differ in poststress plasma levels of corticosterone; NH animals show elevated corticosterone levels for a considerably longer period of time. Thus, the termination of the adrenocortical response to stress in the H animals occurs more efficiently than in NH animals. We had assumed that this difference was associated with the differences in negative-feedback sensitivity between H and NH rats and that the relevant signal was the elevated corticosterone levels achieved during stress. Thus, we believed that the high levels of corticosterone served to provide a strong negative-feedback signal that, in turn, inhibited HPA activity once the drive associated with the stressor had been terminated. However, the adrenal is known to respond to the integrated ACTH signal. The integrated ACTH level determines not only the peak of corticosterone secretion but also the duration of the response; higher levels of ACTH result not only in greater levels of corticosterone but also in a longer period of elevated corticosterone. Therefore, the poststress differences in plasma corticosterone that are observed in the NH animals could occur in response to the amount of ACTH secreted during stress.

Thus, one very interesting question that emerges here concerns the nature of the relevant glucocorticoid feedback signal. There are at least two obvious signals: the basal corticosterone signal prior to stress and the signal associated with the elevated corticosterone levels occurring during stress. Stress-induced elevations in corticosterone could serve as the signal for the termination of the stress response, once the activational effect of the stress has been removed. Alternatively, the increase in plasma ACTH could be associated with differences in the tonic negative-feedback signal associated with basal corticosterone levels.

To examine this question, we (Viau et al. 1993) compared ACTH responses to restraint in H and NH 1) adrenalectomized animals, which lack any glucocorticoid negative-feedback signal, 2) adrenalectomized animals provided the equivalent of a basal corticosterone signal (adrenalectomized + corticosterone), but lacking the negative-feedback signal associated with stress-induced increases in corticosterone, and 3) intact, sham-operated animals that possess both basal and stress-induced glucocorticoid signals. Corticosterone replacement was achieved by implanting fused pellets of corticosterone under the skin of the animal, a procedure that provides a constant level of plasma glucocorticoids (i.e., the animals possessed a basal glucocorticoid signal but were unable to mobilize a glucocorticoid stress response). These animals were studied 5 days following adrenalectomy. At this time the HPA axis has generally stabilized in adrenalectomized + corticosterone animals (see Dallman et al. 1987b). The corticosterone pellets provided circulating hormone levels of about 5 μg/dl, equivalent to the integrated basal level of corticosterone over the diurnal cycle. Adrenalectomy results in a dramatic increase in pituitary ACTH release and in the synthesis of proopiomelanocortin (POMC), which is the precursor for ACTH synthesis. Basal plasma ACTH and anterior pituitary POMC mRNA levels were substantially increased by adrenalectomy in both H and NH rats, and these effects were effectively reversed with corticosterone pellet implants in both groups of animals. Thus, the corticosterone pellet was equally effective in reversing the effects of adrenalectomy on basal HPA activity in H and NH rats.

There were no differences in the plasma ACTH responses to restraint in adrenalectomized/NH vs. adrenalectomized/H animals. This finding is important because it suggests that in the absence of a glucocorticoid negative-feedback signal, ACTH responses to stress are comparable in H and NH rats, thus confirming that the differences in HPA responses to stress observed in intact H and NH animals are associated with differences in glucocorticoid negative-feedback sensitivity. As expected, plasma ACTH levels during and following restraint in the intact NH animals were significantly greater than those in the H animals. Surprisingly, differences in plasma ACTH between H and NH animals were also observed in the adrenalectomized animals that had been provided with basal corticosterone replacement (Figure 3–3). In the adrenalectomized + corticosterone/NH rats, the plasma ACTH response to restraint was comparable to that in the adrenalectomized/NH animals. Thus, basal corticosterone replacement had little effect on the HPA response to stress in NH animals. In contrast, in the adrenalectomized + corticosterone/H rats, the plasma ACTH response to restraint was significantly reduced compared with that in the adrenalectomized/H rats and significantly lower than that in the adrenalectomized + corticosterone/NH animals. Thus, basal corticosterone replacement was sufficient to reinstate the differences between H and NH rats. These data reflect the importance of the increased sensitivity to the negative-feedback effects of glucocorticoids.

It is also important to note the specificity of this effect. The corticosterone replacement regimen used in this study was sufficient to greatly attenuate the adrenalectomy-induced increase in pituitary POMC mRNA, basal ACTH, and plasma CBG in both the H and NH animals, but altered stress-induced ACTH secretion only in the H animals. A number of previous studies have shown that in laboratory rats corticosterone replacement (pellet) of this order of magnitude is sufficient to correct basal ACTH secretion (Akana et al. 1988; Jacobson et al. 1988) and CBG production (Levin et al. 1987), but not stress-induced increases in plasma ACTH; our data with adrenalectomized + corticosterone/NH rats are comparable to these findings. By contrast, basal corticosterone replacement did attenuate the ACTH hypersecretion with stress in adrenalectomized + corticosterone/H rats. The reduced ACTH secretion in response to stress in the adrenalectomized + corticosterone/H animals is consistent with previous data showing increased glucocorticoid negative-feedback sensitivity in H animals. Taken together, these data indicate that differences in HPA response to stress between H and NH animals are dependent upon the presence of glucocorticoids, but are not dependent upon stress-induced elevations in glucocorticoid levels.

These findings also suggest that negative-feedback differences between H and NH animals can occur in response to basal corticosterone levels. These differences appear to be reflected in differences in median eminence content of various ACTH secretagogues. The me-

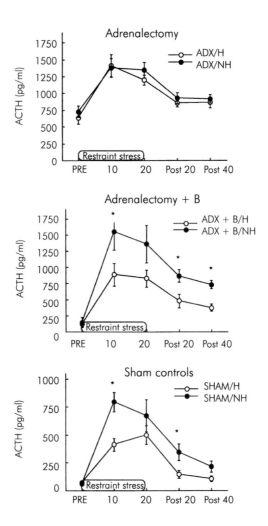

Figure 3–3. Plasma adrenocorticotropin (ACTH) levels before, during, and at various times following a 20-minute restraint in adrenalectomized (ADX), ADX corticosterone–replaced (ADX + B) and intact, sham-operated (SHAM) handled (H) and nonhandled (NH) animals. Asterisk indicates values that differ at *P* < .05. Integrated values (± standard errors of the mean) for plasma ACTH (pg/ml/minute) are as follows: SHAM/H = 326 ± 68; SHAM/NH = 448 ± 83; ADX/H = 1031 ± 61; ADX/NH = 1070 ± 111; ADX + B/H = 609 ± 142; ADX + B/NH = 1091 ± 111.

dian eminence contains the axon terminals of the CRF/AVP neurons of the PVN, and measures of peptide content in this region are assumed to reflect the size of the readily releasable hormone pool. Thus, we found that in rats under resting state conditions, median eminence levels of CRH and AVP (but not oxytocin) were significantly higher in NH compared with H rats (Viau et al. 1993). We also found that hypothalamic CRH mRNA levels were about 2.5-fold higher in NH compared with H animals (Plotsky and Meaney 1993). Thus, under resting conditions, hypothalamic CRH and AVP synthesis appears to be elevated in NH rats, a difference that occurs in the presence of basal glucocorticoid levels.

The differences in median eminence levels of CRH and AVP offer an important insight into understanding the nature of the differences in glucocorticoid negative feedback between H and NH animals. Indeed, we feel that these findings represent a biological basis for individual differences in "responsivity" to stress. Because H and NH animals do not differ in basal levels of ACTH or corticosterone (Meaney et al. 1989, 1992), it seems likely that the differences in CRH and AVP represent differences in readily releasable storage pools of these peptides in axon terminals of PVN neurons located in the median eminence. The excitatory signal at the level of the PVN of the hypothalamus associated with stress likely results in greater CRH and AVP release in the NH animals, which would, in turn, result in a greater plasma ACTH signal. This idea is consistent with the finding that H and NH animals differ in plasma ACTH responses to a wide variety of stimuli. Indeed, the differences in the terminal pools of CRH and AVP suggest that H and NH animals would differ in stressors mediated by either secretagogue. It should be noted that pituitary ACTH responses to both restraint and ether stress appear to be mediated by dynamic variations in both CRH and AVP (e.g., Linton et al. 1985; Nakane et al. 1985). This hypothesis has been at least partially confirmed in one more recent study. Plotsky and Meaney (1993) found that CRH release from the median eminence in response to restraint was significantly greater in NH than in H rats.

It is also important to note that adrenalectomized + corticosterone animals do not differ in corticotroph sensitivity to CRH (Akana et al. 1986) and that differences in ACTH release in response to stress most likely reflect differences in neural regulatory components of ACTH secretion. This idea is also consistent with available information on the role of the hippocampus in mediating glucocorticoid inhibition of HPA activity. Hippocampal lesions result in a prolonged elevation of corticosterone following stress (Sapolsky et al. 1984a). Herman and co-workers (1989) found that hippocampal lesions resulted in increased CRH and AVP mRNA levels in the hypothalamus under basal corticosterone conditions. Moreover, Sapolsky and co-workers (1990) found that portal concentrations of CRH and AVP were negatively correlated with hippocampal glucocorticoid receptor occupancy. Interestingly, hippocampal glucocorticoid receptor occupancy was significantly correlated with resting (prestress) portal concentrations of both CRH and AVP. These findings suggest that an increased glucocorticoid receptor signal at the level of the hippocampus is associated with decreased levels of hypophysial CRH and AVP.

On the basis of these data, it seems reasonable to propose (Figure 3–4) that 1) H and NH animals differ in delayed negative feedback (Meaney et al. 1989) and that this difference is reflected in differential rates of CRH and AVP synthesis in the PVN of the hypothalamus, 2) differences in negative-feedback regulation are apparent even in response to basal corticosterone signals and occur as a result of the increased glucocorticoid receptor density in the hippocampus (and perhaps the medial prefrontal cortex), 3) in response to stress there is a greater release of CRH and/or AVP in the NH animals (Plotsky and Meaney 1993), giving rise to a greater increase in plasma ACTH levels and a greater increase in plasma corticosterone levels, the latter persisting for a longer period of time compared with in the H animals (i.e., higher poststress plasma corticosterone levels in the NH animals). Thus, differences between H and NH animals in HPA activity both during and following stress can occur independently of the stress-induced increase in plasma corticosterone. In our view, the central feature of the handling effect on HPA responsivity to stress involves the changes in hippocampal glucocorticoid receptor gene expression.

Effects of Postnatal Handling on Hypothalamic-Pituitary-Adrenal Responses to Chronic Stress

Thus far, studies on the effects of early environmental regulation of neuroendocrine responses to stress have focused largely on responses to acute stress. The need for studies using chronic stress paradigms is based on the considerations that 1) the more demanding conditions associated with chronic stress are likely to emphasize the differences associated with early environment, revealing underlying vulnerability that may not be apparent with the less challenging conditions of

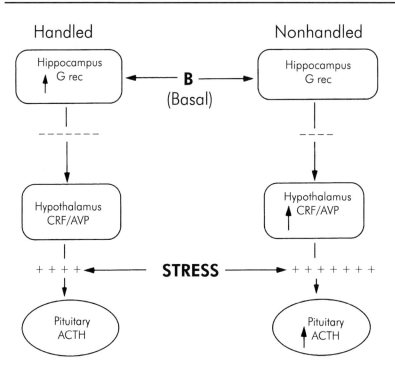

Figure 3–4. A summary of our current understanding of the mechanisms underlying the differences in hypothalamic-pituitary-adrenal (HPA) responses to acute stress in handled and nonhandled animals. The increased glucocorticoid receptor (G rec) levels confer greater sensitivity to corticosterone (B) in hippocampal tissue from handled animals. Therefore, even under basal corticosterone levels (which do not differ in young, adult handled and nonhandled rats), there is a greater tonic inhibitory signal (–) on hypothalamic corticotropin-releasing factor (CRF) and arginine vasopressin (AVP) synthesis in handled rats. In response to the neural signals associated with stress and impinging upon the hypothalamus, there is a greater release of CRF/AVP into portal circulation (+) in the nonhandled rats, resulting in greater adrenocorticotropin (ACTH) release.

acute mild stress, and 2) the chronic stress condition is likely to be more relevant to conditions associated with the development of pathology.

There are two prominent effects of chronic stress on the HPA axis. First, there occurs some adaptation to the stressor with repeated exposure. Some investigators have reported decreased hormone secretion (adaptation) following repeated exposure to the same stressor, depending upon the nature of the stressor and the frequency with which it was applied. Second, there is a potentiation, or facilitation, of the response to a novel stressor (see Dallman et al. 1993). This potentiation/facilitation is reflected in greater hormonal responses in animals that have been exposed to chronic stress than in animals with no recent stressful experience. Thus, animals with a recent background of chronic stress show increased plasma ACTH and corticosterone responses to a novel (i.e., applied for the first time) stressor. This seems to be a more robust effect and one that likely accounts for the clinical finding that chronic stress can compromise our "resistance" to subsequent stress.

In a recent series of studies we (Bhatnagar and Meaney 1995) have examined the HPA response to chronic stress in H and NH animals. In these studies we used daily exposure to a cold (4–6°C) chamber for 4 hours for 21 consecutive days as the chronic stress. Note, this paradigm involves repeated, intermittent chronic stress and not continuous chronic stress (such as 24 hours per day of cold). Animals exposed to the 4 hours per day of cold are able to defend their normal body temperature. The advantage of this form of stress is that it is the only stressor we have found to date that does not allow one to distinguish, on the basis of neuroendocrine response, H from NH animals (i.e., the plasma ACTH and corticosterone response to acute exposure to 4 hours of cold is comparable in H and NH animals). Using this paradigm, we were able to examine the effects of chronic exposure to stress in H and NH animals without the complication of differences in neuroendocrine response on day 1 of testing. Thus, plasma ACTH responses to 4 hours of cold did not differ on day 1 between H and NH animals. However, after the animals were exposed to cold for 21 consecutive days, plasma ACTH responses in H animals had diminished significantly, and to a greater extent than in NH animals. These data suggest that adaptation to repeated, intermittent cold stress was greater in the H animals.

On day 22 of testing, chronically stressed H and NH animals, along with their respective nonstressed controls, were exposed to a novel stressor (i.e., 20-minute restraint). Exposure to chronic stress facilitated HPA responses to restraint in the NH animals, but not the H animals. Thus, NH animals that had been previously exposed to cold stress on days 1 through 21 secreted significantly higher levels of both ACTH and corticosterone compared with NH controls. There were no reliable differences in plasma ACTH and corticosterone responses to restraint between the chronically stressed and control H animals. Thus, chronic stress did not serve to facilitate subsequent HPA responses to acute stress in the H animals.

These data reflect the differences in HPA responses to stress between H and NH animals when the stress was chronic. We should bear in mind that these differences emerged in response to a specific form of chronic stress, and it may well be that the pattern adaptation/ facilitation that occurs is specific to the type of stress. Indeed, in a provocative review on the topic of chronic stress, Dallman and her colleagues (1987a) concluded that the critical neural sites for facilitation are distal to the PVN. If this is indeed true, then we might well expect that different forms of chronic stress might vary in their ability to facilitate HPA responses to novel stressors. Nevertheless, our findings reveal that the differences between H and NH animals are observable within a chronic stress paradigm.

These data also demonstrate how a chronic, background stress can compromise the efficiency of neuroendocrine responses to new stressors. Subsequent experiments have revealed the neural basis for this effect. Bhatnagar and Meaney (1995) found that median eminence CRF content increased following chronic exposure to cold. These findings are consistent with the finding that chronic stress increases hypothalamic CRF mRNA levels (see Harbuz and Lightman 1992). It is important to note that the increase in CRF content was substantially greater (about twofold) in the NH animals. Thus, when stimulation by a novel stressor occurred, there was a greater release of CRF in the chronically stressed NH animals, accounting for the exaggerated plasma ACTH response. At this point it is a matter of speculation as to whether the increased CRF synthesis in the NH animals in response to chronic stress is related to the decreased glucocorticoid negative-feedback sensitivity (although it is an appealing idea).

In addition, these endocrine differences between H and NH animals were associated with differences in the immune function (Bhatnagar and Meaney 1995). When the animals were administered an antigen (sheep red blood cells), the plaque-forming cell response was dramatically suppressed in the chronically stressed NH rats, and suppressed to a significantly less degree in the chronically stressed H rats. Antibody titers showed the same pattern. Thus, chronic stress suppressed immune function (or at least selected measures of immune function) to a substantially greater extent in the NH rats. This finding provides a clear example of how early environment might determine vulnerability to pathology by altering the efficiency of HPA responses to stress.

Effects of Prolonged Periods of Maternal Separation on Hypothalamic-Pituitary-Adrenal Responses to Stress

The aforementioned studies show that the HPA response to stress is modified by early handling. However, handling represents an interesting manipulation. The procedure involves separating the pup from the dam for a period of 3 to 15 minutes (depending upon the laboratory) and exposing the pup to a novel array of sensory stimuli. It is noteworthy that in the course of normal mother-pup interactions the dam is regularly away from the nest, and the pups, for periods of 20 to 30 minutes. Thus, the handling manipulation does not seem to represent any abnormal period of separation or loss of maternal care. But what about much longer periods of separation, in which there is a loss of maternal care (including the nutritional and thermal needs met by the mother)?

Indeed, there seems to be good reason to believe that the effects of short periods of perturbation, such as handling, are *qualitatively* different from more severe forms of maternal separation. Schanberg, Kuhn, and their colleagues (e.g., Kuhn et al. 1990) have found that prolonged periods of maternal separation (>2 hours) result in a suppression of plasma growth hormone. In contrast, brief periods of separation (i.e., 15 minutes) or handling result in an *increase* in plasma growth hormone levels. This finding is of considerable importance, for it suggests that different forms of environmental stimulation can have very different effects on neuroendocrine systems.

What about differences in the long-term consequences of these manipulations? We (Plotsky and Meaney 1993) began our studies on this topic by examining the effects of repeated maternal separation of varying durations. From day 2 until day 14 of life, pups were separated from their mothers once per day for 0, 15, 60, 180, or 360 minutes. The animals were otherwise reared under identical conditions. At 120 days of age the animals were exposed to restraint. The data show, in a manner comparable to that in the Schanberg and Kuhn experiments, that the long-term effects of HPA responses to stress were qualitatively different depending upon the duration of maternal separation. Compared with 0-minute controls (animals reared in the same manner as were NH animals), the 15-minute period of separation (or handling) resulted in animals that showed reduced plasma corticosterone levels during and following stress. In contrast, animals separated for 180 or 360 minutes per day showed *increased* plasma corticosterone levels both during and following stress. Thus, neonatal handling was associated with a 40% reduction in corticosterone secretion as compared with the NH rats, whereas maternal separation was associated with a 40% *increase* in the corticosterone response as compared with the NH group. These findings underscore the very different sequelae associated with handling versus maternal separation. Adult male rats that had been maternally separated for 180 minutes per day also exhibited hypersecretion of ACTH and corticosterone in response to a novel environment as compared with the NH and H groups.

We then compared these animals using a dexamethasone suppression test as an indication of negative-feedback sensitivity. Administration of dexamethasone (10 µg/100 g body weight) at 0900 hours completely suppressed corticosterone secretion (<1 µg/dl) in the H ($n = 6$) and NH ($n = 6$) groups at 3, 6, and 9 hours postadministration. Corticosterone levels of rats in the maternal separation group were also suppressed at 3 hours and 6 hours after dexamethasone administration; however, by 9 hours, circulating corticosterone levels had "escaped" to 4.5 ± 0.3 µg/dl ($n = 6$). These data suggest that the efficiency of glucocorticoid negative feedback was reduced by repeated periods of maternal separation during early life.

Could the effects of maternal separation involve alteration in the regulation of CRF systems? To date, we have demonstrated changes in hypothalamic CRF mRNA and in CRF content in adult rats exposed to handling or maternal separation as neonates. Pups that had experienced maternal separation for 180 minutes per day exhibited a marked increase in hypothalamic CRF mRNA as compared with either H or NH pups. Furthermore, changes in CRF peptide content in the stalk of the median eminence paralleled the changes in hypothalamic mRNA. These preliminary studies are consistent with the idea that the hypothalamic CRF neurons are a target for regulation by neonatal experience and that this regulation results in permanent alteration of the HPA axis. In the case of the study reported above, repeated periods of maternal separation resulted in the development of exaggerated HPA responses to stress, a condition that could render the individual more vulnerable to stress-induced pathology. These findings raise the possibility that inadequate parental care may render the offspring vulnerable to pathology by compromising the development of efficient neuroendocrine (and probably behavioral) responses to stress.

Effects of Neonatal Endotoxin Exposure on Hypothalamic-Pituitary-Adrenal Responses to Stress

In an effort to examine the effects of rather general and common early life events on the development of the HPA response to stress, we (Shanks et al. 1995) examined the effects of early illness. To address this question, we exposed rat pups on days 3 and 5 of life to a low dose of an endotoxin. The dose was chosen to induce illness, but at a level that was not life-threatening (i.e., none of the 100 to 110 pups treated died within the next 2 weeks). The endotoxin treatment elevated plasma glucose levels, severely dampened behavioral activity, and increased body temperature. Thus, the pups were severely ill for most of the first week of life.

When the animals were examined as adults, the results were surprising. The endotoxin-treated animals showed significantly increased plasma ACTH and corticosterone responses to restraint as compared with saline-treated and untreated controls. In following our previous findings, these animals also differed in glucocorticoid negative-feedback sensitivity. An injection of dexamethasone 10 µg/kg body weight 3 hours before restraint completely abolished plasma ACTH responses in the controls (100% suppression). In the endotoxin-treated animals, the plasma ACTH response to restraint was only partially suppressed (~40% suppression). Likewise, resting-state median eminence levels of CRF were significantly higher in the endotoxin-treated animals than in the controls. Thus, endotoxin treatment in early life produced an effect that was functionally the opposite to that of handling. Again, we find evidence of differences in adult hypothalamic CRF activity as a function of early life events.

These findings suggest that a severe illness in early life can alter the development of HPA responses to stress, generally in a manner that is likely to promote vulnerability to pathology in later life. At this time we do not understand the mechanisms by which illness in early life can permanently alter the development of HPA responses to stress. However, these findings are potentially of considerable impact in terms of understanding the relationship between sickness in early life and subsequent vulnerability.

Effects of Prenatal Stress on Hypothalamic-Pituitary-Adrenal Function

In a series of recent studies we (McCormick et al. 1994) have begun to examine the effects of exposure to prenatal stress on the development of HPA responses to stress. In these studies we used a form of prenatal stress that focuses on the third trimester of pregnancy. In these studies pregnant females were exposed to restraint for 1 hour per day for days 15 to 20 of gestation. The offspring were examined as fully mature adults, beginning at 120 days of life.

The effects of prenatal stress were very clearly sexually dimorphic; the effects were far more pronounced on females than on males. Among the adult females, prenatal stress resulted in increased plasma ACTH and corticosterone responses to restraint. There was virtually no effect of prenatal stress on HPA responses in males. Likewise, in females, but not males, resting-state levels of median eminence CRF were greater in the offspring of dams exposed to restraint. Interestingly, these effects are consistent with the effects of prenatal alcohol exposure on HPA development (see Weinberg, in press); in these studies, prenatal alcohol resulted in increased HPA responses to stress in females, but not males.

Following the results of the handling studies, we then exhaustively studied mineralocorticoid and glucocorticoid receptor concentrations in brain and pituitary. The development of the corticosteroid receptor systems was unaffected by prenatal stress. Interestingly, Weinberg and her colleagues have found that prenatal alcohol exposure does not alter corticosteroid receptor development in the brain or pituitary. However, in our studies on prenatal stress, we did find that plasma CBG levels were clearly altered. In females, but not males, plasma CBG levels were elevated by about 50% in the prenatally stressed animals.

This finding suggests that although total (CBG-bound + free) corticosterone levels in the prenatally stressed female animals might be higher in response to stress, the increased CBG levels might serve to offset this difference. Indeed, when we calculated free corticosterone levels on the basis of the plasma CBG levels in these animals, there was little difference in the corticoid response to stress between the prenatally stressed and control groups. Note, it is the free form of the steroid that is biologically active and that determines the level of steroid receptor occupancy (see Figure 3–2).

Such differences in plasma CBG are also likely to account for the increased plasma ACTH response to stress in the prenatally stressed animals. The difference in plasma CBG levels occurs under resting-state conditions. At the same time, there are no apparent differences in basal corticosterone between the prenatally stressed and control animals. Thus, the basal free corticosterone levels in the controls are higher than those in the prenatally stressed animals, and this should provide a stronger resting-state negative-feedback signal in the controls. This difference appears to us as the most likely explanation for the increased hypothalamic CRF synthesis in the prenatally stressed animals and the increased plasma ACTH response to stress.

Individual Differences in Hypothalamic-Pituitary-Adrenal Activity and Brain Aging

Thus far in this chapter we have focused on how early life events can influence the development of HPA responses to stress. In each case, we have some understanding of how early environment can sculpt the individual differences in responses to stress that are so familiar to clinicians. In this section we present clear evidence of how such individual differences can determine vulnerability to neuropathology, in this case age-related hippocampal degeneration.

Endocrine and psychological responses to stress are notoriously variable across individuals of the same species. This variation often emerges as an important predictor of vulnerability to stress-induced pathology. Over the course of the past years we have been attempting to understand the neurobiological mechanisms underlying individual differences in HPA responses to stress, and the importance of these differences in HPA function for age-related pathology.

Increased basal glucocorticoid secretion is often observed in the aged rat (see Meaney et al. 1993; Sapolsky et al. 1990). The increased HPA activity appears to be associated with a loss of hippocampal corticosteroid receptors and decreased glucocorticoid negative-feedback sensitivity (see Meaney et al. 1993; Sapolsky et al. 1990 for reviews). This loss of corticosteroid receptors has important consequences for the hippocampus, which has the greatest density of corticosteroid receptors in the brain and, hence, is very sensitive to changes in circulating glucocorticoid levels. Hippocampal neuron loss is commonly seen in aged rats (Coleman and Flood 1987). In a series of studies Landfield and colleagues (1978, 1981) demonstrated that the occurrence of hippocampal neuron loss was positively correlated with the increase in HPA activity. They then adrenalectomized rats at mid-life (12 months of age) and provided low-level corticosterone replacement. They found that these animals showed little or no evidence of hippocampal neuron loss or of the spatial memory deficits that are common in later life and are closely associated with hippocampal dysfunction. Sapolsky and co-workers (1985) found that young adult rats treated for 3 months with exogenous corticosterone in the upper physiological range (mimicking the elevated basal levels seen in certain old rats) showed profound hippocampal cell loss. Moreover, the pattern of the neuron loss was strikingly similar to that observed in aged animals. This same corticosterone treatment also produces impaired hippocampal long-term potentiation and spatial memory deficits in mid-aged rats (Bodnoff et al., in press).

Aging rats lose hippocampal corticosteroid receptors, become insensitive to glucocorticoid negative-feedback regulation (Sapolsky et al. 1986a, 1986b), and hypersecrete corticosterone under both basal and poststress conditions. Throughout life, however, H animals have significantly higher levels of hippocampal glucocorticoid receptors than do NH animals (Meaney et al. 1988b, 1991, 1992), although both groups do show a loss of receptors. As expected, on the basis of these receptor data, we found that the age-related HPA deficits were far less pronounced in the H rats (Meaney et al. 1988b, 1991). At each age tested, the H animals secreted less corticosterone during restraint stress and terminated corticosterone secretion following stress sooner than did the NH animals.

Moreover, the age-related rise in basal corticosterone levels, often seen in aged rats, was observed in the NH animals, but not the H animals (Meaney et al. 1988b, 1991, 1992). There was about a twofold increase in basal corticosterone levels in the aged NH animals in the P.M. phase of the light cycle and about a 40% increase during the A.M. phase (Meaney et al. 1992). Interestingly, in the rat, glucocorticoid receptor activation has been associated with negative-feedback regulation of P.M., but not A.M., basal ACTH release (see Dallman et al. 1987a). In addition, the difference in the P.M. phase was amplified by the fact that during this time plasma CBG levels in the aged NH animals were significantly lower than in old H animals or young animals. van Eekelen and co-workers (1991) have also found evidence for decreased plasma CBG levels in aged rats. The decrease in CBG in the aged NH animals was associated with a dramatic elevation in free corticosterone to levels ($\sim$2–4 μg/dl over the entire dark phase of the cycle) that approximated those achieved during stress. This is truly an astounding difference. This level of basal free corticosterone suggests that the aged NH rats were exposed to the equivalent of 12 hours of mild stress in terms of glucocorticoid secretion. Aged H animals showed no such decrease in plasma CBG levels and little or no change in basal corticosterone levels. Again, it should be emphasized that these differences in basal corticosterone and CBG between H and NH animals emerge as a function of age; there are no such differences between 6-month-old H and NH animals.

These findings suggested that over the life span, cumulative exposure to the highly catabolic glucocorticoids was greater in the NH animals. We then examined an important neuropathological consequence of this difference. The hippocampus loses neurons with age, particularly in the CA_1 and CA_3 cell fields (Coleman and Flood 1987). The hippocampus has extremely high concentrations of corticosteroid receptors and therefore marked sensitivity to glucocorticoids. Thus, the reduced cumulative exposure to glucocorticoids in the H rats suggested that hippocampal degeneration would be less pronounced in these animals, and this is exactly what we observed. Among NH animals, but not H animals, there occurred a significant ($\sim$40%) loss of neurons with age in both the CA_1 and CA_3 hippocampal cell fields (Meaney et al. 1988b, 1991). Importantly, H and NH rats did not differ in neuron density at 6 months of age. Rather, handling attenuated the loss of hippocampal neurons occurring at later ages.

The difference in hippocampal cell number between the H and

NH animals at the later ages was of functional significance. The hippocampus is known to be of considerable importance in learning and memory, and hippocampal injury profoundly disrupts cognition. These findings suggested that the older H rats, with attenuated cell loss in the hippocampus, should show less evidence of age-related cognitive impairments than the older NH rats. Behavioral testing was performed using the Morris swim maze (Morris 1985), a test of spatial memory in which animals are placed into a large (1.6 meters) circular pool of opaque water and must use distal, spatial cues in order to locate a submerged platform onto which they can climb out of the water. (Rats are proficient, but reluctant, swimmers.) Spatial memory deficits emerged with age in the NH rats such that the 24-month-old NH animals took significantly longer to locate the platform (i.e., 3 to 4 times longer) than the 6-month-old animals on all but the first 3 of 18 trials (Meaney et al. 1988b, 1991). In contrast, among the H rats there were no statistically reliable age differences. The 24-month-old H rats performed as well as did the 6-month-old rats. There were no differences in the performance of the H and NH animals at 6 months of age. It should be noted that in subsequent testing H and NH rats of all ages performed similarly when the platform was made visible by raising it above the water level, indicating that the H/NH differences were due to spatial, rather than motor, skills. These spatial memory deficits in the older NH animals are probably related to the hippocampal damage seen in these animals, because similar deficits are observed after damage to the dorsal hippocampus (see, e.g., Morris 1985).

Several studies have revealed neuroendocrine dysfunction in the aged rat that include glucocorticoid hypersecretion and negative-feedback insensitivity, as well as the loss of hippocampal neurons and glucocorticoid receptors. These deficits form a complex and self-perpetuating cascade (see Sapolsky et al. 1986b): A consequence of glucocorticoid hypersecretion is accelerated neuron loss in the aging hippocampus (including corticosterone-concentrating neurons), and a consequence of hippocampal damage is adrenocortical negative-feedback insensitivity and glucocorticoid hypersecretion. The interaction of these abnormalities occurs with aging in the rat and is accelerated by conditions that further elevate glucocorticoid levels, such as stress. Neonatal handling reduces the HPA response to stress and prevents the age-related increase in basal corticosterone production. Our data show that this effect persists over the life span. Moreover, one of the critical features of this effect, that of reducing gluco-corticoid concentrations under a variety of conditions, appears to prevent the degenerative "glucocorticoid cascade."

The diminished rate of hippocampal neuron loss in aging H rats probably reflects the lower cumulative lifetime exposure to glucocorticoids. It should be noted that this outcome is the product of two apparently opposing trends. While the increased concentrations of hippocampal glucocorticoid receptors are related to the enhanced negative-feedback sensitivity and decreased glucocorticoid secretion in the H rats, the same increased receptor concentrations could conceivably sensitize the hippocampus to the endangering effects of glucocorticoids. In this instance, the decreased secretion apparently outweighs the risk of increased target sensitivity, perhaps by ensuring that the prolonged glucocorticoid exposure necessary for the endangering effects does not occur. It should be noted that under normal resting conditions only about 10% to 15% of the hippocampal glucocorticoid receptor population is occupied by hormone (Meaney et al. 1988a; Reul and De Kloet 1985; Reul et al. 1987). As glucocorticoid levels rise with age, it is the change in hormone levels rather than receptor density that determines the increase in the corticoid signal.

Thus, an environmental manipulation occurring early in life results in a sequence of changes that endure throughout the life span, with dramatic attenuation of some of the deficits typical of aging. These findings demonstrate that relatively subtle individual differences in early experience can profoundly alter the quality of aging years later. This underscores the importance of developmental critical periods and explains a possible source of variability in vulnerability to pathology. It is important that H and NH animals do not differ in hippocampal neuron number and spatial memory ability at 6 months of age. Rather, the difference emerges over time as a function of an interaction with age.

These findings, together with findings from the studies of Landfield, suggest that in a normal population of laboratory rats, individual differences in HPA activity should serve as a predictor of age-related hippocampal pathology. We (Issa et al. 1990) examined this question by screening a large sample of aged (22–28 months) rats using a test of spatial memory. If HPA dysfunction is associated with hippocampal pathology and not merely with advanced age, then we would expect that a sample of aged, cognitively impaired and aged, cognitively unimpaired should differ considerably in HPA activity. We used the Morris swim maze to screen over 100 aged animals in order to select aged animals that were either cognitively impaired or unimpaired (>2 standard deviations or <0.5 standard deviations from the mean performance in 6-month-old animals, respectively). According to these criteria, about 30% of the animals were designated as aged, cognitively impaired and a comparable percentage as aged, cognitively unimpaired (underscoring the extreme variation in cognitive decline in aged rats; see, also, Gage et al. 1984; Gallagher and Pelleymounter 1988). Interestingly, both groups of aged animals showed a loss of hippocampal neurons; however, the decrease in neuron density was substantially greater in the aged, cognitively impaired rats.

The aged, cognitively impaired animals showed increased plasma ACTH and corticosterone levels under both basal and poststress conditions, whereas HPA activity in the aged, cognitively unimpaired animals did not differ from that in 6-month-old controls. As in the aged NH animals, the increase in basal ACTH and corticosterone in the aged, cognitively impaired rats was observed only in the P.M. phase of the cycle. During this period, median eminence levels of both CRH and especially AVP were also significantly higher in the aged, cognitively impaired rats (Sarrieau et al. 1992). It should be noted that although both aged groups showed a loss of hippocampal glucocorticoid receptors (with no change in hypothalamic or pituitary receptor density), the loss was significantly greater in the aged, cognitively impaired animals. The aged, cognitively impaired rats also showed a significant decrease in hippocampal mineralocorticoid receptor density. These findings demonstrate the overall loss of hippocampal corticosteroid receptors in the aged, cognitively impaired animals. The pattern of data in this study was comparable to that in the previous handling studies, with the aged, cognitively unimpaired rats in the study by Issa et al. resembling the aged H animals in the previous studies. Taken together, these data strongly suggest that increased glucocorticoid levels are selectively associated with the occurrence of hippocampal pathology and impaired cognition in later life.

Conclusions

Handling during the early postnatal period leads to increased glucocorticoid receptor binding in the hippocampus and is associated with enhanced negative-feedback control over HPA function. Ultimately, the CRF and CRF/AVP neurons in the PVN of the hypothalamus are the target for these differences in glucocorticoid negative feedback. In turn, the altered hypothalamic CRF/AVP activity serves as the mechanism by which differences in negative feedback are transduced into differences in HPA responses to stress. Likewise, each of the early environmental manipulations studies to date has served to alter resting-state hypothalamic CRF activity, although the changes at the level of the CRF neuron can occur as a result of different processes (i.e., altered hippocampal glucocorticoid receptor density in the case of handling, increased plasma CBG levels in the prenatally stressed females). The changes observed provide a central molecular basis for the differences in HPA function observed in adult rats with differing early life experience.

It is likely that this plasticity reflects a basic process, whereby the early environment is able to "fine tune" the sensitivity and efficiency of certain neuroendocrine systems that mediate the animal's response to stimuli that threaten homeostasis. It is also evident that this fine tuning can occur at different levels of the HPA axis depending upon the nature of the environmental stimulation, as well as the gender and the developmental phase of the animal. Why should such plasticity exist? In responding to this question, it is probably essential to have studied the rat, which, like humans, is found in virtually every ecological niche imaginable. The key for such species is the ability to adapt to varying environmental demands. This includes even rudimentary defense responses, such as those of the HPA axis (or the immune system). Thus, a period of plasticity serves the animal well, and it follows that the environment should have a major role in shaping the developing central nervous system. It also makes sense because most species live their lives within the same region in which they were born. Rats born in the Manhattan underground will live their entire lives under similar conditions. Thus it makes sense that a period of early plasticity "prepares" the brain for the unique challenges of its particular environment. It is also useful that such plasticity occurs early in life, when the animal's mother is present to meet the young animal's basic needs.

Humans are, of course, an exception. We move from rural to urban to residential communities with regularity. And this raises an interesting question. If the processes that we have described above occur within our species, might such migration frustrate the efforts of early development? This is obviously a matter of speculation, but the question does seem to follow from research in developmental psychobiology.

References

Ader R, Grota LJ: Effects of early experience on adrenocortical reactivity. Physiol Behav 4:303–305, 1969

Akana S, Cascio CS, Du J-Z, et al: Reset in feedback in the adrenocortical system: an apparent shift in sensitivity of adrenocorticotropin to corticosterone between morning and evening. Endocrinology 119:2325–2332, 1986

Akana SF, Jacobson L, Cascio CS, et al: Reset in feedback in the adrenocortical system: an apparent shift in sensitivity of adrenocorticotropin to corticosterone between morning and evening. Endocrinology 122:1337–1342, 1988

Antoni FA: Hypothalamic control of ACTH secretion: advances since the discovery of 41-residue corticotropin-releasing factor. Endocr Rev 7:351–370, 1986

Arriza JL, Simerly RB, Swanson LW, et al: Neuronal mineralocorticoid receptor as a mediator of glucocorticoid response. Neuron 1:887–900, 1988

Beaumont K, Fanestil DD: Characterization of rat brain aldosterone receptors reveals high affinity for corticosterone. Endocrinology 113:2043–2051, 1983

Beyer HS, Matta SG, Sharp BM: Regulation of the messenger ribonucleic acid for corticotropin-releasing factor in the paraventricular nucleus and other brain sites of the rat. Endocrinology 123:2117–2123, 1988

Bhatnagar S, Meaney MJ: Hypothalamic-pituitary-adrenal function in handled and non-handled rats in response to chronic stress. J Neuroendocrinol 7:107–119, 1995

Bodnoff SR, Humphreys A, Lehman J, et al: Enduring effects of elevated glucocorticoid levels on spatial memory deficits dampened long-term potentiation and hippocampal neuron loss in mid-aged rats. J Neurosci (in press)

Bradbury MJ, Dallman MF: Effects of type 1 and type 2 glucocorticoid receptor antagonists on ACTH levels in the PM. Society for Neuroscience Abstracts 17:716, 1991

Brindley DN, Rolland Y: Possible connections between stress, diabetes, obesity, hypertension and altered lipoprotein metabolism that may result in atherosclerosis. Clin Sci 77:453–461, 1989

Burnstein KL, Cidlowski JA: Regulation of gene expression by glucocorticoids. Annu Rev Physiol 51:683–699, 1989

Carson-Jurica MA, Schrader WT, O'Malley BW: Steroid receptor family: structure and functions. Endocr Rev 11:201–220, 1990

Coleman PD, Flood DG: Neuron numbers and dendritic extent in normal aging and Alzheimer's disease. Neurobiol Aging 8:521–545, 1987

Dallman MF, Akana SF, Cascio CS, et al: Regulation of ACTH secretion: variations on a theme of B. Recent Prog Horm Res 43:113–173, 1987a

Dallman MF, Akana SF, Jacobson L, et al: Characterization of corticosterone feedback regulation of ACTH secretion. Ann N Y Acad Sci 512:402–414, 1987b

Dallman MF, Levin N, Cascio CS, et al: Pharmacological evidence that the diurnal regulation of adrenocorticotropin secretion by corticosteroids is mediated by type I corticosterone-preferring receptors. Endocrinology 124:2844–2850, 1989

Dallman MF, Akana SF, Scribner KA, et al: Stress, feedback and facilitation in the hypothalamo-pituitary-adrenal axis. J Neuroendocrinol 4:517–526, 1993

Danielson M, Northrup JP, Ringold GM: The mouse glucocorticoid receptor: mapping of functional domains by cloning, sequencing, and expression of wild-type and mutant receptor proteins. EMBO J 5:2513–2522, 1986

Diorio D, Viau V, Meaney MJ: The role of the frontal cortex in the regulation of hypothalamic-pituitary-adrenal activity. J Neurosci 13:3839–3847, 1993

Emadian SM, Luttge WG, Densmore CL: Chemical differentiation of Type I and Type II receptors for adrenal steroids in brain cytosol. J Steroid Biochem Mol Biol 24:953–961, 1986

Evans RM, Arriza JL: A molecular framework for the actions of glucocorticoid hormones in the nervous system. Neuron 2:1105–1112, 1989

Feldman S, Conforti N: Feedback effects of dexamethasone on adrenocortical responses in rats with fornix lesions. Horm Res 7:56–60, 1976

Feldman S, Conforti N: Participation of the dorsal hippocampus in the glucocorticoid negative-feedback effect on adrenocortical activity. Neuroendocrinology 30:52–55, 1980

Fischette CT, Komisurak BR, Ediner HM, et al: Differential fornix ablations and the circadian rhythmicity of adrenal corticosterone secretion. Brain Res 195:373–380, 1980

Funder JW, Sheppard K: Adrenocortical steroids and the brain. Annu Rev Physiol 49:397–412, 1987

Gage FH, Kelly PAT, Bjorklund A: Regional changes in brain glucose metabolism reflect cognitive impairments in age rats. J Neurosci 4:2856–2865, 1984

Gallagher M, Pelleymounter M: Spatial learning deficits in old rats: a model for memory decline in the aged. Neurobiol Aging 9:549–556, 1988

Gibbs DM: Vasopressin and oxytocin: Hypothalamic modulators of the stress response. Psychoneuroendocrinology 11:131–140, 1986

Goldman L, Winget C, Hollinshead G, et al: Postweaning development of negative feedback in the pituitary-adrenal system of the rat. Neuroendocrinology 12:199–211, 1978

Grota LJ: Effects of early experience on the metabolism and production of corticosterone in rats. Dev Psychobiol 9:211–215, 1975

Harbuz MS, Lightman SL: Stress and the hypothalamic-pituitary-adrenal axis: acute, chronic and immunological activation. J Endocrinol 134:327–339, 1992

Herman JP, Schafer MK-H, Young EA, et al: Evidence for hippocampal regulation of neuroendocrine neurons of the hypothalamo-pituitary-adrenocortical axis. J Neurosci 9:3072–3082, 1989

Hess JL, Denenberg VH, Zarrow MX, et al: Modification of the corticosterone response curve as a function of handling in infancy. Physiol Behav 4:109–112, 1969

Hollenberg SM, Weinberger C, Ong ES, et al: Primary structure and expression of a functional human glucocorticoid receptor cDNA. Nature 318:635–641, 1985

Issa A, Gauthier S, Meaney MJ: Hypothalamic-pituitary-adrenal activity in aged cognitively impaired and cognitively unimpaired rats. J Neurosci 10:3247–3254, 1990

Jacobson L, Sapolsky RM: The role of the hippocampus in feedback regulation of the hypothalamic-pituitary-adrenal axis. Endocr Rev 12:118–134, 1991

Jacobson L, Akana S, Cascio CS, et al: Circadian variations in plasma corticosterone permit normal termination of adrenocorticotropin responses to stress. Endocrinology 122:1343–1349, 1988

Jones MT, Gillham B, Greenstein BD, et al: Feedback actions of adrenal steroid hormones, in Current Topics in Neuroendocrinology, Vol 2. Edited by Ganten D, Pfaff D. New York, Springer, 1982, pp 45–68

Keller-Wood M, Dallman MF: Corticosteroid inhibition of ACTH secretion. Endocr Rev 5:1–24, 1984

Kiss JZ, Mezey E, Skirboll L: Corticotropin-releasing factor–immunoreactive neurons of the paraventricular nucleus become vasopressin positive after adrenalectomy. Proc Natl Acad Sci U S A 81:1854–1858, 1984

Kovacs KJ, Makara GB: Corticosterone and dexamethasone act at different brain sites to inhibit adrenalectomy-induced adrenocorticotropin hypersecretion. Brain Res 474:205–210, 1988

Kuhn CM, Pauk J, Schanberg SM: Endocrine responses to mother-infant separation in developing rats. Dev Psychobiol 23:395–410, 1990

Landfield PW, Waymire J, Lynch G: Hippocampal aging and adrenocorticoids: a quantitative correlation. Science 202:1098–1101, 1978

Landfield PW, Baskin RK, Pitler TA: Brain-aging correlates: retardation by hormonal-pharmacological treatments. Science 214:581–583, 1981

Levin N, Shinsako J, Dallman MF: Corticosterone acts on the brain to inhibit adrenalectomy-induced adrenocorticotropin secretion. Endocrinology 122:694–701, 1987

Levine S: Infantile experience and resistance to physiological stress. Science 126:405–406, 1957

Levine S: Plasma-free corticosteroid response to electric shock in rats stimulated in infancy. Science 135:795–796, 1962

Levine S, Haltmeyer GC, Karas GG, et al: Physiological and behavioral effects of infantile stimulation. Physiol Behav 2:55–63, 1967

Lightman SL, Young WS: Vasopressin, oxytocin, dynorphin, enkephalin, and corticotropin-releasing factor in mRNA stimulation in the rat. J Physiol 403:501–523, 1988

Linton EA, Tilders FJH, Hodgkinson S, et al: Stress-induced secretion of adrenocorticotropin in rats is inhibited by antisera to corticotropin-releasing factor and vasopressin. Endocrinology 116:966–970, 1985

McCormick CM, Smythe J, Sharma S, et al: Sex-dependent effects of prenatal stress on the development of brain corticosteroid receptor systems and hypothalamic-pituitary-adrenal responses to stress. Brain Res Dev Brain Res 79:260–266, 1994

McEwen BS, De Kloet ER, Rostene WH: Adrenal steroid receptors and actions in the nervous system. Physiol Rev 66:1121–1150, 1986

Meaney MJ, Aitken DH: The effects of early postnatal handling on the development of hippocampal glucocorticoid receptors: temporal parameters. Developmental Brain Research 22:301–304, 1985

Meaney MJ, Aitken DH, Bodnoff SR, et al: Early, postnatal handling alters glucocorticoid receptor concentrations in selected brain regions. Behav Neurosci 99:760–765, 1985a

Meaney MJ, Aitken DH, Bodnoff SR, et al: The effects of postnatal handling on the development of the glucocorticoid receptor systems and stress recovery in the rat. Prog Neuropsychopharmacol Biol Psychiatry 7:731–734, 1985b

Meaney MJ, Aitken DH, Sapolsky RM: Thyroid hormones influence the development of hippocampal glucocorticoid receptors in the rat: a mechanism for the effects of postnatal handling on the development of the adrenocortical stress response. Neuroendocrinology 45:278–283, 1987

Meaney MJ, Viau V, Bhatnagar S, et al: Occupancy and translocation of hippocampal glucocorticoid receptors during and following stress. Brain Res 445:198–203, 1988a

Meaney MJ, Aitken DH, Bhatnagar S, et al: Postnatal handling attenuates neuroendocrine, anatomical, and cognitive impairments related to the aged hippocampus. Science 238:766–768, 1988b

Meaney MJ, Aitken DH, Sharma S, et al: Postnatal handling increases hippocampal type II, glucocorticoid receptors and enhances adrenocortical negative-feedback efficacy in the rat. Neuroendocrinology 50:597–604, 1989

Meaney MJ, Aitken DH, Sapolsky RM: Environmental regulation of the adrenocortical stress response in female rats and its implications for individual differences in aging. Neurobiol Aging 12:31–38, 1991

Meaney MJ, Aitken DH, Sharma S, et al: Basal ACTH, corticosterone, and corticosterone-binding globulin levels over the diurnal cycle, and hippocampal type I and type II corticosteroid receptors in young and old, handled and nonhandled rats. Neuroendocrinology 55:204–213, 1992

Meaney MJ, Bodnoff SR, O'Donnell D, et al: Glucocorticoids as regulators of neuron survival and repair in the aged brain, in Restorative Neurology, Vol 6. Edited by Cuello AC. Amsterdam, Elsevier, 1993, pp 367–389

Meisfeld R, Okref S, Wikstrom A-C, et al: Characterization of a steroid hormone receptor gene and mRNA in wild-type and mutant cells. Nature 312:779–781, 1984

Merchenthaler I, Vigh S, Petrusz P, et al: The paraventriculo-infundibular corticotropin releasing factor (CRF) pathway as revealed by immunocytochemistry in long-term hypophysectomized or adrenalectomized rats. Regul Pept 5:295–305, 1983

Morris RGM: An attempt to dissociate "spatial-mapping" and "working-memory" theories of hippocampal functioning, in Neurobiology of the Hippocampus. Edited by Seifert W. New York, Academic, 1985, pp 405–432

Munck A, Guyre PM, Holbrook NJ: Physiological functions of glucocorticoids in stress and their relations to pharmacological actions. Endocr Rev 5:25–44, 1984

Nakane T, Aughya T, Kanie N, et al: Evidence for the role of endogenous corticotropin-releasing factor in cold, ether, immobilization, and a traumatic stress. Proc Natl Acad Sci U S A 82:1247–1251, 1985

O'Donnell D, Larocque S, Seckl JR, et al: Postnatal handling alters glucocorticoid, but not mineralocorticoid mRNA expression in adult rats. Brain Res Mol Brain Res 26:242–248, 1994

Partridge WM, Sakiyama R, Judd HL: Protein-bound corticosterone in human serum is selectively transported into rat brain and liver in vivo. J Clin Endocrinol Metab 57:160–166, 1983

Plotsky PM: Regulation of hypophysiotropic factors mediating ACTH secretion. Ann N Y Acad Sci 512:205–217, 1987

Plotsky PM, Meaney MJ: Effects of early environment on hypothalamic corticotropin-releasing factor mRNA, synthesis and stress-induced release. Brain Res Mol Brain Res 18:195–200, 1993

Plotsky PM, Sawchenko PE: Hypophysial plasma portal levels, median eminence content, and immunohistochemical staining of corticotropin-releasing factor, arginine vasopressin, and oxytocin and pharmacological adrenalectomy. Endocrinology 120:1361–1369, 1987

Plotsky PM, Vale WW: Hemorrhage-induced secretion of corticotropin-releasing factor–like immunoreactivity into the rat hypophysial portal circulation and its inhibition by glucocorticoids. Endocrinology 114:164–169, 1984

Plotsky PM, Otto S, Sapolsky RM: Inhibition of immunoreactive corticotropin-releasing factor into the hypophysial-portal circulation by delayed glucocorticoid feedback. Endocrinology 119:1126–1130, 1987

Pratt WB, Sanchez ER, Bresnick EH, et al: Interaction of the glucocorticoid receptor with the Mr 90,000 heat shock protein: an evolving model of ligand-mediated receptor transformation and translocation. Cancer Res 49(suppl):2222–2229, 1989

Ratka A, Sutanto W, Bloemers M, et al: On the role of brain mineralocorticoid (type I) and glucocorticoid (type II) receptors in neuroendocrine regulation. Neuroendocrinology 50:117–123, 1989

Reul JMHM, De Kloet ER: Two receptor systems for corticosterone in rat brain: microdistribution and differential occupation. Endocrinology 117:2505–2511, 1985

Reul JMHM, De Kloet ER: Anatomical resolution of two types of corticosterone receptor sites in the rat brain with in vitro autoradiography and computerized image analysis. J Steroid Biochem Mol Biol 24:269–272, 1986

Reul JMHM, van den Bosch FR, De Kloet ER: Relative occupation of type-I and type-II corticosteroid receptors in rat brain following stress and dexamethasone treatment: functional implications. J Endocrinol 115:459–467, 1987

Ringold GM: Steroid hormone regulation. Annu Rev Pharmacol Toxicol 25:529–566, 1985

Rivier C, Vale WW: Effects of angiotensin II on ACTH release in vivo: role of corticotropin-releasing factor (CRF). Regul Pept 7:253–258, 1983

Rivier C, Brownstein M, Spiess J, et al: In vivo corticotropin-releasing factor–induced secretion of adrenocorticotropin, β-endorphin, and corticosterone. Endocrinology 110:272–278, 1982

Sapolsky RM, Meaney MJ: The maturation of the adrenocortical stress response in the rat. Brain Research Reviews 11:65–76, 1986

Sapolsky RM, Krey LC, McEwen BS: Glucocorticoid-sensitive hippocampal neurons are involved in terminating the adrenocortical stress response. Proc Natl Acad Sci U S A 81:6174-6177, 1984a

Sapolsky RM, Krey LC, McEwen BS: Stress down-regulated cortico-sterone receptors in a site-specific manner. Endocrinology 114:287–292, 1984b

Sapolsky RM, Krey LC, McEwen BS: Prolonged glucocorticoid exposure reduced hippocampal neuron number: implications for aging. J Neurosci 5:1221–1226, 1985

Sapolsky RM, Krey LC, McEwen BS: The adrenocortical axis in the aged rat: impaired sensitivity to both fast and delayed feedback inhibition. Neurobiol Aging 7:331–336, 1986a

Sapolsky RM, Krey LC, McEwen BS: The neuroendocrinology of stress and aging: the glucocorticoid cascade hypothesis. Endocr Rev 7:284–301, 1986b

Sapolsky RM, Armanini MP, Packan DR, et al: Glucocorticoid feedback inhibition of adrenocorticotropic hormone secretagogue release: relationship to corticosteroid receptor occupancy in various limbic sites. Neuroendocrinology 51:328–336, 1990

Sarrieau A, Sharma S, Meaney MJ: Postnatal development and environmental regulation of hippocampal glucocorticoid and mineralo-corticoid receptors in the rat. Developmental Brain Research 43:158–162, 1988

Sarrieau A, Rowe W, O'Donnell D, et al: Increased hypothalamic ACTH secretagogue synthesis in aged impaired vs aged unimpaired rats. Society for Neuroscience Abstracts 18:669, 1992

Selye H: The Physiology and Pathology of Exposure to Stress. Montreal, Acta, 1950

Shanks N, Larocque S, Meaney MJ: Neonatal endotoxin exposure alters the development of the hypothalamic-pituitary-adrenal axis: early illness and later responsivity to stress. J Neurosci 15:376–384, 1995

Sheppard KE, Funder JW: Equivalent affinity of aldosterone and corti-costerone for type I receptors in kidney and hippocampus: direct binding studies. J Steroid Biochem Mol Biol 28:737–742, 1987

Swanson LW, Simmons DM: Differential steroid hormone and neural influences on peptide mRNA levels in CRH cells of the paraventricular nucleus: a hybridization histochemical study in the rat. J Comp Neurol 285:413–435, 1989

Swanson LW, Sawchenko PE, Rivier C, et al: Organization of ovine corticotropin-releasing factor immunoreactive cells and fibers in the rat brain: an immunohistochemical study. Neuroendocrinology 36:165–186, 1983

Tornello S, Orti E, DeNicola AF, et al: Regulation of glucocorticoid receptors in brain by corticosterone treatment of adrenalectomized rats. Neuroendocrinology 35:411–417, 1982

Van Eekelen JAM, Rots NY, Sutanto W, et al: The effect of aging on stress responsiveness and central corticosteroid receptors in the brown Norway rat. Neurobiol Aging 13:159–170, 1991

Van Loon GR, DeSouza EB: Regulation of stress-induced secretion of POMC-derived peptides. Ann N Y Acad Sci 512:300–307, 1987

Viau V, Sharma S, Plotsky PM, et al: Increased plasma ACTH responses to stress in nonhandled compared with handled rats require basal corticosterone levels and are associated with increased levels of ACTH secretagogues in the median eminence. J Neurosci 13:1097–1105, 1993

Weinberg J: The effects of prenatal exposure to ethanol on the development of the hypothalamic-adrenal axis. Ann N Y Acad Sci (in press)

Wilson M, Greer M, Roberts L: Hippocampal inhibition of pituitary-adrenocortical function in female rats. Brain Res 197:344–351, 1980

Wolfson B, Manning RW, Davis LG, et al: Co-localization of corticotropin releasing factor and vasopressin mRNA in neurones after adrenalectomy. Nature 315:59–61, 1985

Young WS, Mezey E, Seigel RE: Vasopressin and oxytocin mRNAs in adrenalectomized and Brattleboro rats: analysis by quantitative in situ hybridization histochemistry. Molecular Brain Research 1:231–241, 1987

Zarrow MX, Campbel PS, Denenberg VH: Handling in infancy: increased levels of the hypothalamic corticotropin releasing factor (CRF) following exposure to a novel situation. Proc Soc Exp Biol Med 356:141–143, 1972

Section II

Sudden Unexpected Trauma

Chapter 4

Coping With Natural Disasters

Thomas M. Haizlip, M.D.
Billie F. Corder, Ed.D.

During the past 7 years, the authors and the staff of the Child Psychiatry Training Program of Dorothea Dix Hospital and the University of North Carolina School of Medicine have been involved in developing interventions for children in communities that have been struck by tornadoes, hurricanes, and devastating fires. In addition, we have helped to develop materials for mental health programs designed to support military families during the Persian Gulf crisis. In this chapter we describe some of the practical problems encountered in delivering mental health services in response to disasters. We then describe our community-based approach to providing support and assistance and elaborate the theoretical basis for our interventions. We also outline some of the materials developed that are now being used nationally in some similar disaster areas by the American Red Cross.

Effects of Stress and Trauma on Children in Disasters

The urgent nature of mental health services delivery in disaster crisis situations has often outweighed priorities for research implementation and objective assessment techniques in our own work. However, significant information for planning and intervention programs has been suggested by a number of studies of children's reactions to hurricanes, tornadoes, floods, blizzards, earthquakes, and brush fires. Pre- and postdisaster functioning has usually been assessed by self-

131

report questionnaires for older children and by parent and teacher interviews and questionnaires for observations of behavior changes in younger children. McFarlane (1987) carried out a longitudinal study of posttraumatic effects of a devastating brush fire on primary school children in Australia. As reported on parent and teacher questionnaires, symptoms (e.g., nightmares, replaying events of the disaster, fears related to reminders of the fire) were noted in 50% of the children 8 months after the fire and in 33% of the children 26 months after the fire. The severity and number of children's symptoms at 26 months were seen as being more closely related to the mother's level of preoccupation and anxiety than to the degree to which the child was directly exposed to the disaster.

Burke and colleagues (1986) analyzed problem areas suggested in fifth-graders' stories that were obtained 10 months after a blizzard and flood disaster. Clinicians' ratings of the content of the stories suggested signs of fears, depression, and anxiety in girls' stories that reflected fear of harm by external forces, preoccupation with death or dying, a sense of being unable to influence one's own fate, frustrating relationships with peers, and anxious, depressed moods. These factors were not reflected at a significant level in stories by fifth-grade boys from the same community. The researchers felt this might be related to "pre-existing differences" on a range of socioeconomic and psychological characteristics of the male and female groups, but lacked pretest data for comparison.

Green and associates (1991) rated psychiatric reports of 179 children aged 2 to 15 for the presence of posttraumatic stress disorder (PTSD) symptoms 2 years after they had been exposed to the Buffalo Creek dam flood disaster. Thirty-seven percent of the children were given a possible diagnosis of PTSD. Of the total sample, 65% of the children showed psychological distress at reminders of the disaster, 37% showed irritability or anger outbursts, 40% showed restriction of social range, and 39% demonstrated a restricted range of affect. Latency-age adolescent girls were more likely than boys to exhibit symptoms. "Family atmosphere" variables were seen as correlated with children's symptoms. The strongest predictors of symptoms in all age groups were the overall functioning of parents and an "irritable atmosphere" in the home.

Terr (1991) outlined definitions of two types of childhood trauma, described typical symptoms and reactions of these types of trauma, and suggested the long-term effects of these events on children. Type I trauma was defined as the mental result of a sudden external negative event that temporarily leaves the child helpless and unable to use ordinary coping and defense mechanisms. The resulting posttraumatic stress disorder seen in children with type I trauma is characterized by behaviors such as repetition (acting out and repeating the events in play), avoidance, hyperalertness, full and detailed memories (unusual ability to report detailed, complete memories despite attempts at suppression), perceptions of "omens" in their environment (retrospective reworking of events), and misperceptions or perceptual distortions. These symptoms seen in Terr's studies of children's acute reactions to type I trauma may also become chronic behaviors in children (Terr 1979, 1983, 1991).

Type II trauma was defined as the mental result of exposure to multiple, variable, or long-standing stressors or repeated, extreme external events, such as chronic physical or sexual abuse. The effects of type II trauma were described as denial and psychic numbing (inability to feel a normal range of emotions, "forgetting" whole segments of childhood life events) and self-hypnosis and dissociation (defined as an ability to remove oneself emotionally and intellectually from chronic harm through techniques such as repeating words or using visual imagery, such as imagining pleasant "scenes"). These behaviors, along with feelings of rage, and other resulting mental changes were hypothesized as forming the basis for a number of types of personality disorders and adjustment disturbances in later periods of development (Terr 1991).

Terr defines general characteristics of all childhood traumas as repeated visualizations or returning perceptions (having detailed memories of the trauma despite attempts at suppression), repetitive behaviors that reflect or are used to act out the actual events of the trauma, fears that appear to be specific to the trauma (worries over bad weather, strangers, separation, etc.), and negative concepts about people, life, and the future. These negative concepts may be characterized by lack of trust in others, lack of feelings of security and protection, and generalized fears and feelings of vulnerability about events that might occur in the future.

Other researchers have reported observations of acute posttraumatic stress symptoms in children exposed to type I trauma that are obvious within weeks of the initial trauma. Pynoos and colleagues (1987; see also Eth and Pynoos 1985) have observed that the severity and number of symptoms reported for these children appear to be related to the degree and extent of the exposure to the threatening trauma. In their study, Pynoos and colleagues (1987) described acute posttraumatic symptoms in children exposed to shootings at a playground that suggested that these children's reactions were similar on some levels to posttraumatic stress reactions seen in adults. Children who were studied following that assault (in which 1 child was killed and 13 others were injured) selected the following test descriptors of themselves: feeling fearful and upset when thinking of the event; having bad dreams and sleep disturbances; experiencing attention problems in school; wishing to avoid feeings or reminders of the event; and having intrusive imagery and thoughts described as threatening visual images and thoughts about the event that returned to the child at inappropriate times. One-half of the children who were exposed to the attack described themselves as losing interest in activities and as having feelings of estrangement and interferences with learning.

Our own clinical observations of children that have been made within a few weeks of the children's having experienced hurricanes, tornadoes, or floods tend to verify the findings from the studies we have described previously. The acuteness and intensity of symptoms reported in children appeared to be related not only to the degree of exposure and injury from the traumatic event but to the child's previous functioning and stress levels. For example, one child whose home and family were in one of the areas less affected by a devastating tornado was identified by counselors as one of the most anxious and symptomatic children in the small community's grammar school. She cried daily in class and constantly asked for extra attention from teachers, asked to call her mother several times a day, and had difficulty staying in class for an entire day. Review of records and interviews revealed that the child's parents had recently separated and the child had been living in a number of different settings during a period that had been both transitional and conflict ridden for the family. The additional stressor of the natural disaster had appeared to magnify the child's previously existing anxieties and lack of structure. Other acute symptoms evident in children we observed within several weeks after a natural disaster are listed in Table 4–1.

The children experienced fears specifically related to the natural disaster such as, in the case of tornadoes or floods, the appearance of dark clouds, high winds, or heavy rain. They feared separation and had unusual concerns about the location of members of their family. Some children became highly anxious and tearful if their parents were only a few minutes late picking them up at school or arriving home from work. Sleep disturbances were reported by parents, who described their children as experiencing difficulty falling asleep and/or having frightening dreams with themes related either directly to the disaster or to fears of separation and loss of their parents.

The children had different reasons for why the disaster occurred. Some children expressed concerns about the disaster's having been some sort of "punishment" for the town's not being a good enough place and having been singled out by God for retaliation.

The children exhibited some hypervigilant behavior and distractibility. When a pencil sharpener was used in a room next to the group interview room, each child present rose out of his or her chair in momentary fear of the sudden, loud, unexpected noise. In addition, lack of ability to attend to structured tasks in the school setting was common. The children were easily distracted and showed poor attention spans for several months following the disaster. Hyperirritability was evident in some children. School staff reported an unusual number of "fights" and confrontations between peers.

Rather than engaging in repetitive play, most of the children appeared anxious to avoid being reminded of and talking about the disaster. They were anxious and upset that the environment was not returned, as soon as they would have liked, to its former state, and often commented on the number of trees still down and on the rubble that had not been removed.

Table 4–1. Acute symptoms seen in children within weeks after exposure to natural disasters

Fears of environmental warning signs

Fears of family separation and safety

Sleep disturbances

Distortions about causes of disaster

Shame and guilt

Hypervigilance

Distractibility

Hyperirritability

Avoidance and suppression

Regression

School reluctance

Some children demonstrated regressive behaviors, demanding help with tasks that they had previously mastered. These demands added to the stressors already experienced by their parents.

Some school reluctance was observed and appeared to be related to the children's fear of separation from their parents and concerns about their family's being separated from and not being able to find one another if a disaster should again occur.

Children sometimes experienced feelings of shame about having to accept help, and they felt ashamed when they were referred to as "Red Cross kids" by other children who did not have to receive housing or other assistance from emergency relief teams. Conversely, some children appeared guilty and reluctant to admit that they had been only mildly affected by the disaster when others were discussing their losses.

Theoretical Framework for Interventions With Children in Disasters: Trauma and the Development of Mastery

Terr (1991) has reported on the long-term effects of children exposed to a single trauma and noted continuing symptoms after the children had undergone 5 to 13 months of brief treatment. She suggested that these symptoms may be related in part to the victim's continuing feelings of having failed at mastery of his or her environment. Erikson (1937) has hypothesized that children's play serves as a mechanism for "hallucinating ego mastery," or creating events in play during which the child is able to overcome difficulties and practice successful handling of tasks. It appears possible that the repetitive play reenactment observed by Terr in the Chowchilla victims may represent their failure in achieving perceived mastery. For these children, reenactment apparently failed to serve an "ego mastery" function, at least on a level that would help to significantly alleviate their symptoms.

In describing short-term treatment for children with less severe physical and sexual abuse (apparently defined as more similar to type I than to the type II trauma of chronically and severely abused children), Sgroi (1982) noted that treatment is related to basic concepts of the development of self-mastery and control. Role modeling, role playing, peer group support, and structured opportunities for practicing independent decisions and choices were listed by Sgroi as techniques that can be focused on self-mastery and control issues, which are in turn critical for the development of independent behavior, accountability, and effective decision making and judgment. Rutter (1978) and Anthony and Koupernick (1974) have described studies of asymptomatic children who, in contrast to the symptomatic, traumatized children's behaviors and impaired coping defenses, have been described as "invulnerable" to chronic life stressors (i.e., type II trauma). These so-called invulnerable children were characterized as showing a high degree of autonomy, as having skills in seeking help from others in the environment, and as actively attempting to master their environment, resulting in a sense of their own power over the environment through a number of techniques, including cognitive relabeling of stressors to lower anxiety levels. Anthony and Koupernick (1974) noted that the asymptomatic, or "invulnerable," children appeared to show high competence on tests of their receptive and organizational skills, suggesting that they were able to create an effective problem-solving frame of reference for dealing with stressors.

Similarly, Garmezy (1976) has outlined "protective factors" that appear to define characteristics of "stress resistant" children—that is, children who appear to be resilient and show adaptive mechanisms for dealing with stress and trauma. These characteristics are outlined as 1) positive self-esteem, 2) positive perception of one's ability to control and handle problems, 3) perception of one's environment as predictable and positive, 4) positive family environments characterized by warmth and cohesion without histories of abuse and neglect, 5) the skills to seek out and receive positive responses from the environment, and 6) a positive school environment.

Rutter, in a verbal consultation with the present authors, suggested that effective treatment efforts for children suffering from type I trauma, if low levels of symptomatology and pathology are present, might be centered on short-term interventions that emphasize development of mastery skills and focus on family involvement to foster continuing development of these skills in these children.

More general guidelines for treatment intervention have been suggested in various manuals used to train mental health professionals working with children who are experiencing disasters. For example, in the National Institute of Mental Health's *Manual for Child Health Workers in Major Disasters* (1978), broad outlines for interventions recommended for children with mild to moderate symptoms included the following: lowering temporarily academic achievement performance requirements; giving increased emotional support and increasing individual time spent with children when possible; providing structured but undemanding responsibilities and activities; encouraging verbal expression of feelings; rehearsing safety measures to be taken in the future; and encouraging older children to participate in environmental and home rehabilitation, cleanup, and rebuilding.

Other disaster intervention guidelines and information have since appeared that emphasize the process of cathartic exploration and verbalization of emotional reactions rather than focus on the development of specific mastery skills for handling these emotional responses (McRee et al. 1984). Those exercises and interventions that might be viewed as mastery skills development appeared limited primarily to rehearsal of safety measures to be followed in the future and to activities focused on involvement in rebuilding the environment.

In our own pilot intervention projects in tornado and hurricane disaster areas, brief interventions and materials have focused on mastery skills building in group settings. The interventions and materials, which will be described in greater detail later in this chapter, generally are aimed at fostering mastery of victims' emotional responses to type I trauma through exercises focused on the following steps:

1. *Discrimination.* Differences between normal and abnormal aspects of weather, wind, lightning, rain, and other environmental conditions connected with the disaster are outlined, along with the necessity for normal environmental changes. The use of intellectualization as a defense mechanism is encouraged by didactic instruction about causes of natural disasters.

2. *Coping.* Cathartic expression of feelings of fears and anxiety is encouraged, and, in conjunction, techniques to compartmentalize, relabel, normalize, and handle these fears through intellectualization, specific steps in keeping oneself safe, and a number of cognitive-behavior modification techniques (e.g., subvocal rehearsal of safety steps, group "chants") are taught.

3. *Restitution.* Activities that help to return the environment to a more normal state, and the roles that each person can take in bringing this about, are discussed.

4. *Dealing with survivor guilt.* Cathartic expression of feelings of guilt over having survived or suffered less than others is encouraged and normalized, and, in conjunction, concrete and symbolic ways to share with others are focused upon.

5. *Reintroduction of structure.* The necessity and expectation for returning to normal activities and schedules as soon as feasible are emphasized. Some transitional changes are outlined to help parents cope with children's reactions in this phase.

6. *Insight into the relationship between symptoms and trauma.* Typical fears, concerns, and behavioral reactions are discussed. In addition to being encouraged to cathartically express these feelings, children are encouraged to use a variety of cognitive-behavioral techniques to deal with their reactions (e.g., relabeling, chants, rehearsal of safety steps).

7. *Reintegration and acceptance of support systems.* The positive aspects of existing support systems are emphasized, and children are encouraged to practice ways to seek out and verbalize their need for this support when necessary.

Through these steps we have attempted to develop some of the mastery skills utilized by "stress-resistant," or "invulnerable," children who have dealt successfully with stress and trauma. More detailed definitions of some of these steps and specific techniques for implementing them are outlined later in this chapter in our discussion of specific short-term intervention groups for children.

Developing a Pilot Project Intervention in a Tornado Disaster

In 1984, the first devastating tornado disaster in almost a century struck a small community in North Carolina. Our state mental health systems struggled to meet service needs that were unusual and atypical for our area. The staff of the Child Psychiatry Training Program, a collaborative program with the University of North Carolina School of Medicine and Dorothea Dix Hospital, began intensive reviews of the literature and existing materials on disaster prevention and initiated a series of consultations with professionals experienced in this work.

General guidelines that emerged from the reviews of existing literature, consultations with others, and from our own program's experiences were as follows:

1. Tailor interventions around the reality that people concerned with immediate survival needs may not be fully aware of mental health concerns.

2. Offer assistance emphasizing objective symptom relief, because families, particularly in a rural, fairly isolated area, might have some difficulty accepting assistance from mental health professionals outside the families' community.
3. Avoid mental illness labels when possible for this population under acute stress.
4. Carry out all service delivery with the blessing of and within the existing community service delivery systems and through their administrative channels.

Since that time, our program has continued to be involved with intervention programs for children and families in a number of natural disasters and a national military action.

Another step in responding to disaster situations comprised complex, detailed, and diplomatic negotiations and communications with the community's service systems. Our staff assisted organizational leaders in outlining their perceived needs and requests for assistance. It became clear that the already overburdened mental health service facilities would need assistance in four general areas:

1. Developing and providing materials and workshops for teachers, day care personnel, and other community caregiving staff. These interventions focused on identifying children's immediate needs and level of stress, suggesting helpful response modes, and offering models for decisions about referring children for further screening.
2. Offering immediate consultation and counseling for children and families who requested these services directly from the local mental health centers and facilities.
3. Providing the personnel for diagnostic and referral screening within the school system for children who had been identified by school counselors as possibly needing further assistance.
4. Providing short-term discussion/intervention groups within the school setting for children who had been identified by counselors as showing mild to moderate concerns and behavior changes. Children with more severe symptomatology or those whose behaviors were more acutely disturbed were referred for more intensive screening at the mental health center.

We have found that these areas of intervention are generally those with which community mental health personnel in other disaster areas request assistance. Outlining the activities involving these areas in advance of a disaster is time- and cost-effective.

In our experience, only a few children were identified by staff screenings as requiring more intensive intervention, and these children were followed by local mental health professionals. As we noted earlier, the children who were identified as showing intense symptoms were more likely to have had a difficult adjustment before the disaster took place or to have come from families that were having greater-than-average problems in reorganizing their lives and environment following the disaster.

Our staff focused on short-term intervention groups for essentially healthy children who had been identified as showing a higher frequency or degree of trauma-related symptoms (e.g., hypervigilance, fears about weather, separation anxiety, inattentiveness, distractibility, regressive behaviors, school reluctance) than classmates. Our observations suggest that this group included approximately 10% of the school population, whereas fewer than 1% of the children displayed intense symptoms.

In addition to focusing on the children, it was necessary to plan informal group meetings that served as a support and discussion group for the community teachers and volunteer caregivers themselves. Many of the teachers and professionals had suffered losses within their own families and homes but had continued to work tirelessly to provide services in their area. Some were approaching exhaustion and had not allowed themselves to examine their own feelings. The informal meetings encouraged cathartic release of shared feelings and emotions, provided a vehicle for exchange of ideas and resources for meeting immediate financial and other needs, and established an arena where these individuals could be rewarded and receive some social reinforcement for their work while being encouraged to recognize the need for perceiving their own physical and emotional limits.

Use of Suggested Materials to Structure Intervention Groups

In our experience, written materials are useful as a means of structuring discussions about natural disasters. For example, simple brochures for three age groups (preschool, elementary school, adolescent) that list common symptoms in children and suggest some responses of adults to help ameliorate these symptoms can be helpful to the community and to any group discussion. These materials should also include an outline of behaviors, including the time frame in which they occur and their duration, that may indicate the need for professional help. We found it helpful to organize brief "workshops" for caregivers focusing on these materials. Reviewing these materials with the groups served two purposes. First, it relayed information, and second, it provided a framework for cathartic exploration of some of the group's own experiences. Most of these caregivers had been affected by the disaster and needed time for cathartic sharing of information about their losses and for exchanging coping strategies and specific information about assistance techniques that had been helpful to them. We termed this process "self-cure" for volunteer caregivers.

Exchange of information for the caregivers included a review of "self-care" guidelines, which involved caregivers realizing their own limitations and finding support for themselves too. Caregivers in this situation must learn to ration their time to consider their own needs and the needs of their families. They must also learn to judge when they themselves need support and to stick to a realistic schedule even when confronted by the enormous needs of others around them. Exhausted people cannot realistically provide effective help for others. Support group discussions such as our own provide "permission" among participants to place limits on the responsibilities assumed. Some role playing can be used to reinforce this perspective and prevent caregivers from promising involvement and effort that are beyond stress limits.

Caregivers are informed of the signs that indicate that they have reached the limits of their energy:

1. Forgetting of large bits of information, or confusion of appointments and details.
2. Exhaustion and stress that may result in either interferences in sleep or falling asleep during some activity.
3. Hyperirritability and extreme impatience.
4. Listlessness and low-level depression that lead to a large number of errors in functioning and may interfere with concentration.
5. Sudden "overflow" of emotions that may be expressed in crying, temper explosions, and so forth.

Although these states would be present to some degree in any group of people involved in a community experiencing a major disaster, caregivers tend to forget to observe, label, and deal with their own reactions while they try to assist others.

Short-Term Intervention Groups for Children

Our own experiences with tornado and hurricane disasters have led us to focus on short-term intervention groups with generally healthy children, from kindergarten to fourth grade, that are held in school settings. Children may be referred to these groups by counselors and teachers, and are screened by mental health volunteers and selected for inclusion in the group on the basis that they exhibit more symptoms than their classmates but appear to function at a level that does not require intensive intervention. Postgroup interviews and follow-up with referral sources are conducted to assess symptom reduction and levels of functioning. Parents and referral sources should be informed of the purposes of the group, which include helping the children to

> develop an intellectual understanding of natural disasters.
> feel control and mastery by developing plans for keeping themselves safe.
> talk about their feelings and understand why they may still have fears and worries.
> learn ways to talk to parents and other helping adults.
> ask for reassurance when they need it.
> remember the positive, good things about their environment.
> "talk to themselves" about fears and worries related to the disaster.

A Model for Short-Term Intervention Groups

Eight-week groups (1 hour weekly) for children in grades kindergarten through third or fourth grade may be organized to include eight children. Pre- and postintervention questionnaires administered by referring teachers, counselors, and parents may be helpful to assess the effectiveness of the group and to identify children who may need more intensive interventions. The groups may be centered on nonthreatening, interesting exercises. For example, our group has developed coloring books focused on building mastery feelings in children. These books contain didactic material about disasters and exercises to encourage cathartic expression of feelings and the development of mastery that are presented in pictures for coloring, following dots, drawing, or gamelike tasks to be shared with a helping adult (Corder and Haizlip 1984).[1] Other structured activities may be developed by the leaders to help to reduce anxiety in the children and to develop a focus on skill building (Corder et al. 1990).

We now describe, session by session, the process that we have experienced in leading these brief intervention groups and provide examples of tasks covered in each session.

Session 1: Discrimination, Intellectualization, Problem Solving, Relabeling

Children and leaders review the goals of the group (described earlier in this section). Each participant may be introduced by exercises such as matching the first letter of each person's name with the first letter of an animal's name (e.g., Betty Bear, Kathy Kangaroo, Tyrone Tiger), and going "around" the group to see who can remember them. The group colors those pages of the coloring book that describe the causes of tornadoes (or hurricanes). These pages also list the good and necessary aspects of changes in weather, emphasize the relative rarity of weather disasters, and describe scientific techniques for predicting such events.

Group discussion can be stimulated by coloring book exercises based on the questions "What would happen if there were no 'good' winds or rain?" and "How do we know when 'bad' winds and rain are coming?" Discussion aims at developing intellectual defenses and promoting both healthy denial and a positive perception of the necessity of weather changes, as well as addressing the relative rarity of disasters and the relative safety offered by early-warning systems.

Along with these coping skills, feelings of mastery are promoted by the use of "homework" following each session. Homework may consist of a series of sentences with blanks to be read and, with the parents, the blanks filled in. The sentences are designed as a review of the

---

[1] One of these coloring books, *After the Tornado: A Coloring Book for Children and Their Parents or Helping Adults,* is available from the American Red Cross or in very limited numbers from the authors.

concepts covered in the group and are such that the child can easily supply answers and fill in the blanks. In addition, exercises may be suggested to encourage intellectualization and healthy denial and to place the probability of occurrence of disasters in a realistic time frame. An example of an exercise is a parent's saying to the child

> Pretend that you are a television reporter who is interviewing your parents for TV. Ask them how old they are and, during the years they have lived, how many tornadoes or hurricanes they have been in. Ask them how they knew when the hurricane or tornado was coming and ask them how they kept safe.

Some cognitive-behavior modification and relabeling skills are encouraged by closing each session with a "chant" or "rap" exercise in which each child repeats a chant while clapping his or her hands with a partner's in complex, "patty-cake" rhythms. For example, the chant may be

Winds can be *good* and winds can be *bad.*
If we never had winds, we'd all be *sad.*
And if a bad wind does come through,   •
We can be *safe* and we *know* what to do!

Session 2: Coping and Mastery, and Problem Solving

After a review of the last week's homework, problem-solving and coping skills are encouraged by using the coloring book pages that describe safety steps to take in a disaster. Family plans and school drill safety exercises are discussed and rehearsed. Cognitive modification and healthy denial are encouraged by rap/chants along with rhythmic handclapping in pairs: "We *know* where to go. We *know* what to do. My *family* will be safe, and *I* will too."

Homework "assigned" in this session consists of outline sheets that encourage parents and children to fill in their own specific home disaster plan, suggestions for practicing a home emergency drill, and a review of questions and suggested answers related to disaster planning for parents and child to discuss together. There are many questions that many children ask their parents. For example, "What if I am at school and you are at work? What will we do if a tornado comes?" A suggested answer is

School has a drill and plan to keep you safe, and we have one at work to keep us safe [describe drill specifically if possible]. Tornadoes do not last very long, and as soon as they are over, and roads are safe, we will come get you. You will not be left alone; teachers will look out for you till we get there. And at work, other workers and police and safety officers will look after us and help us get to school to pick you up.

Session 3: Cathartic Expression of Fears, Along With Suggested Mastery and Coping Techniques and Self-Esteem Building

Some structured exercises and games are used to encourage expression of concerns, anxiety, and fear reactions to the disaster, which are labeled as typical and normal. A set of "Dr. Corder's Faces With Feelings" (or some other commercially available products that illustrate typical feeling reactions in children) is given to each child, and the children are asked to hold up the feeling that fills in the blanks for a story, "Wanda and the Tornado," read by the group leader. Then spontaneous discussion is encouraged and feelings identified as the children respond to a similar story, "Me and the Tornado." Each child is asked to talk about his or her responses to the incomplete sentences as he or she holds up the card illustrating his or her feelings (e.g., "After the tornado was gone, I still felt _____").

The second half of the session is called, "What we can do about these feelings if they keep coming back." Using the coloring book, the group reviews steps such as

● Talking to others who will tell us it is OK to have these feelings, but who will remind us that tornadoes very seldom happen and will go over the ways we will keep safe.
● Learning to talk to ourselves and reminding ourselves that we know how to keep safe.

Some role playing, rehearsal of techniques, and chants close the session (see chant for Session 2).

Homework "assigned" at this session may consist of having group members review Wanda's story, having *parents* fill in story blanks with *their* feelings, normalizing the child's fears and bolstering his or her self-esteem by the realization that grownups must cope with these concerns. Another suggested exercise is for the child to tell his or her parent one thing that he or she still worries about. The parent then gives the child a big hug, telling him or her that those feelings are OK to have, but reminding him or her that tornadoes seldom ever happen. The parent reviews with the child just what the parent would do to keep safe. Remind the child that he or she would always be looked after. This is usually the type of reassurance needed, although the parent may have to repeat this over and over again at different times.

Session 4: Survivor Guilt, Restitution, Coping and Mastery, and Relabeling

Coloring book exercises may be used to review the reasons why winds or rains may injure one house and not another one. The accidental nature of weather development should be stressed, and any myths about other factors causing harm (e.g., punishment for bad deeds) should be explored, along with feelings of guilt about actions that might have been taken to protect the family or others. Some relabeling of guilt feelings is effected. For example, the leader might say, "People don't cause tornadoes, and the weather that causes the tornado may hurt one place and not another. It is not anybody's fault. We wish nobody and no place had been hurt, and it is all right to feel glad if nobody in your house was hurt, or if your house was not hurt. . . ."

Restitution exercises, some symbolic and others concrete examples, are suggested. For example, the leader might say, "After the tornado everyone helps clean up. What are the things you did, and what can children do to help their families? Suggestions may include pick up small limbs, help sweep the house, help find belongings, etc. Sometimes children like to share a small toy with other children who have lost all their toys in the tornado. Draw a picture of a toy you might be able to share."

Sessions may close with chants, added to previous ones practiced, combined with rhythmic clapping such as, "It's *nobody's* fault that a tornado *came*. But we'll *all* help and share, just the *same*." Homework exercises suggested at this session encourage parents to assign small cleaning and repair tasks to children to encourage their sense of control, restitution, and mastery. Parents are also asked to help the children select a small toy to contribute to the Salvation Army or another organization that is distributing items to disaster victims. It might be necessary to purchase a very inexpensive item. Emphasis is placed on the symbolic nature of the act.

Sessions 5 and 6: Insight Into Stress and Trauma, Cognitive-Behavior Modification

Coloring books may be used to focus on children's continuing concerns such as fears at night, heavy rains, and so forth. Children may be helped to make a "diary" of drawings about things that cause them to be concerned. These matters of concern may involve leaving parents in bad weather, hearing loud noises or winds, and so forth. Role playing and practicing in sessions may encourage specific practice of "how to talk to yourself when you feel this way."

> When you are afraid, you need to tell your parents or your teacher, and they will remind you that you will be safe. But you also need to practice talking to yourself. You need to say to yourself that you are afraid because the tornado (hurricane) was a very scary thing, and it is natural to still feel a little afraid when something reminds you of the tornado. But you need to tell yourself that you stayed safe before and you know even more about being safe now, and that there will always be someone to take care of you. Then practice your chants: "That was *then,* but this is *now.* I can keep *safe,* and I know *how.*

Sessions may include going around the group, identifying the concerns and fears in each drawing, and rehearsing with each child some coping strategies, such as discussing what they would tell their parents, how they would ask for reassurance and hugs, and how they would "talk to themselves" about their feelings.

If possible, a small, special stuffed animal toy or hand puppet may be purchased and given to each child as an aid in learning how to "talk to themselves." Using the puppet as a "reminder" of what they learned in the group, children tell the puppet their concerns and have the puppet remind them of the coping techniques suggested in their group. These types of behavior modification techniques using the toys or puppets as "reminders" and transition objects from the group have been helpful in some settings in which children were allowed to keep the toys after the last session.

Homework "assigned" in these sessions may center around sharing of the "feelings diaries" with parents, along with parents' being given sheets of specific suggestions for handling and encouraging their child's sharing of these feelings.

Session 7: Reinstitution of Structure, Self-Esteem Building, Training in Seeking Assistance and Reassurance

Coloring books may be used to structure exercises listing people whom the children feel they can depend on, putting names in a large "heart" to be colored. Role playing, including "asking for hugs," and selecting people with whom feelings can be shared, can be rehearsed with each child. In addition, children are encouraged to view themselves as a resource, perceiving and labeling themselves as "brave survivors." Role-play games may include "I'm My Own Grandpa." In this game children take turns playing themselves as a grandfather, while others in the group take the role of his grandchildren. The child who is playing "Grandpa" describes the "big tornado" when he was a boy and explains how he learned to understand and handle his fears about it, and to know ways to keep safe. The session closes with selected previous chants.

Session 8: Graduation—Rehearsal and Review

In this session a review of completed coloring books and diaries may take place, and a "graduation" celebration is held. Parents, teachers, and counselors may be encouraged to attend, as children march in formally with recorded music to receive their "graduation certificates" that label them as a "Strong Survivor" who knows good ways to handle feelings and keep safe. Refreshments may be shared at a "First Lady Picnic," where leaders take the role of the current First Lady, who would like to learn what the children and their parents would like to broadcast to others in the nation about dealing with tornadoes. Using a television interview technique, the leader reviews with the group a list of the areas that had been covered over the course of the sessions, allowing each child to answer one "question" in the mock interview.

The session closes with chants and presentation of the special puppets as transition objects from the group. Parents can be asked to complete a questionnaire within 2 months of the final session and again 1 year after the intervention.

Summary

Research on the effects of natural disasters (e.g., floods, tornadoes, hurricanes, brush fires) on children's adjustment has suggested that as many as 50% of elementary school–age children in affected areas may show posttraumatic stress symptoms at 8 months following the disaster (McFarlane 1987) and that a significant number of symptoms may persist as long as 10 months (Burke et al. 1986) to 26 months later (McFarlane 1987). Terr's (1983) studies of children who had experienced trauma from a single, unanticipated, frightening event (designated as type I trauma) have suggested that effects on behavior and personality development may be seen as long as 4 years after the event. These studies of posttraumatic effects of disasters and trauma in populations of normal children suggest the need for large-scale mental health interventions for children that can be time- and cost-effective.

We have presented an outline of our experiences and the materials developed for interventions with children who have experienced natural disasters such as those involving a tornado, hurricane, or fire. Short-term group interventions have been described that were used with children who had experienced trauma related to these single, unanticipated events (type I trauma). These groups focused on development of mastery and coping skills similar to those seen in children who have been described as "stress resistant." The intervention consisted of steps defined as discrimination, coping, restitution, dealing with survivor guilt, reintroduction of structure, insight into the relationship between symptoms and trauma, and reintegration and acceptance of support systems.

Anecdotal reports from parents and teachers noted a decrease in symptoms in children who had previously been identified as responding to a disaster with moderate symptoms and behavior difficulties, after their involvement in the short-term intervention groups we have described. The absence of objective measurements of pre- and post-intervention symptom levels and changes related to these interventions are obvious limitations of our work. This type of objective assessment, along with longitudinal studies of children's adjustment following various types of environmental disasters and intervention programs, should continue to be a significant focus for further research.

References

Anthony E, Koupernick A (eds): The Child in His Family: Children at Psychiatric Risk. New York, Wiley, 1974

Burke J, Moccia P, Borus J, et al: Emotional distress in fifth-grade children ten months after a natural disaster. Journal of American Academy of Child Psychiatry 25:536–541, 1986

Corder B, Haizlip T: After the Tornado: A Coloring Book for Children and Their Parents or Helping Adults. Raleigh, NC, American Red Cross, 1984

Corder B, Haizlip T, DeBoer P: A pilot study for a time-limited therapy group for sexually abused pre-adolescent children. Child Abuse Negl 14:243–251, 1990

Erikson E: Configurations in play—clinical notes. Psychoanal Q 6:139–214, 1937

Eth S, Pynoos R (eds): Post-Traumatic Stress Disorder in Children. Washington, DC, American Psychiatric Press, 1985

Garmezy N: Vulnerable and Invulnerable Children: Theory, Research and Implementation. Master Lecture on Developmental Psychology. Washington, DC, American Psychological Association, 1976

Green B, Korol M, Grade M, et al: Children and disaster: age, gender, and parental effects on PTSD symptoms. J Am Acad Child Adolesc Psychiatry 30:945–951, 1991

McFarlane A: Posttraumatic phenomena in a longitudinal study of children following a natural disaster. J Am Acad Child Adolesc Psychiatry 26:764–769, 1987

McRee C, Mullis S, Corder BF, et al: Brief intervention programs for children in a tornado disaster area. North Carolina Journal of Mental Health 20:9–18, 1984

National Institute of Mental Health: Manual for Child Health Workers in Major Disasters. Rockville, MD, National Institute of Mental Health, 1978

Pynoos R, Frederick C, Nader K, et al: Life threat and posttraumatic stress in school age children. Arch Gen Psychiatry 44:1057–1062, 1987

Rutter M: Early sources of security and competence, in Human Growth and Development. Edited by Bruner J, Gaston A. Oxford, UK, Clarendon Press, 1978, pp 254–262

Sgroi S (ed): Handbook of Clinical Intervention in Child Sexual Abuse. Lexington, MA, Lexington Books, 1982

Terr L: Children of Chowchilla: A Study of Psychic Trauma. Psychoanal Study Child 34:547–634, 1979

Terr L: Chowchilla revisited: the effects of psychic trauma four years after a school bus kidnapping. Am J Psychiatry 40:1543–1550, 1983

Terr L: Childhood traumas: an outline and overview. Am J Psychiatry 148:10–20, 1991

Chapter 5

The Avianca Airline Crash: Implications for Community Health Care Response

Victor Fornari, M.D.
Jared Fuss, M.D.
John K. Hickey, D.S.W.
Linda Packman, C.S.W.

On the night of January 25, 1990, Avianca Flight 052 struggled through fog and drizzle over the hamlet of Cove Neck on Long Island, New York. The Colombian airliner had been delayed through various holding patterns and had missed its first landing attempt at JFK Airport.

There were 133 adults and 25 children aboard the plane. A quiet

The authors would like to thank Lenore Terr, M.D., and Sandra Kaplan, M.D., for their ongoing consultations regarding the treatment program; Inez Weinberg, for coordinating the group program and serving as a translator; Jeanette Betancourt, for serving as a translator; Harriet Urgo, for her administrative assistance; Fredi Leisersohn and Jean Duffy, for preparation of the manuscript; and Michael Holland, who supported the project on behalf of Avianca.

Portions of this chapter are reprinted with permission from Fornari V: "The Aftermath of a Plane Crash—Helping a Survivor Cope With Death of Mother and Sibling: Case of Mary, Age 8," in *Play Therapy With Children in Crisis: A Casebook for Practitioners*. Edited by Webb NB. New York, Guilford Press, 1991, pp. 416–434. Copyright 1991, Guilford Press.

The authors would like to dedicate this chapter to the victims of the Avianca airline disaster: those who perished, those who survived, as well as all of their families.

apprehension grew among the passengers, and there was no word of reassurance from the flight crew. The lights began to blink, and then the cabin was plunged into darkness. Quiet apprehension turned to screams of disbelief as the steady roar of the engines gave way to silence. Parents huddled their children, some, unfortunately, on their laps; others strapped their children in their seats. Some passengers began to pray aloud as they realized the inevitable; Flight 052 was going down. Thirty seconds later, the Boeing 707 was a mass of twisted wreckage on a wooded hillside. There was no fire or explosion because, as was later realized, the aircraft had run out of fuel.

Of the 158 people aboard Flight 052, 73 were killed in the crash, including 69 adults and 4 children. Among the 85 survivors were 21 children and adolescents.

The actual experience of a plane crash from a child's point of view can only be surmised by his or her drawings, play, and occasional statements as well as by descriptions from adults on the plane. At 9:45 at night, many children were exhausted from the 9-hour trip, and some were asleep. Some were seat-belted into their seats for the second landing attempt; others were held by their parents on their parents' laps.

The first phase of the children's trauma took less than 1 minute. Many were awakened by the screams of the adults when the cabin lights flickered and then went out completely. When the engines failed, parents did not know what to do. There were no instructions from the crew. Some assumed the crash position; others unstrapped their children and held them. Within 30 seconds, the aircraft slammed into the hillside at close to 200 miles per hour, splitting into sections of twisted wreckage. Many children were catapulted at high velocity, some still strapped in their seats. Some miraculously escaped severe injury or death by being thrown clear of the aircraft. One boy was found hanging by his clothes in a tree. Another child was found sitting on top of the fuselage, still strapped in her seat. Some children were found, later on, lying in the mud in the dark or hidden among the trees. One girl, who had part of her brain exposed, was placed in the field morgue. She was later heard moaning and was removed to a hospital where she survived. Other children were wedged among wreckage and bodies.

From impact onward, these children were hurled into a world of darkness, mass destruction, mutilation, and physical pain. At the time parental comforting was needed the most, the whereabouts of their parents were unknown. When the children were found by rescuers, they were placed in the care of strangers who did not speak the children's language. The children were carried down the hillside to waiting ambulances and helicopters, by which they were rushed to the emergency rooms of nearby community hospitals.

Four children died in the wreckage, but 21 others survived their injuries. All of the surviving children were injured and were hospitalized. For these children, their significant stressors were experienced over time and included severe injuries; death or hospitalization of parents, siblings, and/or relatives; and the horrifying experience of the crash itself (Figure 5–1).

Another group of children were not on the plane but were awaiting the arrival of their relatives at JFK Airport. Many families had one parent and several children returning from Colombia on the plane. They had been waiting for several hours because of the plane's delay in landing. Finally, this group and their accompanying relatives were gathered together at the Avianca office and bussed to the relatives' staging area at the Nassau County Medical Center. Here, the children gathered in the auditorium while their relatives went through morgue photos and, in some cases, eventually identified bodies in the morgue.

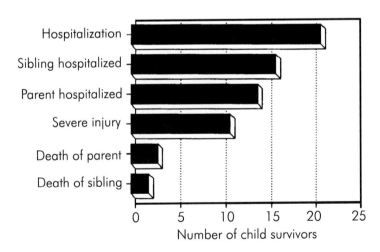

Figure 5–1. Significant stressors for child survivors of the crash of Avianca Flight 052.

Some children were more fortunate and were reunited with family members located in nearby hospitals.

Another, indirectly affected group of children were those living in the community who had no direct relationship with those on the plane. These were children who lived near the crash site or who watched the graphic, unedited film on local television stations. Some of these children came with their parents to the community outreach center, and others attended group meetings sponsored by the children's library.

Crash Site and Community Response

Without any forewarning, in the middle of the night, the crash of Avianca Flight 052 made immediate demands upon the resources, strength, and resolve of Nassau County. This disaster in our midst challenged the dedication, caring, and giving of countless rescue workers and volunteers. As bodies were placed in the field morgue and the injured were being rushed to community hospitals by ambulance and helicopter, relatives were anxiously waiting at JFK Airport for news about the fate of their loved ones. These were the pending challenges to be met by the Nassau County Mental Health Service.

Fortunately, a disaster mental health plan had been drawn up by the Nassau County Department of Mental Health, Mental Retardation and Developmental Disabilities 2 years earlier and had been integrated into the county's Civil Preparedness Plan. The plan called for the provision of crisis intervention for survivors, crisis intervention for relatives of victims and survivors, referral of survivors and relatives to community mental health services, and treatment of rescue workers beyond their critical incident stress debriefing. A roster of potential mental health responders was developed from among the various crisis programs in the county that were licensed by the State Office of Mental Health. While this cadre was activated, it was essential to recruit an additional 125 Spanish-speaking mental health workers from state psychiatric centers, community clinics, and Hispanic service agencies.

The most intensive mental health intervention took place at the Nassau County Medical Center auditorium, located near the medical examiner's office. This became the staging area for relatives, many of whom were bussed in from JFK Airport, where they had gathered to greet their loved ones. By early afternoon on Friday, January 26,

18 hours after the crash, there was a sea of emotionally drained, tired, and hungry people. Most of them had been up all night; many spoke no English. The children who had accompanied their relatives to the airport and continued on to the medical center slept on chairs, snacked on doughnuts, and tiredly clung to their parents.

The mental health responders in the auditorium attempted to work with entire families, but the emphasis at that point was upon the adults who were there to learn the fate of their relative(s) or friend(s). Information was sparse. There had been no assigned seating on the plane. Some passengers had traveled under other family names, and many lost their identification in the crash. Emotions were quite intense. Some relatives felt the urgent need to search area hospitals on their own. As the list of located survivors was read off, expressions of joy and relief from one family only lessened the hopes of the other families there.

For some, the sudden loss of a loved one was becoming increasingly probable. Morgue photographs were set up in the chaplain's office. Relatives reluctantly formed a line across the auditorium so that they could slowly file past the pictures displayed in the room. Each person was accompanied by a mental health responder. Later on, those who identified photos would be expected to view those bodies in the morgue for positive identification. For each child or adult, survivor or relative, each new unfolding incident was yet another step in a series of traumatic events.

Dr. Lenore Terr (1991) has defined childhood trauma as "the mental result of one sudden, external blow or a series of blows, rendering the young person temporarily helpless and breaking past ordinary coping and defensive operations" (p. 11). A major airplane crash has sufficient impact to overwhelm the victim's usual effective ability to cope. It presents overwhelming stressors that overload the ability of the mind to handle the impact of the event. Most disasters confront their victims with a series of traumatic events over a period of time rather than a singular incident. In the Avianca accident, the primary victims were passengers who were killed or injured in the crash. No one escaped without injury. For those who survived, their physical injuries were compounded by psychic trauma resulting from overwhelming stressors, including the devastating scene, threats of the unknown, and the sudden loss of loved ones who had perished in the crash.

The task of the disaster mental health responder was to actively assist victims through their psychic trauma as they experienced it and as they coped with its aftermath. The desired result of the intervention was a decrease of external stressors acting upon the victim and an increase in the victim's ability to cope with the traumatic situation. Achieving this goal required the close-in support and consistent presence of mental health clinicians who possessed crisis intervention skills, the recognized authority to negotiate systems, and prior training in working in settings involving multiple psychic trauma.

The major effort of the disaster mental health response team took place in the first 8 days after the crash and fell into three distinct phases of operation: emergency, recovery, and community support (Figure 5–2). Although each phase required specific tasks of the mental health responders, the general functions of responders could be categorized as follows:

1. *Outreach/engagement.* Responders presented themselves as persons who had the authority to be there, could help survivors and relatives with specific needs, would listen empathically to them, and would provide a strong, consistent presence throughout their ordeal. Engagement of family members was accomplished primarily at the staging area. Outreach and home-based crisis intervention were provided to some family members in the area, particularly children, who were unable to come to the staging area. Other persons were reached through the establishment of a neighborhood drop-in center near the crash site.

2. *Emotional support.* Responders provided a strong emotional shoulder to lean upon. They encouraged persons to verbalize their experiences, fears, and anxieties as well as information about their deceased or missing relatives, no matter how gruesome or horrible the information sounded. Responders remained emotionally available for the relatives as the latter were confronted with a series of traumatic experiences. These included determination of the status of their relative, identification through morgue photos, identification of the body in the morgue, and arrangements for care of the deceased. In situations involving positive identification of a body, relatives were encouraged to talk about the victim until they could do so in the past tense. They were later, at the hotel, supported in their grieving process through visits by the clergy and by representatives from Hispanic organizations, from the American Red Cross, and from social agencies.

Days 1, 2, and 3	Days 4, 5, and 6	Days 7 and 8
Phase of operation		
Emergency phase	Recovery phase	Community support phase
Tasks of mental health response team		
Outreach/Engagement		
Engage family members at the staging area and the hotel. Visit homes of relatives who are unable to come to staging area. Establish neighborhood drop-in center near crash site. Engage injured in community hospitals.	Engage survivors who are returning from hospitals to the hotel. Engage newly arrived relatives. Maintain neighborhood drop-in center.	Make public announcements regarding mental health resources for those persons in need.
Emotional support		
Provide consistent, close support Learning status of relative. Identification through morgue photos. Identification of bodies at the morgue. Arrangements for care of the deceased. Ongoing grieving process.	Maintain emotional support of survivors and families at the hotel. Conduct formal CISD for mental health responders.	Prepare persons to leave the hotel and return home or arrange for alternative resource.
Assessment		
Assess symptom development, coping ability, and functioning of victims and relatives. Assess needs of families.	Continue assessment of symptom development, coping ability, and functioning of victims and relatives.	Assess victims' and relatives' ability to travel and to carry out necessary details.
Assurance and education		
Provide assurance to victims and relatives that their reaction is normal and their symptoms, if any, are normal and expectable in response to an abnormal experience. Educate victims and families as to what reactions and symptoms could be expected to occur.	Continue the process of assurance and education begun in the emergency phase and include new arrivals in the process. Keep victims and relatives informed of impact of the event on the public.	Continue information on community impact.
Organization and advocacy		
Assist persons in locating injured or deceased relatives. Assist victims and relatives in planning a course of action. Refer victims and relatives to other services when required.	Accompany relatives to hospitals to meet with injured family members.	Meet with community agencies to plan for housing and support of families while they remain in the area to be near injured relatives. Refer victims and relatives to community mental health resources.
Social support		
Begin peer interaction at drop-in center and in dining room at the hotel.	Encourage peer interaction and identify leadership potential.	Include leadership in planning conferences.

Figure 5–2. Mental health response to crash of Avianca Flight 052, January 25, 1990, the week following the crash. CISD=critical incident stress debriefing.

3. *Assessment.* Responders assessed the ability of each person to cope and to function. Some relatives presented in a confused, bewildered, and immobilized state, while others responded with boundless energy. The degree of involvement and the specific tasks of the responder were influenced by this assessment.

4. *Education and assurance.* Responders assured relatives that many of the symptoms they were experiencing were normal reactions to an abnormal experience. The relatives were advised about other reactions or symptoms that they might later experience and were assured that these too were normal and to be expected.

5. *Organization and advocacy.* Whenever it was possible to do so, responders encouraged persons to function to the best of their ability and to make critical decisions. Responders provided updated information and attempted to clarify conflicting or confusing statements. Family members were helped to define their immediate needs and to develop a course of action. Responders assisted, when such assistance was required, in negotiating the various systems involved and acted as direct advocates for the families.

6. *Social support.* It is often the nature of airline crashes that a group of survivors suddenly find themselves in a foreign environment that, although protective and caring, is devoid of other healing factors such as presence of family and friends, and customs. In the case of the crash of Avianca Flight 052, most relatives lived outside the area. Within hours, they began to arrive from other parts of the United States and, a short time later, from Colombia. They were deprived of their natural social support system at a time when they needed it most. The initiation of peer interaction and the development of a mutually supportive organization were encouraged by the responders as the emergency phase was completed.

The literature speaks of the need to create an artificial, nurturing environment for persons who become victims of mass trauma away from their natural setting (Sloan 1988). This environment has been characterized as a "libidinal cocoon" (Black 1987). A libidinal cocoon was created at the local hotel by the Nassau Chapter of the American Red Cross. In the cocoon were housed the headquarters for the Red Cross, the Disaster Mental Health Team, funeral directors, disaster services, and governmental units. On the floor below, individual families were housed in 24 rooms where their needs for privacy, food, shelter, and emergency clothing were met. Those families who wanted to sleep or be alone closed the door to their room. Those who were receptive to visits from the mental health responders, clergy, and Red Cross representatives left their doors open. Red Cross headquarters became the central gathering place for relatives. There, they could have a cup of coffee, get updated information, and meet with other families. This was the beginning of a social support network that grew over the next several days.

The extent to which interpersonal support can serve a mediating role during times of high stress has not been consistently determined (Cook and Bickman 1990; Murphy 1988). Following the immediate trauma, however, it was apparent that the Avianca survivors and their relatives were drawn to those who understood their language and their culture. Gradually, a kinship developed at the hotel among the crash survivors. There was a feeling that "you had to be there" to understand what they had gone through. One survivor, a little girl, observed that another child survivor could not have been on the plane because she did not have a scar across her forehead. The scar was her symbol for belonging to the group.

Thirty-six hours after the crash, all the families were assigned to individual tables in the hotel dining room. A mental health responder joined each family at the table for breakfast and remained with that family throughout the day, as the family either searched for relatives in the local hospitals or traveled to the morgue to identify family members whose photos had been viewed earlier. Some families needed to return to the morgue more than once because they had lost more than one relative or because of their inability to identify their loved one the first time.

Some children in the community also required the services of a mobile response team. For example, an adolescent boy, upon learning of the death of his father, locked himself in his room and refused to get out of bed or accept any food. A mobile team with Spanish-speaking responders from the county children's psychiatric hospital was able to help the boy cope with his traumatic loss.

Other mobile teams went to the community hospitals, at their invitation, to work with children who were separated from their families. These teams served as a link to parents and siblings who were in other hospital units or had been released to the hotel. In one situation, a mobile team supported a young man as he told family members about the death of his mother and the injuries to his son, who was in another hospital. The deaths of children were difficult for the mental health responders to handle; one responder accompanied a father on three visits to the morgue before the father was able to identify his son's body. In another situation, a team accompanied a mother on leave from her hospital bed to attend her son's funeral.

Deploying mobile teams in the community was far more effective than offering urgent clinic appointments. Only one family attended a clinic session; this was a young woman and her three children, ages 4, 5, and 6 years. The family had to fly back to Colombia on Avianca 5 days after the crash in which the father was killed. The mother was terrified to fly and the children were upset by their father's pending cremation, believing that their mother was going to have their father "burned." After two sessions involving art therapy and play therapy, the family was able to make their flight.

At the end of the emergency intervention phase, the team received a call from the medical examiner, who asked for a responder to come to the morgue to meet with a family. A late-adolescent boy and his uncle berated the medical examiner for misidentifying the body of their relative. Although the medical examiner was certain of the body's identity, the family had the funeral home return the body to the morgue. After considerable grief work with the responder, the family members were ready to view the body for a second time. This time, the boy identified the body as his mother. The family became distraught because they had not recognized their own relative. They were helped by the mental health responder to understand the nature of the mind's defense against pain and that this reaction is a common occurrence. The adolescent had lost not only his mother in the crash but his brother as well.

Although the primary effort focused upon persons directly traumatized by the sudden loss of a loved one, we were aware, also, of the effects of such a large-scale disaster upon the entire community. The Mental Health Association established a community outreach center near the site of the crash. Mental health workers maintained a presence there for 1 week. Community residents, particularly those who had gone to the crash site or were involved in the rescue operation, were able to meet with counselors and neighbors in small groups. Several children who lived near the crash site visited the outreach center with their parents.

Mental Health Practice in the Disaster Environment: Effect Upon the Mental Health Responder

The nature of the Avianca crash resulted in mental health intervention with both the 85 injured survivors and the relatives of the 73 deceased victims. Generally, many of the 125 mental health responders worked at the relatives staging area, hospital emergency rooms, and the medical examiner's office, where they were exposed to shocking images and overwhelming numbers of persons experiencing intensive suffering. These on-site interventions put the mental health responders in the role of emergency services personnel and exposed them to the same emotional impact experienced by other emergency responders. Other responders focused their attention on survivors and relatives at the hotel and were further removed from the more tragic scenes. This distancing did not ensure protection against being emotionally affected, however. McCann and Pearlman (1990) speak of the "vicarious traumatization" of therapists as a consequence of and a normal reaction to exposure to clients who present shocking verbal images of horror and suffering.

The impact of a large-scale disaster or a particularly tragic incident upon rescue workers has long been noted (Genest et al. 1990; McCammon et al. 1988). A pioneer in this field, Jeff Mitchell, developed a methodology for group debriefing of emergency services personnel termed "critical incident stress debriefing," or CISD (Mitchell 1985). The symptoms experienced by rescue workers have been well documented by Mitchell and others and include generalized anxiety, depression, anger, irritability, sleep disturbances, and intrusive visual images. Emergency workers are also prone to withdrawal from others who did not experience the event. Such withdrawal serves to protect the emergency worker's spouse or significant other from the horrors he or she has experienced, but it also serves as an attempt to suppress unpleasant memories.

These symptoms were noted among some of the mental health responders to the Avianca crash. Although there were no reports of severe reactions among the mental health responders, there were indications that, for some, the "traumatic imagery" was "too overwhelming, emotionally or cognitively, to integrate" (McCann and Pearlman 1990). Some found it difficult to talk with anyone other than their own peers who would "understand" them. Nightmares and sleep disturbances were frequently reported symptoms. One responder was plagued by numbers running through his head when he attempted to fall asleep after spending 18 hours on the job. The next day, back at the morgue, he found the origin of his symptom. Each relative who had identified a photograph was given a number that was called out when it was his or her turn to view the body. It was generally noted that the mental health responders tended to work "nonstop" for long hours with little signs of fatigue or emotional impact. These conditions would catch up with them later.

In the postoperation critique, it was decided to incorporate the following protocol into the county disaster mental health plan:

1. On-site critical incident stress debriefings will be used to monitor the stressors experienced by the mental health responders, and these debriefs will be made available to these individuals whenever necessary (Talbot et al. 1992).
2. Besides on-site CISD activity, formal group debriefing of mental health responders will be provided by neighboring CISD teams that are not involved in the particular event.
3. A drop-in center will be established nearby where emergency rescue workers, mental health workers, Red Cross representatives, clergy, and others can meet informally over a cup of coffee for a well-needed "time out."

Emergency Room and Hospital Care

Immediately following the crash of Avianca Flight 052, 9 children were brought to North Shore University Hospital–Cornell University Medical College for emergency medical care. All of the patients who had previously been receiving treatment in the North Shore–Cornell emergency room were either transferred to the cafeteria (where a temporary emergency room was set up), admitted to the hospital, or discharged home. Thus, the emergency room was evacuated and prepared to receive an unknown large number of injured crash victims. Prior to the arrival of any of the crash victims, several hundred physicians, nurses, social workers, and other health care providers were called in as part of a disaster plan to prepare for receiving the crash victims. Nearly 25 members of the

Department of Psychiatry were called into the emergency room.

There was a high degree of anxiety and uncertainty in the emergency room before the arrival of the first crash victim. No one knew quite what to expect. No one had ever experienced the emergency room in this heightened sense of readiness. As the first crash victims were helicoptered to the landing pad and wheeled by stretcher through the emergency room doors, the grim reality of the crash became vivid to all who heard the cries, moans, and screams of the injured survivors. The helpless injured were covered with blood and were wheeled on stretchers to examining rooms surrounded by five or six health care professionals. Initially, a sense of helplessness pervaded the emergency room.

Despite the large number of staff, the emergency procedures went quite smoothly, and each staff member seemed to find his or her role. As the first child was wheeled into the emergency room, it seemed clear that one of the roles that would be critical was to speak to each conscious child and try to calm him or her down in an effort to ease his or her anxiety while the emergency medical care was being provided. Many of the children sustained fractured bones, and they were in a high degree of pain.

After treatment in the emergency room, many of the survivors were transferred to the medical and pediatric floors. Teams of mental health providers began to make rounds on the pediatrics unit to visit the children and to talk with the medical house officers and nursing staff. These rounds served several important functions: 1) an opportunity for mental health responders to support health care providers on the medical floors, 2) an opportunity for mental health responders to assess the mental health issues of the survivors, and 3) an opportunity for mental health responders to support one another during this critical period. Emotions were intense: children crying in pain and fear; nurses, interns, and residents overwhelmed by their own feelings; mental health responders attempting to remain calm and supportive while feeling the enormity of human suffering.

Several immediate challenges faced the mental health responders, including how to answer questions such as "Is my daddy dead?" and how to be supportive when feeling overwhelmed. A calm approach was adopted. Children and staff were reassured that as information was made available it would be transmitted. But what should be done when it was learned that a child survivor's parent or sibling had died? Who would convey the news to the child survivor and when? These issues were addressed on an individual, case-by-case basis depending upon the age of the child, the severity of the physical injuries sustained, and the availability of surviving next-of-kin.

Within 12 hours of the crash, therapists were assigned to each surviving child through the child and adolescent psychiatry consultation–liaison service. Each therapist met with each child and available family members on a daily basis. Spanish-speaking therapists were assigned to non-English-speaking children. Coordination between health care providers at other hospitals was a critical piece of work that bridged survivors cared for in different hospitals, as survivors had been transported to 10 different hospitals. The Department of Social Work led this coordination effort. In some instances, survivors were transferred to other hospitals, when medical conditions permitted, so as to be close to their relatives. The Child Life Program provided intensive bedside activities for the youngsters that offered them an invaluable opportunity to discharge their creative energy at a time of extreme stress. These activities included drawing, playing games, storytelling, video games, and, as clinically appropriate, classroom instruction. Although some reports have tended to minimize the impact of trauma on children, we believe it is helpful to assist children to recall their memories of a terrifying event close to the time that the trauma actually occurred.

During our work with these hospitalized children, many concerns and issues were raised:

> A 10-year-old boy who had been traveling with his newly adoptive father worried that after living in an orphanage for 5 years, his chance of having a family life had come to an end. While he was in traction and in considerable pain, he asked, "Is my poppy dead?"

> A 6-year-old boy whose father had been violently killed 2 years earlier, when the child was 4 years of age, was traveling from Colombia with his 18-year-old mildly mentally retarded sister. His sister had been killed in the crash, and he was told of her death. The boy initially refused to believe that she had died. Family members insisted that he be convinced of her death.

> Another youngster, with two broken legs, asked repeatedly, "Will I ever walk?" Despite daily reassurances, she continued to ask, "Are you sure I will walk again?"

The work done by the child therapists is exemplified in the following case vignette:

> An 8-year-old girl was traveling from Colombia to the United States, accompanied by her mother and 5-year-old brother. They were to reunite with her father, who had come to New York 10 days earlier on business. He worked for a pharmaceutical company. This was their first trip to the United States. They were anticipating 5 days in New York and then 1 week in Orlando, Florida, where they were to visit Disney World, the anticipated highlight of their trip.
>
> The child reported that she had had some apprehension about her trip to the States, as this was to be her first ride on an airplane. Throughout the 9-hour flight, she and her brother played, ate, and rested in preparation for their reunion with their dad. Just before the plane crashed, she reported, the lights went out. There was a lot of screaming as the plane lost altitude and ultimately crashed. She recalled being awake and seeing her mother and brother either asleep or dead.
>
> The child sustained multiple fractures of her legs but no other serious injuries and no apparent loss of consciousness. She required traction, and both of her legs were casted. She worried about her own survival as well as the uncertain condition of her mother and brother, whom she feared dead. Her mother and brother had indeed perished in the crash.
>
> It appeared that this girl was a mature, sensitive, and particularly polite girl. Her father informed her of the death of her brother and mother. She told the therapists of these losses.
>
> During the days following the child's disclosure of her mother's and brother's death, the therapist met with her daily. She regularly greeted her therapist with enthusiastic and energetic exclamations, as though she was rooting for a team at a football game. Ten days after the crash, her dad left for Colombia to accompany the remains of his deceased wife and son. Her separation from her dad during this critical period in her recovery and mourning process intensified her attachment to her therapist.

The following is excerpted from a therapy session with this child, 5 weeks after the crash:

> **Child:** Doctor—I had a bad dream last night. I've had it before, but I never remember the whole thing.
> **Doctor:** Tell me about your dream.
> **Child:** I am on a plane. I see God's face. I think he's wearing

a long white beard. I ask to see my mommy. I don't remember anymore.

Doctor: What do you think about your dream?

Child: I don't know why I was on a plane, I will never take
a plane even if I have to walk back home to Colombia.

Doctor: The idea of taking a plane must be very scary.

Child: It is. (*pause*)

Doctor: What else about the dream?

Child: I remember seeing God's face.

Doctor: What about God's face?

Child: I wonder if my mommy is with him. I want to tell him
to take care of her and ask him how she is. I miss her so
much. It's not fair that he has her and I don't. Doctor, do
you know if you can drive from New York to Colombia? I'm
never going to fly!

Doctor: Right now flying seems so scary—but you don't have
to decide about this now.

The intensity of this child's fear of airplanes became increasingly apparent as she began to think about her long-awaited release from the hospital and eventual return home to Colombia.

During the weeks that followed, much time was spent reviewing
the crash, talking as well as drawing, in order to begin to help her
to master flying and the trauma of the crash.

After 50 days in the hospital, the child was to be released. She
was apprehensive about losing the security of her friends and the
hospital routine. She was to go to a home in the community with
her dad for several months for further rehabilitation and physical
therapy. Separation and loss remained as sensitive themes.

The girl had made many close friends while in the hospital. Her
kindness and gentle innocence attracted caring and concern. She
was discharged to a home in the community, where she and her dad
resided for nearly 2 months before their return to Colombia. The
therapist remained in contact with her and her father.

The therapist accompanied this child, her dad, and a family
friend to the orthopedist's office when she was to have her casts
removed. She would walk for the first time in 10 weeks. Later, in
the physical therapist's office, the therapist met with the child, her
dad, the family friend, and the physical therapist. The girl was
walking and pleased with her progress. Before departing for
Colombia, she and the therapist shared a warm goodbye. Four
months after the crash, she and her father returned to Colombia.

The therapist later heard conflicting stories about the return trip to Bogotá. First it was reported that the girl had refused to fly. A family friend called to say that she and her father had taken a train from New York to Miami, Florida. From there, they went by boat to a South American port, where they continued their return to Colombia by train, bus, and then car.

Subsequently, it was told that the trip proceeded differently. In actuality, they drove by car from New York to Miami. The reason for this arrangement was that the girl's dad had not made the necessary arrangements in time to fly. (Perhaps he was afraid to fly or to let her fly.) However, once in Miami, they traveled by plane to Bogotá. The child expressed fear about flying, but after being comforted by her dad while on the plane, she was able to relax during the return flight home.

Child Art Therapy Group Program

During the months following the crash, a collaborative effort was undertaken between the Nassau County Department of Mental Health and the Division of Child and Adolescent Psychiatry at North Shore University Hospital–Cornell University Medical College, in cooperation with and underwritten by Avianca. The goal of this project was provision of mental health follow-up for the child and adult survivors and their families.

Continuing psychiatric treatment and follow-up for the children of Flight 052 presented many challenges to the treatment team. The potential child patient population would consist of child survivors and their child relatives, as well as child relatives of adult survivors and deceased victims. There would be diversity in terms of age and "primary language" (Spanish vs. English) in the patient population. In addition, financial, geographic, and temporal factors would have to be considered in the design of the treatment plan.

To meet these logistical issues, as well as to address presented symptomatology challenges, the treatment team designed a program that combined elements of two types of psychotherapy. Terr (1989) noted that group therapy following traumatic experiences, despite possible problems, is an excellent preventive mode. The group therapy format outlined by Terr was combined with the techniques of art therapy. The literature supports group therapy (Bartone and Wright 1990; Terr 1989) and art therapy (Johnson 1987), as well as combined therapy, in the treatment of traumatized children.

The outpatient child art therapy group program was led by a psychiatric social worker and a child psychiatrist. The child psychiatrist had prior experience working with some of the crash victims via consultations at North Shore University Hospital following the crash. The social worker had expertise in the treatment of traumatized children and specialty training in art therapy. Both of the co-therapists had experience working with children in various group therapy programs. As there were several group members who spoke only Spanish (and as neither of the co-therapists was fluent in Spanish), a translator was also present during each group session.

An invitation was extended to all survivors and their families. The groups were composed of child survivors of the crash, their child-age relatives, and children who were related to adult survivors, representing great diversity. The ages of the group members ranged from 3 years to 11 years. As noted earlier, the experiences of the children in relation to the airplane crash were varied. Each group member had had different experiences with mental health professionals; some group members were already in individual psychotherapy, some were in family psychotherapy, and others had had no contact with mental health professionals apart from the group sessions. Some of the children had no apparent symptomatology; others were seen as highly anxious, plagued by bad dreams, intrusive traumatic visualizations, and dysphoric cognitions. These symptoms have been reported in traumatized children (Terr 1991).

There have been 16 art therapy group sessions between October 1990 and November 1992. There was a different number of children and, in fact, a varying population present during each session. The attendance varied from 2 children to 10 children. One child attended eight sessions, and another child attended six sessions. The remainder of the children attended from one to three sessions. Thus, some children were seen on a continuous, longitudinal basis, and others were seen on a discontinuous, "cross-sectional" basis.

The sessions began with a gathering of all adults and child survivors and their relatives. In addition to the patient population, both the adult and child therapists were present during the large group meeting. Lunch was served to facilitate the therapeutic process. There was a general discussion of the participants' functioning. Following this "combined group," the children and adults separated into two groups along with the designated therapists.

In the child group therapy sessions, the children continued to have snack foods available to help relieve anxiety. In addition, the children were given free access to drawing paper, pencils, crayons, and markers. Following the large combined group meeting, the children were keenly aware of the nature of the sessions. Each group session was structured according to the "projective free drawing and story telling" technique outlined by Pynoos and Eth (1986). According to these authors, this format, proceeding "from projective drawing and story telling, to discussion of the actual traumatic situation and the perceptual impact, to issues centered on the aftermath and its consequences" (p. 306), allows for "a sense of immediate relief and a reestablishment of human relatedness" (p. 318). Although the "child interview" was defined by Pynoos and Eth as a single session, we have adapted their interview technique to an ongoing group therapy format. (However, for those children who attended only one session, the format was used as a de facto single-session format.)

As the sessions progressed, three themes emerged among the children's drawings and stories. First, there was the fear of flying and of airplane crashes, as well as a generalized fear of other accidents (i.e., train crashes, automobile crashes). Second, several children expressed their worries "of a dangerous world, fear of abandonment, of uncertainty who to turn to for guidance and safety." Last, there were reports of intrusive visualizations of the crash. According to Terr (1991), these themes, respectively, are similar to three (of four) characteristics that she has suggested as being related to childhood trauma: "trauma-specific fears," "changed attitudes about people, aspects of life, and the future," and "strongly visualized or otherwise repeatedly perceived memories" (p. 12).

The course of the intervention with and the artwork of the following three children exemplify these themes as well as some of the therapeutic process of the art therapy group program.

A 10-year-old Colombian boy was traveling to the United States with his 11-year-old sister and his adoptive father (referred to earlier in a clinical vignette). He and his sister were orphaned when he was 4 years old. Their parents were killed in a mud slide subsequent to an earthquake. He had reportedly witnessed the death of his parents. Following their traumatic loss, this boy and his sister were raised in an orphanage in Colombia. He and his sister had been adopted by an American couple, and they were coming to the United States, for the first time, with their adoptive father on Flight 052. The boy suffered severe lacerations and bruises but he did not sustain life-threatening injuries during the crash. His adoptive father and sister, likewise, did not sustain life-threatening injuries. Although initially separated and sent to different hospitals, they were eventually reunited to begin their life together in the United States.

Upon interview during his first group session, the boy's adoptive parents reported that he did not exhibit any psychiatric symptoms of trauma. During his first group therapy session, at age 11 years, 10 months after the crash, he produced two especially noteworthy drawings. The first depicted a volcanic eruption, replete with lava, flames, and jungle background (Figure 5–3). The boy's accompanying story revealed the theme of a "prehistoric jungle" with (unseen) "dinosaurs trapped in the jungle." This drawing could be thought of as a visualization of this child's loss of his parents. In a study of the spontaneous drawings of 200 school children between the ages of 3 and 15 years, it was observed that pictures of fire and volcanoes are produced by children with acute emotional conflicts (Brick 1978). Certainly, even apart from the crash, this boy's development was replete with psychic trauma.

A subsequent drawing from that session (Figure 5–4) focused on

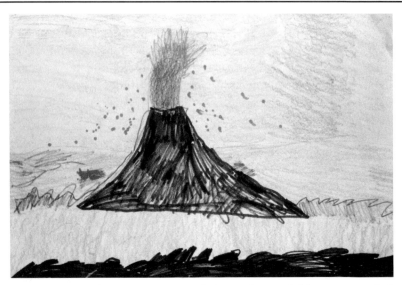

Figure 5–3. Volcanic eruption; drawing by a child survivor of the crash of Avianca Flight 052, at 11 years of age, 10 months after the crash.

a ship on the ocean. The boy's accompanying story was the following: "It's a Colombian boat with a lot of people. High waves swept over the boat. People were cold, wet, and many people died. Then, some people made it to land . . . to a house. They were saved."

During the session, the boy was able to report several experiences of intrusive, traumatic visualizations. Reportedly, he had not told his adoptive parents about these symptoms. These data were shared with his parents, and individual psychotherapy, in addition to group therapy, was recommended.

A 2-year-old girl had been traveling back to the United States, with her mother, on Flight 052. She and her family had been on a family visit in Colombia. She and her family escaped the crash with moderate lacerations and bruises. The child's primary language at home was Spanish, although she had some understanding of both Spanish and English.

At the time of her first group session, 9 months after the crash, the child was 2¾ years old. She reportedly had been "nervous and jumpy" and had been "different" since the crash. During her first ses-

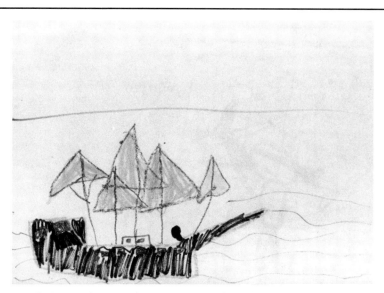

Figure 5–4. A ship on the ocean; another drawing by the child survivor of the crash of Avianca Flight 052 whose earlier drawing was presented in Figure 5–3, from later in the same session in which the drawing in Figure 5–3 was made.

sion and with the aid of a translator, she was able to draw a picture and relate her thoughts regarding the crash (Figure 5–5).

This girl drew a picture of seemingly random, multicolored dots, lines, circles, and squiggles. However, in the accompanying story, she revealed that her picture was not a random design at all. She stated that her drawing represented "a lot of people . . . all of the people who were not on the airplane." She went further, elaborating on the theme of who was present on the plane. She pointed to a small scar on her forehead, stating it was "proof she was on the plane" and that other children in the group, without such scars, could not have been on the plane at all. It should be remembered that "children are *never* the same after psychic trauma. Their lives are marked by their traumatic experiences as before or after the event (Fornari 1991, p. 433). This girl had developed this particular cognition about people based on her traumatic experience.

As this child was followed in group therapy, her cognitive and motor skills matured. At the time of the fifth group therapy session, 18 months after the crash, she, at the age of 3½ years, was able to

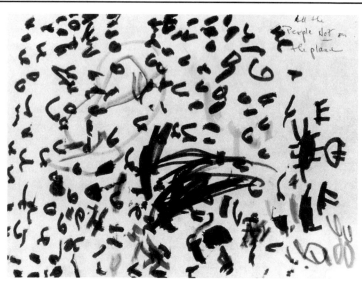

Figure 5–5. Seemingly random squiggles; drawing by another child survivor of the crash of Avianca Flight 052, at 2¾ years of age, 9 months after the crash.

represent her experiences in a more realistic fashion. Her drawing at this time was a clearer representation of an airplane with a well-defined figure (Figure 5–6). The accompanying story revealed memories of "flying and confusion on the plane" and of a "man helping people out of the plane." This drawing highlights Terr's thoughts (1991) about the power of visualization, even for toddlers. Over time, this girl had become less symptomatic.

A 5-year-old girl had been traveling with her parents and 12-month-old sister, after a visit to Colombia, on Flight 052. Fortunately, she and her family escaped life-threatening injury during the crash. However, her father suffered a significant leg injury that necessitated physical therapy and use of a cane. At her first session, 9 months after the crash, the child, who was then 5¾ years old, reported bad dreams and intrusive thoughts. She drew several pictures. Although her drawings and her stories alluded to the airplane crash, she did not draw a picture directly related to the crash. For example, she drew a girl standing beneath a rainbow (Figure 5–7). The accompanying story was as follows: "I was going on the plane, and it was a sunny day. That is

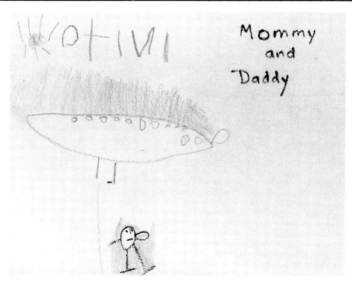

Figure 5–6. An airplane and a man; another drawing by the child survivor of the crash of Avianca Flight 052 whose earlier drawing was presented in Figure 5–5, at 3½ years of age, 18 months after the crash.

why I saw the rainbow. The little girl is me, and she's happy. I never wanted to go to Colombia."

By the fifth group session, 18 months after the crash, this child, at the age of 6½ years old, drew a picture of an airplane with emerging smoke, falling into the ocean (Figure 5–8). She added that she could not

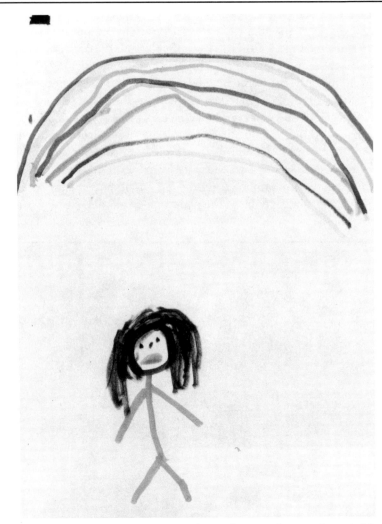

Figure 5–7.   A girl beneath a rainbow; drawing by another child survivor of the crash of Avianca Flight 052, at 5¾ years of age, 9 months after the crash.

draw the real crash—that "this was an imaginary crash." She related a story of how she warned the pilots of the danger on the plane and of her single-handed rescue of her parents and sister from the crash. In this text, no one sustained any injuries. Throughout the sessions, this child has also expressed a sense of helplessness, that no one could keep her safe from danger.

This girl's psychic experiences, as displayed in her artwork, revealed her progression toward her formulation of "inner plans of action" (Pynoos and Eth 1986). As Pynoos and Eth (1986) have pointed out, these "inner plans of action," or "cognitive reappraisals," often "seek to alter the precipitating events, to undo the violent act, to reverse the lethal consequences, or to gain safe retaliation" (p. 310). Terr (1983) has stated that therapy can help the child formulate appropriate and realistic plans. This girl has participated in individual and family psychotherapy as well as in the art therapy group program. She continues to be somewhat symptomatic, although reportedly less so over time.

We believe that the art therapy group program described above has represented a unique opportunity for psychiatric intervention and follow-up. The program has combined the techniques of projective drawing and story-telling within the group therapy format. Despite the heterogeneity of the population as well as the presence of a translator, this therapeutic intervention was very fruitful. We were able to recognize many of the psychological processes that had been identified in previous reports of childhood psychic trauma. We also were able to provide both direct therapeutic intervention by means of group support and abreaction through drawing to counteract the powerlessness of the traumatic experience (Pynoos and Eth 1986; Terr 1989). In addition, we were able to identify several children in need of more intensive psychotherapeutic interventions. These children were referred for these services. Having witnessed the process and, indeed, the power of our therapy program, we feel that the creative arts therapies do indeed have great potential as a psychologically reparative force.

Conclusions

Following the tragic crash of Avianca Flight 052, a large number of mental health professionals collaborated to provide mental health services to the survivors, their families, and the families of the deceased victims.

Working with child survivors of psychic trauma soon after the traumatic event, as in our interventions with the hospitalized child survivors of the crash of Avianca Flight 052, offers an opportunity to observe the initial coping responses of the children. The therapist is thus allowed a direct opportunity to experience the trauma with the

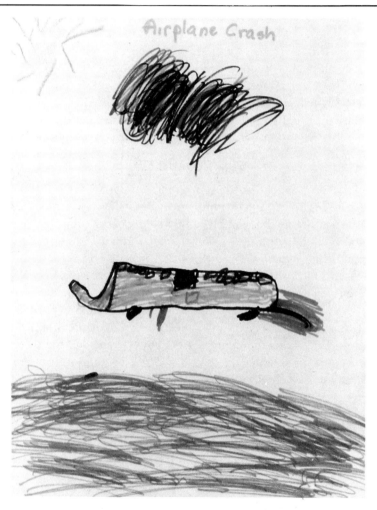

Figure 5–8. An imaginary crash; another drawing by the child survivor of the crash of Avianca Flight 052 whose earlier drawing was presented in Figure 5–7, at 6½ years of age, 18 months after the crash.

child, rather than attempting to reconstruct it in the consulting room many years later. This offers the rare and unique opportunity of early intervention and the possibility of prevention of a variety of symptoms that might otherwise develop.

The outpatient group therapy program has represented an ongoing reappraisal of the needs of the survivors of the crash of Avianca Flight 052 and their families, and has provided a flexible program to meet these needs. We hope that our future efforts, and those of other mental health professionals, will include the use and refinement of structured instruments to better define these needs and to follow the progress of these families as well as survivors of other forms of psychic trauma.

In any case, the collaboration between the Nassau County Office of Mental Health, the Mental Health Association, the psychiatry departments at multiple community hospitals, and volunteers and dedicated therapists has been an opportunity for mental health professionals to respond to a large-scale disaster within their own community. It is clear that a team of responders who can quickly and flexibly address the needs of the victims and their families and reassess these needs as the recovery process moves on is necessary and can perhaps provide a model for the entire mental health community.

References

Bartone PT, Wright KM: Grief and group recovery following a military air disaster. Journal of Traumatic Stress 3:523–539, 1990

Black JW Jr: The libidinal cocoon: a nuturing retreat for the families of plane crash victims. Hosp Community Psychiatry 38:1322–1326, 1987

Brick M: Mental hygiene value of children's art work. Am J Orthopsychiatry 14:136–146, 1978

Cook JD, Bickman L: Social support and psychological symptomatology following a national disaster. Journal of Traumatic Stress 3:541–556, 1990

Fornari V: The aftermath of a plane crash—helping a survivor cope with death of mother and sibling: case of Mary, age 8," in Play Therapy With Children in Crisis: A Casebook for Practitioners. Edited by Webb NB. New York, Guilford, 1991, pp 416–434

Genest M, Levine J, Ramsden V, et al: The impact of providing help: emergency workers and cardiopulmonary resuscitation attempts. Journal of Traumatic Stress 3:305–313, 1990

Johnson DR: The role of creative arts therapies in the diagnosis and treatment of psychological trauma. The Arts in Psychotherapy 14:7–13, 1987

McCammon S, Durham TW, Ellison EJ Jr, et al: Emergency workers' cognitive appraisal and coping with traumatic events. Journal of Traumatic Stress 1:353–372, 1988

McCann IL, Pearlman LA: Vicarious traumatization: a framework for understanding the psychological effects of working with victims. Journal of Traumatic Stress 3:131–149, 1990

Mitchell JT: Healing the helper, in Role Stressors and Supports for Emergency Workers. Rockville, MD, National Institute of Mental Health, 1985, pp 105–118

Murphy SA: Mediating effects of interpersonal and social support on mental health 1 and 3 years after a natural disaster. Journal of Traumatic Stress 1:155–172, 1988

Pynoos R, Eth S: Witness to violence: the child interview. Journal of the American Academy of Child Psychiatry 25:306–319, 1986

Sloan P: Post-traumatic stress in survivors of an airplane crash-landing: a clinical and exploratory research intervention. Journal of Traumatic Stress 1:211–229, 1988

Talbot A, Manton M, Dunn PJ: Debriefing the debriefers: an intervention strategy to assist psychologists after a crisis. Journal of Traumatic Stress 5:45–62, 1992

Terr LC: Play therapy and psychic trauma: a preliminary report, in Handbook of Play Therapy. Edited by Schaefer C, O'Connor K. New York, Wiley, 1983

Terr LC: Treating psychic trauma in children: a preliminary discussion. Journal of Traumatic Stress 2:3–20, 1989

Terr LC: Childhood traumas: an outline and overview. Am J Psychiatry 148:10–20, 1991

Chapter 6

Exposure to Catastrophic Violence and Disaster in Childhood

Robert S. Pynoos, M.D., M.P.H.

Over the past 15 years, our research group has conducted a planned series of studies concerning children exposed to catastrophic violence and disaster. These studies have included traditional epidemiological surveys in which we examined the prevalence and course of symptom reactions in children exposed to large-scale disasters, to catastrophic community violence, or to war and occupation. For example, we have completed studies of school-age children directly exposed to a 1984 sniper attack on their school playground in South Central Los Angeles (Nader et al. 1990; Pynoos et al. 1987), the 1988 Spitak earthquake in Armenia (Pynoos et al. 1993a), and the 1991 Iraqi invasion of Kuwait (Nader et al. 1993). In other studies we have obtained detailed clinical material from several cohorts of children who witnessed different forms of extreme interpersonal violence—for example, the homicide or rape of a parent or a parent's suicide attempt (Pynoos and Eth 1985; Pynoos and Nader 1988a). Recently, our group has collaborated in studies of young children exposed to life-threatening illness and life-endangering medical procedures (Stuber et al. 1991).

In addition to systematic assessment of clinical symptoms, these studies have included in-depth interview material that permits exploration of children's subjective experiences (see Pynoos and Eth 1986), microanalysis of their memory operations, and examination of developmental processes. More recently, these investigations have also included pilot examination of potential neurophysiological disturbances

181

and their developmental implications (Ornitz and Pynoos 1989). In addition, we are currently examining strategies of intervention, from school-based public health methods of psychological first aid to principles of brief and long-term therapy (Pynoos and Nader 1988b, 1993). We have been especially interested in strategies of pulsed interventions over the course of the child's further development.

Exposure to Violence and Disaster

The dose-of-exposure experimental model, with the use of cotemporaneous comparison groups, provides one scientific procedure for examining the causal relationship between a traumatic stress and its psychiatric sequelae. In this model, subjects are sorted by their relative exposure to a similar traumatic stress on a continuum from high exposure to nonexposure. Examination of the relatively homogeneous subgroups, based on stress criteria, permits a more accurate assessment of relative risk due to exposure or to other covariables at differing levels of exposure. Large-scale studies of adults exposed to disaster, criminal victimization, and combat have documented a direct relationship between dose of exposure and severity of the posttraumatic stress reaction. In our own studies we have demonstrated a similar relationship for children and adolescents exposed to violence and disaster (Pynoos 1991).

Paralleling the progress in the study of adult traumatic stress has been the development of more refined descriptions of the nature and degree of children's exposure to traumatic events. The result has been a more precise identification of the specific features of traumatic experiences that are associated with risk for posttraumatic stress disorder (PTSD) and other reactions. For example, recent studies of disasters and transportation accidents have indicated that factors such as being exposed to direct life threat and injury to self, witnessing mutilating injury or grotesque death (especially of family members or friends), and hearing unanswered screams for help and cries of distress are strongly associated with the onset and persistence of PTSD in children and adolescents (Gleser et al. 1981; Pynoos et al. 1993a; Yule and Williams 1990).

The literature related to violence has identified additional objective risk factors (Pynoos 1993), which include the following:

Proximity to violent threat

The unexpectedness and duration of the experience(s)

The extent of violent force and the use of a weapon or injurious object

The number and nature of threats during an episode

The witnessing of atrocities

Relationship to the assailant and other victims

Use of physical coercion

Violation of the physical integrity of the child

Degree of brutality and malevolence

The post-trauma viewing of graphic details, such as photographs of atrocities or the mutilated corpse of a family member or friend, may constitute an important secondary source of risk (Nader et al. 1993).

In recent studies investigators have begun to examine the contribution of children's subjective perception of threat to findings of intraexposure group differences in severity of post-trauma distress (Schwarz and Kowalski 1991; Yule et al. 1992). Guilt over acts of omission or commission that are perceived as having endangered others has been found to be associated with increased severity and persistence of posttraumatic stress reactions (Pynoos et al. 1987, 1993a; Yule and Williams 1990). Investigators have also suggested that the generation of other negative emotions (e.g., shame and rage) may play a similar role (Lansky 1990).

Measuring the dose of exposure to catastrophic violence at an elementary school, Pynoos and co-workers (1987) found that 1) there was a correlation between *degree* of exposure to the violence and *severity* of the posttraumatic stress reaction; 2) the *symptom profile* among the most severely distressed children was similar to that in adults, and 3) there was a pattern of *symptom accrual,* suggesting that specific symptoms are accumulated as exposure and severity of the reaction increase. Mild reactions were associated with general apprehension and anxiety; moderate reactions included more intrusive phenomena as well as a wish to avoid feelings; severe reactions included the full range of posttraumatic stress symptoms. In the most severe reactions, estrangement and interference with learning became more prominent. A pattern of symptom improvement was evident over the first year, with the rate of recovery primarily dependent on the severity of the posttraumatic stress reaction reported at the end of the first month (Nader et al. 1990).

Proximal posttraumatic stress–related psychopathology in children and adolescents has been reported to include symptoms of PTSD,
depressive disorders, phobic disorders, new onset or exacerbation of
existing attention-deficit disorder, dissociative disorders, obsessive-
compulsive disorder, sleep disorders, somatization disorder, disorders
of attachment and conduct, and substance abuse (Pynoos 1990a).

Developmental Psychopathology Model of Traumatic Stress

As PTSD has become a less controversial diagnosis, there has been
a trend for this concept to be reified and for clinicians and researchers to lose sight of the intimate union of traumatic stress and
child development. Recently, I offered an expanded conceptual
scheme to characterize the complex interaction of child development
with traumatic stress and its sequelae (Pynoos 1993) (Figure 6–1).

Viewing traumatic stress from the perspective of developmental
psychopathology suggests important areas of clinical assessment and
intervention and new avenues for future research. Examining traumatic stress from this perspective involves the use of more rigorous
descriptive typologies of traumatic exposures, reminders, and secondary stresses as these relate to proximal and distal risks of stress-
related psychopathology, developmental disturbances, and maladaptive
adjustment.

The conceptual schema incorporates a tripartite model of the etiology of the distress consequent to traumatic experiences in which the
distress derives not only from the nature of the experience itself
but also from the subsequent traumatic reminders and secondary
stresses. Such a model would indicate that a proper assessment of all
three categories—traumatic exposure, traumatic reminders, and secondary stresses—is essential to the evaluation of a child, particularly
in clarifying the relative contribution of each etiological factor to subsequent psychiatric symptoms and comorbid conditions.

Over the past several years, researchers studying childhood traumatic stress have developed refined typologies of childhood traumatic
experiences that are supplanting earlier conceptual frameworks that
typically referred to acute, cumulative strain (Khan 1974) and chronic
traumatic circumstances (Terr 1991). Researchers are beginning to
consider the interaction of traumatic exposure to single or recurring

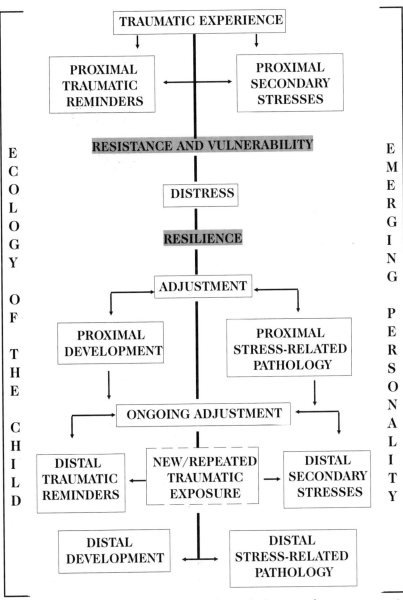

Figure 6–1. Developmental psychopathology and posttraumatic stress disorder. *Source.* Adapted from Pynoos RS: "Traumatic Stress and Developmental Psychopathology in Children and Adolescents," in *American Psychiatric Press Review of Psychiatry,* Vol. 12. Edited by Oldham JM, Riba MB, Tasman A. Washington, DC, American Psychiatric Press, 1993, pp. 205–238.

extrafamilial violence within an environment of chronic danger, the impact of acute or repeated intrafamilial traumatic experiences within the context of a more general pathogenic family environment, and the potential interaction over time of these extra- and intrafamilial traumatic experiences and their associated ecologies (Bell and Jenkins 1991; Cicchetti and Carlson 1989; Garbarino et al. 1991; Macksoud and Dyregrov 1993; Martinez and Richters 1993; Richters and Martinez 1993). The typology of trauma should also include characterization of the developmental cycle of the family, which involves assessing the current developmental phase of each family member as well as the developmental phase of the family as a whole (Brown 1980).

These refined typologies have permitted more precise characterization and have brought attention to the contribution of multiple traumatic experiences within a child's environment. For example, in situations of child abuse, additional exposures to spousal abuse and/or to parental suicidal and homicidal behavior (at different points in the child's life) influence the form and content of subsequent developmental disturbances. A developmental perspective contributes to a more complete characterization of traumatic stress by including consideration of the changing developmental context even within a particular type of traumatic stress. For example, the nature and circumstances of repeated physical or sexual abuse or witnessing of violence necessarily changes over time, as both the child and the circumstances develop. A parent's expressed reason or threat, the child's attribution of meaning, and the content of retaliatory rage, protection, and escape fantasies will vary with developmental maturation (Mones 1991).

The Complexity of Traumatic Experience(s) in Children and Adolescents

Empirical studies of acutely traumatized school-age children and adolescents have increased clinical awareness of the complexity of their traumatic experiences. The clinical understanding of the subjective experience of the child entails recognition of the interrelated components of the experience (Pynoos 1993).

First, one must understand the context of the child's life and, in specific, those factors that contribute to the acute affective state, cognitive preoccupations, and developmental concerns at the onset of the traumatic stress.

Second, a traumatic experience involves intense moment-to-moment perceptual, kinesthetic, and somatic experiences accompanied by appraisals of external and internal threats. The child is challenged by the intensity and duration of the physiological arousal, affective responses, and psychodynamic threats and, at the same time, makes continuous efforts to address the situation in behavior, thought, and fantasy and to manage the physiological and emotional reactions.

Third, the vantage point of concern or attention in the child may vary. Children may have their attention drawn away from (or suppress fear for) their own safety when there is imminent danger to (or actual injury of) a parent, sibling, or friend, and experience unalleviated empathic distress (Hoffman 1979). Alternatively, when faced with an immediate threat or injury, a child may experience a moment of unconcern for, and even estrangement from, other family members who may also be under threat. When injury to self or other occurs, children may become suddenly preoccupied with concerns about the severity of injury, rescue, and repair. In violent circumstances, children may also feel compelled to inhibit wishes to intervene or to suppress retaliatory impulses out of fear of provoking counterretaliatory behavior.

Fourth, a more radical change in the child's attention and concerns occurs when his or her physical integrity or autonomy begins to be compromised, at which time the child's attention becomes directed more toward fears and fantasies of the nature and extent of psychic and physical harm than intervention. The child may try to use self-protective mechanisms to meet the internal threats, including "dissociative responses" that allow the child to feel a physical distancing from what is happening, to feel it is not happening to him or her, to control autonomic arousal and anxiety, to protect certain ego functions, and to decrease any sense of active participation (Rose 1991). During incestuous violation or hostage situations, there may be attempts either to disclaim or to invoke affiliative needs and desires as a means of warding off any sense of active participation or mitigating awareness of the physical menace, psychological abasement, and the accompanying distress (Bernstein 1990; Strenz 1982).

Fifth, traumatic stress may include additional traumatic moments that occur after cessation of violence or threat, including staying by an injured or dead family member until help arrives, trying to stop bleeding or giving resuscitation, witnessing the arrival and activities of the police or paramedics and subsequent emergency room care or surgery, or waiting for information about the condition of a family member or friend.

Sixth, a traumatic experience is often multilayered. Worry about the safety of a family member or friend, whether he or she is in the next room or at a different location, adds an additional source of extreme stress. The danger may also remind a child of a previous situation, renewing old fears and anxieties that influence the immediate appraisal of threat and exacerbate physiological and psychological responses. Witnessing the death of an attachment figure or peer evokes concurrent acute reactions to the loss, even while the life threat continues.

Lastly, a salient developmental impact of the experience may involve specific disruptions in evolving developmentally conditioned expectations associated with efforts to appraise and address external dangers. These may include the failure of alarm reactions (H. Krystal 1991), social referencing (Emde 1991), or a protective shield; the inability to resist coercive violation (Murray 1938); the betrayal of basic affiliative assumptions; the failure of emerging catastrophic emotions to protect against harm (Rangell 1991); the disruption of a belief in a socially modulated world; and the acknowledgment of having to surrender to an unavoidable moment of danger (H. Krystal 1991).

Traumatic Reminders and Secondary Stresses

Traumatic reminders, which are ubiquitous in the aftermath of trauma, refer to specific traumatic features of the external and internal threats and subjective reactions of the child and constitute an additional source of ongoing distress. An individual's responsiveness to these reminders contributes to the periodic or phasic nature of renewed traumatic anxiety or avoidant behavior. The unexpected nature of the reminders may reevoke a sense of unpreparedness and lack of control. Because of the complexity of a traumatic experience and its occurrence in a natural setting, there may be a large number of cues whose previously more neutral or even positive associations are now superseded by associations with the traumatic experience(s).

The influence of distal traumatic reminders may depend on the extent to which, later, they become embedded in the circumstances of everyday life. The more these reminders involve intricacies of interpersonal interactions, bodily sensations, and internal affective states, the more difficult they are to identify as sources of renewed hypervigilance or other arousal behavior, anxiety, or avoidance. The influence of traumatic reminders may become apparent only in quite specific, future challenging adult situations, and the troubling aspects of the exposure are variable over time.

Traumatic events are commonly associated with secondary stresses and adversities that may vary considerably with both the type of trauma and the environmental responsiveness to the child. These secondary stresses constitute additional sources of distress and increase the risk of initial comorbidity of posttraumatic stress reactions with other adverse reactions. These secondary stresses complicate efforts at adjustment and may interfere with normal opportunities for developmental maturation. They may substantially interfere with the availability and/or effectiveness of support to the child from parents, family, school, and community.

Distal secondary stresses may be a continuation of stresses that occurred in the immediate aftermath of the trauma, or they may arise out of new developmental challenges or life circumstances. These new developmental challenges or life circumstances may include the need for future medical treatment and accommodations to disabilities, involvement in criminal or civil proceedings, renewed apprehension at the release of an assailant from prison, contact of an abusive parent or relative with children of the next generation, or the need to acquire social skills to explain trauma-related behavior to intimate persons in one's later life, including spouse, children, selected colleagues, and friends.

Traumatic Stress and Proximal Development

By their very nature and degree of personal impact, traumatic experiences tend to skew an individual toward extreme expectations about the world, the safety and security of interpersonal life, and one's sense of personal integrity. In childhood these traumatic expectations impinge on the course of proximal and distal development. Children face the risk of premature trauma-induced foreclosure of a vital process of ongoing developmental and experiential revisions (Pynoos 1993).

There may be a developmental tendency for viridical and nonviridical representations of traumatic exposures to initiate the formation of co-existing, frequently incompatible working models (Bowlby 1979a). These internal models, once organized, tend to operate outside of conscious awareness and to resist dramatic change (Cicchetti et al. 1990). Their inclusion in traumatic expectations changes forecasts about the future that, in turn, may alter current and later behavior by limiting the range of constructive plans for the future (Bowlby 1979a).

Traumatic stress interacts with emerging personality in the following areas:

- Achievement of psychological and physiological maturation
- Hierarchical integration of competencies
- Intrapsychic structure of internal and external dangers
- Inner representation of self and other and mechanisms of cognitive and emotional regulation
- Schematization of security, safety, risk, injury, loss, protection, and intervention
- Behavioral attributes of fear, courage, and fearlessness
- Evolving intervention fantasies and their relationship to internal scripts, constructive actions, and creativity

Trauma may also have a transgenerational legacy in that these disturbances may influence future generations, perhaps, through effects on parental character and competence.

The assessment of posttraumatic distress in children and adolescents should include consideration of proximal developmental tasks that fall into three main categories: the ontogenesis of developmental competencies (Cicchetti 1989); interpersonal and intrafamilial developmental transitions (Rutter 1988); and biological plasticity and consolidation (Ornitz 1991). Recently acquired developmental achievements may be particularly vulnerable to disruption (Rutter 1988). Specific developmental areas to be assessed are presented in Table 6–1 and have been elaborated elsewhere (Pynoos 1993).

Neurobiology of Traumatic Remembrances and Expectations

The neurobiology of posttraumatic stress reactions includes neurophysiological, neurohormonal, and memory operations that differ from those associated with generalized anxiety or depressive reactions (Charney et al. 1993; Yehuda et al. 1990). These biological systems govern the immediate response and appear to become vulnerable to acute reactivity and slow biological recovery in response to future traumatic reminders or subsequent stress. Trauma-induced release of stress hormones in early childhood may influence the process of selection and formation of neuronal networks that extends throughout the school-age years and into adolescence (Chugani et al. 1987). For example, one trial of aversive training, which is associated with novel situations, may explain resistance to extinction of traumatic expectations by marking memories as important through a mechanism of neural convergence (see Garcia et al. 1986).

The startle reaction provides a good example of potential vulnerability during a critical developmental period of neurophysiological consolidation. This reaction involves a well-elucidated neuroanatomical and biochemical pathway with known developmental maturation (Ornitz 1991). Prestimulation-induced startle amplitude and latency modulation do not reach mature value until sometime between 6 and 8 years of age. Ornitz and Pynoos (1989) have provided preliminary evidence that consolidation of the inhibitory control of the startle reflex may be interfered with by traumatic exposure, leading to a "neurophysiological regression" to an earlier pattern of startle

---

Table 6–1.   Areas of proximal development

Selective attention/cognition/learning

Generation of intense negative emotions

Self-attributions

Autonomous strivings

Perceptions of self-efficacy

Specific psychodynamic/psychosocial/narcissistic concerns

Impulse control

Moral development

Awareness/sense of historical continuity

Representation of self and others

Biological maturation

Interpersonal and intrafamilial transitions

Ontogenesis of competencies

---

modulation. The central nucleus of the amygdala regulates fear-enhanced startle (Ornitz 1991) and, perhaps, the heightened reactivity to novel stimuli of inhibited children (Kagan 1991). The loss of inhibitory control over the startle reflex may interfere with the acquisition of a number of latency skills, such as increased control over activity level and the capacity for reflection, academic learning, and focused attention.

Similar changes in brain-stem modulation may underlie other posttrauma arousal symptoms including parasomnia, hypervigilance, dysregulation of aggression, and irritability. There is evidence to suggest a relationship between startle and sleep phenomena. Children appear to be especially prone to non–rapid eye movement (non-REM) posttrauma sleep disturbances (Pynoos 1990b). There may be increases in the percentage of time in stage 2 and stage 4 sleep, and in the occurrence of non-REM sleep phenomena, including parasomnia symptoms of somnambulism, vocalization, motor restlessness, and night terrors. These disturbances can be intermittent and associated with the occurrence of traumatic reminders at night, indicating a fear-enhanced proneness to increased awakenings.

Persistent hypervigilance and exaggerated startle may alter a child's usual behavior by leading to constant efforts to ensure personal security or the safety of others. These recurrent "bouts of fear" may seriously affect the child's emerging self-concept. In addition, temporary or chronic difficulty in modulating aggression can make children more irritable and easy to anger. This difficulty in modulating aggression may result in reduced tolerance of the normal behaviors and slights of peers and family members, followed by unusual acts of aggression or social withdrawal (Pynoos et al. 1991). A chronic sleep disturbance may be associated with disturbances in attention and learning. Chronic symptoms of hyperarousal and phasic reactivity have been shown to be associated with more severe and chronic posttraumatic responses (Pynoos et al. 1993b).

Trauma-induced changes in the reactivity of central catecholaminergic systems may produce a biological analogue of altered expectations by modulating the level of response of the central nervous system (CNS) with regard to specific trauma-related information, including reminders. Such trauma-induced changes in the reactivity of the central catecholinergic systems may also change the regulation of attentional balance between interoceptive (internal) and exteroceptive (environmental) cues, increasing focused attention on external stimuli to detect danger and make appropriate defensive response (J. H. Krystal et al. 1989). These changes may initiate "anticipatory bias," a "state of preparedness" for extremely negative emotions, and "anxiety of premonitions" (Kagan 1991). These changes are commonly accompanied by increased autonomic and sympathetic reactivity (e.g., heart rate, blood pressure, and skin conductance) that may have long-term implications for the physical health of the child (Perry 1994).

Developmental maturation may govern a progressive capacity to integrate unimodal sensory information, affective valence, and spatial representation of threat in the interactive neuroprocessing system of the amygdala, hippocampus, and cortical feedbacks. This system tends toward stimulus completion (Rolls 1989), whereby one sensory, affective, or cognitive reminder tends to elicit the fuller range of associated stimuli, affects, and meanings. Working at the interface of psychoanalysis and neurobiology, Freud first proposed that suppression, repression, and lack of integration and fragmentation of stimuli in young children may constitute efforts to interrupt stimulus completion when the child is presented with a frightening reminder (Freud 1900/1953). In latency, the combined maturation in cortical inhibitory control (Shapiro and Perry 1976) and capacities for increased contextual discrimination and affective tolerance may begin to reduce the engagement of these protective mechanisms.

Of special importance, traumatic experiences appear to activate neuromodulatory systems that enable their "personal consequentiality" (Conway 1993), as well as their novelty, to influence both remembrance and expectation (McGaugh 1988). In terms of remembrance, traumatic experiences initiate neurohormonal responses that appear to enhance and extend the period of reappraisal. From an evolutionary perspective, this period of reappraisal can facilitate a more accurate discrimination of potential dangers. At the same time, this "reworking" memory may incorporate other forms of mental modification that mediate the adaptational response, not only acutely but over time. From a developmental perspective, the child may be vulnerable to immature appraisals of future dangers and disturbances in future appraisal processes because of continued reliance on earlier forms of mental modifications. Young children, especially, may also be highly vulnerable to inadequacies and incompleteness in these processes.

Memory Markers, Episodic Memory, and the Trauma Narrative

Our findings confirm earlier formulations regarding the recall of episodic, autobiographical memory as a reconstruction, rather than a reproduction, of the event (Bartlett 1932). In unassisted recall, the narrative is shortened, and certain features become central, apparently serving as anchor points for remembering. Some details are emphasized and others are omitted. Three central findings have emerged from our examination of the nature and content of these anchor points in school-age children (Pynoos and Nader 1989).

First, when children are trying to remember life-threatening situations, recall is not organized as a single episode. Spatial and temporal registrations, affective and cognitive responses, and sets of perceptions differ for each memory anchor point. The organization of memory and the strategy of recall differ as children focus on different memory anchor points and their meaning, such as personal life threat, worry about a sibling, or cues of distress. Of special importance are significant interactive moments, including not only the moment of harm or protective intervention but also affective and verbal exchanges with others, including appraisal of facial expressions and verbal tone. Because of previous life experiences, children may emphasize certain details and attribute special meaning to certain aspects of the traumatic situation.

Second, each of these memory anchor points is associated with imagined or intended actions that are inextricably part of the memory network associated with the experience. Such "inner plans of action," as Lifton (1980) referred to them, invariably accompany recall. Some are associated with contemplated actions that occurred during the episode and/or in the immediate aftermath. They represent complex mental activities, influenced by maturity, gender, and life experience, that demonstrate a developmental hierarchy in children's efforts to address the convergence of external and internal threats (Pynoos and Nader 1993).

Third, and perhaps least considered in prior literature, the role of the acute consultation interview in providing a strategy of recall for the child, and how that strategy may also become part of the child's memory network, must be considered (Pynoos and Nader 1988b). Laboratory studies of young children's memory have demonstrated that it is often immaturity in children's strategy of recall, rather than any deficit in memory retention, that accounts for difficulties in memory tasks (Johnson and Foley 1984). It has been our consistent observation that the manner in which the child is assisted in both remembrance and the construction of a trauma narrative becomes incorporated as part of any ongoing memory processing. This finding parallels Solnit's (1989) discussion of the role of clinician and family in "memory as preparation" in the early and later adaptational responses of children who were exposed to medical procedures and hospitalization.

Because of the extended period of reappraisal, ongoing parental responsiveness is critical. Parental responsiveness to the child in assisting cognitive and emotional reappraisals may facilitate the child's adjustment by providing a co-construction of the contextual situation and meaning, as well as an empathic legitimization of the child's emotional experience. Parents, however, may be reluctant to respond to the child because they may feel too challenged by the traumatic material and by certain revelations that raise issues of accountability or call for interventions that they are not prepared to undertake.

Children may be under pressure from adult caregivers to disregard their own attribution of meaning to a traumatic experience because of misleading explanations, prohibitions, threats, or a covert conspiracy of silence. These responses from caregivers tend to curtail efforts at adjustment and lead to impaired cognitive and emotional processing and failure to address issues of accountability (Bowlby 1979b; Cain and Fast 1972; Kestenberg 1972).

Developmental Hierarchy of Response to External and Internal Dangers

We have identified five types of intervention fantasies involving efforts to 1) alter the precipitating events, 2) interrupt the traumatic action, 3) reverse the lethal or injurious consequences, 4) gain safe retaliation, and 5) prevent future trauma and loss (Table 6–2). The intervention fantasies may vary as the child focuses on different moments of the experience, including the circumstances preceding the experience and its aftermath (Pynoos and Nader 1993).

In their conscious fantasies children demonstrate a developmental hierarchy in their appraisal and responses to external and internal danger (Pynoos and Nader 1993). For example, preschool-age children may desperately envision the need for outside help while invoking fantasies of superhuman powers primarily to protect themselves against attack. School-age children who entertain conscious fantasies of intervening (e.g., taking the gun out of the assailant's hand) may evoke fantasies of special powers in order to intervene without fear of harm, or may employ phase-appropriate fantasies of rescue and exile to seek safety for themselves or others. With maturity and appreciation of the surrounding circumstances, adolescents envision more opportunities for intervention. They can imagine themselves or peers taking direct action, sometimes reckless or endangering, while maintaining a sense of narcissistic invulnerability.

Revenge fantasies are a form of protective action after the fact and serve as often overlooked indications of how children are attempting, belatedly, to address an admission of helplessness. Revenge fantasies challenge the child's emerging impulse control and contribute to posttrauma dysregulation of aggression. These fantasies also show a developmental progression. For example, a preschool-age child may envision the police tearing an assailant limb from limb while in prison. A latency-age child may envision joining other family members in delivering vigilante justice. An adolescent actually may contemplate taking revenge into his or her own hands, either directly or by eliciting peer assistance.

Of curiosity is the correspondence of the maturation of the neurophysiological pathways with the changing nature of intervention fantasies. For example, the faciliatory nature of the startle mechanism

---

Table 6–2.   Intervention fantasies in response to traumatic event

To alter the precipitating events.

To interrupt the traumatic action.

To reverse lethal or injurious consequences.

To gain safe retaliation (fantasies of revenge).

To prevent future trauma.

Source. Adapted from Pynoos RS, Nader K: "Issues in the Treatment of Post-Traumatic Stress in Children and Adolescents," in *The International Handbook of Traumatic Stress Syndromes.* Edited by Wilson JP, Raphael B. New York, Plenum, 1993, pp. 535–549.

found in preschool-age children enhances avoidant or escape behavior and corresponds to children's conscious thoughts of turning away from and seeking out external protection and intervention. The inhibitory modulation of the startle evolves developmentally at a stage when children can be observed to engage in fantasies of personally addressing, disarming, or directly harming the source of the danger, and in more constructive fantasies of anticipating dangerous situations in order to change them. By adolescence, when the inhibitory startle is likely to be more permanently consolidated, the adolescent not only fantasizes about intervention but struggles with decisions about taking direct action or engaging the assistance of peers.

The slow maturation of the startle mechanism in childhood serves an evolutionary function in regard to fearful situations, serving to enhance the search for protective intervention at an early age when turning toward the danger would be most ineffectual, and permitting the child to "face the danger" as the capacity to intervene potentially can be more protective of self and others. This process raises developmental questions about the evolution of self-concepts of cowardliness, courage, and fearlessness, and the adolescent theme of hero and anti-hero.

A key indicator of how children are addressing trauma-specific features is the content and evolution of intervention fantasies (Pynoos and Nader 1993). Changes in the form and content of intervention fantasies over time reflect increasing maturity, access to additional outside information, and future life experiences. Intervention fantasies may incorporate new reappraisals as well as revised intrapsychic conflicts and narcissistic accommodations. Psychodynamic considerations are particularly germane in understanding the progressive developmental modifications of intervention fantasies as children attempt both to maintain a reality-based viridical memory representation and to modify that representation to be more internally tolerable (Pruett 1984).

The evolving intervention fantasies, with embedded traumatic elements, can be instrumental in the construction of specific internal scripts that guide expectations and goals as well as real interpersonal interactions (Emde 1991). These fantasies may direct a child's attention toward future constructive actions, both short- and long-term, and may serve as an ongoing source of creativity in career or artistic pursuits. On the other hand, unaddressed or maladaptive revenge fantasies may contribute to a chronic pattern of dangerous reenactment behaviors. Compensatory fantasies of omnipotence and underestimation of the degree of threat may interfere with the development of appropriate self-protective capabilities and caution. Mental modification in the form of spatial misrepresentation of threat may, if incorporated into an evolving mental schema, increase the risk of further victimization. Lack of adequate schematization of protective intervention may compromise self-preservative and self-caring functions in children (Hartman and Burgess 1989) and may interfere with adult protective behavior (Wyatt et al. 1992).

Issues of Accountability

Addressing or resolving issues of human accountability is among the most difficult challenges to adjustment. This issue varies depending on whether the perpetrator is considered inside or outside the family or group affiliation (Pynoos 1993). Intrafamilial accountability causes profound disturbances in the family matrix by creating intense conflicts of loyalty, different attributions of blame by family members, severe challenges to basic affiliative assumptions, and difficulties in resolving feelings of shame and guilt and rage, hatred, and revenge. Extrafamilial agencies can provoke extreme, conscious fantasies of retaliation and counterretaliation that can be terrifying and, at the same time, deeply challenging to the child's emerging sense of moral and social conscience. Family, group, or society may attempt to mobilize these intense retaliatory wishes into group hatreds, persecution, and armed violence.

Implications for Treatment Strategies

The foci of therapeutic intervention correspond to key elements of the developmental psychopathology model of traumatic stress. For example, the alleviation of distress requires attention to each component of the tripartite etiology: the traumatic experience(s), traumatic reminders, and secondary stresses. Specialized interview and therapeutic approaches may be required to assist the child in exploring his or her moment-to-moment subjective experiences and in working through his or her attribution of causation and meaning.

Delineation of a typology of reminders for a particular child and attention to the ongoing occurrence of such reminders will be important in promoting appropriate family and school support to assist the child in gaining increased tolerance and understanding of their traumatic reference. Understanding these trauma-related behavioral precipitants can help the child, family, and school to minimize negative self-attributions or deviant labeling of otherwise unexplained aggressive or avoidant behavior. Addressing, anticipating, and ameliorating secondary stresses often require a proactive stance in regard to family, peers, school, and social agencies. By remaining attentive to secondary changes in the child's life, the clinician can continue to help the child and family in posttrauma decision making.

Treatment strategies needed to address proximal developmental disturbances vary and differ from those employed in the clinical assessment and treatment of posttraumatic stress–related psychopathology. For example, redressing an interruption in learning to read subsequent to the witnessing of violence may require remedial educational assistance along with therapeutic attention to the disturbance in visual information processing. Prevention of the secondary repercussion of academic failure with attendant loss of self-esteem and disturbances in peer relations may reduce the risk of other subsequent development disturbances and psychopathology.

In the treatment of posttraumatic stress–related psychopathology, we have previously described five levels of intervention for children and adolescents (Pynoos and Nader 1993) (Table 6–3).

1. *Psychological first aid* can provide important emotional relief through the provision of acute psychological and social services and age-appropriate interventions (Pynoos and Nader 1988b). Differing theoretical approaches recognize that the traumatic cues, the emotional meaning of the event, and the personal impact of the event are embedded in the details of the experience.
2. The *initial consultations* promote a shared understanding of the child's complex experience.
3. *Brief therapy* permits contextual understanding of the traumatic experience(s) within the circumstances and culture of the individual, family, and community. It facilitates ongoing emotional and cognitive reworking of the succession of traumatic moments and the interplay of traumatic reminders and secondary stresses. Cognitive-behavioral and psychodynamic approaches share a number of goals (Marmar et al. 1993) (Table 6–4).

Cognitive-behavioral approaches rely on learning theories of fear acquisition, and the role of reexposure and cognitive restructuring in reducing the intensity and frequency of fear and anxiety reactions. These approaches take into account the complicated hierarchy of fearful moments that emerge or evolve from traumatic events (Saigh 1988) and the need to include reworking of the meaning of the event as dangerous (Foa and Kozak 1986). *Psychodynamic approaches* emphasize a hierarchy of internal dangers and the complex affective states that characterize the child's experience and subsequent response. In these approaches is the recognition that meaningful associations are linked to each moment of the traumatic event and its aftermath and that these associations recruit unconscious conflict from earlier developmental issues and emerging self-regulatory mechanisms. In these approaches the focus is on the emerging mental schemas of danger, protection, and intervention, and concerns regarding safety, risk, injury, loss, and parental protection or supervision, including transference and countertransference issues. Evolving intervention fantasies are addressed therapeutically to help resolve conflicts over traumatic helplessness and viridical and nonviridi-

Table 6–3.	Levels of intervention in the treatment of posttraumatic stress–related psychopathology in children and adolescents

Psychological first aid

Initial consultations

Brief therapy
    Individual therapy
    Pharmacotherapy
    Family therapy
    Group therapy
    School-related interventions

Pulsed interventions

Long-term therapy

Source. Adapted from Pynoos RS, Nader K: "Issues in the Treatment of Post-Traumatic Stress in Children and Adolescents," in *The International Handbook of Traumatic Stress Syndromes.* Edited by Wilson JP, Raphael B. New York, Plenum, 1993, pp. 535–549.

cal representations, and to intervene in pathological narcissistic and psychosexual disturbances.

Pharmacotherapy targets psychobiological mechanisms underlying hyperarousal, cue-specific hyperreactivity, sleep distur-

---

Table 6–4. Goals of cognitive-behavioral and psychodynamic approaches in the treatment of posttraumatic stress–related psychopathology

---

To increase the capacity to respond to threat with realistic appraisal rather than exaggerated or minimized responses.

To maintain normal levels of arousal rather than hypervigilance or psychic numbing.

To facilitate return to normal development, adaptive coping, and improved functioning in work and interpersonal relations.

To restore personal integrity and normalize traumatic stress response, in part by validating the universality of stress symptomatology and by establishing a frame of meaning.

To conduct treatment in an atmosphere of safety and security to ensure that the threat of retraumatization is modulated.

To regulate level of intensity of traumatic aspects to facilitate cognitive reappraisal.

To increase capacity to differentiate remembering from reliving of the trauma, for both external reminders and internal cues.

Neither to eradicate the memories of the trauma nor to avoid and overreact rigidly to reminders, but rather to place trauma in perspective and regain control over life experiences.

To attend to early risk factors that shape trauma response.

To intervene actively to address secondary adversities and prevent future complications, including the risk for spreading comorbidities.

To regard self-concept as impacted by changes in dynamic, cognitive, behavioral, and neurobiological systems.

To facilitate a transformation from a victim identity to a sense of constructive engagement in daily life and future goals.

To enhance a sense of personal courage in approaching the memories and reminders of the trauma.

Source. Adapted from Marmar CR, Foy D, Kagan B, et al.: "An Integrated Approach for Treating Posttraumatic Stress," in *American Psychiatric Press Review of Psychiatry,* Vol. 12. Edited by Oldham JM, Riba MB, Tasman A. Washington, DC, American Psychiatric Press, 1993, pp. 239–272.

bances, and comorbid anxiety and depressive disorders. Amelioration of intense and persistent arousal symptoms (e.g., those associated with non-REM sleep disturbances) may be essential to
restore a sense of restfulness and daytime concentration and attention. The reduction of tonic and phasic physiological arousal
may contribute to the therapeutic process by permitting fuller
registration and tolerance of traumatic reminders and improved
cognitive discrimination.

The family provides a key context for reinstating a sense of
safety and security. This goal is inherently jeopardized when the
agent and victim of the violence are family members. Other family
members may require their own therapeutic intervention before
they can adequately provide ongoing support to a spouse, parent,
child, or sibling who was the immediate victim. A primary goal of
family therapy is to help family members validate and legitimize
one another's psychological tasks, thereby facilitating continued
mutual support. Because of different degrees of exposure, family
members may experience estrangement or impatience with one
another. The skills of family members can be enhanced through
education regarding posttraumatic stress reactions, realistic expectations about the course of recovery, differing psychological
agendas, management of temporary behavioral alterations or regressions, and the importance of encouraging open communications.

Likewise, *group therapy* offers the opportunity to reinforce
the normative nature of reactions and recovery, to share mutual
concerns, to address common fears and traumatic reminders and
avoidant behaviors, to increase tolerance for disturbing emotions, to provide early attention to depressive reactions, and to
aid recovery through age-appropriate and situation-specific problem solving.

4. A developmental model of traumatic stress would suggest that an
optimal intervention strategy would include as one of its components *pulsed interventions* that include planned periods of consultation after an acute phase of treatment. After initial
treatment, the child is seen at certain critical junctures, determined by anticipated or reported reminders, including judicial
proceedings, and at important life transitions or challenges that
may be compromised by the child's experiencing renewed symptoms. These interventions assist the child with future experiential

and maturational reappraisals in an effort to maintain normal developmental progression (Budman and Gurman 1988).

5. In long-term treatment, clinical attention is directed to trauma-related intrapsychic schemas or conflicts, narcissistic accommodations, and traumatic influences on emerging personality. However, recognition that emotional meaning remains embedded in the traumatic experience remains a constant feature of therapeutic work. Intrafamilial violence requires attention to the preexisting relationship with the perpetrator, to issues of identification and conflict of loyalty, to vulnerabilities secondary to a chronic impulse-ridden environment, and to the stigma and legacy of domestic violence. When the trauma is violent and massive, a central goal is to alleviate dangerous unconscious reenactment behavior and to address conscious and unconscious intervention fantasies, especially unresolved revenge fantasies and accompanying preoccupations with rescue or reparative roles. Resolution of associated psychosexual disturbances also may require more extended therapeutic intervention.

References

Bartlett FC: Remembering. Cambridge, UK, Cambridge University Press, 1932

Bell CC, Jenkins EJ: Traumatic stress and children. Journal of Health Care for the Poor and Underserved 2:175–186, 1991

Bernstein AE: The impact of incest trauma on ego development, in Adult Analysis and Childhood Sexual Abuse. Edited by Levine HB. Hillsdale, NJ, Analytic Press, 1990, pp 65–91

Bowlby J: The Making and Breaking of Affectional Bonds. London, Tavistock, 1979a

Bowlby J: On knowing what you aren't supposed to know and feeling what you are not supposed to feel. Can J Psychiatry 24:403–408, 1979b

Brown SL: Developmental cycle of family: clinical implications. Psychiatr Clin North Am 3:369–381, 1980

Budman SH, Gurman AS: Theory and Practice of Brief Therapy. New York, Guilford, 1988

Cain A, Fast I: Children's disturbed reactions to parent suicide: distortion and guilt, communication and identification, in Survivors of Suicide. Edited by Cain A. Springfield, IL, Charles C Thomas, 1972, pp 93–111

Charney DS, Deutch AY, Krystal JH, et al: Psychobiologic mechanisms of posttraumatic stress disorder. Arch Gen Psychiatry 50:294–305, 1993

Chugani H, Phelps ME, Mazziotta JC: Positron emission tomography study of human brain functional development. Ann Neurol 22:487–497, 1987

Cicchetti D: How research on child maltreatment has informed the study of child development: perspectives from developmental psychopathology, in Child Maltreatment: Theory and Research on the Causes and Consequences of Child Abuse and Neglect. Edited by Cicchetti D, Carlson V. New York, Cambridge University Press, 1989, pp 377–431

Cicchetti D, Carlson V (eds): Child Maltreatment: Theory and Research on the Causes and Consequences of Child Abuse and Neglect. New York, Cambridge University Press, 1989

Cicchetti D, Cummings M, Greenberg M, et al: An organizational perspective on attachment beyond infancy: implications for theory, measurement and research, in Attachment in the Preschool Years. Edited by Greenberg M, Cicchetti D, Cummings M. Chicago, IL, University of Chicago Press, 1990, pp 3–49

Conway MA: Emotion and memory. Science 261:369–370, 1993

Emde RN: Positive emotions for psychoanalytic theory: surprises from infancy research and new directions. J Am Psychoanal Assoc 39:5–44, 1991

Foa EB, Kozak MD: Emotional processing of fear: exposure to corrective information. Psychol Bull 99:20–35, 1986

Freud S: The interpretation of dreams (1900), in Standard Edition of the Complete Psychological Works of Sigmund Freud, Vols 4 and 5. Translated and edited by Strachey J. London, Hogarth Press, 1953

Garcia J, Lasiter PS, Bermudez-Rattoni F, et al: A general theory of aversion learning. Ann N Y Acad Sci 43:8–21, 1986

Garbarino J, Kostelny K, Dubrow N: What children can tell us about living in danger. Am Psychol 46:376–383, 1991

Gleser G, Green B, Winget C: Prolonged Psychosocial Effects of Disaster: A Study of Buffalo Creek. New York, Academic, 1981

Hartman CR, Burgess AW: Sexual abuse of children: causes and consequences, in Child Maltreatment: Theory and Research on the Causes and Consequences of Child Abuse and Neglect. Edited by Cicchetti D, Carlson V. New York, Cambridge University Press, 1989, pp 95–128

Hoffman ML: Development of moral thought, feeling, and behavior. Am Psychol 34:959–966, 1979

Johnson MK, Foley MA: Differentiating fact from fantasy: the reliability of children's memory. Journal of Social Issues 40:33–50, 1984

Kagan J: A conceptual analysis of the affects. J Am Psychoanal Assoc 39(suppl):109–130, 1991

Kestenberg JS: How children remember and parents forget. International Journal of Psychoanalytic Psychotherapy 1:103–123, 1972

Khan MMR: The Privacy of the Self. New York, International Universities Press, 1974

Krystal H: Integration and self-healing in post-traumatic states: a ten year retrospective. American Imago 48:93–117, 1991

Krystal JH, Kosten TR, Perry BD, et al: Neurobiological aspects of PTSD: review of clinical and preclinical studies. Behavior Therapy 20:177–198, 1989

Lansky MR: The screening function of posttraumatic nightmares. British Journal of Psychotherapy 6:384–400, 1990

Lifton RJ: The broken connection. Evaluation and Change (special issue) 1980, pp 55–70 [excerpts from Lifton RJ: The Broken Connection. New York, Simon & Schuster, 1979]

Macksoud MS, Dyregrov A: Traumatic war experiences and their effects on children, in The International Handbook of Traumatic Stress Syndromes. Edited by Wilson JP, Raphael B. New York, Plenum, 1993, pp 625–633

Marmar CR, Foy D, Kagan B, et al: An integrated approach for treating posttraumatic stress, in The American Psychiatric Press Review of Psychiatry, Vol 12. Edited by Oldham JM, Riba MB, Tasman A. Washington, DC, American Psychiatric Press, 1993, pp 239–272

Martinez P, Richters J: NIMH Community Violence Project, II: children's distress symptoms associated with violence exposure. Psychiatry 56:22–35, 1993

McGaugh J: Involvement of hormonal and neuromodulatory systems in the regulation of memory storage. Ann Rev Neurosci 12:255–287, 1988

Mones P: When a Child Kills: Abused Children Who Kill Their Parents. New York, Pocket Books, Simon & Schuster, 1991

Murray HA: Explorations in Personality. London, Oxford University Press, 1938

Nader K, Pynoos RS, Fairbanks LA, et al: Childhood PTSD reactions one year after a sniper attack. Am J Psychiatry 147:1526–1530, 1990

Nader K, Pynoos RS, Fairbanks LA, et al: Acute post-traumatic reactions among Kuwait children following the Gulf crisis. Br J Clin Psychol 32:407–416, 1993

Ornitz EM: Developmental aspects of neurophysiology, in Child and Adolescent Psychiatry: A Comprehensive Textbook. Edited by Lewis M. Baltimore, MD, Williams & Wilkins, 1991, pp 38–51

Ornitz EM, Pynoos RS: Startle modulation in children with post-traumatic stress disorder. Am J Psychiatry 147:866–870, 1989

Perry BD: Neurobiological sequelae of childhood trauma: PTSD in children, in Catecholamine Function in Posttraumatic Stress Disorder: Emerging Concepts. Edited by Murburg MM. Washington, DC, American Psychiatric Press, 1994, pp 233–255

Pruett K: A chronology of defensive adaptations to severe psychological trauma. Psychoanal Study Child 39:591–612, 1984

Pynoos RS: Children's adjustment following a sniper incident in Los Angeles. Paper presented at Community Violence & Children's Development: Research & Clinical Implications, a conference sponsored by the National Institute of Mental Health, Washington School of Psychiatry, and The MacArthur Foundation, Washington, DC, November 1990a

Pynoos RS: Post-traumatic stress disorder in children and adolescents, in Psychiatric Disorders in Children and Adolescents. Edited by Garfinkel BD, Carlson GA, Weller EB. Philadelphia, PA, WB Saunders, 1990b, pp 48–63

Pynoos RS: The dose exposure model in the study of child PTSD. Paper presented at the annual convention of the Association of the Advancement of Behavior Therapy, International Research on Childhood PTSD Symposium, New York, November 1991

Pynoos RS: Traumatic stress and developmental psychopathology in children and adolescents, in The American Psychiatric Press Review of Psychiatry, Vol 12. Edited by Oldham JM, Riba MB, Tasman A. Washington, DC, American Psychiatric Press, 1993, pp 205–238

Pynoos RS, Eth S: Children traumatized by witnessing acts of personal violence: homicide, rape, or suicide behavior, in Post-Traumatic Stress Disorder in Children. Edited by Eth S, Pynoos RS. Washington, DC, American Psychiatric Press, 1985, pp 17–43

Pynoos RS, Eth S: Witness to violence: the child interview. Journal of the American Academy of Child Psychiatry 25:306–319, 1986

Pynoos RS, Nader K: Children who witness the sexual assaults of their mothers. J Am Acad Child Adolesc Psychiatry 27:567–572, 1988a

Pynoos RS, Nader K: Psychological first aid and treatment approach for children exposed to community violence: research implications. Journal of Traumatic Stress 1:445–473, 1988b

Pynoos RS, Nader K: Children's memory and proximity to violence. J Am Acad Child Adolesc Psychiatry 28:236–241, 1989

Pynoos RS, Nader K: Issues in the treatment of post-traumatic stress in children and adolescents, in The International Handbook of Traumatic Stress Syndromes. Edited by Wilson JP, Raphael B. New York, Plenum, 1993, pp 535–549

Pynoos RS, Frederick C, Nader K, et al: Life threat and posttraumatic stress in school-age children. Arch Gen Psychiatry 44:1057–1063, 1987

Pynoos RS, Nader K, March J: Post-traumatic stress disorder, in The American Psychiatric Press Textbook of Child & Adolescent Psychiatry. Edited by Weiner J. Washington DC, American Psychiatric Press, 1991, pp 339–348

Pynoos RS, Goenjian A, Karakashian M, et al: Posttraumatic stress reactions in children after the 1988 Armenian earthquake. Br J Psychiatry 163:239–247, 1993a

Pynoos RS, Sorenson SB, Steinberg AM: Interpersonal violence and traumatic stress reactions, in Handbook of Stress: Theoretical & Clinical Aspects, 2nd Edition. Edited by Goldberger L, Breznitz S. New York, Free Press, 1993b, pp 573–590

Rangell L: Castration. J Am Psychoanal Assoc 39:3–23, 1991

Richters J, Martinez P: NIMH Community Violence Project, I: children as victims of and witnesses to violence. Psychiatry 56:7–21, 1993

Rolls E: Functions of neuronal networks in the hippocampus and neocortex in memory, in Neural Models of Plasticity: Experimental and Theoretical Approaches. Edited by Byrne J, Berry W. San Diego, CA, Academic, 1989, pp 240–265

Rose D: A model for psychodynamic psychotherapy with the rape victim. Psychotherapy 28:85–95, 1991

Rutter M: Epidemiological approaches to developmental psychopathology. Arch Gen Psychiatry 45:486–495, 1988

Saigh PA: The use of an in vitro flooding package in the treatment of traumatized adolescents. J Dev Behav Pediatr 10:17–21, 1988

Schwarz ED, Kowalski JM: Malignant memories: PTSD in children and adults after a school shooting. J Am Acad Child Adolesc Psychiatry 30:936–944, 1991

Shapiro T, Perry R: Latency revisited. Psychoanal Study Child 31:79–105, 1976

Solnit A: Memory as preparation, in Dimensions of Psychoanalysis. Edited by Sandler J. Madison, CT, International Universities Press, 1989, pp 193–217

Strenz T: The Stockholm syndrome, in Victims of Terrorism. Edited by Ochberg F, Soskis D. Boulder, CO, Westview, 1982, pp 149–164

Stuber ML, Nader K, Yasuda P, et al: Stress responses after pediatric bone marrow transplantation: preliminary results of a prospective longitudinal study. J Am Acad Child Adolesc Psychiatry 30:952–957, 1991

Terr LC: Childhood traumas: an outline and overview. Am J Psychiatry 148:10–20, 1991

Wyatt GE, Guthrie D, Notgrass CM: The differential effects of women's child sexual abuse and subsequent sexual assault. J Consult Clin Psychol 60:167–173, 1992

Yehuda R, Southwick SM, Perry BD, et al: Interactions of the hypothalamic-pituitary-adrenal axis and the catecholaminergic systems in posttraumatic stress disorders, in Biological Assessment and Treatment of Posttraumatic Stress Disorder. Edited by Giller EL Jr. Washington, DC, American Psychiatric Press, 1990, pp 115–134

Yule W, Williams RM: Post-traumatic stress reactions in children. Journal of Traumatic Stress 3:279–295, 1990

Yule W, Bolton D, Udwin O: Objective and subjective predictors of PTSD in adolescence. Presentation at the World Conference of the International Society for Traumatic Stress Studies, Amsterdam, The Netherlands, June 1992

Section III

Relationship Between Medical Illness and Stress

Chapter 7

Emotional Stressors and the Onset of Asthma

David A. Mrazek, M.D., F.R.C.Psych.
Mary Klinnert, Ph.D.

Although the effects of emotional stressors on somatic processes have been frequently observed, the mechanisms that underlie these linkages have remained elusive. Most individuals have a personal intuitive appreciation of the effects of stress on their own physiological processes. One individual may have the perception of his or her heart pounding when he or she experiences increased anxiety, whereas another may feel a tightening knot in his or her stomach when he or she experiences conflict. Asthmatic children have airways that have an increased sensitivity to a variety of stimuli. For them, intense anxiety is often accompanied by a sudden sensation of tightening in their chest that can soon be followed by a growing fear that they will become unable to breathe. The use of an inhaler with a wide range of bronchodilators usually brings rapid relief, but the emotional process by which their bronchoconstriction was initiated can leave a somatic memory. With repeated asthmatic experiences, asthmatic children can develop anxiety about the possibility of experiencing intense conflicts in the same way that allergic children can develop a fear of, for example, coming into

This work was supported through grants from the W. T. Grant Foundation (Grant No. 88-1013-85), the National Institute of Mental Health (Grant No. 2KO2-MH00430), the Hasbro Children's Foundation, and the Developmental Psychobiology Research Group.

contact with cats or inadvertently eating a shrimp.

In this chapter we explore the role of a specific class of emotional stressors in the precipitation of asthma. The mechanisms by which stressors exert an effect could include direct influence on airway receptor sensitivity or more indirect effects that induce changes in the somatic reactions to infection or exposure to antigenic stimulation in such a way that the threshold necessary for these triggers to precipitate an asthmatic attack is lowered. Although there is considerable evidence to document that stressors can exacerbate chronic asthma, there has been little empirical evidence to demonstrate that intense chronic emotional distress can play a role in the initial onset of asthma in children who have a genetic vulnerability for a hyperreactive airway. One premise of this thesis is that a genetic predisposition for asthma is a necessary but not sufficient condition for developing the illness. There is little doubt that asthma is familial, and although the specific gene loci have yet to be identified, a number of possible genetic mechanisms have been put forward (Mrazek and Klinnert 1991).

The most straightforward evidence for the importance of both genetic and environmental factors in the etiology of asthma comes from twin studies. However, difficulties with diagnostic criteria have led to a variety of estimates of the relative monozygotic versus dizygotic concordances. Despite some conflicting results, a clear pattern of moderate heritability is derived from the majority of studies that have examined these monozygotic and dizygotic twins correlations. Hopp and co-workers (1984) have shown this to be the case with bronchial reactivity as assessed by methacholine challenge, which suggests that this sensitivity may represent one of the underlying genetic traits of primary interest in the development of asthma (Mrazek et al. 1991).

Pediatric asthma tends to begin early in life. Considering only children who develop asthma, 75% of those who develop the disease will experience their initial symptoms before the age of 5 years (Falliers 1971). Consequently, if the effects of stressors on disease onset are to be considered, these stressors must be defined within a developmentally salient context. Given that these emotional stressors are associated with the initial expression of airway reactivity, some understanding of the mechanism by which the stressor actually "turns on" the genes responsible for bronchoconstriction becomes an area of central scientific interest. These methodological issues were addressed in the design of the W. T. Grant Asthma Risk Project, which will be the central focus of this chapter.

The W. T. Grant Asthma Risk Project

Study Design

The only research design that can adequately test the hypothesis that emotional stressors are associated with the onset of asthma is a prospective longitudinal study of a "high risk" sample. Although asthma is the most common chronic disease in childhood, it still affects only approximately 7% of children (Smith 1988). To study a general population sample would be inefficient and minimally informative, because more than 90% of the children being studied would never develop asthma. A more practical method that can be used to identify children at risk for the onset of asthma is to study the children of asthmatic parents. Considerable variability in estimates of familial risk have been reported. However, a synthesis of the results of multiple studies suggests that if both parents have the illness, the risk for their children's developing asthma is about 50% (Zeiger 1988). If only one parent has asthma, the risk for the parents' offspring developing the disease drops to about 20%. If in addition to one parent with asthma there are other first- and second-degree relatives within the pedigree who have asthma, the risk for development of asthma is expected to be between 30% and 40%. In the future, genetic mapping will allow clinicians to precisely identify children who have affected genes that are associated with the illness, and it is these children who will be studied. However, at this stage in the development of our understanding of the illness, pedigree studies provide a methodology for exploring the interrelationship of etiological factors.

The families in the Asthma Risk Project were selected based on the criterion that at least one of the parents had been diagnosed as having asthma. In total there were 150 at-risk families. In 90 families the mother had asthma, but neither the father nor any of his first-degree relatives had the disease. In 32 families, the mother had asthma, and her husband also had a first-degree relative with the illness, but he did not have the disease himself. In 28 families, both parents had asthma. Additionally, a comparison sample of 30 families was studied in which neither the mother nor the father had asthma.

A prospective design was used in the Asthma Risk Project because of the need to prevent retrospective bias. It is a well-known phenomenon that once a symptom appears, it is human nature to look back in time and search for a likely stressor that preceded the symptom that could plausibly have played a role in the origin of the disease. Similarly, the potential impact of severe stressors that have been successfully managed tends to be minimized if exposures to these stressors do not actually result in wheezing. Only by regularly measuring the occurrence and intensity of stressors using a method that is independent of the identification of their hypothesized results can "after the fact" reconstruction of plausible but fictitious scenarios be avoided.

A longitudinal design was used in this study because the chronology of both the independent variables (i.e., the risk factors) and the dependent variable (i.e., the onset of asthma) required ongoing surveillance. Given that asthma often occurs in the first year of life, the beginning of the study had to precede the first plausible time of onset. Consequently, every family was recruited during the pregnancy with the index child. Furthermore, parental risk factors were assessed during the third trimester of the pregnancy, at the time of delivery, and during a 1-hour home visit when the index child was 3 weeks of age. All of these time points preceded the onset of any episodes of wheezing for any of the children. These families were subsequently followed at regular intervals over the duration of the study, but subsequent measurements necessarily followed the onset of wheezing for some children.

The longitudinal nature of the study also allowed the sequential documentation of the time of onset of the disease to be carefully recorded, thus permitting analyses designed to examine the impact of emotional stressors at specific sensitive periods in the development of the children. During the home visit when the child was 3 weeks of age, specific measures of the parents' adaptation to the infant were rated after a 1-hour semistructured interview with the mother and direct observation of the mother with the infant (Mrazek et al. 1995). In addition to assessing the presence of parenting difficulties, investigators made judgments as to the quality of the mother's marriage and the presence and severity of postpartum depression.

Methodology

Diagnostic Criteria

Asthma, defined in straightforward terms, is a lung disease that is characterized by 1) airway obstruction (i.e., narrowing) that is reversible, 2) airway inflammation, and 3) airway hyperresponsiveness to a variety of stimuli or triggers (Department of Health and Human Services 1991). This is, however, a deceptively simple definition. Furthermore, the diagnostic criteria implicit in this definition have rarely been used to identify asthmatic children in epidemiological surveys.

The key symptom associated with the bronchoconstriction and inflammation that occur during an asthmatic attack is an *expiratory wheeze*. A wheeze is a high-pitched, whistlelike breath sound that usually occurs during exhalation. Despite the explicit admonition that "every wheeze is not asthma," epidemiological studies identify "a case" based upon a positive response to one of two questions: 1) "Have you been diagnosed as having asthma?" or 2) "Have you ever wheezed?"

Use of this methodology clearly leads to an inflated estimate of the prevalence of asthma as well as creates some confusion regarding the role of risk factors that can lead to the expression of asthma. To avoid this problem of false positive diagnosis, investigators involved in the design of the Asthma Risk Project developed a specific set of diagnostic criteria for use in the study. These diagnostic criteria initially included the requirement that there be two distinctly separate periods of reported wheezing and that at least one of these episodes of wheezing occur in the absence of a bronchial infection. This latter criterion was included because of the realization that although potentially asthmatic children would have more difficulty with viral infections, nonasthmatic children also often experience wheezing during the course of a severe respiratory syncytial virus (RSV) infection. A separate diagnostic category, "infectious wheezing," was utilized for children who had multiple episodes of wheezing but had never experienced respiratory symptoms in the absence of infection. Although these children were felt to be at high risk for the development of asthma, no generalized reactivity to a broader range of environmental stimuli could be documented.

During the initial 2 years of the study, the documentation of wheezing was established by either *maternal report* of the child's symptoms or documented reports of wheezing symptoms in the *medical record* of the child as assessed by the child's pediatrician. On review of each of the initial cases, a concern developed about the accuracy of some of the maternal reports. Consequently, the diagnostic criteria were modified to require documentation of wheezing by the child's physician that was recorded within the medical record. This recoding effort led to changing the recorded times of onset for some of the children who had originally been classified as asthmatic. However, this better-documented method of establishing the diagnosis virtually eliminated the possibility of false positive designation.

Determination of What Constitutes an Emotional Stressor in Infancy

Of all the methodological dilemmas presented by this research, the measurement of *salient* emotional stressors for children in the first 2 years of life was the most central for this study. The measurement of stressors for adult subjects remains problematic. A quantitative estimate is usually based on the documentation of life events that can then be discussed with the subjects to obtain corroborative evidence of their subjective perception of stress (Brown and Harris 1978). Similar corroboration is not possible for infants.

From a more positive perspective, the range of adaptive responses of infants is far more limited, and infants' potential universe of experience is more circumscribed. Given our interest in the role of emotional stressors on gene function in very young children, we postulated that only the most "proximal" emotional stressors would be salient for these young children. Furthermore, we hypothesized that the single most critical factor related to the stressfulness of their early experience would be the effectiveness of their primary attachment figure in the modulation of their early experience. In this regard, family stressors such as the father's losing his job or a sibling's developing cancer would result in a negative impact on the child only through the influence of these events on the capacity of the parent to care for the infant. In one family, the death of a paternal grandmother could precipitate a maternal depression that might result in considerable disequilibrium in the emotional experience of the infant. In another family the mother may either have little emotional response to the death of her mother-in-law or be able to manage her parental interactions in a sensitive manner despite her grieving. Although the mother's decision to inhibit her own emotional responses in the best interest of her child may be a risk factor for her own emotional well-being, we hypothesized that it would be a protective factor for the well-being of her infant. The focus of the assessment of stressors was consequently aimed at measuring the impact of life stressors on the ability of the parents to care for the index child.

Another consideration was that for an emotional stressor to have an impact, it was hypothesized that it would have to result in a change in parenting over a substantial period of time. For instance, a car accident occurring when the infant was 3 months old that resulted in no medical consequences and led promptly to the replacement of the car with a new vehicle was considered to have much less impact than a persistently problematic pattern of parenting based on the presence of a chronic stressor such as a serious medical illness.

Rating of Parenting Risk

Given the focus of the Asthma Risk Project, a new rating system was developed to specifically quantify the presence of substantial risk for problematic parenting. This rating was conceptually based on a scoring scheme developed during a longitudinal study of children of depressed mothers (Radke-Yarrow et al. 1992). The first parenting risk ratings in the Asthma Risk Project were completed 3 weeks after the birth of the index child. The ratings were made by a mental health clinician after an hour-long interview conducted during a home visit. During the same visit, the interactions between the mother and the child were observed. Three levels of risk were conceptualized:

1. The designation of "adequate parenting" was made if there was no overt evidence of parenting disturbance. Two-thirds of the mothers in the asthma risk sample ($n = 100$) received this rating.
2. The designation of "parenting concerns" was made on the basis of evidence that a pattern of caregiving was occurring that could negatively impact the child's development. This designation could be made based on the observation of overt parental disturbance such as maternal depression that seemed to be sufficiently severe to indicate that the symptoms of the illness might interfere with the parent's care of the child. Alternatively, a rating of parenting concern could be scored if the mother evidenced some insensitivity to the child's needs, but was generally committed to appropriate care. Approximately one-quarter of the mothers in the asthma risk sample ($n = 37$) were categorized as having this level of problematic parenting.
3. The designation of "parenting difficulties" was made when overt difficulties in parenting were evident. Although a wide range of behaviors could qualify a parent for this rating, general areas of

difficulty included a lack of knowledge about appropriate infant care, a lack of concern for the child's physical or emotional well-being, overt psychopathology that directly affected the welfare of the child, or serious marital conflicts that directly interfered with the care of the child. One-tenth of the mothers ($n = 15$) in the asthma risk group were scored to be at high risk for parenting because of the presence of parenting difficulties.

The reliability of these judgments was calculated to 76% for coding the dichotomy of "no risk" versus "some risk" (Mrazek et al. 1991). However, some clinical experience and training are required to make this subjective rating reliably. The interviewer must have the ability to explore a superficial response such as "everything is fine" in order to identify those mothers who will reveal more concerns only after sensitive probing. The design of the interview allowed the evaluator to raise each particular area of interest and then follow up the original probe with a series of specific questions. A particular rating issue is that the experience of being a parent oneself is helpful in making these ratings. Although it is not essential to be a parent to make this judgment, it would be misleading to suggest that it is not an advantage. What is necessary to develop these assessment skills is considerable exposure to the range of parenting issues and problems that arise in the course of caring for young children. Experienced child mental health clinicians, who have never been parents themselves, become adept at assessing parenting over the course of their training through their involvement with dozens of families. As a consequence of this process, they slowly come to appreciate the skills that parents require to successfully deal with temperamentally difficult infants, as well as how to facilitate the development of more easygoing children. For the Asthma Risk Project, all of the parenting risk ratings that were made during the critical home visit assessment period when the index child was 3 weeks old were completed by one of two experienced clinical social workers, both of whom had successfully completed doctoral training.

Findings

Risk Factors for the Onset of Asthma

Several biological risk factors have been believed to be associated with the onset of asthma. Specifically, viral infections, exposure to highly antigenic substances, and excessive exposure to passive smoking have been implicated in the onset of the disease (Busse 1989; Frick et al. 1979). In this chapter we do not discuss these important physical factors but instead focus on the relationship between emotional stressors on the onset of the illness.

Although previous reports have linked psychiatric crises to the onset of an individual case of asthma, it has been difficult to conduct a study to prospectively demonstrate this relationship across a number of individuals. However, the Asthma Risk Project has provided evidence that parenting risk as defined in this chapter is associated with a greater incidence of asthma by the time children from high-risk families reach 2 years of age. Furthermore, it is postulated that parenting risk is the most salient form of emotional stress for an infant, in part because it is a sufficiently broad construct to capture the wide range of disturbances that are plausibly relevant to the pathophysiology of asthma. The only other recent study that has prospectively addressed the question of whether social stressors are associated with asthma did not show a relationship (Horwood et al. 1985). Our explanation for the absence of an association in that study is that no plausible measure of salient stress was included in the design of the study. In the analyses by Horwood and colleagues (1985), difficult temperament scores and a maternal depression rating scale score did not predict the onset of the disease. However, for this relationship to have been demonstrated it would have required that these very discrete measures act as very specific markers for a much wider range of disturbance. Not surprisingly, this was not the case.

Parenting Difficulties and the Prediction of Asthma

The incidence of asthma in the genetically at-risk children whose mothers had been observed, when their infant was 3 weeks old, to have had parenting difficulties was shown to be significantly increased when compared with the incidence in children with similar genetic risk but whose mothers had been judged to have been parenting adequately (Mrazek et al. 1991). Initially, when a maternal report of wheezing was considered to be sufficient documentation for establishing the designation of a case of asthma, 21 children were designated as asthmatic by 24 months of age. When far more restrictive diagnostic criteria were used, requiring documentation of wheezing to have been made by the child's physician in the medical record, only 9 children were classified as asthmatic by the age of 24 months (Table 7–1). However, regardless of which of the two diagnostic criteria sets for asthma was used, those genetically at-risk children who were exposed to early parenting difficulties were significantly more likely to develop problems than those who did not. When the criteria set requiring documentation by the pediatrician in the medical record was used, the level of significance actually rose (to $P < .005$).

An alternative way to consider the relationship between these variables is to examine how many of these children with the very earliest onset of asthma actually came from families in which there were parenting difficulties. Interestingly, the first two children in the study were from such families, as were 78% of all children who developed asthma by the end of the second year of life (Table 7–2). Only two children in the comparison sample met the conservative (i.e., more restrictive) illness criteria for asthma, despite 40% of the families in the comparison sample having been coded as having early parenting difficulties. Interestingly, both of these two "comparison" children had an asthmatic grandparent.

The only other familial risk factor measured during the home visit when the index child was 3 weeks old that showed even a trend of an association with asthma was serious maternal depression (Table 7–3). However, all of the severely depressed mothers whose infants had developed asthma by 2 years of age had also been coded as having parenting difficulties. None of the children of severely depressed mothers who had not been coded as having parenting difficulties had developed asthma by 2 years of age. In the future, it will be possible to examine the incidence of parenting difficulties in children with later onset of asthma. This approach will clarify whether this early association occurs only in infancy or is true throughout early childhood.

Table 7–1.   Number of children in the W. T. Grant Asthma Risk Project who developed asthma per year

Age	Children with asthma	
	Defined by medical records	Defined by maternal report alone
1st Year	2	5
2nd Year	9	21

Effect of Stress on the Onset of Asthma

The role of emotional stressors in the management of children who have asthma has been described elsewhere (Mrazek 1988). Furthermore, complex psychoneuroimmunological interactions have been postulated and, to a limited extent, demonstrated (Mrazek and Klinnert 1991). The mechanism by which parenting difficulties effect the *initial* expression of the disease probably works at the level of gene regulation as opposed to the level of either regulation of an immunological process or control of the autonomic nervous system. Three plausible mechanisms for a genetic hypothesis are supportable based on indirect evidence. The first possible mechanism is that poor parenting leads to increased exposure to a wide range of physical environmental risk factors that subsequently alter gene function. This hypothesis can eventually be definitively tested by the simultaneous assessment of multiple risk factors, but preliminary appraisal of those factors included in the Asthma Risk Project data set does not provide support for this explanation. The second possible mechanism is that neurotransmitters and/or neuropeptides associated with intense stress have a direct effect on the genome at the level of the nucleotide sequences, resulting in the "switching on" of a gene product that subsequently alters the reactivity of the airway receptors. Clarification of this hypothesis must await the development of methodologies that can identify the control of switching mechanisms. The third possible mechanism is that parenting is a largely genetically controlled behavior and that, like their parents, these children have a sensitivity to emotional distress (Scarr 1992). This speculative but plausible hypothesis would be supported by the identification of two genes (i.e., a gene

Table 7–2. Percentage of asthmatic children with parenting risk in the W. T. Grant Asthma Risk Project

Age	Number of children with asthma[a]	Percentage with parenting risk[b]
1st Year	2	100
2nd Year	9	78

[a]As defined by documentation by pediatrician in medical record.
[b]As defined at 3 weeks' visit.

for bronchial reactivity and a gene for autonomic hyperreactivity) that are closely linked on the same chromosome. For individuals with normal alleles at both sites, neither asthma nor emotional reactivity would be likely. If only the gene for bronchial reactivity were present, the possibility of developing overt asthma would require another triggering mechanism that could be genetically controlled such as immunological hyperreactivity, or the asthma could result from exposure to environmental factors such as a viral infection. Children with a normal allele for bronchial reactivity but with exaggerated autonomic reactivity would not be asthmatic but might well have difficult or impulsive temperaments. Finally, children with both bronchial and emotional hyperreactivity would be hypothesized to have a form of asthma that would be quite labile and prone to precipitation by emotional distress.

Further evidence is required before it will be possible to differentiate which, if any, of these explanations is valid. However, the importance of the role of emotional state during infancy and the consideration that emotional stressors may affect gene expression are supported by the described association between early parenting difficulties and the early onset of asthma. Further evidence is likely to be derived from two types of investigations. The first set of illuminating studies would be randomly controlled trials of preventive intervention, targeted to modify specific risk factors, that successfully result in achieving a decreased incidence of asthma in those children receiving the intervention. The second set of required studies would be genetic analyses that reveal specific sites of relevant genes and the full range of salient alleles.

Table 7–3.   Association of other risk factors with the onset of asthma at 2 years

Risk factors[a]	Significance (P values)
Maternal depression	.180
Marital adjustment	.225
Stress	.260
Coping	.418

[a]Risk factors assessed by home visit when the index child was 3 weeks old.

References

Brown GW, Harris T: Social Origins of Depression: A Study of Psychiatric Disorder in Women. New York, Free Press, 1978

Busse WW: The relationship between viral infections and onset of allergic diseases in asthma. Clin Exp Allergy 19:1–9, 1989

Department of Health and Human Services: Executive Summary: Guidelines for the Diagnosis and Management of Asthma. Bethesda, MD, National Institutes of Health, 1991

Falliers C: Treatment of asthma in a residential center. Ann Allergy 28:513–521, 1971

Frick OL, German DF, Mills J: Development of allergy in children, I: association with virus infections. J Allergy Clin Immunol 63:228–241, 1979

Hopp DO, Bewtra AK, Watt GD, et al: Genetic analysis of allergic disease in twins. J Allergy Clin Immunol 73:265–270, 1984

Horwood L, Fergusson D, Hons B, et al: Social and familial factors in the development of early childhood asthma. Pediatrics 75:859–868, 1985

Mrazek DA: Asthma: psychiatric considerations, evaluation, and management, in Allergy: Principles and Practice, 3rd Edition. EdIted by Middleton E, Reed CE, Ellis EF. St Louis, CV Mosby, 1988, pp 1176–1196

Mrazek DA, Klinnert M: Asthma: psychoneuroimmunologic considerations, in Psychoneuroimmunology II. Edited by Ader R, Felten DL, Cohen N. Orlando, FL, Academic, 1991, pp 1013–1035

Mrazek DA, Klinnert MD, Mrazek P, et al: Early asthma onset: consideration of parenting issues. J Am Acad Child Adolesc Psychiatry 30:277–282, 1991

Mrazek DA, Mrazek P, Klinnert MD: Clinical assessment of parenting. J Am Acad Child Adolesc Psychiatry 34:272–282, 1995

Radke-Yarrow M, Nottelmann E, Martinez P, et al: Young children of affectively ill parents: a longitudinal study of psychosocial development. J Am Acad Child Adolesc Psychiatry 31:68–77, 1992

Scarr S: Developmental theories for the 1990's: development and individual differences. Child Dev 63:1–19, 1992

Smith JM: Epidemiology and natural history of asthma, allergic rhinitis and atopic dermatitis (eczema), in Allergy: Principles and Practice, 3rd Edition. Edited by Middleton E, Reed CE, Ellis EF. St Louis, CV Mosby, 1988, pp 891–929

Zeiger RS: Development and prevention of allergic disease in childhood, in Allergy: Principles and Practice, 3rd Edition. Edited by Middleton E, Reed CE, Ellis EF. St Louis, CV Mosby, 1988, pp 930–968

Chapter 8

Stress, Depression, Mood, and Immunity

Jacqueline A. Bartlett, M.D.
Melissa K. Demetrikopoulos, M.S.
Steven J. Schleifer, M.D.
Steven E. Keller, Ph.D.

Psychoneuroimmunology is the study of interactions among psychological factors, the central nervous system (CNS), and the immune system. More recently this field has begun to expand into health outcome research. The scope of psychoneuroimmunology studies has included in vitro and in vivo investigations in both animal and human models. In this chapter, after providing a brief introduction to the immune system, we review some of the highlights of animal and adult human psychoneuroimmunology studies as well as present available information concerning children and adolescents.

The Immune System

The primary function of the immune system is to defend the body against disease. The immune system of humans and other mammals consists of several specialized cell types. These cells have two main lineages: the lymphoid and the myeloid cell lines.

The lymphoid lineage produces lymphocytes and the myeloid lineage produces phagocytes. There are three main types of lymphocytes: T cells (CD3+), B cells (CD19+), and natural killer (NK) cells (CD56+). T cells are subdivided into several types, including T helper

(CD4+) cells and T cytotoxic/suppressor (CD8+) cells, which are further subdivided by surface markers and function. T cells are involved in cellular immune response, while B cells are the antibody-producing cells. NK cells function in immune surveillance for tumor cells and virally infected cells. For a review of the immune system and its cell types and functions, we refer the reader to Stites et al. 1987.

The myeloid lineage produces monocytes and polymorphonuclear granulocytes (PMNs). Monocytes act both to remove particulate antigens by phagocytosis and as antigen-presenting cells involved in initiation of the immune response. PMNs are subdivided into neutrophils, eosinophils, and basophils. Neutrophils are the predominant subtype of PMNs and are important in acute inflammation because of their ability to phagocytize microorganisms. Eosinophils are important modulators of the inflammatory response, and basophils play an important role in controlling parasitic infections (Roitt et al. 1989).

There are several methods commonly used in psychoneuroimmunology research to measure immunity. These include both enumerative and functional assays. Cell counts, expressed as either total number or percentage of the total peripheral blood white cell count, are measured by flow cytometry. The functional measures include skin testing and induction of antibody production de novo or in sensitized organisms. T and B cell function can both be measured by use of mitogen stimulation assays. Mitogens will polyclonally (i.e., nonselectively) stimulate lymphoid cells to enter the cell cycle and divide. Different cell types are preferentially stimulated by specific mitogens. Commonly utilized mitogens include pokeweed (PWM), phytohemagglutinin (PHA), and concanavalin A (Con A). NK cell activity is commonly measured with a chromium release assay that measures the NK ability to lyse virally infected or cancerous target cells. There are various procedures used to measure the function of PMNs; these include measures of the ability to adhere to, ingest, and/or kill microorganisms. Both functional and enumerative measures have been investigated in studies of stress effects on the immune system. Further, some studies have investigated how these changes in the immune system affect health.

Animal Studies

Although it is beyond the scope of this chapter to thoroughly review the psychoneuroimmunology literature on nonhuman studies, it is compelling to examine at least a few illustrative examples for background to the work with humans (for reviews, see McKinney 1986 and Coe et al. 1988a).

Maternal Separation and Immunity

Early repeated parental separation has been documented as a significant stress for children. It is well documented that early life experiences can have lasting psychological consequences, and there is a growing literature which suggests that these early experiences have both immediate and lasting physiological consequences, including alterations in immune function and effects on health outcome.

Animal psychoneuroimmunology research has explored models that may be relevant both to understanding the potential immunological consequences of this phenomenon and to finding ways to minimize this effect. An early study by Laudenslager and co-workers (1982) demonstrated that a 2-week maternal separation caused suppressed lymphocyte response to Con A and PHA in both the mother and infant pigtail monkeys. Ackerman and co-workers (1988) examined the immunological consequences of early maternal separation in Wistar rats. Rat pups who were prematurely and permanently separated from their mothers at 15 days of age showed decreased peripheral blood lymphocyte response to PHA mitogen at 40 days of age. Furthermore, an attempt to investigate longer-term (100-day) effects of premature separation was precluded by an opportunistic respiratory infection in the colony. Although this outbreak necessitated premature termination of the study, it proved to be instructive because pneumonitis was evident almost exclusively in the prematurely separated animals and especially in prematurely weaned males. This chance occurrence suggested that the decreased lymphocyte function may be a marker for, if not causally related to, real health consequences.

The possible role of lymphocyte function as a marker for real health consequences was also suggested by an earlier study that examined the ability of infant squirrel monkeys to respond to viral challenge after maternal separation (Coe et al. 1987). Some infant monkeys were separated from their mothers at 6 months of age for 7 days. The monkeys who were separated had diminished ability to develop antibodies following exposure to a benign virus compared with those who remained with their mothers. This effect of maternal separation could be ameliorated by either leaving the infant in its home environment or providing familiar social companions in the novel environment. For those monkeys who were left in familiar surroundings or with familiar companions, antibody response to the virus was not different from that in the control monkeys. This finding suggests that it was not maternal separation per se that was the key mediating variable, but rather the lack of "social support" in a potentially hostile environment.

Coe and co-workers (1988b) further examined the immunological consequences of maternal separation by examining macrophage function. They tested the killing ability of peripheral blood monocytes following zymosan stimulation by measuring chemiluminescence (a measure of the oxidative bursts that produce microbicidal intracellular factors). Following a 24-hour separation, both the mother and the infants had increased chemiluminescence that was apparent for 2 weeks postseparation, with the chemiluminescence returning to normal levels by 2 months postseparation. An elevated cortisol response following separation was also found, but this did not appear to account for the increased chemiluminescence because the cortisol levels had normalized by 2 weeks postseparation. Coe et al. noted that increased macrophage activity is not necessarily a positive change, because it can be associated with suppression of other immune responses. This underscores the need to recognize that up-regulation of one immunological component can result in overall suppression of immunological function.

Rearing and Immunity

To expand on their earlier findings with maternal separation, Coe and co-workers (1989) examined the effects of a variety of rearing conditions on later immunological functioning. One group of juvenile rhesus monkeys were separated from their mothers at birth and raised in a nursery. When these nursery-raised monkeys were studied immunologically at 1 year and 2.5 years of age, they were found to have elevated responses to Con A when compared with monkeys raised by their mothers. They also had increased response to PHA and to PWM at 1 year of age, with the response returning to normal by 2.5 years of age. Additionally, Coe and co-workers studied a group of monkeys that were weaned prematurely from their mothers at 6 months of age, as opposed to the normal 12 months. These investigators found that the early-weaned monkeys had mitogen response intermediate to those of the nursery-raised and the normally raised monkeys. This effect was evident regardless of the later housing conditions of the monkeys (i.e., whether they were later individually or socially housed). This study also examined a group of monkeys who had experienced multiple brief (either daily or 2 days per week) maternal separations between 3 and 7 months of age. These subjects showed decreased rather than increased mitogen responses after living undisturbed for 1 year in a pair-housing condition. This finding suggests that the different effects on the immune system (measured by mitogen response) may be related to differences between acute, short-lived stressful episodes and chronic stress. Finally, these authors found that, in contrast to the effects of rearing on mitogen response, there were no differences among any of the groups in NK cell activity.

Human Studies

Adult Stress and Immunity

Behavioral and psychological states have been shown to influence immunity. Research on life stress and immunity in adult humans has identified several conditions in which altered, primarily suppressed, immunity occurs. The death of a spouse is among the most stressful of commonly occurring life events and has been associated with increased medical mortality (Helsing et al. 1981) and suppressed lymphocyte function (Bartrop et al. 1977; Schleifer et al. 1983). The links between bereavement and suppressed immunity are complex and may be related to indirect effects resulting from alterations in activity, sleep, and diet. Direct CNS effects, possibly mediated by hypothalamic processes associated with psychological states such as depression or anxiety, may also be involved. For a review of possible mechanisms of stress-induced immune function, see Ader et al. 1991.

There have been several studies of the effects of other types of stress on immunity in young adults. Glaser, Kiecolt-Glaser, and coworkers conducted a series of experiments examining changes in immunological status during final examination week in medical students. In their first study (Kiecolt-Glaser et al. 1984), they found decreased NK cell activity following exam stress in first-year medical students. Further, intercurrent life stress and loneliness were found to contribute additionally to the suppressed NK cell function. A subsequent study (Glaser et al. 1985) demonstrated diminished percentages of total T cells, T helper cells, and T suppressor cells in response to exam stress in a group of second-year medical students. These students also had diminished response to PHA and Con A following the exam.

That stressful events may suppress immunity at least transiently has been suggested by other investigations similar to those of Glaser, Kiecolt-Glaser, and co-workers. Locke and co-workers (1984) found evidence for decreased NK cell activity in college students experiencing high levels of life stress together with emotional distress. However, another study of examination stress found decrements in some immune measures and elevation of others (Dorian et al. 1986). This latter finding further supports the concept that down-regulation of one immune measure, either enumerative or functional, may occur in conjunction with, be the result of, or contribute to up-regulation of other immune parameters.

Adult Depression and Immunity

Bereaved subjects characteristically manifest depressed mood, and a subgroup of the bereaved have symptom patterns consistent with major depressive disorder (MDD) (Clayton et al. 1972; Helsing et al. 1981). This led investigators to hypothesize that depression might also be associated with alterations in immunity. Cappel and co-workers (1978) reported that PHA responses were lower in psychotically depressed patients during the acute phase of their illness than following clinical remission. Kronfol and co-workers (1983) found that depressed patients had lower mitogen responses than nonmelancholic psychiatric patients and normal control subjects. Diminished NK cell activity has been reported in depressed adults compared with control subjects by several investigators (Irwin et al. 1990; Nerozzi et al. 1989; Urch et al. 1988).

Schleifer, Keller, and Stein conducted a series of studies to investigate whether depressive disorders are associated with altered immunity. In these authors' initial studies, severely depressed hospitalized patients with MDD were found to have significantly lower lymphocyte mitogen responses and decreased T and B cells compared with matched control subjects (Schleifer et al. 1984). In contrast, decreased mitogen responses were not found in less severely depressed and younger ambulatory patients with MDD (Schleifer et al. 1985). In a more recent study, involving 91 drug-free patients with MDD, unipolar subtype, these authors demonstrated that the altered lymphocyte function in depression is related to the age of the depressed subjects, with differing immune effects in younger and older depressed patients. Older depressed patients had lower mitogen responses to PHA, Con A, and PWM compared with control subjects, whereas younger adult depressed patients had elevated mitogen responses compared with control subjects. Similar age-related alterations in T helper cell (CD4+) number were also found (Schleifer et al. 1989).

Additional studies have further underscored the specificity of behavioral effects on immunity in relation to specific psychosocial conditions and immune functions. In contrast to the findings in patients with MDD, no changes in lymphocyte function were found in young to middle-age patients hospitalized for schizophrenia or in patients hospitalized for elective herniorrhaphy (Schleifer et al. 1985). Linn (1983) similarly found no overall changes in immunity in patients awaiting elective surgery, but found surgical-stress effects on lymphocyte function in the subgroup of older patients.

In sum, studies with adults have revealed evidence of both up- and down-regulation of immune function in relation to stress and depression. The complex relationships between different stressors and immunity are just beginning to be understood. In the remainder of this chapter we examine these relationships in children and adolescents.

Child Depression and Endocrine Function

That psychoimmunological processes may be operative in children is suggested by a variety of findings. The hypothalamus modulates both humoral and cell-mediated immunity (Cross 1982; Keller et al. 1980; Stein et al. 1982), and alterations in the hypothalamic-pituitary adrenal (HPA) axis have been described in pediatric as well as adult patients with MDD (Asnis et al. 1981, 1982; Carroll et al. 1976; Cytryn et al. 1974; Doherty et al. 1986; Livingston et al. 1984; Poznanski et al. 1982; Sachar et al. 1973; Stokes et al. 1984; Weller et al. 1984).

The breadth of the literature on endocrine function in children and adolescents who are under conditions of stress and depression is well beyond the scope of this chapter. Interested readers are referred to a recent review on the neuroendocrine aspects of depression in children by Puig-Antich (1987). The following brief overview may aid in the consideration of possible mediating variables of the effects of depression on immunity. Cortisol, thyroid-stimulating hormone (TSH), and growth hormone (GH) are important neuroendocrine markers of *adult* depression and have documented effects on immunity (Ader et al. 1991). The apparently conflicting findings in the child literature on the role of these markers as mediators of depressive symptoms may result from procedural differences among the studies. Future research is necessary to understand how these subtle differences in neuroendocrine markers are potential important mediators of depressive somatic symptoms.

Cortisol.   Corticosteroids have important immune effects, including suppression of lymphocyte proliferation (Cupps and Fauci 1982) and redistribution of T-helper cells (Cupps et al. 1984). Further, adults with MDD have been reported to hypersecrete cortisol as measured by an increase in plasma levels, an increase in secretion per episode, and an earlier rise in plasma levels during sleep. Additionally, dexamethasone often does not produce suppression of plasma cortisol in depressive adult patients (Puig-Antich et al. 1989).

The data concerning cortisol secretion and suppression by dexamethasone in children and adolescents are not as well investigated nor as clear. Some studies have suggested that the dexamethasone suppression test (DST) is useful in detecting depression in prepubertal children (Fristad et al. 1988; Weller et al. 1984). Others have not shown differences in cortisol secretion in prepubescent children with MDD (Puig-Antich et al. 1989). Similarly conflicting findings are evident in the adolescent literature. Some authors suggest that the DST is abnormal in this age group (Appelboom-Fondu et al. 1988; Hsu et al. 1983; Khan 1987), whereas several investigators found no differences in cortisol secretion in depressed adolescents (Kutcher et al. 1991). It is important to note, however, that cortisol secretion and dexamethasone suppression do not necessarily measure the same neuroendocrine construct.

Thyroid-stimulating hormone.   The response of TSH to thyroid-releasing hormone (TRH) may be important in depression because there is evidence for a negative relationship between amelioration of depression and enhanced TSH response. Puig-Antich (1987) reported no differences in TSH response to TRH in depressed prepubertal children.

This finding was replicated by Garcia, Puig-Antich, and co-workers (1991). However, after examining the subjects' results in terms of aggression, Garcia et al. demonstrated that depressed subjects who scored high on aggression showed lower TSH response. Similarly, there was a trend for a blunting of the TSH responses for children with serious suicidal ideation. These findings suggest that impulsive and aggressive mood states may be more important in relation to this variable. Further research is, however, necessary.

The adolescent literature concerning TSH and depression is less consistent. Several investigators found no differences in response to TRH (Brambilla et al. 1989; Khan 1987; Puig-Antich 1987), whereas in a recent study investigators demonstrated increase TSH secretion under basal conditions (Kutcher et al. 1991). Future research is necessary to understand the significance of these differences.

Studies of TSH and thyroid hormone effects on immunity have tended to demonstrate that thyroid hormones have positive effects in sustaining immune function (Ader et al. 1991). Impaired thyroid function may therefore result in a down-regulation of immune activity.

Growth hormone.   Growth hormone has been shown to enhance immune function (Snow 1985). GH is normally secreted in response to growth hormone–releasing hormone (GHRH) from the hypothalamus. Puig-Antich (1987) found that prepubescent depressed children showed hypersecretion of GH during sleep and hyposecretion of GH in response to insulin-induced hypoglycemia. However, neither of these effects was found in an adolescent sample, which led Puig-Antich to suggest that estrogens may mask (ameliorate) this effect. Additionally, he found no effect of depression on GH response to desmethylimipramine in either prepubescent children or adolescents. Brambilla and co-workers (1989) demonstrated an increase in GH secretion in response to TRH in five of eight depressed subjects from 9 to 16 years of age. Unlike Puig-Antich (1987), Kutcher and co-workers (1991) found that basal GH secretion was the best differentiator between depressed and nondepressed adolescents. GH therefore remains a putative mediator of the link between depression and immunity, possibly having differentiating effects in children and adolescents.

Sex steroids.   Differences in immunity are associated with the estrous cycle, which suggests that estrogens or other circulating sex steroids may influence immune measures. Evans and co-workers

(1992) found differences in circulating lymphocytes and NK cell activity in depressed adult males, but not females, when compared with matched control subjects. In a study of prepubescent children with MDD, we found that female gender was associated with lower numbers of CD8+ cells (Bartlett et al., in press). Further, there was a trend for lower numbers of lymphocytes and B cells to be associated with female gender. These data suggest that gender may mediate immune alterations associated with depression or stress.

Neonatal Stress and Neutrophil Function

A series of studies have examined neutrophil function in newborn infants who have undergone a stress experience. In these studies, stress was generally defined as a condition requiring assisted ventilation such as noninfectious respiratory illness or birth asphyxia (i.e., the stress was physiological). Harris and co-workers (1983) demonstrated that polymorphonuclear leukocytes of newborns had increased phagocytosis of Group B Streptococcus compared with adults irrespective of stress condition, but found no differences between the stressed and healthy newborns. In a subsequent study, these authors examined the killing of Group B Streptococcus by polymorphonuclear leukocytes in a similar population (Stroobant et al. 1984) and again found differences between neonates and adults but not between the stressed and healthy neonates. The authors concluded that the bactericidal capacity of neonates is lower than that of adults and that stress does not add to this effect. However, methodological factors may explain the lack of a difference between the stressed and healthy subjects: blood from healthy control subjects was obtained from cord segments at delivery, whereas blood from the "stressed" subjects was drawn from indwelling arterial or venous catheters at approximately 3 days of age. The process of birth might also have constituted a stressor for the control group. Furthermore, clearly it is not known whether there are subtle maturational differences over the first 3 days of life that may mask the stress effects. Additionally, cord blood may differ from peripheral blood.

A later study, by Krause and co-workers (1986), controlled for these potential problems by sampling both groups of neonatal subjects at a similar age (1–88 days of age for the stressed subjects and 3–88 days of age for the control subjects). These authors examined polymorphonuclear leukocyte chemotaxis (i.e., the process of phagocytic cells moving toward the pathogen site) and adherence (i.e., the ability to adhere to vascular endothelium) in stressed and health neonates compared with each other and with adults. In findings similar to the above, the neonates had decreased adherence compared with adults irrespective of the stress condition. However, the authors demonstrated a significant decrease in polymorphonuclear leukocyte chemotaxis in the stressed neonates as compared with control neonates or adults. They suggested that the impaired chemotaxis found in stressed neonates may, in part, explain the increased susceptibility to bacterial infection found in this group.

Although these studies suggest that stress influences immunity early in life in humans, these stressors were primarily physiological and the subjects were physically ill. Whether early psychological distress in the absence of physical illness would produce similar immune alterations is a matter of speculation, as no such studies have been reported.

Child Life Events and Immunity

There are considerable data associating life events with immunological processes and health outcomes (see early reviews by Rabkin and Struening [1976] and Rahe and Arthur [1978]). LeShan (1966) examined the early life histories of children with cancer and their siblings, who did not have cancer. The cancer patients had a shorter duration of being the youngest child compared with their siblings without cancer. LeShan suggested that the birth of a younger sibling is a traumatic event because of the perceived loss of the parent and that a child is less able to cope with this event the earlier in life it happens. This is reminiscent of the findings from some animal studies in which premature weaning is associated with negative health outcome.

In a more recent study, Jacobs and Charles (1980) reexamined the relationship between life events and cancer in children. The subjects were cancer patients, with a mean age of 9.5 years (range of 3–17 years of age). The control group was drawn from a general pediatric clinic and was matched for sex, age, and socioeconomic background. The Holmes and Rahe Life Schedule of Recent Events was used to investigate life events. There were two factors associated with the birth of the children that differentiated between the cancer patients and the control subjects. Fewer of the patients were the result of a planned pregnancy, and more had experienced difficult births. Furthermore, the cancer subjects had both higher number of life events and higher weighted scores that took into account the emotional significance of the event. Life events that were much more common in the patient group included moving and parental marital separation. Although the authors stressed that their data do not demonstrate a causative modality, the data suggest that life events are in some way related to the occurrence of cancer.

Heisel (1972) examined life changes as being a possible etiological factor in the development of the autoimmune disorder juvenile rheumatoid arthritis. They modified the life event scale of Coddington and studied children from 1 to 15 years of age. The control subjects were drawn from a population of healthy children and matched by age, sex, race, religion, and parents' education level. The children with juvenile rheumatoid arthritis had significantly higher life change units compared with the control subjects. However, the patients with polyarticular onset had low scores. This led Heisel to suggest that there may be more than one type of juvenile rheumatoid arthritis, with only monoarticular onset being related to premorbid stress. These results were essentially replicated in another study that demonstrated increased life events prior to the onset of juvenile rheumatoid arthritis (Heisel et al. 1973). The investigators in this latter study also found a slight increase in life events for general pediatric patients and fewer events for hemophiliac patients. It is of interest that many of the complaints by the general pediatric patients were of immunological consequence such as respiratory disease, infections, and allergic conditions.

In a case report, Morillo and Gardner (1979) described possible effects of bereavement on Graves' disease, an autoimmune disease with marked hyperthyroidism. Four children were studied, ranging in age from 8 to 14 years. All of the subjects had experienced loss of a loved one (three the death of a close relative, and the fourth a sudden and permanent separation from the mother figure). The children all first developed depressive symptoms and then displayed Graves' disease. Although predisposition to Graves' disease appears to have a strong genetic component involving a defect in immunological surveillance, the expression of the disease may be more likely following a stressful experience. In these cases the acute event, or the subsequent depression, may have served to alter immune surveillance, triggering the Graves' disease.

Boyce and co-workers (1977) examined the effects of life events on respiratory illness. Their subjects ranged in age from 1 to 11 years, with a mean age of 4.3 years. The children were observed 5 days per week for 1 year at a day care–elementary school complex. Additionally, biweekly nasopharyngeal cultures for bacteria, mycoplasmas, and viruses were conducted. Four dependent illness variables were measured: number of illnesses, average duration, average severity, and a composite sickness score. Life change scores were calculated based on Coddington's modification of the Holmes and Rahe schedule. A measure of family routines was also administered. The authors found that life change scores predicted illness duration such that more life events were associated with an increase in the average illness duration. Although the authors had originally postulated that family routines are protective during times of high life events stress, they found that the severity of the illness was predicted by combined high scores on both life events and family routines. They suggested that as the life events increase there may be a breakdown in established routines, or, alternatively, that the ongoing minor uncertainties in a non-routine family may offer protection against later larger disruptions.

It is important to note that the relationship between life events and illness is not invariable. Steinhausen (1983) did not find an association of life events with either cystic fibrosis or inflammatory bowel disease. Although an autoimmune mechanism may be possible for these two diseases, there is considerable controversy concerning their etiology. Inflammatory bowel disease may be an expression of poor nutrition (Taylor and Thomas 1987), and cystic fibrosis is known to have a strong genetic component. Also, whereas Heisel (1972) found increased life events for general pediatric patients, Bailey and Garralda (1987) did not find a relationship between life events and attendance at a health care service. It is of note that the experimental group in Bailey and Garralda's study was similar to the control group in the study by Jacobs and Charles (1980) that assessed the effects of life events on cancer. The data, in sum, seem to suggest that life events do not predict generalized health-seeking behavior but may predict risk of specific illnesses with significant immunological components.

There are no published studies of stress-related immune alterations in children and adolescents. We have reported preliminary data from a study of inner city adolescents that assessed past year life events (Coddington Life Events Scale [CDLES]), distress (Perceived Stress Scale [PSS]), and immune function (Bartlett et al. 1992). The data on 306 healthy adolescents (mean age of 15.9 ± 1.7) were analyzed. Regression analyses were used to test the associations of immunity with age, sex, race, life events (based on CDLES scores), and, concurrently, perceived stress (based on PSS scores). These analyses revealed an independent association of PSS scores with increased white blood cell counts and CD4+ (T-helper) cells. CDLES scores predicted increased percentage of T cells, T-helper cells, activated T cells, T inducers of help, and T inducers of suppression, along with decreased percentage of B cells. These data demonstrated that stressful life events and, to a lesser extent, perceived stress were associated with increased circulating T lymphocyte subtypes.

Child Family Composition and Immunity

It is well documented that the presence of social support can act as a mediating variable in health and disease (see, e.g., review by Broadhead and co-workers [1983]). Graham and co-workers (1990) examined the relationship of maternal stress and social support with acute respiratory illness in children. Mothers of 22- to 23-month-old children participated in the study. Approximately half of the children were prone to respiratory distress and the other half were specifically not prone. The respiratory proneness of the children was evaluated by the frequency of respiratory-related illnesses and symptomatology in the past year. Maternal stress was measured by life events (Life Events Inventory) and psychological distress (General Health Questionnaire). Social support was measured by the Maternal Social Support Index, and family function was measured by the Family APGAG. Moderate and high levels of maternal stress were associated with proneness to respiratory illness in the children. Although maternal social support per se was not associated with respiratory illness, respiratory distress–prone children were more likely to come from dysfunctional families. These findings suggest that the dynamics of the family environment may be an important variable in the health of children.

Although there are no published data on stress and/or social support and immunity in children, we have found in one study that family composition is associated with immunological functioning. We examined granulocyte function in prepubescent children 8 to 12 years of age. Using regression models controlling for sociodemographic and psychosocial variables, we found that granulocytes in children from nonintact families had decreased killing activity of *Staphylococcus aureus* (Staph A). Although depression, which was more common in nonintact families, also tended to predict decreased killing, prior marital separation in the family was the strongest predictor of decreased granulocyte function.

Child Depression and Immunity

Shain and co-workers (1991) examined NK cell activity in hospitalized 13- to 18-year-olds with MDD and in health volunteer control subjects. Severity of depression was measured with the Reynolds Adolescent Depression Scale and the Children's Depression Rating Scale—Revised. NK activity was significantly correlated with age in both patients and control subjects. Although the authors did not find an effect of MDD diagnosis per se on NK cell activity, they did find a negative correlation between NK cell activity and scores on the Reynolds Adolescent Depression Scale.

We studied immunity in association with prepubescent MDD in otherwise healthy children. The children were 8 to 12 years of age and at Tanner stage I (prepubescent). The diagnosis of depression was made according to DSM-III-R (American Psychiatric Association 1987), and severity of depression was measured by the Children's Depression Rating Scale (CDRS) and the Children's Depression Inventory (CDI). The depressed children were compared with healthy age-, sex-, socioeconomic-, and race-matched control subjects. Both the depressed children and the control subjects were drug-naive for neuroleptics and antidepressants.

Five of the 18 subject/control pairs were female; 13 were Caucasian, non-Hispanic; 3 were Hispanic; and 2 were African American. The control subjects had no anxiety, mood, or other DSM-III-R disorder and were in good physical health. The depressed children met the criteria only for unipolar depression (major depression).

Lymphocyte counts were within normal ranges for the depressed subjects and the control subjects. There were no differences between the depressed subjects and the control subjects with respect to total number of lymphocytes or lymphocyte subsets, and no correlations between age or gender and lymphocyte counts were found. Regression analyses controlling for age, gender, and diagnostic group (MDD) were undertaken to explore the effects of severity of depressive symptoms (as measured by scores on the CDI or CDRS) on the enumerative measures. These analyses revealed an independent, inverse relationship between levels of depressive symptoms and the total number of lymphocytes. Greater severity was also associated with lower numbers of B cells and CD8+ cells, with a trend for lower total T cell counts. Furthermore, and of note, when the severity of symptomatology was also considered, a significant independent association of the diagnosis of MDD with *higher* numbers of lymphocytes, B cells, and CD8+ cells was found. The immune effects for diagnostic group were therefore opposite those for the symptomatology measure.

With respect to the functional immune measures, there was little evidence for an association between childhood depression and lymphocyte mitogen responses for PHA or PWM. Responses to Con A demonstrated significant depressive diagnosis by mitogen dose interaction, suggesting possible differences in the dose response in depressed children. No effects of depressive symptomatology in relation to mitogen response were revealed in regression analysis.

For NK cell activity, lower responses were found in the depressed children at the highest (100:1) effector:target (E:T) ratio. Regression analyses revealed that severity of symptomatology tended to predict lower NK cell activity at each E:T ratio. When severity of symptomatology was also considered, a trend for MDD diagnosis to be independently associated with *increased* response at the lowest E:T ratio was also revealed. This effect for diagnostic group was opposite that of the symptomatology measure and comparable to the relationship found for the quantitative lymphocyte measures. These findings suggest that alterations in regulatory lymphocyte subsets may account for altered NK cell activity in depressed children. Such effects could contribute to health risk.

Stress, Immunity, and Health

Cohen and co-workers (1993) examined the effect of psychological stress on respiratory infection and the induction of the common cold in subjects experimentally exposed to respiratory viruses. In this study the authors used three measures of psychological stress—life events, perceived stress, and a negative-affect scale—and then combined them into a single index. The subjects were exposed to virus by the use of nasal drops in doses that mimic normal transmission. They demonstrated that stress predicted risk of respiratory illness and increased rates of infection. This study represents an important step in examining the effect of stress on health outcome measures.

We investigated 226 healthy inner city adolescents to examine the relationship between psychological and immune functioning. These subjects were screened for MDD with the revised Diagnostic Interview Schedule for Children and for severity of depression with the Hamilton Rating Scale for Depression. Thirty-six adolescents met the criteria for MDD and were followed longitudinally at 6-month intervals. In preliminary analysis (Keller et al. 1992) it was found that syndromal depression at time one was related to minor illness as well as to decreased B and T cell function at time two. These data suggest that affective alterations may lead to immune dysfunction that then leads to increased illness.

Conclusions

Preclinical studies and those with adult humans strongly suggest that psychological factors such as stress and depression influence immunity. The available data also suggest that the immune system is altered in children with MDD who are under stress. The patterns of immune change in children share some similarities with those seen in depressed young adults. Altered immunity in association with childhood MDD, as with adult MDD, is likely influenced by age, gender, and especially severity of symptomatology. The different effects of MDD and of severity of symptomatology in depressed children, as well as in adults, suggest that the mechanistic influences on the immune system associated with the syndromal state (i.e., depressive disorder) are different from those associated with the symptomatology typical of depression. These data also suggest that there may be a biological continuum between childhood and adult depressive disorders as expressed in age-dependent immune system changes. An immunological interaction between depression and age may involve developmental and/or aging processes influencing immune alterations. Whether the immune alterations in depressed children are state dependent, antedate the first episode, or persist between depressive episodes requires study.

That health too is influenced by stress and other psychological factors is also suggested by the available literature. Whether these effects are mediated by psychoimmune interactions remains to be investigated.

References

Ackerman SH, Keller SE, Schleifer SJ, et al: Brief communication: premature maternal separation and lymphocyte function. Brain Behav Immun 2:161–165, 1988

Ader R, Felten DL, Cohen N (eds): Psychoneuroimmunology II. San Diego, CA, Academic, 1991

American Psychiatric Association: Diagnostic and Statistical Manual of Mental Disorders, 3rd Edition, Revised. Washington, DC, American Psychiatric Association, 1987

Appelboom-Fondu J, Kerkhofs M, Mendlewicz J: Depression in adolescents and young adults—polysomnographic and neuroendocrine aspects. J Affect Disord 14:35–40, 1988

Asnis GM, Sachar EJ, Halbreich U, et al: Cortisol secretion in relation to age in major depression. Psychosom Med 43:235–242, 1981

Asnis GM, Halbreich V, Halbreich U, et al: Relationship of dexamethasone (2 mg) and plasma cortisol hypersecretion in depressive illness: clinical and neuroendocrine parameters. Psychopharmacol Bull 18:122–126, 1982

Bailey D, Garralda ME: Children attending primary health care services: a study of recent life events. J Am Acad Child Adolesc Psychiatry 26:858–864, 1987

Bartlett JA, Schleifer SJ, Eckholdt H, et al: Stress and immunity in adolescents, in 1992 New Research Program and Abstracts, 145th annual meeting of the American Psychiatric Association, Washington, DC, May 1992, NR312, p 124

Bartlett JA, Schleifer SJ, Demetrikopoulos MK, et al: Immune changes associated with depression in children. Biol Psychiatry (in press)

Bartrop RW, Luckhurst E, Lazarus L, et al: Depressed lymphocyte function after bereavement. Lancet 1:834–836, 1977

Boyce WT, Jensen EW, Cassel JC, et al: Influence of life events and family routines on childhood respiratory tract illness. Pediatrics 60 (No 4, Part 2):609–615, 1977

Brambilla F, Musseti C, Tacchini C, et al: Neuroendocrine investigations in children and adolescents with dysthymic disorders: the DST and clonidine tests. J Affect Disord 17:279–284, 1989

Broadhead WE, Kaplan BH, James SA, et al: Reviews and commentary: the epidemiologic evidence for a relationship between social support and health. Am J Epidemiol 117:521–537, 1983

Cappel R, Gregoire F, Thiry L, et al: Antibody and cell mediated immunity to herpes simplex virus in psychotic depression. J Clin Psychiatry 39:266–268, 1978

Carroll BJ, Curtis GC, Mendels I: Neuroendocrine regulation in depression, II: discrimination of depressed from nondepressed patients. Arch Gen Psychiatry 33:1051–1058, 1976

Clayton PJ, Halikas JA, Maureice WL: The depression of widowhood. Br J Psychiatry 120:71–78, 1972

Coe CL, Rosenberg LT, Fischer M, et al: Psychological factors capable of preventing the inhibition of antibody responses in separated infant monkeys. Child Dev 58:1420–1430, 1987

Coe CL, Rosenberg LT, Levine S: Immunological consequences of psychological disturbance and maternal loss in infancy, in Advances in Infancy Research, Vol 5. Edited by Rovee-Collier C, Lipsitt LP. Norwood, NJ, Ablex Publishing, 1988a, pp 97–134

Coe CL, Rosenberg LT, Levine S: Prolonged effect of psychological disturbance on macrophage chemiluminescence in the squirrel monkey. Brain Behav Immun 2:151–160, 1988b

Coe CL, Lubach GR, Ershler WB, et al: Influence of early rearing on lymphocyte proliferation responses in juvenile rhesus monkeys. Brain Behav Immun 3:47–60, 1989

Cohen S, Tyrrell DAJ, Smith AP: Negative life events, perceived stress, negative affect, and susceptibility to the common cold. J Pers Soc Psychol 64:131–140, 1993

Cross RJ: Hypothalamic-immune interaction: effect of hypophysectomy on neuroimmunomodulation. J Neurol Sci 53:557–566, 1982

Cupps TR, Fauci AS: Corticosteroid-mediated immunoregulation in man. Immunol Rev 65:134–155, 1982

Cupps TR, Edgar LC, Thomad CA, et al: Multiple mechanisms of B cell immunoregulation in man after administration of in vivo corticosteroids. J Immunol 132:170–175, 1984

Cytryn L, McKnew DH Jr, Logue M, et al: Biochemical correlates of affective disorders in children. Arch Gen Psychiatry 31:659–661, 1974

Doherty MD, Madansky D, Kraft J, et al: Cortisol dynamic and test performance of the DST in 97 psychiatrically hospitalized children aged 3–16. Journal of the American Academy of Child Psychiatry 25:400–408, 1986

Dorian BJ, Garfinkel PE, Keystone EC, et al: Stress, immunity and illness (abstract). Psychosom Med 48:304–305, 1986

Evans DL, Folds JD, Petitto JM, et al: Circulating natural killer cell phenotypes in men and women with major depression: relation to cytotoxic activity and severity of depression. Arch Gen Psychiatry 49:388–395, 1992

Fristad MA, Weller EB, Weller R, et al: Self-report vs biological markers in assessment of childhood depression. J Affect Disord 15:339–345, 1988

Garcia MR, Ryan ND, Rabinovitch H, et al: Thyroid stimulating hormone response to thyrotropin in prepubertal depression. J Am Acad Child Adolesc Psychiatry 30:398–406, 1991

Glaser R, Kiecolt-Glaser JK, Stout JC, et al: Stress-related impairments in cellular immunity. Psychiatry Res 16:233–239, 1985

Graham NMH, Woodward AJ, Ryan P, et al: Acute respiratory illness in Adelaide children, II: the relationship of maternal stress, social supports and family functioning. Int J Epidemol 19:937–944, 1990

Harris MC, Stroobant J, Cody CS, et al: Phagocytosis of group B streptococcus by neutrophils from newborn infants. Pediatr Res 17:358–361, 1983

Heisel JS: Life changes as etiologic factors in juvenile rheumatoid arthritis. J Psychosom Res 16:411–420, 1972

Heisel JS, Ream S, Raitz R, et al: The significance of life events as contributing factors in the diseases of children, III: a study of pediatric patients. Behavioral Pediatrics 83:119–123, 1973

Helsing KJ, Szklo M, Comstock GW: Factors associated with mortality after widowhood. Am J Public Health 71:802–809, 1981

Hsu GLK, Molcan K, Cashman MA, et al: Brief communications: the dexamethasone suppression test in adolescent depression. Journal of the American Academy of Child Psychiatry 22:470–473, 1983

Irwin M, Patterson T, Smith TL, et al: Reduction of immune function in life stress and depression. Biol Psychiatry 27:22–30, 1990

Jacobs TJ, Charles E: Life events and the occurrence of cancer in children. Psychosom Med 42:11–24, 1980

Keller SE, Stein M, Camerino MS, et al: Suppression of lymphocyte stimulation by anterior hypothalamic lesions in the guinea pig. Cell Immunol 52:334–340, 1980

Keller SE, Schleifer SJ, Bartlett JA, et al: Affective processes and immune dysfunction have health consequences. Poster presentation at the annual meeting of the Society of Biological Psychiatry, Washington, DC, December 1992

Khan AL: Biochemical profile of depressed adolescents. J Am Acad Child Adolesc Psychiatry 26:873–878, 1987

Kiecolt-Glaser JK, Garner W, Speicher C, et al: Psychosocial modifiers of immunocompetence in medical students. Psychosom Med 46:7–14, 1984

Krause PJ, Herson VC, Boutin-Lebowitz J, et al: Polymorphonuclear leukocyte adherence and chemotaxis in stressed and healthy neonates. Pediatr Res 20:296–300, 1986

Kronfol Z, Silva J Jr, Greden J, et al: Impaired lymphocyte function in depressive illness. Life Sci 33:241–247, 1983

Kutcher S, Malkin D, Silverberg J, et al: Nocturnal cortisol, thyroid stimulating hormone, and growth hormone secretory profiles in depressed adolescents. J Am Acad Child Adolesc Psychiatry 30:407–414, 1991

Laudenslager ML, Reite M, Harbeck R: Suppressed immune response in infant monkeys associated with maternal seperation. Behav Neural Biol 36:40–48, 1982

LeShan L: An emotional life-history pattern associated with neoplastic disease. Ann N Y Acad Sci 125:780–793, 1966

Linn BS: Age and immune response to a surgical stress. Arch Surg 118:405–409, 1983

Livingston R, Reis CJ, Ringdahl IC: Abnormal dexamethasone suppression test results in depressed and nondepressed children. Am J Psychiatry 141:106–108, 1984

Locke SE, Kraus L, Leserman J, et al: Life change stress, psychiatric symptoms, and natural killer cell activity. Psychosom Med 46:441–451, 1984

McKinney WT: Primate separation studies: relevance to bereavement. Psychiatric Annals 16:281–287, 1986

Morillo E, Gardner LI: Bereavement as an antecedent factor in thyrotoxicosis of childhood: four case studies with survey of metabolic pathways. Psychosom Med 41:545–555, 1979

Nerozzi D, Santoni A, Bersani G, et al: Reduced natural killer cell activity in major depression: neuroendocrine implications. Psychoneuroendocrinology 14:295–301, 1989

Poznanski EO, Carroll BJ, Barnegas MC, et al: The dexamethasone suppression test in prepubertal depressed children. Am J Psychiatry 139:321–324, 1982

Puig-Antich J: Sleep and neuroendocrine correlates of affective illness in childhood and adolescence. Journal of Adolescent Health Care 8:505–529, 1987

Puig-Antich J, Dahl R, Ryan N, et al: Cortisol secretion in prepubertal children with major depressive disorder: episode and recovery. Arch Gen Psychiatry 46:801–809, 1989

Rabkin JG, Struening EL: Life events, stress, and illness. Science 194:1013–1020, 1976

Rahe RH, Arthur RJ: Life change and illness studies: past history and future directions. Journal of Human Stress 3:3–15, 1978

Roitt I, Brostoff J, Male D: Immunology. New York, Grower Medical Publishing, 1989

Sachar EJ, Hellman L, Roffwarg HP, et al: Disrupted 24-hour patterns of cortisol secretion in psychotic depression. Arch Gen Psychiatry 28:19–24, 1973

Schleifer SJ, Keller SE, Camerino M, et al: Suppression of lymphocyte stimulation following bereavement. JAMA 250:374–377, 1983

Schleifer SJ, Keller SE, Meyerson AT, et al: Lymphocyte function in major depressive disorder. Arch Gen Psychiatry 41:484–486, 1984

Schleifer SJ, Keller SE, Siris SG, et al: Depression and immunity: lymphocyte function in ambulatory depressed patients, hospitalized schizophrenic patients, and patients hospitalized for herniorrhaphy. Arch Gen Psychiatry 42:129–133, 1985

Schleifer SJ, Keller SE, Bond RN, et al: Major depressive disorder and immunity: role of age, sex, severity, and hospitalization. Arch Gen Psychiatry 46:81–87, 1989

Shain BN, Kronfol Z, Naylor M, et al: Natural killer cell activity in adolescents with major depression. Biol Psychiatry 29:481–484, 1991

Snow EC: Insulin and growth hormone function as minor growth factors that potentiate lymphocyte action. J Immunol 135(suppl): 776S–778S, 1985

Stein M, Schleifer SJ, Keller SE: The role of the brain and neuroendocrine system in immune regulation: potential links to neoplastic disease, in Biological Mediators of Behavior and Disease. Edited by Levy S. New York, Elsevier/North-Holland, 1982, pp 147–174

Steinhausen H: Life events in relation to psychopathology among severely and chronically ill children and adolescents. Child Psychiatry Hum Dev 13:249–258, 1983

Stites DP, Stobo JD, Wells JV (eds): Basic and Clinical Immunology, 6th Edition. Norwalk, CT, Appleton & Lange, 1987

Stokes PE, Stoll PM, Koslow SH, et al: Pretreatment DST and hypothalamic-pituitary-adrenocortical function in depressed patients and comparison groups: a multicenter study. Arch Gen Psychiatry 41:257–267, 1984

Stroobant J, Harris MC, Cody CS, et al: Diminished bactericidal capacity for group B streptococcus in neutrophils from "stressed" and healthy neonates. Pediatr Res 18:634–637, 1984

Taylor KB, Thomas HC: Gastrointestinal and liver diseases, in Basic and Clinical Immunology. Edited by Stites DP, Stobo JD, Wells JV. Norwalk, CT, Appleton & Lange, 1987, pp 457–480

Urch A, Muller C, Aschauer H, et al: Lytic effector cell function in schizophrenia and depression. J Neuroimmunol 18:291–301, 1988

Weller EB, Weller RA, Fristad MA, et al: The dexamethasone suppression test in hospitalized prepubertal depressed children. Am J Psychiatry 141:290–291, 1984

Chapter 9

Stress and Pediatric Medical Technology

Margaret L. Stuber, M.D.
Beth Houskamp, Ph.D.

The past two decades have brought almost miraculous advances in the technology of pediatric care. Acute lymphoblastic leukemia, a previously universally fatal illness, can now be treated so that 60% of diagnosed children become long-term survivors (Pui and Rivera 1991). Replacement of defective or failed body parts has extended from kidneys to bone marrow, livers, hearts, and lungs, allowing children to grow up despite severe congenital abnormalities or overwhelming childhood illness. Technological assist devices provide total parenteral nutrition for children without gastrointestinal tracts and ventilation for children with paralysis of their own breathing mechanism. Preterm newborns can now survive despite extremely small size and extreme organ immaturity.

There are several major drawbacks to most of these technological rescues of dying children. First, almost all of the advances require extremely aggressive interventions. Multiple invasive procedures, mutilative surgery, prolonged intensive care, and highly toxic drugs are relatively common aspects of the new treatments. Although these approaches have unquestionably improved the overall prognosis for

This work was supported in part by a National Institute of Mental Health (NIMH) Academic Career Development Award (MH-01604) and a NIMH National Research Service Award (MH-16381).

many pediatric illnesses, the progress has been costly. The new technology is extremely expensive, requiring highly trained personnel, many hospital days, and elaborate machinery to administer treatments and to evaluate the results. The cost is so high that many insurance companies and state Medicaid agencies have questioned the widespread availability of many of these aggressive types of treatment. Health care reforms, prompted by rapidly escalating costs, will be closely scrutinizing the cost-effectiveness of these approaches and beginning the difficult task of prioritizing the health care dollar.

Second, the price of "high-tech" pediatrics is not just financial. There are significant physical and psychological costs associated with these aggressive new treatments, for both the pediatric patients and their families. Much of this impact can be understood under the general heading of stress. These acute stressors and the resulting stress responses will be a major focus of this chapter.

Third, although these technologically advanced treatments rescue the child from certain death, they rarely are truly curative. For example, children who undergo organ transplantation usually survive what would otherwise be a fatal disease. However, they must remain on immunosuppressive drugs for the rest of their lives. Consequently, they are at increased risk of infectious disease, as well as subject to the side effects inherent with all medications. In essence, the child and family have traded a fatal disease for a chronic illness. The ongoing care is expensive: drugs like cyclosporin A cost in the range of $10,000 a year. Chronic medication and ongoing medical risk are also sources of physical and psychological stress for children and parents. In addition to focusing on the acute stress of technologically advanced intensive treatment for life-threatening illness in children, in this chapter we examine the long-term impact for survivors and their families.

Language is a problem in any consideration of stress. Is the word "stress" appropriately used to describe an event, such as an invasive procedure; the physical response, such as an increase in serum cortisol; or the psychological reaction to the event? The confusion engendered by common use of the term in English runs throughout the literature. In the interests of clarity, whenever possible, in this chapter we refer to specific events or describe events as stressful events, or *stressors*. Physical or psychological responses to such events will be referred to as *stress responses*.

Acute Stressors and Acute Stress Responses

To understand acute stress responses in children undergoing aggressive treatment for life-threatening illness, we must examine what is known about 1) children's responses to invasive procedures and 2) children's responses to life threat. We can then examine the areas of acute stress introduced by these new procedures.

Newborns and Stress

Recent careful studies of behavioral, physiological, and neuroendocrine responses to common procedures such as heelstick or circumcision have demonstrated that even newborns have clear and measurable stress responses to noxious stimuli (Anders et al. 1970; Field and Goldston 1984; Franck 1986; Grunau and Craig 1987; Gunnar et al. 1988). Preterm newborns in neonatal intensive care units experience invasive procedures (and the consequent stress responses) many times each day. Additionally, investigators have found that procedures that are not as obviously painful also elicit stress responses. These procedures include seemingly benign events such as weaning from the incubator and neonatal behavioral assessments (Field 1987).

Attempts to diminish stress for children in neonatal intensive care have demonstrated the utility of limiting the number of invasive procedures and of restricting procedures to specific periods of the day (Long et al. 1980). Providing pacifiers during procedures (Field and Goldston 1984), gently placing hands on the infant when not doing procedures (Jay 1982), and massaging the infant (Field et al. 1986; Scafidi et al. 1990) have also been found to be effective in reducing acute stress responses.

Variations in Stress Responses

Despite a number of interesting studies, it is not yet clear why some children appear to have more severe stress responses when subjected to the same procedures. Two major theoretical constructs have been used in these investigations: temperament and coping style. Because temperament is seen as to some extent determining coping style, these constructs often overlap. An extensive literature includes a number of studies that have examined the differences between children who respond to stressful procedures by either actively seeking or

avoiding information about the procedures (Burstein and Meichenbaum 1979; Field 1987; Knight et al. 1979; Siegel 1977). Although there appear to be behavioral differences between what have been called "sensitizers" (i.e., children who are resistant, expressive, active, and protesting) and "repressors" (i.e., children who are cooperative and stoic), it is not clear whether these behavioral differences predict differences in the severity of stress responses in children (Field 1987). The intensity of response appears to be related to an interaction between a child's temperament (i.e., dispositional tendencies to respond or cope in a certain way), situational opportunities to use a particular coping approach, and the child's flexibility in choosing a strategy (Miller 1990; Miller et al. 1989). Previous negative experiences, especially with similar procedures, will also alter the severity of stress responses, increasing arousal and anticipatory anxiety (Dahlquist et al. 1985; Onufrak 1989).

Temperament appears to have biological as well as behavioral dimensions that may alter the intensity of stress response. Vagal tone and exaggerated cardiovascular reactivity appear to be directly related to children's behavioral responses to stimuli (Boyce and Jemerin 1990). These biological differences may lead to clinically significant medical differences. For example, temperamental dimensions such as activity level, reactivity, and biological regularity appear to be predictors of good versus poor control of juvenile diabetes (Rovet and Ehrlich 1988).

Parental Response to Procedures

Understanding stress responses in children undergoing invasive procedures is complicated by the need to factor in parental responses to procedures. Researchers have found that anxiety in children undergoing medical procedures may be indirectly influenced by their mothers' attitudes, behaviors, and autonomic arousal while they are interacting with health care providers (Manne et al. 1990; Melamed and Ridley-Johnson 1988; Routh and Sanfilippo 1991). It has long been hypothesized that maternal anxiety is communicated both verbally and nonverbally to children (Escalona and Corman 1974). Further investigations have identified parental behavior as the salient variable, finding that disorganized parental behavior in response to stress correlated with increased anxiety and less effective coping strategies in the children (Kaplan et al. 1973). Generalizations from

these findings must be made with caution, however, because most of the studies have been of small numbers of subjects largely from intact, white families. However, the findings clearly suggest that stress responses in children are responses not only to the procedure itself but to the behavior of the adult present immediately before and after the procedure (Blount et al. 1989).

Interventions

Interventions to reduce stress responses to invasive pediatric procedures have included hypnosis (Katz et al. 1987; Zeltzer and LeBaron 1982), behavioral interventions (Dahlquist et al. 1985; Jay et al. 1985; Redd et al. 1979), and combined pharmacological and cognitive-behavioral approaches (Jay and Elliott 1990; Jay et al. 1987). Behavioral interventions with parents have also been successful in decreasing children's stress responses (Jay et al. 1991; Manne et al. 1990). Most of these interventions have been designed to reduce the anxiety and pain associated with procedures. Because the anxiety and pain subjectively experienced during a procedure will be influenced by the perception and experience of previous procedures, interventions very early in the treatment (e.g., before the first invasive procedure) can serve a major prophylactic function (Jay et al. 1983). In addition to experiencing increased stress responses during the procedure, children who have been traumatized by a procedure may manifest anticipatory symptoms that are very similar to those experienced during the procedure (Katz et al. 1980). Behavioral interventions can also be used to decrease these conditioned responses (Redd et al. 1979). Alternatively, as with the newborns, the actual procedures may be modified to diminish the acute stress. The potential for severe, acute stress responses to result in chronic or posttraumatic stress responses is discussed in the next section.

Psychological Sources of Acute Stress

The discussion thus far has focused on one source of stress responses in children, the multiple invasive procedures common to the new aggressive pediatric treatment of life-threatening illness. These are probably the most obvious sources of stress for the effected children and families, and may have the greatest potential for modification or reduction. However, the psychological sources of stress are also significant. Some of these have to do with the life threat faced by the child and family. In many cases it is not only the underlying diagnosis but also the treatment that is potentially lethal. Other psychological sources of stress involve choosing to move beyond conventional medicine and into a world where children become news items and their case becomes the topic of ethical or financial debates. Although more amorphous and less studied than children's responses to invasive procedures, each of these areas of psychological stress has a significant body of literature that is worthy of consideration.

Life Threat

Only in the past 30 years has children's ability to comprehend life threat been acknowledged and cognitive developmental theory used to help children talk about death (Kübler-Ross 1969, 1983). Because their focus was a more qualitative assessment of the process of dying, these descriptive studies did not attempt to quantify the specific psychiatric responses to life threat experienced by pediatric survivors. To understand the stress responses of children to life threat and violations of body integrity, it is useful for the clinician to look beyond the pediatric literature and into the more recent research on childhood trauma (Lyons 1987). Children who have survived sniper attacks (Nader et al. 1990; Pynoos et al. 1987), physical or sexual abuse (Nader et al. 1990; Pynoos et al. 1987), and kidnapping (Terr 1981) have reported symptoms very similar to those described in adults after trauma. These symptoms have been described and labeled in various ways. The most commonly used models are the *stress response syndrome* (Horowitz and Kaltreider 1979) and *posttraumatic stress disorder* (PTSD) (American Psychiatric Association 1994). Diagnostic criteria for PTSD include intrusive memories of the event, avoidance of reminders or numbing of responses, and increased autonomic arousal and vigilance. As in studies of traumatized adults (Foy et al. 1987), the severity of symptoms seen in traumatized children correlates with the child's physical proximity to the life threat, or to the perception of actual life threat (Briere et al. 1988; Friedrich 1990).

A traumatic stress model of understanding life threat and response to physical assault has only recently been applied to children who are undergoing intensive treatment for life-threatening illness. Examining the experience of pediatric oncology patients, Nir (1985) suggested that posttraumatic stress appeared to be an appropriate model for understanding the response of the children who were under-going treatment. A study of psychiatric symptoms in pediatric bone marrow transplant patients, although not specifically looking for PTSD, found that a number of the symptoms at the time of treatment, and 6 and 12 months after the transplant, were suggestive of post-traumatic stress (Pot-Mees 1989). A prospective longitudinal study of posttraumatic stress symptoms found that 35% of the children in the sample studied ($N = 34$) reported mild to moderate stress response symptoms at the time of admission for bone marrow transplantation. There was a significant correlation between degree of perceived life threat and severity of stress response symptoms reported ($r = .42$, $P < .02$) (M. L. Stuber, K. Nader, B. M. Houskamp, R. S. Pynoos, un-published manuscript, 1990). When asked about what they found most difficult, and the source of their stress response symptoms, chil-dren cited hospitalization, anticipation of the bone marrow trans-plant, and memories of past treatment. It is noteworthy that the events children reported as traumatic were not necessarily seen by the medical providers as the most serious or invasive aspects of the treat-ment they had received. It appears that the responses of children fac-ing the possibility of death from disease and the responses of children encountering violent life threat, although not identical, can be under-stood using similar models (Nader et al. 1991). Catastrophic illness, like other catastrophic events, can be traumatic for children. The im-plications of this finding for long-term stress in survivors of intensive pediatric interventions will be considered later in this chapter.

Choice of Highly Technological Interventions

An additional psychological source of stress for recipients of the new aggressive pediatric interventions is the element of choice. Although the majority of these treatments are no longer experimental, they are often new enough to have few long-term follow-up data for families to consult when making a decision. Often more has been published by the popular press than in the medical literature (Chang 1991). In addition to the relative lack of information available with which to make the decision, financing the procedure is often a problem. Insur-ance companies may not yet have approved the procedure for cover-age, leaving families to raise money or begin a letter-writing or political campaign to change the rating of the procedure. Either fundraising or campaigning takes time and energy, which are often in short supply when families are trying to manage the physical and psychological demands of a critically ill child. Friends and relatives often inadvertently add to the stress by taking adamant stances for or against the intervention, based on their own experiences or attitudes toward technology or invasive procedures.

Families bombarded with well-meaning but uninformed advice from laypeople often feel they receive little guidance from the medical personnel. Unless the procedure is clearly the best possible option, members of the medical team may be divided in their own opinions about the advisability of aggressive treatment and about the point at which they would recommend moving from attempts at cure to ensuring the child's comfort. If the procedure is indeed still experimental, the doctors are obliged to remain neutral about the recommendations for treatment and to explain every possible complication of the experimental treatment. Parents may be required to read and sign documents, of 10 pages or more, detailing a host of medical catastrophes and reminding the parents that both the disease and the treatment threaten the child's life (Ruccione et al. 1991).

Parental responses to limited information and guidance about intensive interventions for otherwise fatal conditions fall into one of two general categories, with some parents moving from one to the other at different times. One view is that the treatment would be needless torture for all concerned and that the most loving thing parents can do for their child is to provide protection from painful and intrusive experiences. The other view is that if a treatment offers a possibility for survival, it must be tried. Parents endorsing the latter perspective generally do not see that there is a choice, because they see the pursuit of survival as the only real option (Stolberg 1993). Either way, encountering such momentous decisions is extremely stressful for many parents, resulting in anxiety, insomnia, disturbances of appetite, and irritability (Patenaude et al. 1979; Pfefferbaum et al. 1977).

Children are also involved in the decision to pursue treatment. In the case of procedures that are experimental, children as young as 7 years of age must give informed assent to the procedure. Consequently, the child must be informed of the risks and side effects of treatment and sign a paper agreeing to undergo the treatment (Thurber et al. 1992). Significant conflicts, with resulting stress, occur when parents do not want their children informed of the risks of a procedure or when pediatric patients and their parents disagree about pursuit of a particular line of treatment. Although the law is clear about the necessity of a pediatric patient's informed assent to a procedure, there is considerable controversy about the impact of this policy (Holder 1985). Pediatric studies have demonstrated that open communication and honesty between parent and child lead to better psychological outcome for the critically ill child (Fergusson 1976; Spinetta and Deasy-Spinetta 1981; Stehbens and Lascari 1974). Pediatricians generally seek to respect their patient's growing capacity for involvement and choices (King and Cross 1989). However, children's responsivity to suggestion (Hilgard and LeBaron 1984) and the growing belief in the lay press and some portions of the medical community that negative emotions hamper recovery (Cousins 1979; Simonton et al. 1992) lead some pediatricians to conclude that there should be little emphasis on pain or death in presenting a treatment plan.

Disagreement between patient and family about treatment decisions is likely to produce stress responses in all parties. It is clear that a mentally competent 18-year-old can legally make an autonomous decision regarding a particular line of treatment, and that parents legally make the decision for younger children. However, the relative contribution of children under age 18 to the decision making varies widely. Determinants of how much input the child has include the child's age and temperament and the family style of decision making. Clinical experience leads many pediatricians to give significant weight to the preferences of adolescents, knowing that the patient's cooperation and commitment during and after the procedure will influence the outcome of the treatment. Patients who are actively opposed to undergoing a lengthy, invasive treatment often do not do well, both physically and psychiatrically (Leikin 1989).

While the decisions involved in innovative care are often difficult, encountering the lack of choice inherent in randomization to specific treatment protocols is also a source of stress for parents and children. The enormous advances in pediatric care have been achieved by conducting repeated comparisons between the current standard care and promising new protocols. The new alternatives vary in terms of components such as medications, length of treatment, or intensity of treatment. Often these alternatives appear promising but need evaluation as to whether they actually represent an improvement over what is currently considered the treatment of choice. Patients and families are asked to allow themselves to be randomly assigned to one of the types of treatment. The difficulty for most families in understanding the rationale for randomization is not simply unfamiliarity with scientific method but discomfort in accepting that the doctors genuinely do not know which alternative is best. Parents uncomfortable with this lack of control often decide to arbitrarily choose one treatment protocol, rather than to let random chance determine something that is potentially so important. This has become a significant enough problem that it is being researched by a national cancer study group (Children Cancer Group Study 1993).

The Setting

University hospitals, where most innovative pediatric therapies are offered, have the triple task of providing treatment, training medical personnel, and discovering new ways of thinking about or treating disease. Although these tasks are designed to be complementary, prioritizing these tasks inevitably creates occasional conflict. The choice of an innovative treatment generally requires that families leave their familiar pediatrician and begin dealing with multiple teams in an unfamiliar hierarchy. A child may be examined by more than 3 individuals at the time of admission and be seen by as many as four teams of 2 to 15 persons daily. Doctors rotate on and off service at intervals, creating a need for the patient and family to develop new relationships and leading to confusion over the different approaches of the new persons. Knowing that the person performing an invasive procedure is a student, under supervision, can increase the stress response of the child and family, as can the suspicion that something is being done more for the benefit of the doctor's research than for the patient's clinical well-being.

Physicians working in hospitals that pride themselves on being state of the art must frequently make decisions about attempting something that has not been done before. The motivations for such decisions are complex (see Stuber and Reed 1991) but spring partially from the belief that technology exists to respond to almost any situation if the clinician is sufficiently skilled and innovative to choose and apply the appropriate technology. This attitude, while obviously useful in fostering hope and encouraging new treatment approaches, can also increase the stress experienced by patients and families who have chosen to pursue aggressive treatment. Once a decision has been made to pursue cure, it is difficult to determine the point at which one may wish to change the goal to comfort or dignity. As a particular type of treatment moves from experimental to standard care, the medical personnel often become less invested in aggressive innovation and are more able to assist the families in determining the points at which they can reassess their initial decision to pursue aggressive treatment.

Recent examples of dilemmas concerning use of available technology include the use of organs from anencephalic donors for infants (Holzgreve et al. 1987) and the use of reduced size or partial livers for small children (Broelsch et al. 1990). Both approaches were designed to provide alternatives for the 10% to 20% of children who die while waiting for a suitable organ donor (United Network for Organ Sharing, personal communication, 1990). Use of partial lungs from related donors is just being pioneered. The use of organs from anencephalic donors has temporarily been discontinued, because the neurology of the newborn with anencephaly precludes the use of a brain-death definition until after the internal organs are no longer viable for transplantation. The use of partial livers has advanced from an experimental procedure to the option of using hepatic lobes from living related donors. These adult relatives (usually parents) undergo a partial hepatectomy. The lobe removed is surgically altered to function as an intact liver for the pediatric recipient (Broelsch et al. 1990). Because the liver regenerates, the liver in both the donor and recipient grow and provide all necessary functions. There appear to be no disadvantages of this procedure for the recipient. The donor, however, undergoes a major surgical procedure, with its attendant morbidity and potential mortality. Although reducing the stress of the powerless wait for a donor organ, the availability of this new option creates a number of potential stressors. How is a family to decide whether to subject a family member to such a procedure? If there are multiple potentially suitable donors in a family, how is one chosen? What practical problems are raised by having one parent recovering postoperatively while the other parent or other family members care for the patient and other needs of the family? None of these questions are entirely new, as similar stresses are inherent in living–related kidney donation (Simmons et al. 1977). The major difference is the availability of alternative technologies for prolonging the life of the child with renal failure (i.e., hemodialysis or peritoneal dialysis). Although dialysis does not eliminate the need to consider various transplant options for the child with renal failure, it reduces the urgency of the decision-making process. Additionally, because living–related donation of kidneys is a well-established procedure, the uncertainty inherent in deciding about procedures is reduced.

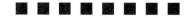

The acute stresses of the new innovative treatments for life-threatening pediatric illness are significant. Studies in the pediatric and trauma literature provide an understanding of expected symptoms and suggestions for reducing stress responses. In the remainder of this chapter we examine the long-term impact of these new procedures.

Long-Term Stress Associated With Pediatric Medical Interventions

As we mentioned in the opening of this chapter, the stress produced by pediatric interventions does not end with the conclusion of treatment. Successful treatment, although life-saving, does not result in "cure" in the sense in which most families interpret the word. Cure implies wellness or the absence of disease. For the majority of pediatric patients and their families, continued medical care will be necessary. Although the demands are almost always less intense and problematic than those that were placed on the patient before the intervention, children may be prescribed medications taken several times daily for life and there may be the necessity for periodic intrusive procedures (e.g., heart biopsies) and for alterations of daily habits, such as diet (Zitelli et al. 1987). Each medical intervention provides regular reminders of the original illness and treatment, and some interventions (e.g., heart biopsies) are potentially traumatic in their own right.

In addition to the continued medical care, many children have specific residual medical problems as a consequence of the underlying illness or the life-saving treatment (Li and Stone 1976; Simmons et al. 1977; Zitelli et al. 1987). Graft-versus-host disease, cardiac complication of antibiotics, and pulmonary fibrosis secondary to radiation are life-altering and sometimes life-threatening sequelae of aggressive treatment. An increased risk of second malignancies in children who have received intensive oncologic treatment and accelerated graft atherosclerotic disease in the coronary vessels of heart transplant recipients mean that, however much they may wish to forget, survivors must be watchful. Rather than experiencing a return to normalcy, most pediatric survivors of life-threatening illness have won continued life at the price of both short-term acute trauma and long-term chronic medical problems.

Medical and psychological sequelae have been extensively investigated for pediatric cancer survivors (Holmes and Holmes 1985; Koocher and O'Malley 1981; Li and Stone 1976; Mulhern et al. 1989; Wasserman et al. 1987); children undergoing kidney (Simmons et al. 1977), bone marrow (Stuber et al. 1991b), liver (Stewart et al. 1989), or heart transplants (Bailey et al. 1989); and survivors of serious burns (Stoddard et al. 1989) or neonatal intensive care (Cohen et al. 1982, 1986). Most of the early studies examined global adjustment and found that the majority of survivors did not manifest major psychiatric problems. However, clinicians noted that the subset with difficulties was large (e.g., 47% of the Koocher and O'Malley [1981] sample of cancer survivors reported adjustment problems).

Psychological problems were initially seen as responses to the medical sequelae of the illnesses and treatment. The focus of long-term follow-up clinics became "late effects," or the long-term medical consequences, of toxic treatments. Neuropsychiatric outcome was carefully monitored, as it became apparent that cognitive deficits were directly related to the amount of radiation administered to the head (Mulhern et al. 1992). However, research with a number of types of illness survivors has found that medical and psychological outcomes are not necessarily correlated. The actual severity or type of illness was not the best predictor of the psychiatric outcome for preterm infants, for pediatric cancer survivors, or for adolescents with serious burns. More important contributors were home environment, in the case of preterm infants (Cohen et al. 1982, 1986); parental attitude, in the case of cancer survivors (Fritz et al. 1988); and peer support, in the case of adolescent burn survivors (Orr et al. 1989). In an assessment of 38 families 6 months postpediatric liver transplant, Kennard and co-workers (1990) found that those with the most successful adaptation to the transplant had intact marriages, private insurance coverage, less subjective financial stress, and children with higher intellectual and developmental functioning. Post-transplant complications were most frequently found in single-parent families who had no preevaluation involvement with liver transplant organizations and whose child had lengthy postoperative hospital stays (Kennard et al. 1990).

One of the most perplexing and dangerous responses to the stress of continued medical needs is nonadherence to recommended treatment. Failure to take immunosuppressive drugs as prescribed is the major reason for failure of kidney transplants, especially in adolescents (Didlake et al. 1988; Ettinger et al. 1991; Korsch et al. 1978). There are many specific reasons for this common behavior, but the central focus appears to be a judgment by the patient that the benefits of adherence are not worth the price. This price may be measured in terms of medical consequences of adherence, such as hirsutism on cyclosporin, or truncal obesity on steroids. Other children are seeking to avoid the daily reminders of their brush with death, or the way in which they will never quite be "normal." Discontinuation of immuno-suppression for an organ transplant recipient threatens the survival of the transplanted organ and of the recipient, particularly organs for which backup technology such as dialysis does not exist. Nonadher-ence is so prevalent among adolescents that some transplant teams have considered making adolescence a relative contraindication for organ transplantation (Stuber 1993).

To understand this seemingly self-destructive behavior, it is again useful to consider the stress response model. If indeed a child has been traumatized by the life-threatening illness and/or the intrusive treatment, further medical procedures, clinic visits, or even medica-tions may serve as traumatic reminders, reawakening anxiety and arousal symptoms or triggering avoidance and numbing. Rather than becoming accustomed to medical interventions, these children expe-rience traumatic stress symptoms whenever they are exposed to re-minders, far beyond the acute phase of treatment.

There is evidence to suggest that survivors of pediatric life-threat-ening illnesses do experience posttraumatic stress symptoms even years after the end of the intensive phase of treatment. Using struc-tured interviews (Diagnostic Interview for Children and Adolescents, Child and Parent Versions), Stoddard and co-workers (1989) evaluated 30 children and adolescents ages 7 to 19 who had been severely burned a number of years previously (approximately half had been burned at age 2 or younger). At the time of interview, 6.7% met the criteria for PTSD, and 30% met the criteria for having had PTSD some-time in their lives. Overanxious disorder was diagnosed in 30% (33% lifetime), phobias in 47% (both current and lifetime), and major de-pression in 3% (27% lifetime).

It could be argued that burns constitute a trauma more than ill-nesses such as cancer because they are the result of external, violent assaults on body integrity. However, even more striking results have been noted in several recent studies of pediatric cancer patients. Six children who were evaluated before and 3, 6, and 12 months after bone marrow transplantation reported mild to moderate symptoms of posttraumatic stress up to a year after the bone marrow transplantation. The highest number of symptoms were reported at 3 months after the bone marrow transplantation. Severity then decreased but did not return to the pretransplantation levels within the year. Two of the children met the criteria for PTSD at 3 months post-transplant (Stuber et al. 1991a, 1991b). Similar symptoms were noted in pediatric bone marrow transplantation survivors in England (M. L. Stuber, K. Nader, B. M. Houskamp, R. S. Pynoos, unpublished manuscript, 1990). Preliminary results of an ongoing study found that of 61 childhood cancer survivors, 39% met the criteria for PTSD by self-report 2 to 12 years after concluding successful treatment (Kazak et al. 1992). The presence and severity of symptoms were not related to the time since treatment ended. Very similar findings were reported by Alter and co-workers (1992) and by Pelcovitz and Kaplan (1992) in a study done as part of the DSM-IV field trials. In this study, approximately one-third of 25 adolescent cancer survivors met the criteria for a PTSD diagnosis.

Parents of pediatric cancer survivors also report symptoms of posttraumatic stress. In the Kazak et al. (1992) study, 37% of the mothers ($n = 63$) and 26% of the fathers ($n = 46$) reported having symptoms consistent with severe posttraumatic stress; 25% of the mothers and 24% of the fathers met the criteria for a diagnosis of PTSD. The DSM-IV field trials reported a current PTSD prevalence of 30% in the mothers of 25 adolescent cancer survivors. Although stress responses in parents during the acute phase of treatment have been widely observed and documented in clinical papers (Patenaude et al. 1979; Pfefferbaum et al. 1977), these are the first studies to look specifically at long-term stress responses.

An anecdotal case illustrates this point. Unaware of any research on parental stress response to organ transplantation, a mother of a liver transplant recipient did her own literature search to investigate the symptoms she was experiencing. She then wrote to her gastroenterologist:

> I believe PTSD is an important component within the larger dynamic of psychological issues surrounding pediatric organ transplantation. In recalling my own experiences and that of my family,

as well as recounting numerous informal conversations with other transplant parents, it became obvious to me that many parents were displaying symptoms of PTSD. (N. D. Sullivan, personal communication, 1992)

These studies suggest that the intensive treatment and life threat experienced by children (and, by proxy, their parents) may be experienced as a traumatic, rather than merely stress-producing, event and result not only in acute stress responses (which have been well documented) but posttraumatic stress symptoms. Broadening "criterion A," or the definition of a traumatic event, for a PTSD diagnosis is not supported by all researchers in the field (March 1993; McNally 1993). The recent data from studies of pediatric cancer survivors require duplication with larger numbers of subjects and with other medical populations. However, the posttraumatic stress model has clear heuristic value in understanding certain behaviors of survivors and parents, such as the nonadherence discussed earlier in this chapter. We know from the trauma literature that traumatized individuals are likely to demonstrate avoidance of traumatic reminders and hypervigilance for danger. One might expect survivors to show avoidance of medical personnel or hypervigilance for medical problems, resulting in either under- or overutilization of medical services. Either mode of coping has potentially serious consequences for health care delivery for a population known to be at risk, as well as for the survivor's physical and psychological well-being.

A post-trauma model would also lead to the hypothesis that survivors of intensive pediatric interventions for life-threatening illness would experience alterations in psychological development. Developmental psychopathology has been described in traumatized children, with the severity of pathology related to characteristics of the child and the family, as well as of the trauma itself (Pynoos 1993). Alterations in developing personalities that have been suggested to occur as a result of trauma include diminished expectations for the future (including a sense of shortened life expectancy), dissociative disturbances, disturbances in attachment, and inability to regulate boundaries between self and other (James 1989; Pynoos and Nader 1993; Terr 1990). Evidence of dissociative symptoms in childhood cancer survivors in a range similar to that found in survivors of childhood sexual abuse was found in a study of 8- to 18-year-olds currently 2 to 12 years off treatment and in whom there was no evidence of disease

(Kasiraj 1992). The DSM-IV field trials found that over 25% of adolescent cancer survivors and their mothers reported difficulties in sexual functioning, feelings of despair and hopelessness, and somatic complaints (Pelcovitz and Kaplan 1992). Such findings have obvious implications for the long-term care of pediatric patients who have been exposed to potentially traumatic illness or treatment.

The post-trauma model also provides a new perspective on existing data on survivors of life-threatening pediatric illness and intensive treatment. For example, among the criteria for PTSD is difficulty remembering or concentrating. Saigh's studies with traumatized children suggest that children who meet the criteria for PTSD may also have clinically significant learning disabilities (Saigh 1992). Intellectual impairment following cancer treatment has long been recognized and has been attributed to intensity of toxic treatment regimens (Ochs et al. 1991). Similarly, pediatric liver transplant recipients are recognized as having some learning difficulties, which are considered minimal when compared with their pretransplant mental states (Zitelli et al. 1988). Application of a trauma model suggests that children who have had a posttraumatic stress response to their illness and treatment might have concentration and memory problems that are secondary to the psychological stress and that may prove additive to the biological toxic response.

In summary, stress responses are not limited to the acute phase of treatment for life-threatening medical conditions. Continuing medical interventions and residual medical complications can present ongoing sources of stress for survivors and their families. In addition, there is evidence that a significant number of children experience the illness and treatment as traumatic and develop posttraumatic stress symptoms. A post-trauma model raises questions about personality development and learning difficulties for survivors traumatized by life-threatening illness and/or invasive treatment.

Interventions

Psychological interventions for pediatric patients with life-threatening illness have been multiple and varied. As mentioned earlier in this chapter, relatively simple and effective interventions for children undergoing the acute stress of treatment have included touch, hypnosis, distraction, and parent training. In some cases the actual treatment has been changed, as when the schedule for procedures done in the neonatal intensive care unit is consolidated. Most pediatric inpatient units now have play facilities for children, allow parents 24-hour visitation, and employ child development specialists to provide preparation for procedures and opportunities for distraction. Many pediatric centers employ consulting psychiatrists or psychologists. These are all fairly recent innovations in pediatric care.

Psychological interventions offered after the acute phase of treatment, however, are rare. The common advice to parents and children has been to follow medical advice but otherwise try to live "normally" and forget that all this ever happened. Eager to restore some sense of order to their lives, and wishing to normalize their child's development, parents embrace this advice.

However appropriate it might be for some, achieving "normalcy" by forgetting is not a realistic goal for all pediatric survivors and their families. Recent studies strongly suggest that there are some children and parents who are traumatized by their experience and who have ongoing difficulties. The data are not yet available, however, to tease out which aspect constitutes the traumatic event. There is some suggestion that perception of severity of life threat is a predictor of severity of symptoms ($r = .42$, $P < .02$ for a group of 34 children awaiting bone marrow transplantation) (M. L. Stuber, K. Nader, B. M. Houskamp, R. S. Pynoos, unpublished manuscript, 1990). It is not yet clear whether the child's perception may be primarily an indirect measure of the actual intensity of the treatment or the life threat, or an independent factor.

Clarification of the traumatic event has important implications for intervention because pediatric treatment need not be traumatic. When a combination of established, effective interventions to reduce acute stress responses and carefully considered protocols designed to eliminate all unessential sources of acute stress is used, treatment-related trauma could be significantly diminished. The unavoidable sources of stress, such as the life-threat of the underlying illness, could be approached psychotherapeutically immediately and over time, rather than ignored once the acute episode is past.

There is a precedent for having psychological outcome influence both acute and long-term treatment for life-threatening pediatric illness. The almost miraculous improvement in survival for pediatric leukemia is the result of intensive cytotoxic treatment, including chemotherapy and radiation. Continued follow-up of early survivors revealed that children were manifesting learning disabilities 2 to 4 years after treatment. Initially the learning disabilities were attributed to prolonged school absences or indulgent parents, but careful studies revealed a correlation between intensity of cranial irradiation and degree of impairment. Two types of intervention were instituted: 1) children who had undergone cranial irradiation were followed with neuropsychological evaluations and provided with appropriate tutoring as indicated, and 2) protocols were devised to examine whether the amount of cranial irradiation could be decreased without decreasing the efficacy of the treatment (Ochs et al. 1991). If the consequences of a specific intervention are significantly negative, that intervention must be evaluated as to whether the benefit outweighs the cost.

Summary

The trauma model has the potential to supply the conceptual framework needed to apply what is known about reducing acute stress responses in children undergoing aggressive medical treatment. Interventions based on such a model would also serve to prevent clinically significant long-term post-trauma responses. Much further study is needed to clarify specific predictors of stress response and individual differences in response. Working with children who have survived life-threatening illness offers an exciting opportunity to effect primary as well as secondary prevention of stress in a group of high-risk children and families, as well as to gain further understanding of the importance of temperament and coping in children.

References

Alter CL, Pelcovitz D, Axelrod A, et al: The identification of PTSD in cancer survivors. Paper presented at the annual meeting of the Academy of Psychosomatic Medicine, San Diego, CA, October 1992

American Psychiatric Association: Diagnostic and Statistical Manual of Mental Disorders, 4th Edition. Washington, DC, American Psychiatric Association, 1994

Anders TF, Sachar EJ, Kream J, et al: Behavioral state with plasma cortisol response in human newborn. Pediatrics 46:532–537, 1970

Bailey LL, Wood M, Rassork A, et al: Heart transplantation during the first 12 years of life. Arch Surg 124:1221–1226, 1989

Blount R, Sturges J, Powers S, et al: Adult's influence on children's coping and distress during painful medical procedures. Behavior Therapy 20:585–601, 1989

Boyce WT, Jemerin JM: Psychobiological differences in childhood stress response, I: patterns of illness and susceptibility. J Dev Behav Pediatr 11:86–94, 1990

Briere J, Evans D, Runtz M, et al: Symptomatology in men who were molested as children: a comparison study. Am J Orthopsychiatry 58:457–461, 1988

Broelsch CE, Whitington PF, Emond JC: Evolution and future perspectives for reduced size hepatic transplantation. Surg Gynecol Obstet 171:353–360, 1990

Burstein S, Meichenbaum D: The work of worrying in children undergoing surgery. J Abnorm Child Psychol 7;121–132, 1979

Chang I: Baby girl's bone marrow transplanted into sister. Los Angeles Times, 1991

Children's Cancer Group Study (Wiley FM, Study Chairman), Protocol Number 9-891, 1993

Cohen SE, Sigman M, Parmelee AH, et al: Perinatal risk and developmental outcome in preterm infants. Semin Perinatol 6:334–339, 1982

Cohen SE, Parmelee AH, Beckwith L, et al: Cognitive development in preterm infants: birth to eight years. J Dev Behav Pediatr 7:102–110, 1986

Cousins N: Anatomy of an Illness as Perceived by the Patient. New York, WW Norton, 1979

Dahlquist LM, Gil KM, Armstrong D, et al: Behavioral management of children's distress during chemotherapy. J Behav Ther Exp Psychiatry 16:325–329, 1985

Didlake RHJ, Dreyfus K, Kerman RH, et al: Patient noncompliance: a major cause of late graft failure in cyclosporin-treated renal patients. Transplant Proc 20:63–69, 1988

Escalona SK, Corman MH: Early life experiences and the development of competence. International Review of Psycho-Analysis 1–2:151–168, 1974

Ettinger RB, Rosenthal JT, Mark JL, et al: Improved cadaveric renal transplant outcome in children. Pediatr Nephrol 5:137–142, 1991

Fergusson JH: Later psychologic effects of a serious illness in childhood. Nurs Clin North Am 11:83–93, 1976

Field T: Alleviating stress in the NICU neonate. J Am Osteopath Assoc 87:646–650, 1987

Field T, Goldston E: Pacifying effects of nonnutritive sucking on term and preterm neonates during heelstick procedures. Pediatrics 74:1012–1015, 1984

Field T, Schanberg S, Scafidi F, et al: Tactile/kinesthetic stimulation effects on preterm neonates. Pediatrics 77:654–658, 1986

Field T, Alpert B, Vega-Lahr N, et al: Hospitalization stress in children: sensitizer and repressor coping styles. Health Psychol 7:433–445, 1988

Foy D, Carroll E, Donahue C: Etiological factors in the development of PTSD in clinical samples of Vietnam combat veterans. J Consult Clin Psychol 43:17–27, 1987

Franck L: A new method to quantitatively describe pain behavior in infants. Nurs Res 35:28–31, 1986

Friedrich WN: Psychotherapy of Sexually Abused Children and Their Families. New York, WW Norton, 1990

Fritz G, Williams J, Amylon M: After treatment ends: psychosocial sequelae in pediatric cancer survivors. Am J Orthopsychiatry 58:552–561, 1988

Grunau RVE, Craig KD: Pain expression in neonates: facial action and cry. Pain 28:395–410, 1987

Gunnar M, Connors J, Isensee J, et al: Adrenocortical activity and behavioral distress in newborns. Dev Psychobiol 21:297–310, 1988

Hilgard JR, LeBaron S: Hypnotherapy of Pain in Children With Cancer. Los Altos, CA, William Kaurmann, 1984

Holder AR: Legal Issues in Pediatric and Adolescent Medicine. New Haven, CT, Yale University Press, 1985

Holmes H, Holmes F: After ten years, what are the handicaps and life styles of children treated for cancer? Clin Pediatr (Phila) 14:819–823, 1985

Holzgreve W, Beller FK, Bucholz B, et al: Kidney transplantation from anencephalic donors. N Engl J Med 316:1069–1070, 1987

Horowitz MJ, Kaltreider MD: Brief therapy of the stress response syndrome. Psychiatr Clin North Am 2:365–377, 1979

James B: Treating Traumatized Children. Lexington, MA, Lexington Books, 1989

Jay S: The effects of gentle human touch on mechanically ventilated very short gestation infants. Matern Child Nurs J 11:199–256, 1982

Jay S, Elliott CH: A stress inoculation program for parents whose children are undergoing painful medical procedures. J Consult Clin Psychol 58:799–804, 1990

Jay SM, Ozolins M, Elliott CH, et al: Assessment of children's distress during painful medical procedures. Health Psychol 2:133–147, 1983

Jay SM, Elliott CH, Olson R, et al: Behavioral management of children's distress during painful medical procedures. Behav Res Ther 23:513–520, 1985

Jay SM, Elliott CH, Katz E, et al: Cognitive-behavioral and pharmacologic interventions for children's distress during painful medical procedures. J Consult Clin Psychol 55:860–865, 1987

Jay SM, Elliott CM, Woody P, et al: An investigation of cognitive behavior therapy combined with oral Valium for children undergoing painful medical procedures. Health Psychol 10:317–322, 1991

Kaplan DM, Smith A, Grobstein R, et al: Family mediation of stress. Soc Work 18:60–69, 1973

Kasiraj JM: Predicting residual trauma symptoms in child and adolescent cancer survivors. Unpublished doctoral dissertation, California School of Professional Psychology, Fresno, CA, 1992

Katz ER, Kellerman J, Siegel SE: Behavioral distress in children with cancer undergoing medical procedures: developmental considerations. J Consult Clin Psychol 48:356–365, 1980

Katz ER, Kellerman J, Ellenberg L: Hypnosis in the reduction of acute pain and distress in children with cancer. J Pediatr Psychol 12:379–394, 1987

Kazak A, Stuber M, Torchinsky M, et al: Childhood cancer survivors and parents: anxiety after treatment ends. Paper presented at the annual meeting of the American Psychological Association, Washington, DC, August 1992

Kennard BD, Petrik K, Stewart SM, et al: Identifying factors in postoperative successful adaptation to pediatric liver transplantation. Soc Work Health Care 15:19–33, 1990

King NMP, Cross AW: Children as decision makers: guidelines for pediatricians. J Pediatr 115:10–16, 1989

Knight RB, Atkins A, Eagle C, et al: Psychological stress, ego defenses, and cortisol production in children hospitalized for elective surgery. Psychosom Med 1:40–90, 1979

Koocher G, O'Malley J: The Damocles Syndrome. New York, McGraw-Hill, 1981

Korsch BM, Fine RN, Negrete VF: Noncompliance in children with renal transplants. Pediatrics 61:872–876, 1978

Kübler-Ross E: On Death and Dying. New York, Macmillan, 1969

Kübler-Ross E: On Children and Death. New York, Macmillan, 1983

Leikin S: A proposal concerning decisions to forgo life-sustaining treatment for young people. J Pediatr 115:17–22, 1989

Li F, Stone R: Survivors of cancer in childhood. Ann Intern Med 84:551–553, 1976

Long J, Alistair G, Philip AGS, et al: Excessive handling as a cause of hypoxemia. Pediatrics 65:203–207, 1980

Lyons JA: Posttraumatic stress disorder in children and adolescents: a review of the literature. J Dev Behav Pediatr 8:349–356, 1987

Manne SL, Redd WH, Jacobsen PB, et al: Behavioral intervention to reduce child and parent distress during venipuncture. J Consult Clin Psychol 38:565–572, 1990

March JS: What constitutes a stressor? The "Criterion A" issue, in Posttraumatic Stress Disorder: DSM-IV and Beyond. Edited by Davidson JRT, Foa EB. Washington, DC, American Psychiatric Press, 1993, pp 37–54

McNally RJ: Stressors that produce posttraumatic stress disorder in children, in Posttraumatic Stress Disorder: DSM-IV and Beyond. Edited by Davidson JRT, Foa EB. Washington, DC, American Psychiatric Press, 1993, pp 57–74

Melamed BG, Ridley-Johnson R: Psychological preparation of families for hospitalization. J Dev Behav Pediatr 9:96–101, 1988

Miller SM: To see or not to see: cognitive informational styles in the coping process, in Learned Resourcefulness: On Coping Skills, Self-Regulation and Adaptive Behavior. Edited by Rosenbaum M. New York, Springer, 1990, pp 95–126

Miller SM, Combs L, Stoddard E: Information, coping, and control in patients undergoing surgery and stressful medical procedures, in Stress, Personal Control and Health. Edited by Steptoe A, Appels AD. Chichester, UK, Wiley, 1989, pp 107–129

Mulhern RK, Wasserman AL, Friedman AG, et al: Social competence and behavioral adjustment of children who are long-term survivors of cancer. Pediatrics 83:18–25, 1989

Mulhern RK, Fairclough D, Ochs J: Deterioration of intellect among children surviving leukemia: IQ test changes modify estimates of treatment toxicity. J Consult Clin Psychol 60:477–480, 1992

Nader K, Pynoos RS, Fairbanks LA, et al: Childhood PTSD reactions one year after a sniper attack. Am J Psychiatry 147:1526–1530, 1990

Nader K, Stuber M, Pynoos RS: Posttraumatic stress reactions in pre-school children with catastrophic illness: assessment needs. Comprehensive Mental Health Care 1:223–239, 1991

Nir Y: Post-traumatic stress disorder in children with cancer, in Post-Traumatic Stress Disorder in Children. Edited by Eth S, Pynoos RS. Washington, DC, American Psychiatric Press, 1985, pp 121–132

Ochs J, Mulhern RK, Fairclough D, et al: Comparison of neuropsychologic functioning and clinical indicators of neurotoxicity in long-term survivors of childhood leukemia given cranial radiation or parenteral methotrexate: a prospective study. J Clin Oncol 9:145–151, 1991

Onufrak EJ: Effect of coping style and quality of previous medical experience on children's response to hospital information. Unpublished master's thesis, University of Florida, Gainesville, 1989

Orr DA, Reznikoff M, Sith GM: Body image, self-esteem, and depression in burn-injured adolescents and young adults. J Burn Care Rehabil 10:454–461, 1989

Patenaude AC, Szymanski L, Rappeport J: Psychological costs of bone marrow transplantation in children. Am J Orthopsychiatry 49:403–422, 1979

Pelcovitz D, Kaplan S: Disorders of extreme stress and PTSD in cancer survivors. Paper presented at the annual meeting of the International Society for Traumatic Stress Studies, Los Angeles, CA, November 1992

Pfefferbaum B, Lindamood M, Wiley FM: Pediatric bone marrow transplantation: psychosocial aspects. Am J Psychiatry 134:11–15, 1977

Pot-Mees C: The Psychosocial Effects of Bone Marrow Transplantation in Children. The Netherlands, CW Delft, 1989

Pui C, Rivera GK: Childhood leukemias, in American Cancer Society Textbook of Clinical Oncology. Edited by Holleb AI, Fink DJ, Murphy GP. Atlanta, GA, American Cancer Society, 1991, pp 433–452

Pynoos RS: Traumatic stress and developmental psychopathology in children and adolescents, in The American Psychiatric Press Review of Psychiatry, Vol 12. Edited by Oldham JM, Riba MB, Tasman A. Washington, DC, American Psychiatric Press, 1993, pp 205–238

Pynoos RS, Nader K: Issues in the treatment of post-traumatic stress in children and adolescents, in The International Handbook of Traumatic Stress Syndromes. Edited by Wilson JP, Raphael B. New York, Plenum, 1993, pp 535–549

Pynoos RS, Frederick C, Nader K, et al: Life threat and posttraumatic stress in school-age children. Arch Gen Psychiatry 44:1057–1063, 1987

Redd WH, Porterfield A, Andersen B: Behavior Modification. New York, Random House, 1979

Routh DK, Sanfilippo MD: Helping children cope with painful medical procedures, in Children in Pain: Clinical and Research Issues From a Developmental Perspective. Edited by Bush JP, Harkins SW. New York, Springer-Verlag, 1991

Rovet JF, Ehrlich RM: Effect of temperament on metabolic control in children with diabetes mellitus. Diabetes Care 11:77–82, 1988

Ruccione K, Krame RF, Moore LK, et al: Informed consent for treatment of childhood cancer: factors affecting parents' decision making. J Ped Onc Nurs 8:112–121, 1991

Saigh P: PTSD in children. Workshop presented at the annual meeting of the International Society for Traumatic Stress Studies, Los Angeles, CA, October 1992

Scafidi F, Field T, Schanberg S, et al: Massage stimulates growth in preterm infants: a replication. Infant Behavior and Development 13:167–188, 1990

Siegel L: Therapeutic modeling as a procedure to reduce the stress associated with medical and dental treatment. Paper presented at the annual meeting of the Association for the Advancement of Behavior Therapy, Atlanta GA, December 1977

Simmons RG, Klein SD, Simmons RL: The Gift of Life: The Psychological and Social Impact of Organ Transplantation. New York, Wiley, 1977

Simonton OC, Henson R, Hampton B: The Healing Journey. New York, Bantam Books, 1992

Spinetta JJ, Deasy-Spinetta P (eds): Living With Childhood Cancer. St Louis, MO, CV Mosby, 1981

Stehbens JA, Lascari AD: Psychological follow-up of families with childhood leukemia. J Clin Psychiatry 30:394–397, 1974

Stewart SM, Vavy R, Waller D, et al: Mental and motor development, social competence, and growth one year after successful pediatric liver transplantation. J Pediatr 114:574–581, 1989

Stoddard FJ, Norman DK, Murphy JM, et al: Psychiatric outcome of burned children and adolescents. J Am Acad Child Adolesc Psychiatry 28:589–595, 1989

Stolberg S: Historic living transplant draws a mixed reaction. Los Angeles Times, February 11, 1993, A1

Stuber ML: Psychologic care of adolescents undergoing transplantation, in Textbook of Adolescent Medicine. Edited by McAnarney ET, Kriepe RD, Orr DP, et al. Philadelphia, PA, WB Saunders, 1993, pp 1138–1142

Stuber ML, Reed G: Never been done before: consultative issues in innovative therapies. Gen Hosp Psychiatry 13:337–343, 1991

Stuber ML, Davidson RB, Nader K, et al: Long-term impact of pediatric transplantation. Paper presented at the annual meeting of the American Psychiatric Association, New Orleans, LA, May 1991a

Stuber ML, Nader K, Yasuda P, et al: Stress responses following pediatric bone marrow transplantation: preliminary results of a prospective, longitudinal study. J Am Acad Child Adolesc Psychiatry 30:952–957, 1991b

Terr LC: Psychic trauma in children: observations following the Chowchilla school-bus kidnapping. Am J Psychiatry 138:14–19, 1981

Terr LC: Too Scared To Cry: Psychic Trauma in Childhood. New York, Harper & Row, 1990

Thurber FW, Deatrick JA, Grey M: Children's participation in research: their right to consent. Journal of Pediatric Nursing 7(June):165–170, 1992

Wasserman A, Thompson E, Williams J, et al: The psychological status of survivors of childhood/adolescent Hodgkins disease. Am J Dis Child 141:626–631, 1987

Zeltzer L, LeBaron S: Hypnosis and nonhypnotic techniques for reduction of pain and anxiety during painful procedures in children and adolescents with cancer. J Pediatr 101:1032–1035, 1982

Zitelli BJ, Gartner JC, Malatack JJ, et al: Pediatric liver transplantation: patient evaluation and selection, infectious complications and life-style after transplantation. Transplant Proc 19:3309–3316, 1987

Zitelli BJ, Miller JW, Gartner JC, et al: Changes in life-style after liver transplantation. Pediatrics 82:173–180, 1988

Chapter 10

The Intense Stress of Childhood Cancer: A Systems Perspective

Anne E. Kazak, Ph.D.
Dimitri A. Christakis, M.D.

During the family meeting of a child who has been newly diagnosed with cancer, the health care team empathically imparts the clear message: Your child has cancer, and without treatment, your child will die. With treatment, while there is no promise of long-term survival, there is reason to remain hopeful. Most parents have vivid memories of the day when they were told their child's diagnosis, and many identify it as the worst day of their lives. It is undeniably the point at which an unexpected severe stressor enters their family and world, and its multiple reverberations continue throughout their child's treatment, and potentially much longer. In this chapter we discuss the stressors associated with the diagnosis and treatment of cancer, for children and families. A better understanding of the stresses of cancer, one of the most traumatic experiences that can impinge on childhood, may enhance understanding of intense childhood stress generally.

Pediatric cancers are increasingly treatable conditions, with survival rates among children with these cancers as high as 65%. Accordingly, what was once an acute disease ending in death is now a stressful chronic process replete with toxic treatments, painful procedures, hospitalizations, long-term sequelae, and lingering fears of recurrence. Changes in prognosis and medical interventions limit the applicability of much of the earlier literature, which focused heavily upon cancer as a terminal disease. Indeed, more recent research addresses issues of quality of life during and after treatment. Unfortunately, a conceptual understanding of the stresses of childhood cancer and their implications for psychological interventions has received little attention.

The effects of these stressors transcend the boundary of the family and include interactions with medical and educational systems. Our orientation is guided by family systems and social ecological theories. In this chapter we discuss stressful aspects of pediatric cancer across these systems. We also present, from family and systems perspectives, findings from research and interventions for understanding and ameliorating the stress.

Family and Systems Approaches to Serious Childhood Illness

Consideration of children in the context of the family is basic to the practice of pediatrics. Pediatric patients rarely come unaccompanied to a physician and usually cannot give informed consent for treatment. These patients' levels of development may hamper their comprehension of diseases and treatments. They usually must rely upon adults to provide medical care, particularly when it is intense, long-term, and complex. The relevant caregiving system for an ill child is broader than the family. Ideally, children and their families have a relationship with the pediatrician who provides their care. This enables the practitioner to appreciate the impact of disease-related stressors as experienced by the patients and to understand the resources that are available to help the patients cope with these stressors.

Although this optimal relationship may be attainable for routine health problems, serious pediatric conditions such as cancer often require referrals to outside, distant, tertiary-care facilities. Therefore, care is frequently received away from a family's relatives and the familiar health care setting, and in the absence of community support. At the tertiary-care facility, the family meet medical, nursing, and psychosocial staff who are unaware of the family's history but yet will be intensely involved with them as they struggle with diagnosis and treatment.

Pediatric tertiary-care cancer centers usually have a strong family orientation. But there are ways in which the reality of the highly technological and aggressive treatments may compromise a family-centered approach and increase the inherent stress of the situation.

First, the distance between the pediatric oncology center and a family's home may present obstacles to comprehensive family-based interventions. The logistics of travel and accommodations away from home necessarily increase the disruption to family routine during treatment and heighten concerns about siblings at home.

Second, despite the presence of diverse psychosocial resources at tertiary-care centers, children and families often feel isolated. Feelings of isolation can arise when children are at the center separated from families and friends at home. Alternatively, as they become increasingly connected with the center, children can feel isolated at home, away from the expertise of their health care team.

Third, the most intense emphasis in care for a child with cancer is on the acute stages of illness and treatment, and tertiary-care facilities often maintain less contact with the family as their child's disease stabilizes or remits. Longer-term concerns (particularly with respect to psychological impact on the child and the family) can receive appreciably less attention. In particular, the message that life can (or should) return to "normal" when treatment ends may indirectly invalidate psychological reactions to the treatment experience that may be beginning to surface.

Fourth, while the family is probably the single most important context for the ill child, other systems (e.g., schools, hospital) have an impact on the child's and the family's adjustment and are often overlooked. The ways in which families and community systems interact with one another to ensure continuity of medical, educational, and psychosocial care should be a focus of professionals in the communities to which these children and families return.

We emphasize these four points to highlight the need for mental health services for children with cancer and their families to be provided throughout the course of treatment and to be focused not only on the affected children but also on their families and the broader systems in which they are embedded. Ultimately, many chronic medical and psychosocial needs of seriously ill children and their families must be addressed within local communities together with tertiary-care facilities. These aspects of family interventions for pediatric cancer patients receive little attention in the literature. McDaniel and co-workers (1992) have provided excellent illustrations of ways of treating families with medical problems and a careful and insightful balance of family and system dynamics in their work. However, there have been few efforts to link family, hospital, and community in providing psychosocial care for children with serious life-threatening chronic disease.

Social Ecology

Social ecology (Bronfenbrenner 1979) provides a useful model for understanding the ways in which childhood cancer reciprocally impacts on individuals and systems internal and external to the family (Kazak 1989; Kazak and Nachman 1991). The child is typically considered at the center of nested concentric spheres of influence (Figure 10–1).

Social Ecological Levels of Analysis

The Microsystem

The *microsystem* is the "patterns of activities, roles, and interpersonal relations experienced by the developing person" in the context of the immediate family. The social ecological model thereby emphasizes the importance of individual development and the implications of developmental processes for coping and adapting. The disease itself, because it places particular demands on a child and family, is part of the microsystem. "Putting the illness in its place" and treating it as a present, although unwelcome, force has been suggested as a coping strategy (Gonzalez et al. 1989).

Within the microsystem, one can examine parent-child interactions and the development of sibling bonds. These are areas of inherent interest in families with ill children. Understanding parent-child or sibling interactions explains ways in which these families are both similar to and different from families without ill children.

The microsystem is also the level of analysis utilized by most empirical research on childhood chronic illness. The impact of childhood illness on families, and on mothers and fathers specifically, has been addressed in research, although few conclusions can be drawn from this literature.

The Mesosystem

The *mesosystem* comprises interrelated microsystems. For children, at the mesosystemic level of analysis, one explores the relationships between families and schools or families and hospitals. Although these relationships are prominent for any child or family, families with a chronically ill child often have particular educational needs that accentuate the importance of family/school relationships. Moreover, the chronically ill child and family members have long-term relationships with the health care team that change with the nature and demands of treatment.

Many professionals interact with chronically ill children and their families (Figure 10–1). The density of individuals and systems within the mesosystem conveys the large number of professionals active in the lives of children with special health care needs. One important

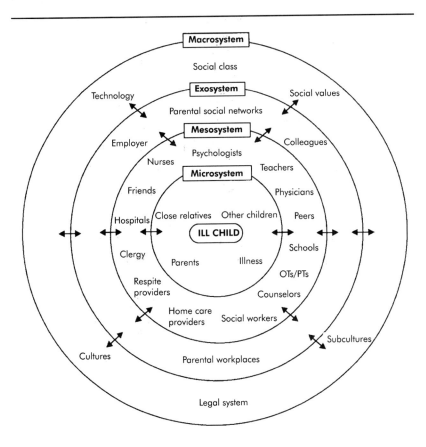

Figure 10–1. A social ecological model of pediatric oncology. OTs = occupational therapists; PTs = physical therapists.

system of professionals, often overlooked in the literature, is composed of home-care providers. The increasing use of highly technical home care (e.g., intravenous antibiotics and chemotherapies) has made these professionals an important adjunct system for the child and family.

Implicitly important in consideration of mesosystems are the values, beliefs, and policies that guide interactions with the ill child and the family. Health care providers must examine their own attitudes about illness and death, their assumptions about particular coping strategies (e.g., Is denial an adaptive coping style?), and the extent to which their own families of origin and experiences shape their professional identities and behaviors.

Moreover, it is interesting and informative to reflect upon the values, beliefs, and resultant policies that are supported in particular cultures at different points in time. For example, whereas it was once considered inappropriate to tell a child that he or she has cancer, open communication (after first consulting with parents) is now standard practice. Similarly, many services provided today for children with special health care needs are guided by a family-centered model, advocated by the Association for the Care of Children's Health (ACCH) and other groups. Bolstering programs that support families, this model reflects the current gestalt of our health care and social services systems. It reveals a circularity and return to the ethos of home- and family-centered human services.

The Exosystem

The *exosystem* is an environment that does not affect the child directly but has profound indirect effects. Typically, research in this area has considered the impact of parental social networks and employment on children. Given the importance of caregiving for chronically ill children and the fact that the vast majority of caregiving is provided by parents, understanding the social context in which parents function is critical. For example, the extent to which family and friends are supportive of caregiving demands impacts the child and family. Similarly, health care needs of children with cancer can demand parental absences from work. The extent to which parental employers are flexible in this respect may affect the child indirectly through increased or decreased parental stress associated with work.

The Macrosystem

Finally, at the outermost level, is the *macrosystem,* that is, the impact of subculture, culture, and general belief patterns on the entire system. The values of our society, and the attitudes toward persons with disabilities particularly as they are manifested in laws and policies, must be evaluated in a thorough and thoughtful understanding of caregivers. The ways in which caregiving is valued or devalued may affect caregivers' self-concept and the nature of the care that is ultimately provided. A lack of supportive local, state, and federal policies and services (e.g., education, transportation) can have direct effects on caregiving styles and the level of stress that caregivers face.

Other Social Ecological Components

Other important components of social ecological theory include reciprocity and the importance of change in the natural progression of development. Emphasizing the interactive rather than the linear nature of development and relationships, *reciprocity* is a cornerstone of contextual theory. Children's temperament and the nature of their illness impact on their caregivers just as caregivers' style and resources impact on their interactions with their children. Transitions are critical as well and can be either expected or unexpected. Developmentally expected (e.g., starting school, leaving school) and unexpected (e.g., accidents, recurrence of illness) transitions affect families and warrant further attention.

Microsystems

The Disease

Pediatric cancer itself is a broad and diverse diagnostic category including illnesses with different peak ages of incidence, treatments, prognosis, and medical sequelae. Moreover, the stage of therapy itself can be a critical variable. Many studies of pediatric cancer survivors' adjustment include children with different diseases and at different points in treatment (e.g., in active therapy, in early remission, or many years out of treatment). The stressors faced at each phase are different. Therefore, study results based on small heterogeneous samples must be interpreted conservatively.

There are many types of pediatric cancers, with broad variability

Table 10–1. Summary of some pediatric cancers and treatment alternatives for children younger than 15 years of age

Type of cancer	Annual incidence (per million)	Five-year survival	Chemotherapy	Radiotherapy	Surgery	BMT	Treatment length (months)
Acute lympho-blastic leukemia	30–50	65%	X	(X)		(X)	24–36
Acute myelogenous leukemia	5	25%	X			(X)	6–12
Hodgkin's disease	8	60%–85%	X	(X)	(X)	(X)	6–12
Non-Hodgkin's lymphoma	7	70%	X	(X)	(X)	(X)	6–18
Osteosarcoma	2–3	50%	X		X		3–5
Brain and nervous system cancer	25	58%	X	X	X		4–12
Rhabdomyosarcoma	4	47%	X	(X)	(X)		6–18
Wilms' tumor	7	83%	X	(X)	(X)		3–15
Retinoblastoma	3	90%	(X)	(X)	X		1–8
Neuroblastoma	8	50%	(X)	(X)	(X)	(X)	1–6
Ewing's sarcoma	3	64%	X	X	X	(X)	12

Note.   X = always part of therapy; (X) = can be part of therapy depending on patient's disease and its course. BMT = bone marrow transplantation.

Source.   United States incidence/survival data from the National Cancer Institute (compiled by the SEER Program).

in disease and treatment (Table 10–1). Families face different prognoses, treatments, toxicities, and treatment lengths. Despite the variability in rates of long-term survival, it is dangerous to characterize cancers as "good" or "bad" to patients and parents. There are no "good" cancers, and individual children die even from those cancers associated with the best overall survival rates. For all pediatric cancers, learning to live with these uncertainties, on top of the illness and treatment demands, is one of the most challenging aspects of the stress of childhood cancer (Comaroff and Maguire 1981). Conceptually, chronic health problems in children can be explored noncategorically or specifically. A "noncategorical" approach to the stresses of chronic illness emphasizes commonalities across conditions (Stein and Jessop 1982). Although it is important to identify common stressors and coping strategies across illnesses, efforts to delineate parameters of illnesses that may affect coping and adjustment are also critical.

Rolland (1984, 1987) has proposed a model for understanding psychosocial characteristics of illnesses. The four dimensions outlined are onset, course, outcome, and degree of incapacitation. Similarly, Jacobs (1992) has outlined five aspects of illness in terms of the impact on the family: unpredictability, disability, stigma, monitoring, and uncertainty in prognosis.

Each of these characteristics has implications specifically related to the stress to systems of a child with cancer. The disease itself carries a unique stigma. Unlike some other childhood diseases, cancer also affects adults. For many adults, cancer in children can jar fears they harbor about their own health.

Furthermore, cancer diagnosis and treatment proceed in phases. During the *acute phase*, immediately after diagnosis, parents confront the possibility of losing a previously healthy child. Then, during the *toxic treatment phase*, parents and children must cope with the stress of procedures, chemotherapy, and hospitalizations. Finally, there is *a prolonged period of medical uncertainty* after treatment has ended when parents and children grapple with the possibility of relapse. Even in the absence of relapse, sequelae of treatment (such as learning difficulties, growth abnormalities, or organ damage from treatment) may be unfolding, each associated with its own uncertainty and stressors. Unlike other serious childhood medical conditions (e.g., mental retardation, cystic fibrosis, diabetes, AIDS) in which there are no "cures" and a more predictable course can be expected (even if it includes death), pediatric cancer follows an often unpredictable course. Affording no assurances while offering prospects of death or cure, pediatric cancer has stressors that change with time.

The particular course of a child's cancer evokes other stressors throughout the system. For example, in a family with a terminally ill child, stress may intensify with time. During this period caregivers must cope with their grief and loss while providing more intense care for the dying child. In contrast, children whose cancer follows a more stable course may demand a steadier level of caregiving and require family reorganization, but major changes and emotional upheaval are not anticipated.

The Ill Child

Although a higher incidence of psychiatric problems has been reported in children with chronic diseases (see Cadman et al. 1987), psychiatric disturbances are not inevitable. Children with chronic health conditions can be considered "at risk" for psychological difficulties. Much remains to be understood in terms of identifying child and family predictors of psychological outcome, given the risk factor of illness.

Despite the potential differences in the impact that different illnesses and treatments have on children, examination of the relationship between illness severity in childhood chronic illness and adjustment yields inconsistent data. Some investigators have found an association between the degree of children's disabilities and their psychiatric problems (Cadman et al. 1987; Daniels et al. 1987; Steinhausen et al. 1983), whereas others have found none (Breslau 1985; Wallander et al. 1989).

Much of the research seeking to correlate severity of illness with degree of psychiatric disturbance has examined children with disabilities and not necessarily those facing death. Although it might be expected that children experiencing the stress of a life-threatening illness would experience feelings of sadness and depression, research using standardized paper-and-pencil measures of depression in children with cancer and survivors report extremely low rates of depression (Greenberg et al. 1989; Kaplan et al. 1987; Worchel et al. 1988). These low levels of depression have been interpreted primarily in three ways: 1) resilience, coping skills, and support may eradicate depression; 2) depression may be denied; and 3) methodological difficulties of self-report scales preclude obtaining accurate data on the types of depression experienced by children with cancer. Indeed, in an interview study, Kashani and Hakami (1982) reported that 17% of their sample of children with cancer met DSM-III criteria for a major depressive episode.

Consideration of anxiety in children with cancer has been limited primarily to situational anxiety related to invasive medical procedures and to chemotherapy-related nausea and vomiting (Jay et al. 1983; Zeltzer and LeBaron 1982; Zeltzer et al. 1984). As with depression, there is evidence that generalized anxiety may be denied (Fife et al. 1987). Akin to depression is the strong possibility that methodologically rigorous and relevant research examining aspects of anxiety related to treatment, for the child and the entire family, is lacking in the literature.

There has been an increase in the amount of research on survival and the psychological ramifications of survival (generally of leukemia), paralleling the increase in the number of children who survive childhood cancer. We review, below, the earlier psychological data on survival. In a later section of this chapter we discuss other emerging models for understanding the impact of survival and identify areas for further research.

The best described individual psychological implications of survival are declines in intellectual ability related to cranial irradiation. At the dose of 24 Gy, clear effects on short-term memory, attention, and cognitive processing have been identified (cf. Eiser 1991; Meadows et al. 1981; Pfefferbaum-Levine et al. 1984). To balance survival with psychological morbidity (IQ decline), radiation doses have been reduced when no compromise in efficacy has been documented. The impact of lower doses (18 Gy) on intellectual ability is less, although specific learning deficits are being identified (Mulhern et al. 1988, 1991). The effects of other treatments, such as methotrexate, on later cognitive functioning are also being described (Ochs et al. 1992). Detailed discussions of methodological complications in this literature can be found in Madan-Swain and Brown (1991).

The first psychological study on social and emotional adjustment after childhood cancer, *The Damocles Syndrome* (Koocher and O'Malley 1981), continues to be one of the best known. Over the following decade a group of studies on long-term survivors were published (Fritz et al. 1988; Greenberg et al. 1989; Kazak and Meadows 1989; Mulhern et al. 1989; Spirito et al. 1990). These reports were generally of survivors of leukemia or Hodgkin's disease, tended to include a wide age range, and were based on self-report scales assessing adjustment and/or psychopathology. These studies presented overall normative levels of adjustment for long-term survivors. There is also consistent evidence that a significant subset of this population has psychological difficulties that cannot be fully understood from the measures that were employed in these studies.

Siblings

Serious illness and its treatment have many direct effects on siblings. Whereas parents frequently worry about the impact of their child's illness on their other children, investigators have focused relatively little research and clinical attention on siblings. Early studies looked at responses to the death of a sibling and focused on serious psychiatric or behavioral disorders as evidence of maladjustment. Literature on siblings across a range of medical conditions has shown these individuals to be at risk for adjustment problems, although more recent studies have called such conclusions into question. Furthermore, current studies have addressed differential effects of age and sex of the siblings. For example, Bristol and co-workers (1988) studied the effects of developmental disability in male children on adaptation and family roles of both parents. These authors noted that fathers of disabled children assumed less responsibility for child care than comparison fathers even in mother-employed families and, more important, that this decrease in child involvement was specific to the disabled children and not their siblings. In a study of 25 preschoolage siblings of children with cancer and a matched group of comparison families, Horwitz and Kazak (1990) examined the ways in which mothers viewed siblings as similar to or different from the ill child. Mothers of children with cancer were more likely to view the sibling similarly to the way they viewed the child with cancer than were comparison mothers, who rated their two well children.

The Family

Concern for the parents and family of the child with cancer is longstanding, based in part on the strong tradition of social work in pediatric oncology and, before improvement in prognoses, the necessity of preparing families for the death of their child. The existing empirical literature on family adjustment to childhood cancer provides use-

ful data. However, refinements in methodology and careful consideration of methodological and developmental issues are important
emerging trends (see Kazak and Nachman 1991).

Kupst and her colleagues have reported on a longitudinal study of
childhood cancer that substantiates the notion that positive long-
term adjustment can be predicted (Kupst and Schulman 1988; Kupst
et al. 1982, 1984). In this study, adjustment was related to social support, marital satisfaction, fewer concurrent stressors, and open communication. All these factors parallel clinical experiences with
families.

One of the most important questions concerning family adaptation has to do with the course of adjustment over time. Several research groups have confirmed that the most intense levels of parental
distress are at time of diagnosis, with a gradual decrease over the first
year of treatment (Fife et al. 1987; Kupst et al. 1982, 1984). Although
these findings endorse clinical experiences with respect to coping
with stress (i.e., cancer), important questions remain. The range of
adaptation in coping with chronic childhood illness is broad (see
Kazak 1989). Differentiation of predictors of more and less positive
adaptation is needed. The small sample sizes and the heterogeneity of
disease types in previous research also hinder our understanding of
potentially important variables such as age and severity (e.g., staging,
type of treatment) on the course of family adjustment. Indeed, the
course of illness is unpredictable and often seems idiosyncratic, with
events occurring that can change the nature of the experience. In
a later section of this chapter we discuss some of these additional
stressors.

A strong, early tradition in research on family adjustment to
chronic illness has been the comparison of families with and without
an affected child. This design serves an important function but also
has some unintended effects and potential complications. To select
measures that are applicable to both groups, one often cannot ask
important questions about the very experience of interest (the illness!). More general measures of either adjustment or psychopathology may fail to identify important aspects of family experience that
may have little to do with psychopathology. Furthermore, use of comparison groups usually is accompanied by hypotheses that predict that
families with a child with a chronic medical condition will often exhibit more pathology than the comparison families. Although reasonable methodologically, this orientation may promote a deficit

orientation. Finding no differences between groups translates to a failure to reject the null hypothesis and may be viewed as unreportable or uninteresting because the null hypothesis could not be rejected. A recent group of studies supporting findings of "no differences" between target and control groups in this field highlights the importance of examining positive coping strategies and a competency-based approach in research.

Mesosystems

Peers

In a study comparing children with cancer with a carefully matched sample of healthy peers, on the basis of teacher ratings, the children with cancer were more isolated and were perceived as having less leadership potential than their peers (Noll et al. 1990). This finding itself substantiates parents' concerns that knowledge of their child's illness will adversely affect the perception and treatment of their child at school. Peers' reactions to knowledge of the child's illness are troubling because they lead some parents to withhold information regarding their child's illness from schools and thereby hamper the requisite open communication between family and school systems. Thorough and thoughtful consideration of peer issues for chronically ill children can be found in the discussion by Spirito and co-workers (1991).

Schools

Serious illness disrupts children's participation in routine school activities, with potentially disruptive effects on academic achievement and social development. Besides increased school absence during serious illnesses such as cancer, the child is often physically different upon return (e.g., without hair, weaker). The resultant short-term issues around successful return to school have been addressed quite comprehensively (Kazak and Meadows 1989). However, other educational concerns remain less well understood.

For example, the ways in which schools as systems interact with families and hospitals over time in terms of addressing the short- and long-term educational needs of patients often remain problematic. Many children cured of cancer have long-term medical and psychological sequelae that may not be well understood. In one study, children who had had leukemia that had been treated with 24 Gy were achieving at an average of two grade levels below the grade level typical for their age, with particular difficulties in math and reading (Peckham et al. 1988). Special education placements and retention in a grade were common. Other questions regarding rather subtle aspects of learning problems in children who received cranial irradiation (even at relatively low doses) may arise several years after treatment ends.

Parents and schools need collaborative partnerships in assessing difficulties, determining if problems may be related to treatment, and charting an educational program. Thus, learning problems and educational progress and placement can be considered long-term stressors that accumulate on top of the initial stressors associated with diagnosis and treatment. Interventions must be guided by an appreciation of the entire range of stressors faced by long-term survivors.

The Health Care System

The ways in which health care systems interface with family systems have been largely unexplored. Social ecological and general systems models predict that as a family with a child with cancer joins these larger systems, components of these systems will affect one another. Research has looked at unidirectional aspects of these systems, such as what parents think or feel about medical care (Chesler and Barbarin 1984; Mulhern et al. 1981; Patno et al. 1988), but has not addressed these issues over time or described attributes of the systems themselves. Although research in this area is difficult to conduct, there are conceptualizations that can be useful in looking at similarities and fit between systems (see Schwartzman and Kneifel 1985).

Surprisingly, data on linkages between pediatric and mental health care systems and professionals point to a general lack of referral of children and families for mental health services, despite understanding of the potential for psychological difficulties related to childhood illnesses (Sabbeth and Stein 1990; Weiland et al. 1992). Although mental health professionals in pediatric cancer centers offer a great deal of diverse assistance to families, much of their work is directed at crisis intervention, and many significant mental health needs may go unnoticed. As the focus during cancer treatment narrows (to treat the cancer successfully), other problematic psychosocial concerns may not be expressed by patients and families. Much work remains to enhance mental health utilization for these families.

There are some issues that have been described primarily at the level of the individual child or family that can be understood as broader systems concerns. For example, compliance with treatment can be thought of as reflecting, in part, the fit between the family and the health care system (Kazak and Rostain 1989) and encompasses more obvious family interactions that can influence compliance. Thinking about compliance in this way allows for consideration of ethnic differences and provokes examination of the fit among families, professionals, and settings.

Another practical treatment concern that has been investigated primarily at the level of the individual child is the pain and anxiety associated with invasive medical procedures during childhood cancer treatment. Behaviorally oriented interventions have proven effective in decreasing child distress. However, linkages between behavioral distress in a specific treatment situation (procedures) with family adaptation are just beginning to be acknowledged (Kazak et al. 1995). At levels beyond the family, clarification is needed concerning the ways in which multidisciplinary staff attitudes toward children's pain and associated interventions (both pharmacological and psychological) affect child behavior before, during, and after procedures.

Exosystems: Parental Social Support Networks

The people and places that children with cancer encounter clearly exert direct influence on their adjustment, but there are also many indirect influences that moderate or exacerbate their stress and can affect psychosocial outcomes of families. Prime among these are the social support networks and resources available to parents. Although the potential social isolation in families facing serious chronic illness has been long acknowledged, investigation of social support allows for a detailed understanding of the types of persons available to parents for support and of the ways in which help is provided.

Research that examines social support networks in families with and without children with disabilities suggests that differences in size of the networks are not apparent, although professionals (primarily members of the child's health care team) constitute a significant portion of the network (Kazak 1987; Quitner et al. 1990). Network characteristics such as density (the extent to which members of the network know and interact with one another) and the timing of support offered have been identified as important components of social support (Hobfoll and Lerman 1988; Kazak 1991).

Intervention at the level of parental social support networks is warranted in light of evidence that "the relationship between social relationships and health increasingly approximates the evidence in the 1964 Surgeon General's report that established cigarette smoking as a cause or risk factor for mortality and morbidity from a range of diseases" (House et al. 1988, p. 543). It is possible to enhance the provision of social support in many ways. Strengthening of relationships with extended family members, old friends, and new friends, and utilization of community resources are ways in which social support can be mobilized.

There are also personal characteristics of parents that warrant consideration. For example, some parents often feel unwilling to ask for help and feel uncomfortable about the imbalance that help seeking may create in relationships in which reciprocity is desired. Others are aware that social support can be both negative and positive and may shun available supports. Lane and Hobfoll (1992) have documented ways in which the anger that chronically ill adults experience affects, in turn, their relationships with sources of support. Parents' anger at support network members' discomfort about pediatric cancer is an overlooked factor in determining the level of support available in chronic childhood illness as well. Many parents accurately perceive the general discomfort that the public feels about children with cancer, but some may overlook the ways in which their own feelings and actions may make it difficult to receive support.

Course and Process of Childhood Cancer

Parents frequently ask for reassurance with respect to their child's and their own emotional reactions to the cancer with the question "Will things get better?" Assuring parents and children that, one way or another, they will cope with what is ahead reinforces the very important sense of hope. As noted earlier, the empirical literature on child and family adjustment to serious illness has focused on the identification of potential psychopathology. Other studies document a wide range of adaptation and support the notion that most families do well, despite severe stress and periods of distress, a finding consistent with clinical observation.

These points do not detract from an appreciation of the severe stress associated with childhood cancer and its treatment. Rather, they necessitate the development of different models for understanding the nature of the stressors associated with the diseases and their treatments. For example, from an empirical perspective, relatively little is actually known about predicting points of particular stress during (and after) treatment.

In the following subsections we discuss the stages of treatment and points that can be considered stressors over the course of childhood cancer. Stressors can be organized into two general categories. *Initial stressors* are those associated with the diagnosis and early stages of treatment (such as diagnostic procedures, learning of the diagnosis, and early treatment). These stressors, despite variability in diseases and in coping resources of patients and families, are experienced by *all* pediatric oncology patients. *Later stressors* are those that are less frequent and are specific to certain treatments or to particular outcomes of a disease and the corresponding treatment. These stressors are not experienced by all families of childhood cancer patients, although most families of these patients will experience some of these stressors. Later stressors include serious acute episodes, bone marrow transplantation, relapse, terminal care and death, and survival (cure) of childhood cancer.

Initial Stressors: Diagnosis and Treatment

One important way in which parents cope with the early stress is by putting faith in their physicians (Martinson and Cohen 1988). Initial stress in parents is derived in part from the loss of control that a life threat to their child poses. The medical team presents the only realistic hope of controlling this threat, and parents frequently (and understandably) invest tremendous faith and hope in them. There is often attendant guilt upon the initial diagnosis when parents fault themselves for missing or dismissing earlier signs of the disease. Often these feelings of guilt are persistent and can have an almost magical quality. For example, the father of a child who was several years into remission blamed the cancer on a wrist X-ray that he, the father, had had years earlier, after the child had been born.

One factor that is not given adequate consideration in research of familial responses to childhood cancer is the extent to which responses are affected by the premorbid psychological state of the individuals and the members of the system involved. Studies of individual and collective coping of necessity begin at the point of diagnosis. Obviously a prospective study of families with children who go on to develop cancer is impossible to design. Consequently, the premorbid condition of families under study is frequently assessed retrospectively. Such analysis is fraught with confounding factors. Moreover, often neglected are past familial encounters with illness or significant life stressors. Responses to the present crisis are surely mediated by responses to past ones.

Beyond the distress associated with diagnosis and the upheaval related to treatment in a tertiary-care hospital, the family of a newly diagnosed child frequently feels the accelerated pace that is characteristic of the hospital and inherent in the accompanying treatment decisions, including decisions about participating in clinical research studies. There is little time for reflection. Parents must quickly assume an active role in familiarizing themselves with the members of the health care team and their roles, the hospital systems, and the details of treatment (e.g., what medications are given when, and how it will be decided if they have efficacy). Simultaneously, parents must reorganize their families to care for other children and their jobs. These tasks must be accomplished while supporting the ill child and communicating the diagnosis and the imminent side effects of treatment.

Although there is minimal empirically based research to guide parents (and staff) in coping with some of these early stressors, the general tenets of individual and family assessment apply. Effective interventions often hinge on a balance of a problem-solving approach with one that supports and encourages ventilation of feelings. That is, the family must be helped to cope with the stressor(s) with which they are confronted, without allowing the enormity and anxiety of the situation to paralyze them. Validation of feelings and support for expressing the disbelief, sorrow, and anger that may emerge are helpful.

Many children with cancer experience some anxiety and/or pain during early stages of treatment, associated with procedures such as bone marrow aspirates, lumbar punctures, and chemotherapy. Behavioral interventions for procedural pain and anticipatory nausea and vomiting are among the most clearly efficacious treatments found in this literature (Jay and Elliott 1990; LeBaron and Zeltzer 1984). Although this commonly reported efficacy reflects in part the nature of behavioral interventions and the empirical evaluation built into the intervention, these approaches remain helpful ones that patients, parents, and staff can use.

Later Stressors: Ongoing Treatment and Its Sequelae

Serious acute episodes.   Serious acute episodes represent abrupt shifts in treatment and can be a source of tremendous emotional upheaval. The associated stressors range from the common (e.g., fever signaling infection coupled with neutropenia brought on by chemotherapy that requires immediate hospitalization for intravenous antibiotics) to the life-threatening (e.g., fulminating sepsis requiring admission to an intensive care unit [ICU]).

Research that assesses stress associated with specific episodes is limited. A study comparing levels of stress in mothers of previously healthy children admitted to the ICU with those in mothers of previously healthy children admitted to the general hospital found ICU admissions to be considerably more stressful than a general ward admission and capable of inducing anxiety, depression, and anger (Berenbaum and Hatcher 1992). For parents of children with cancer, the stress of an ICU or hospital admission can rekindle fears that their child could die. However, unlike the parents of previously healthy children in Berenbaum and Hatcher's study, parents of pediatric cancer patients have seen their children very sick and are familiar with both hospitals and intensive treatments. How these experiences affect their response to acute episodes is unknown. With their familiarity of the hospital, the stress of acute episodes may be mitigated. The prognosis, not the event itself, may guide their responses.

Bone marrow transplantation.   Bone marrow transplantation is an intense form of treatment for childhood cancer that has been used increasingly to enhance the chances of survival for children with specific types of cancer. In some ways, transplant treatments are similar to, but more intense than, more routine types of treatment. That is, chemotherapy protocols associated with bone marrow transplantation are very intense, radiation of the whole body is often necessary, and concerns about infection demand rigid control of the child's environment, including periods of isolation. As such, components of the transplantation experience are stressors much like other stressors associated with treatment for childhood cancer.

In other ways, however, transplantation may be a different type of stressor than are more routine types of treatment in that it is still often viewed as a "last chance" for survival, and the child has already undergone these more routine types of cancer treatment. Thus, transplantation requires the child and family to prepare for another round of treatment—one that is highly toxic and is associated with increased rates of mortality. In addition, siblings and parents may be screened to determine their suitability for donating marrow. There are many, largely unexplored, issues related to the donor's feelings associated with giving marrow and the eventual outcome of the child's disease (survival or death).

Many interventions with the child who is undergoing transplantation and his or her family are helpful, although much of the literature is based upon clinical evidence rather than empirical research. The intense stress experienced by the family has been described (Hare et al. 1989), as have difficulties in psychosocial adaptation after transplant (Freund and Siegel 1986) and compliance issues related to the intensified medication regimen (Phipps and DeCuir-Whalley 1990). Other data are beginning to appear that document the effects of total body irradiation with respect to learning ability (Kramer et al. 1992).

A promising model for understanding the psychological impact of intense stressors associated with childhood cancer is posttraumatic stress. Two studies have reported data on children within the first year after transplant that suggest high levels of symptoms consistent with a diagnosis of posttraumatic stress syndrome (Pot-Mees 1987; Stuber et al. 1991). Intense medical stressors are common traumatic events associated with life threat. The symptoms themselves provide opportunities for psychological intervention, and analyzing transplant and other medical stressors from this perspective is promising in terms of enhancing our knowledge of how children and families cope with intense stress in general.

Relapse.   Relapses, even those that are not likely to result in death, are extraordinarily difficult times for children and families. The stress of "starting over," usually with a more intense treatment protocol and with the odds for long-term survival reduced, can be overwhelming. Although familiarity with treatment and the hospital can be comforting, families of relapsed patients generally warrant higher levels of psychosocial support.

Terminal care and death.   It is no longer the case that all children with cancer die. However, as we can rightfully celebrate the increasing rates of survival from pediatric cancers, the anguish experienced by the many families who still must face their child's death cannot be neglected. Indeed, it may be all the more important to focus our energies on assisting patients with terminal illness and their families, because either path (survival or death) is common.

With relapse, or with multiple relapses, the child may reach a point at which the goal of treatment is no longer cure, but to assure quality of life over the course of terminal illness. Here the relationships among the patient, family, and health care team are paramount in terms of grappling with difficult issues regarding palliative chemotherapy, home care for terminally ill children, and discontinuation of life-sustaining treatment. Freyer (1992) has provided an articulate overview of the issues related to discontinuation of life-sustaining treatments that are specific to pediatric oncology, including consideration of the fact that the child can continue to live for an extended period while terminally ill.

Providing the child with a supportive environment and helping the family in communicating their love and support to the child are of critical importance as the child's death approaches. The family should be encouraged to discuss death and beliefs about afterlife in ways that are comfortable to them. Continued support to parents during these difficult times is important. Bolstering the survivors' feelings of competency, in terms of having done all that could be done, is key to their adjustment to the loss of the child.

It is beyond the scope of this chapter to discuss bereavement in detail. The stages of loss outlined by Kübler-Ross (1969) continue to guide much of the field, although the work of Wortman and Silver (1989) provides alternatives to a stage model and underscores unique aspects of grief for individuals.

Survival.   Stressors associated with childhood cancer do not end with the end of treatment. The implications of having had cancer continue, throughout the levels of the social ecological model, to impact on the patient and family. Ironically, the sense of ambiguity continues. There is an uncertainty even about defining "survival."

Medically, children are considered "cured" of a cancer if their remission lasts for at least 5 years. At this point, they can rightfully be considered "survivors" of childhood cancer. But what are we to call patients between the end of their treatment and that 5-year mile-stone? Are they survivors yet? And what of patients who live beyond the 5-year mark free of cancer but who still show cognitive or emotional effects of their treatments. Can their disease be considered cured? Increasingly, "surviving" cancer must be looked at as a lifelong process much like surviving incest or recovering from alcoholism. Cancer survivors and their parents see their lives as fundamentally changed by their experience.

A recent study of pediatric leukemia "survivors" ages 7 to 19 who had been off treatment for at least 2 years assessed implications of the experience using a posttraumatic stress model. The investigators found that 28% of children, 26% of their fathers, and 30% of their mothers manifested levels of posttraumatic stress that were considered to be in the "severe" range (Stuber et al., in press). Many of these individuals had symptomatology that would meet the DSM-III-R criteria for posttraumatic stress disorder (American Psychiatric Association 1987). The purpose of this preliminary and ongoing research is not to pathologize the patients or their responses to the illness; rather it is to develop a model by which we can better understand and hopefully relieve the stress of pediatric cancer diagnosis and treatment.

Unlike other stressful events capable of inducing posttraumatic stress disorder symptomatology in children (e.g., violence, abuse), the stressors of childhood cancer occur under relatively controlled and controllable conditions. This makes early interventions as well as later ones feasible. Longer-term psychosocial support extending well beyond the time of completion of treatment and perhaps even beyond the time of "medical cure" should be coupled with a better understanding of the effects of the "process" of treatment for cancer and its attendant stresses.

Conclusions

Cancer is one of the most stressful events that can affect children and families. The ways in which patients, families, and broader systems organize and function in response to the life threat of cancer provide valuable insight into coping with intense childhood stress. Childhood cancer imposes a series of stressors on children and families for which further research and development of clinical interventions are needed.

References

American Psychiatric Association: Diagnostic and Statistical Manual of Mental Disorders, 3rd Edition, Revised. Washington, DC, American Psychiatric Association, 1987

Berenbaum J, Hatcher J: Emotional distress of mothers of hospitalized children. J Pediatr Psychol 17:359–372, 1992

Breslau N: Psychiatric disorder in children with physical disabilities. Journal of the American Academy of Child Psychiatry 24:87–94, 1985

Bristol M, Gallagher J, Schopler E: Mothers and fathers of young developmentally disabled and nondisabled boys: adaptation and spousal support. Developmental Psychology 24:444–451, 1988

Bronfenbrenner U: The Ecology of Human Development. Cambridge, MA, Harvard University Press, 1979

Cadman D, Boyle M, Szatmari P, et al: Chronic illness, disabilities and mental and social well-being: findings of the Ontario Child Health Study. Pediatrics 79:805–813, 1987

Chesler M, Barbarin O: Relating to the medical staff: how parents of children with cancer see the issues. Health Soc Work 9:59–65, 1984

Comaroff J, Maguire P: Ambiguity and the search for meaning: childhood leukemia in the modern clinical context. Soc Sci Med 15:115–123, 1981

Daniels D, Miller JJ, Billings AG, et al: Psychosocial functioning of siblings of children with rheumatic disease. J Pediatr 109:379–383, 1987

Eiser C: Cognitive deficits in children treated for leukemia. Arch Dis Child 55:164–168, 1991

Fife B, Norton J, Groom J: The family's adaptation to childhood leukemia. Soc Sci Med 24:159–168, 1987

Freund B, Siegel K: Problems in transition following bone marrow transplantation: psychosocial aspects. Am J Orthopsychiatry 56:244–252, 1986

Freyer D: Children with cancer: special considerations in the discontinuation of life sustaining treatment. Med Pediatr Oncol 20:136–142, 1992

Fritz G, Williams J, Amylon M: After treatment ends: psychosocial sequelae in pediatric cancer survivors. Am J Orthopsychiatry 58:552–561, 1988

Gonzalez S, Steinglass P, Reiss D: Putting the illness in its place. Fam Process 28:69–87, 1989

Greenberg H, Kazak A, Meadows A: Psychological adjustment in 8- to 16-year-old cancer survivors and their parents. J Pediatr 114:488–493, 1989

Hare J, Skinner D, Kliewer D: Family systems approach to pediatric bone marrow transplantation. Children's Health Care 18:30–36, 1989

Hobfoll S, Lerman M: Personal relationships, personal attributes, and stress resilience: mothers' reactions to their child's illness. Am J Community Psychol 16:565–589, 1988

Horwitz W, Kazak A: Family adaptation to childhood cancer: sibling and family systems variables. Journal of Clinical Child Psychology 19:221–228, 1990

House J, Landis K, Umberson D: Social relationship and health. Science 241:540–545, 1988

Jacobs J: Understanding family factors that shape the impact of chronic illness, in Family Health Psychology. Edited by Akamatsu J, Stephens M, Hobfoll S, et al. Philadelphia, PA, Hemisphere, 1992, pp 111–128

Jay S, Elliott C: A stress inoculation program for parents whose children are undergoing painful medical procedures. J Consult Clin Psychol 58:799–804, 1990

Jay S, Ozolins M, Elliott C, et al: Assessment of children's distress during painful medical procedures. Health Psychol 2:133–147, 1983

Kaplan S, Busner J, Weinhold C, et al: Depressive symptoms in children and adolescents with cancer. J Am Acad Child Adolesc Psychiatry 26:782–787, 1987

Kashani J, Hakami N: Depression in children and adolescents with malignancy. Can J Psychiatry 27:474–477, 1982

Kazak A: Families with disabled children: stress and social networks in three samples. J Abnorm Child Psychol 15:137–146, 1987

Kazak A: Families of chronically ill children: a systems and social ecological model of adaptation and challenge. J Consult Clin Psychol 57:25–30, 1989

Kazak A: The social context of coping with childhood chronic illness: family systems and social support, in Advances in Pediatric Psychology: Stress and Coping With Pediatric Conditions. Edited by La-Greca A, Siegel L, Wallender J, et al. New York, Guilford, 1991, pp 263–278

Kazak A, Meadows A: Families of young adolescents who have survived cancer: social-emotional adjustment, adaptability, and social support. J Pediatr Psychol 14:175–191, 1989

Kazak A, Nachman G: Family research on childhood chronic illness: pediatric oncology as an example. Journal of Family Psychology 4:462–483, 1991

Kazak A, Rostain A: Systemic aspects of family compliance in childhood chronic illness. Newsletter of the Society of Pediatric Psychology 13:12–17, 1989

Kazak A, Boyer B, Brophy P, et al: Parental perception of procedure related distress and family adaptation in childhood leukemia. Children's Health Care 24:143–158, 1995

Koocher G, O'Malley J: The Damocles Syndrome. New York, McGraw-Hill, 1981

Kramer J, Crittenden M, Halberg F, et al: A prospective study of cognitive functioning following low dose cranial radiation for bone marrow transplantation. Pediatrics 90:447–450, 1992

Kübler-Ross E: On Death and Dying. New York, Macmillan, 1969

Kupst M, Schulman J: Long-term coping with pediatric leukemia: a six-year followup study. J Pediatr Psychol 13:7–22, 1988

Kupst M, Schulman J, Honig G, et al: Family coping with leukemia: one year after diagnosis. J Pediatr Psychol 7:157–174, 1982

Kupst M, Schulman J, Mauer J, et al: Coping with pediatric leukemia: a two-year followup. J Pediatr Psychol 9:149–163, 1984

Lane C, Hobfoll S: How loss affects anger and alienates potential supporters. J Consult Clin Psychol 60:935–942, 1992

LeBaron S, Zeltzer L: Assessment of acute pain and anxiety in children and adolescents by self report, observer reports and a behavior checklist. J Consult Clin Psychol 52:729–738, 1984

Madan-Swain A, Brown R: Cognitive and psychosocial sequelae for children with acute lymphocytic leukemia and their families. Clinical Psychology Review 11:267–294, 1991

Martinson IM, Cohen MH: Themes from a longitudinal study of family reaction to childhood cancer. Journal of Psychosocial Oncology 6:81–98 1988

McDaniel S, Hepworth J, Doherty W: Medical Family Therapy: A Biopsychosocial Approach to Families with Health Problems. New York, Basic Books, 1992

Meadows A, Gordon J, Massari D, et al: Declines in IQ scores and cognitive dysfunctions in children with acute lymphocytic leukemia treated with cranial irradiation. Lancet 2:1015–1016, 1981

Mulhern R, Crisco J, Camitta B: Patterns of communication among pediatric patients with leukemia, parents, and physicians: prognostic disagreements and misunderstandings. J Pediatr 99:480–483, 1981

Mulhern R, Wasserman A, Fairclough D, et al: Memory function in disease free survivors of acute lymphocytic leukemia given CNS prophylaxis with or without 1800 cGy cranial irradiation. J Clin Oncol 6:315–320, 1988

Mulhern R, Wasserman A, Friedman A, et al: Social competence and behavioral adjustment of children who are long-term survivors of cancer. Pediatrics 83:18–25, 1989

Mulhern R, Fairclough D, Ochs J: A prospective comparison of neuropsychologic performance of children surviving leukemia who receive 18 Gy, 24 Gy, or no cranial irradiation. J Clin Oncol 9:1348–1356, 1991

Noll R, Bukowski W, Rogosch F, et al: Social interactions between children with cancer and their peers: teacher ratings. J Pediatr Psychol 15:43–56, 1990

Ochs J, Mulhern R, Fairclough D, et al: Comparison of neuropsychologic functioning and clinical indicators of neurotoxicity in long-term survivors of childhood leukemia given cranial irradiation or parenteral methotrexate: a prospective study. J Clin Oncol 9:145–151, 1992

Patno K, Young P, Dickerman J: Parental attitudes about confidentiality in a pediatric oncology clinic. Pediatrics 81:296–300, 1988

Peckham VC, Meadows AT, Bartel N, et al: Educational late effects in long-term survivors of childhood acute lymphocytic leukemia. Pediatrics 81:127–133, 1988

Pfefferbaum-Levine B, Copeland D, Fletcher J, et al: Neuropsychological assessment of long-term survivors of childhood leukemia. Am J Pediatr Hematol Oncol 6:123–128, 1984

Phipps S, DeCuir-Whalley S: Adherence issues in pediatric bone marrow transplantation. J Pediatr Psychol 15:459–475, 1990

Pot-Mees C: Beating the burn-out. Nursing Times 83:33–35, 1987

Quitner A, Glueckauf R, Jackson D: Chronic parenting stress: moderating versus mediating effects of social support. J Pers Soc Psychol 59:1266–1278, 1990

Rolland J: Towards a psychosocial typology of chronic and life threatening illness. Family Systems Medicine 2:245–262, 1984

Rolland J: Chronic illness and the life cycle: a conceptual framework. Fam Process 26:203–221, 1987

Sabbeth B, Stein R: Mental health referral: a weak link in comprehensive care of children with chronic physical illness. J Dev Behav Pediatr 11:73–78, 1990

Schwartzman H, Kneifel A: Familiar institutions: how the child care system replicates family patterns, in Families and Other Systems. Edited by Schwartzman J. New York, Guilford, 1985, pp 87–107

Spirito A, Stark L, Cobiella C, et al: Social adjustment of children successfully treated for cancer. J Pediatr Psychol 15:359–371, 1990

Spirito A, DeLawyer D, Stark L: Peer relations and social adjustment of chronically ill children and adolescents. Clinical Psychology Review 11:539–564, 1991

Stein J, Jessop D: A noncategorical approach to childhood chronic illness. Public Health Rep 97:354–362, 1982

Steinhausen H, Schindler H, Stephan H: Correlates of psychopathology in sick children: an empirical model. Journal of the American Academy of Child Psychiatry 22:559–564, 1983

Stuber M, Nader K, Yasuda P, et al: Stress responses after pediatric bone marrow transplantation: preliminary results of a prospective longitudinal study. J Am Acad Child Adolesc Psychiatry 30:952–957, 1991

Stuber M, Christakis DA, Houskamp B, et al: Posttraumatic stress in childhood cancer survivors. Psychosomatics (in press)

Wallander J, Feldman W, Varni J: Physical status of psychosocial adjustment in children with spina bifida. J Pediatr Psychol 14:89–102, 1989

Weiland S, Pless I, Roghamann K: Chronic illness and mental health problems in pediatric practice: results from a survey of primary care providers. Pediatrics 89:445–449, 1992

Worchel F, Nolan B, Willson V: Assessment of depression in children with cancer. J Pediatr Psychol 13:101–112, 1988

Wortman C, Silver R: The myths of coping with loss. J Consult Clin Psychol 57:349–357, 1989

Zeltzer L, LeBaron S: Hypnosis and nonhypnotic techniques for reduction of pain and anxiety during painful procedures in children and adolescents with cancer. J Pediatr 101:1032–1035, 1982

Zeltzer L, LeBaron S, Zeltzer P: The effectiveness of behavioral intervention for reduction of nausea and vomiting in children and adolescents receiving chemotherapy. J Clin Oncol 2:683–690, 1984

Chapter 11

Coping With Chronic Medical Illness: Lessons From Working With Children and Adolescents With Diabetes Mellitus

William T. Garrison, Ph.D.

D iabetes mellitus is one of the more prevalent chronic diseases in childhood, with estimates ranging from 1.2 to 2.0 per 1,000 persons. Epidemiological surveys in the United States indicate that up to 1 per 600–800 children of school age are affected by diabetes mellitus, with a resulting prevalence of 166 per 100,000 school-age children (Gortmaker and Sappenfield 1984; Kohrman et al. 1987). It has also been estimated that nearly 100,000 new cases are diagnosed each year in the U.S. Diagnosis of the disease is more common as children near adolescence, though there appears to be a smaller peak incidence point between 5 and 6 years of age.

The disease is more common in Caucasian populations than in minority groups. Males and females are affected in similar proportions. Little evidence exists that might suggest a socioeconomic effect in observed prevalence rates of the disease, though there has been suggestion in a number of empirical studies that sociodemographic factors interact to affect rates of psychological and compliance problems that can, in turn, create difficulties in the successful management of the disease (Anderson et al. 1990; Gavin and Goodwin 1990; Hanson et al. 1987).

Diabetes is a lifelong physical condition that has the potential to shorten the life expectancy of affected individuals. The daily regimen required for good control of the disease requires blood glucose monitoring, regular administration of insulin at the proper dose, attention to diet, and regular exercise. Failure to adhere to the regimen, and resulting poor glycemic control over time, have been linked with significantly reduced longevity in adult patients with diabetes.

A portion of those persons diagnosed with the disease are known to present with a difficult-to-manage profile that may be at least partially physiological in origin, giving rise to their being described as so-called brittle diabetic patients. The majority of patients with poor metabolic control, however, have been viewed as being in relative noncompliance with the medical and lifestyle regimen required for control of the disease.

The range and types of psychologically related problems seen in juvenile diabetes include denial of the disease or of its seriousness by the child or parents, noncompliance with medical prescriptions regarding the disease regimen, poor adjustment as evidenced by new onset or exacerbation of behavioral or emotional problems, and potential interference with normal developmental progress and family milieu. Less obvious problems can include the child's learning to use deception as a coping mechanism in his or her dealings with adult authority figures, a child's evolving sense of alienation from peers unaffected by the disease, delayed social maturation, subtle learning and neuropsychological problems, increased family conflict related to disease management, and an inability to comprehend known associations across behavioral compliance, disease control during the childhood period, and serious medical complications that can arise during adulthood.

The primary interventions for children with diabetes and their parents in medical settings have been largely *educational* in nature (Court 1991). Where available, systematic training of child and parents about diabetes care is typically provided immediately following clinical diagnosis. In more specialized medical care of the disease, the child is followed by his or her physician every 3 months and receives developmentally appropriate education during each visit. The diabetes education interventions that are offered vary widely across different medical settings, however, because the majority of young patients with diabetes are followed medically by primary-care physicians without benefit of or access to more specialized diabetes educators or mental health personnel with expertise in this area.

Generally, *clinical* or mental health–related interventions for younger children have been behaviorally oriented, with the practical and reasonable goal of improving child or adolescent compliance with the medical regimen (Johnson 1980; Stark et al. 1987). More recently, though, there has been growing emphasis on family-based treatments for both the child and the adolescent with diabetes (Anderson et al. 1990; Johnson 1985). Only a handful of contemporary researchers have reported on psychodynamic or ego-psychological views of the impact of diabetes on child development and personality. This work has been especially helpful in treating older children with adjustment problems that are related to their chronic disease. In a similar vein, diabetes has become a primary focus for studies of processes of psychological coping with chronic stress (see La Greca et al. 1992).

Juvenile diabetes is clearly one of the more widely researched chronic physical conditions in children that is also directly relevant to issues and questions about psychological and developmental outcomes associated with disease onset during childhood and adolescence. Diabetes has been referred to by some as an "invisible" disease, because its manifestations are not visually detectable in childhood or adolescence. And, because of its often complicated medical regimen, diabetes has been portrayed by at least one researcher as creating an "achievement" context within an otherwise normal childhood—an atypical life context that can present the child and family with considerable challenges and stress (Delamater 1992). These additional stresses, in turn, may set the child and family on an atypical developmental trajectory, with eventual outcomes or sequelae made evident later in the child's life.

Despite the potential of diabetes to be well controlled medically, certain psychosocial variables have been suspected to exert considerable influence on actual clinical outcomes in the disease, in terms of both physical and psychological status (Drash and Berlin 1985). These variables include the family milieu and attitudes, individual factors such as intelligence and psychological adjustment, and external factors such as stressful life events and chronic conditions.

Because of the growing literature examining the impact of diabetes on children and their family members, this particular disease entity provides an excellent paradigm for exploring and understanding broader implications of stressful chronic conditions and their effects on child and family development.

Global Versus Specific Disease Effects

At this juncture it is important to note that controversy exists concerning the importance of research and clinical practice remaining attuned to the *disease-specific* characteristics of various chronic conditions, versus combining chronic physical conditions through an essentially *noncategorical* approach—one that minimizes the importance or specific effects of individual disease entities. In this chapter, however, I attempt to describe those findings and insights derived from studies of children with diabetes and apply them to the broader and more heterogeneous population of children exposed to chronic sources of stress such as physical disease.

What is clear across the literature on serious chronic illness and psychosocial outcomes in children is that at least two dimensions of chronic conditions are likely to be significant in determining the risk status for any one child or adolescent with a particular disease or condition. In chronic conditions 1) the range and severity of effects on *brain* or *neurological* functioning are directly correlated to psychological outcomes, and 2) the degree of *physical incapacitation* is directly associated with increased risk of social and psychological problems (Breslau 1985; Garrison and McQuiston 1989).

Aside from these two major dimensions within chronic illness, findings concerning the impact of more disease-specific characteristics have been equivocal across various studies in the research literature. It is important to remember, however, that certain disease entities have been researched in a limited or rather cursory manner or have not been investigated at all using a mental health or psychosocial frame of reference. Consequently, the specific effects of less prevalent or exotic chronic diseases on psychological or psychiatric outcomes are largely unknown in any scientific sense and can only be surmised via anecdotal case reports or through generalizations based on studies of other disease types.

In this chapter I selectively review a number of empirical studies and conceptual ideas that pertain to psychological factors in diabetes mellitus. Through such a review, as noted previously, I hope to derive important lessons from a body of work that serves to inform a broader conceptual understanding of stress and coping with chronic diseases during childhood. Finally, I seek to inform clinical interventions for psychiatric problems in those children, adolescents, and families affected by chronic diseases, regardless of the particular theoretical orientation that might be employed.

Juvenile Diabetes and Psychological Disturbances

Those studies that have attempted to estimate the rates of psychiatric and psychological comorbidity in diabetic youth have reported a range between 15% and 50%, depending on the specific measurement approach employed (Garrison and McQuiston 1989; Johnson 1980; Stein and Jessop 1984). Several studies have associated sociodemographic, family milieu, and compliance behaviors to metabolic control and adjustment to the disease (Anderson et al. 1990; Grey et al. 1991). Some clinical studies have focused primarily on the relationship between depression and childhood diabetes (Barglow et al. 1986; Hauser et al. 1986; Jacobson et al. 1986; Kovacs et al. 1986; Simonds 1977). The more conceptually sophisticated mental health studies of diabetic children and adolescents have focused on the effects of the disease on normal, personal, or family development (Anderson et al. 1990; Hauser et al. 1990; Kovacs et al. 1986) and the presence or absence of subclinical depression and anxiety symptoms in response to diabetes onset and the aftermath of the diagnosis (Kovacs et al. 1986).

Each of these approaches at measuring comorbidity of childhood-onset diabetes with mental disorders has suggested that *risk likelihoods* for significant disorder and/or deviations in development may be greater than rough estimates of these measures provided by surveys based solely on the current presence of behavioral problems or psychiatric symptoms. That is, there is some suggestion that a more subtle process may be operating in childhood-onset diabetes that predisposes affected youth to problems not easily discerned soon after disease onset, or even during the initial years postonset, because its nature is not well described by current approaches to psychiatric nosology or behavioral disorders. It is clear, however, that depressive symptomatology is rather common in newly diagnosed children and parents, though a good number of those affected resolve these problems within a year postdiagnosis. The residual effects of these depressive phenomena and the ongoing stress of coping with a chronic disease such as diabetes are less clear.

Although prospective-longitudinal studies of children with diabetes have been few, the data that do exist suggest that the effects of diabetes over the longer term appear to be subject to developmental influences as well as to premorbid functioning and the array of environmental and individual factors already mentioned. For example, compliance problems appear to increase with adolescence and then improve in early adulthood. Also, the child's knowledge base about diabetes, as well as his or her ability to problem-solve in the face of the disease's challenges, is a factor very much influenced by developmental status (Garrison and Biggs 1990). Ongoing studies of diabetic youth with sufficiently large samples across the childhood age span (Hanson 1992) promise to answer some very basic questions about the longitudinal effects of disease onset, as well as cross-age differences in outcome.

In any assessment of the psychological coping of the child and family in response to the onset of the disease, or as psychological coping relates to daily living with diabetes, it is important to separate *direct* effects of the condition from *indirect* effects. The most obvious direct effects include the addition of daily challenges related to management of the disease that can place the child, and to some degree his or her family as well (Kazak 1989), on a differential developmental trajectory as compared with unaffected children or adolescents. In addition, the onset of a chronic condition can act as a catalyst for previously existing problems in the child or family—in effect, serving as yet another stressor that must be dealt with amid an array of additional problems or concerns in people's lives.

As was stated earlier in this chapter, clinicians and researchers familiar with childhood diabetes have likened it to an "achievement context" (Delamater 1992) that is imposed by virtue of the difficult and often multifactorial regimen it can require of the child. Also, it has been called an "invisible disease" because its effects are largely undetectable in children or adolescents. This lack of overt symptomatology may not be a positive factor in facilitating coping, however, because several studies in the research literature on coping with chronic disease would suggest that the overt manifestation of a disease or handicapping condition can sometimes lead to *better* coping processes, by virtue of there being a broader social awareness of the child's true situation by peers and adults in his or her everyday life.

Studies of psychological coping mechanisms and strategies become highly relevant to understanding which children will be likely to adjust well, and which poorly, to this lifelong disease. Similarly, normal variation in children as a function of their unique blend of characteristics has been implicated in children's ability to meet the "tasks" of diabetes mellitus.

The literature on individual differences in children, or the concept of *temperamental variation,* would also suggest that reactions to diabetes onset and ongoing management can be significantly mediated by the inherent diversity in human personality or behavioral style (Garrison 1992; Garrison et al. 1990). This is true at both the *individual* level of analysis (i.e., the child) and the *parental* level (i.e., parent characteristics and parenting style). For example, several studies have reported that characteristics of temperament such as "activity level" and "attention-span" (Garrison et al. 1990), or "negative mood," "rhythmicity," and "distractibility" (Rovet and Ehrlich 1988), are related directly to the child's metabolic control, although it is likely they are mediated by behavioral compliance. In a similar vein, children's cognitive and intellectual status has been related to outcomes in diabetes, both from the perspective of the individual resources available to buffer or enable the child (Delamater 1992) and in terms of the disease's potentially causing or coexisting with deficits or reduced cognitive function (Ryan 1988; Rovet et al. 1988).

One of the most important factors for estimating psychological coping in the child affected by diabetes is, as was alluded to earlier, the family context in which the child lives day to day. It is clear that parental coping with disease onset and management is entwined to a major degree with the child's capacity to adjust to diabetes. Not only do general family milieu factors affect the child's ability to cope with the disease, but also more specific patterns, such as who takes responsibility for the medical and lifestyle monitoring of the child, are important (Anderson et al. 1990). The majority of studies in this area have employed questionnaire measures of family functioning or milieu (Compas et al. 1992), although in some, investigators have chosen to observe directly and describe family interaction patterns as a method for distinguishing between normal and affected families (Hauser et al. 1986).

In general, increased amounts of family conflict, a lack of cohesiveness among family members, the presence of mental health problems in the parents, and parental inability to cope with the child's disease have all been correlated with poorer outcomes in diabetes. These patterns of findings may not be surprising, but they do serve to reinforce the fact that child coping appears to be firmly implanted within the context provided by the family and their broad ability to deal with stressful life events or conditions.

Research has also provided some interesting and clinically valuable distinctions between at least two types of psychological coping strategies relevant to children with diabetes, or any chronic or acute life stress for that matter. Compas and colleagues (1992) have reviewed the literature that examines the differences between children who employ "problem-focused" versus "emotion-focused" coping techniques. In problem-focused coping, the child actively makes efforts to alter or control a stressful situation. For example, in diabetes, the child who attempts to follow a structured and consistent schedule for monitoring blood glucose and insulin administration would be seen as evidencing a problem-focused style to coping. In emotion-focused coping, the child attempts to deal directly with the negative emotions associated with stressful situations, perhaps by showing avoidant, denying, or emotion-reduction behaviors. Again, in the case of diabetes, the child who pretends not to have a disease, or who avoids the unpleasant aspects of care, may be "coping" with the situation, in a sense, but the implications of this coping style for his or her ability to master the regimen that diabetes requires are of concern. Similarly, the child who only tries to relax himself or herself or minimize his or her affective reactions to the disease, in the absence of proactive, problem-solving responses, may have poorer outcomes with the disease and adjustment to it.

Compas and colleagues (1992), based on their review of the literature, concluded that problem-focused strategies to coping appear to be more beneficial generally, although the "controllability" of stressful events or conditions can mediate this tendency. For example, coping with a disease such as cystic fibrosis might become more emotion-focused as a function of the fact that much of the physical deterioration associated with that disease cannot be controlled completely. Thus, the role of psychological denial in the face of unrelenting and immutable stressful events or conditions should not be viewed as necessarily maladaptive or psychologically *primitive,* given that some things in life simply cannot be changed and there may be a limit to our ability to significantly alter what may be inevitable outcomes.

In addition, there is evidence to suggest that emotion-focused coping may increase as the child ages, perhaps as a function of ongoing and relatively dramatic affective development during later childhood and adolescence, and despite the fact that active, problem-focused coping strategies can be more pragmatically valuable in many stressful situations.

From a related perspective, the concepts of the child's sense of *personal control,* his or her *causal attributions* about internal versus external locus of control, and his or her *perceptions of controllability* of events or conditions appear to be central to observed differences in psychological coping across individuals.

For example, two studies have reported that the child's particular attributional style is associated with variation in metabolic control and compliance in diabetic youth (Brown et al. 1991; Kuttner et al. 1990). One style, characterized by the child's making internal, stable, and global attributions related to negative life events, has been linked with *better* metabolic control and behavioral compliance. For example, a child who employs such a coping strategy would take a certain amount of personal responsibility for disease status and would do so with consistency and a broader applicability, and even in some situations in which they were not in complete control or wholly responsible for preventing negative events. However, when this particular coping style is accompanied by feelings of helplessness, hopelessness, and/or depressive affect—a "depressive" attributional stance, as some researchers have called it (Brown et al. 1991)—such children may also show problems in adjusting adequately to their disease status (Kuttner et al. 1990). Taken as a whole, findings from these studies suggest that "[children's taking] responsibility for controllable negative events but not for uncontrollable negative events associated with their illness is most adaptive" (Brown et al. 1991, p. 924).

In the special case of diabetes, however, personal control can, at times, be somewhat illusory. For example, many children, when first diagnosed with the disease, will have a "honeymoon" period during which their bodies continue to produce an appreciable amount of insulin that helps to keep them in better glycemic control and, despite what they do behaviorally, helps them to manage the disease. Consequently, the connection early on between what they do in response to the disease and actual physical outcomes may not appear to be either direct or significant. This false sense of personal control can set the child with diabetes up for major problems as his or her disease becomes less manageable in subsequent months or years. On the other hand, some children can attempt to manage their disease by almost obsessive adherence to the stipulated medical regimen and still manifest problems with glycemic control because of factors outside their control. Because the disease process is multifactorial, predictability and control will be far from complete.

Models of Stress and Clinical Outcomes in Juvenile Diabetes

Studies of the effects of stress on diabetes outcomes have primarily focused on two lines of inquiry. In the first, the direct effects of stress-induced states have been measured in relation to metabolic control. These studies have been reviewed elsewhere (Delamater 1992), but the current consensus appears to be that the direct metabolic effects of stress on diabetes control are not significant for most individuals affected by the disease (Kemmer et al. 1986). However, it is still not clear whether or not certain subgroups of persons, such as those with the type A personality constellation for example, may demonstrate metabolic alteration as a function of life stress (Stabler et al. 1987). It may be that other subgroups of children or adolescents will show such effects as they are defined and compared with other children with diabetes.

Developmental changes in the child's capacity to deal with stress are important to take into account in both theory and practice. There are likely to be important differences in stress effects in the early childhood period, when children are largely dependent on and refer-ent to parents and their reactions or behavior, compared with in ado-lescence, when the teenager's cognitive and affective development has dramatically matured and their transactions with family members and the external world have altered in complicated and significant ways. Weist and co-workers (1991) have suggested that treatment targets for children with chronic illnesses such as diabetes should be develop-mentally appropriate and not uniform for children of various ages or developmental levels:

> Primary issues for diabetic infants and toddlers are to learn to cope with disrupted home routines, separation from parents, painful medical procedures, and dealing with strangers. For middle-aged children, important themes are the development of independent management abilities, coping with feelings of being different from other children, and dealing with embarrassing informa-

tion-seeking from peers. Particular issues for adolescents are body image problems, noncompliance to illness management routines, and controlling alcohol intake. (p. 532)

New Directions

Studies of outcomes associated with psychosocial factors in juvenile diabetes have tended to employ laboratory-derived indices of metabolic control via assays of glycosylated hemoglobin (Bacon et al. 1986; Nathan et al. 1984). These values, taken from blood samples typically collected at 3-month intervals, are presumed to measure the patient's glucose regulation broadly and have been portrayed as a useful, though imperfect, index of compliance with medical regimen and actual control of the disease.

Most psychological research in juvenile diabetes has used ratings of behavioral compliance, either globally determined through case review or more specifically measured via separate ratings of several important components of the medical regimen, including insulin administration, blood glucose monitoring and logging of values, frequency of exercise, and attention to dietary restrictions or guidelines.

The critical relationship between these two indices must be clarified more fully or the field will continue to be plagued by methodological problems. In addition, a certain amount of controversy exists about both the actual representativeness of glycosylated hemoglobin assays for all children and the inherent and thorny methodological problems associated with various measures of behavioral compliance in diabetes.

From a clinical perspective, continued attempts to broaden the traditional purview of mental health beyond a pathology model, to one that includes psychological adaptation in adults, children, and families affected by chronic physical illnesses or conditions, can lead to major strides in prevention. Current nosological approaches that do not allow for adequate diagnosis of reactions to chronic stress caused by disease or physical conditions hamper our ability to intervene when necessary. In a similar vein, insurance companies and managed care systems need to see the value in preventive work with such children and their families, in terms of both psychological health and reduction of future medical costs.

Deception in self-monitoring by children with diabetes, and the degree to which parents collude or encourage such practices, constitute a relatively unstudied but widely known phenomenon in juvenile diabetes (Garrison and Biggs 1990). Studies in children and adults have suggested that 40% to 50% of patients with diabetes falsify blood glucose testing in some manner (Mazze et al. 1984; Wilson and Endres 1986). This pattern of deception and impression management may be one fruitful avenue for exploring the implications of a chronic disease for variations in individual development.

Many researchers have called for more attention to family communication and group behavior related to management of a chronic condition such as diabetes (Anderson et al. 1990). They argue that in research or clinical work, neglecting the sharing of responsibilities and the communication patterns around such illness or condition-related duties is a mistake and can lead to less effective interventions.

Another attempt to "reframe" the diabetes management regimen to render it more acceptable by children and adolescents has been work that looks at the child's ability to distinguish differences in blood glucose levels as a function of symptom or cue awareness (Ruggiero et al. 1991). Treatment would be geared toward not only increasing compliance with blood glucose monitoring on a regular basis but also enhancing the child's ability to self-monitor physical symptoms. This approach has the added value of empowering the child in his or her own care and also makes the testing more relevant from the child's own perspective, in that testing sometimes occurs when the child prompts himself or herself, rather than in response to adult demands or expectations.

Each of these different approaches to the management of diabetes and to facilitating psychological coping with the disease may act to diminish the longer-term effects on development and health that have been discussed in the research literature. Many writers in the area of stress and coping with acute or chronic conditions have pointed out that stressful life events can actually strengthen individuals, and not only render negative effects on psychological or psychiatric health. Aside from personal and social protective factors, such as intelligence level, personality characteristics, family resources, and so on, it is likely that the affected person's ability to exert control over a stressful situation, as well as his or her cognitive appraisal concerning the seriousness and implications of the stress, is also an important factor in eventual coping and adjustment.

Final Comments

Much of the research on children and adolescents with diabetes has informed a broader inquiry into the nature of stressful life events, chronic conditions, and psychological outcomes in individuals. It is clear that diabetes is unique in some ways, when compared with other types of life stressors, in that the initial effects of the disease are largely or wholly unseen to observers, a complex and sometimes difficult daily regimen is required, alterations in lifestyle are required to maintain the necessary metabolic control, and the disease has the potential to seriously threaten both the quality and the longevity of an affected person's life through an insidious and prolonged process (Geffner et al. 1983).

Still, those individual or family characteristics and coping strategies that appear to buffer affected children and families from life stress in diabetes contain remarkable similarities to the techniques reported from psychological studies of other disease entities and the research literature on loss and bereavement and on stressful life events. In addition to the more predictable finding that preexisting problems can be worsened by the onset of diabetes, and that diabetes itself will induce particular types of behavioral or adjustment problems, there are both clinical and research data which suggest that the disease—and perhaps any chronic disease—also causes more subtle but important changes in the more typical developmental trajectories, and perhaps even the ego-psychological makeup, of these children and adolescents.

The diabetes literature, in combination with clinical experience with many children and adolescents affected by the disease, bolsters the view that the family provides the crucial context or background in which child coping and adjustment will take place. Children not only model parental responses to stressful events or conditions but also rely on their parents to teach them the skills they will need to manage or even fight disease and handicapping conditions. More work on family systems and the nature of interactions and transactions within families affected by a childhood chronic disease holds the most promise for future clinical work. That line of research, however, should be parallel to ongoing studies of the possible developmental and personal alterations in individuals that can be attributed to the onset of a disease, and the ongoing stressors that the disease entails within the context of a life.

There is reason to hope that a medical cure for diabetes may be at hand within the next few decades and that a time may come in which the longer-term significance of the disease will be diminished greatly. If this actually occurs, however, efforts to treat and manage the disease will have left a positive legacy. Diabetes in children, especially, has been a major focus for some of the best conceptual and clinical thinking about children's reactions and adjustment to chronic sources of stress and the often profound effects that childhood diseases can exert on the more typical and expected developmental course.

References

Anderson BJ, Auslander WF, Jung KC, et al: Assessing family sharing of diabetes responsibilities. J Pediatr Psychol 15:477–492, 1990

Bacon GE, Ladu C, Shein HE, et al: Evaluation of glycosylated hemoglobin in the management of young patients with insulin-dependent diabetes mellitus. Journal of Adolescent Health Care 7:187–190, 1986

Barglow P, Berndt D, Burns W, et al: Neuroendocrine and psychological factors in childhood diabetes mellitus. Journal of the American Academy of Child Psychiatry 25:785–793, 1986

Breslau N: Psychiatric disorder in children with physical disabilities. Journal of the American Academy of Child Psychiatry 24:87–94, 1985

Brown RT, Kaslow NJ, Sansbury L, et al: Internalizing and externalizing symptoms and attributional style in youth with diabetes. J Am Acad Child Adolesc Psychiatry 30:921–925, 1991

Compas BE, Worsham NL, Ey S: Conceptual and developmental issues in children's coping with stress, in Advances in Pediatric Psychology: Stress and Coping in Child Health. Edited by La Greca AM, Siegel LF, Wallander JL, et al. New York, Guilford, 1992, pp 7–24

Court J: Outpatient-based transition services for youth. Pediatrician 18:150–156, 1991

Delamater AM: Stress, coping and metabolic control among youngsters with diabetes, in Advances in Pediatric Psychology: Stress and Coping in Child Health. Edited by La Greca AM, Siegel LF, Wallander JL, et al. New York, Guilford, 1992, pp 191–211

Drash A, Berlin N: Juvenile diabetes, in Issues in the Care of Children With Chronic Illness. Edited by Hobbs N, Perrin JM. San Francisco, CA, Jossey-Bass, 1985, pp 211–220

Garrison WT: The conceptual utility of the temperament construct in understanding coping with pediatric conditions, in Advances in Pediatric Psychology: Stress and Coping in Child Health. Edited by La Greca AM, Siegel LF, Wallander JL, et al. New York, Guilford, 1992, pp 72–84

Garrison WT, Biggs D: On the subjective reports of young children about their diabetes mellitus. Diabetes Educator 16:304–308, 1990

Garrison WT, McQuiston S: Chronic Illness During Childhood and Adolescence: Psychological Aspects. Newbury Park, CA, Sage, 1989

Garrison WT, Biggs D, Williams K: Temperament characteristics and clinical outcomes in young children with diabetes mellitus. J Child Psychol Psychiatry 31:1079–1088, 1990

Gavin JR, Goodwin N: Diabetes in black populations: current state of knowledge. Diabetes Care 13(suppl):1139–1208, 1990

Geffner ME, Kaplan SA, Lippe BM, et al: Self-monitoring of blood glucose levels and intensified insulin therapy. JAMA 249:2913–2916, 1983

Gortmaker SL, Sappenfield W: Chronic childhood disorders: prevalence and impact. Pediatr Clin North Am 31:3–18, 1984

Grey M, Cameron ME, Thurber FW: Coping and adaptation in children with diabetes. Nurs Res 40:144–149, 1991

Hanson CL: Developing systemic models of the adaptation of youths with diabetes, in Advances in Pediatric Psychology: Stress and Coping in Child Health. Edited by La Greca AM, Siegel LF, Wallander JL, et al. New York, Guilford, 1992, pp 212–241

Hanson CL, Henggeler SW, Burghen GA: Race and sex differences in metabolic control of adolescents with IDDM: a function of psychosocial variables? Diabetes Care 10:313–318, 1987

Hauser ST, Jacobson AM, Wertlieb D, et al: Children with recently diagnosed diabetes: interactions with their families. Health Psychol 5:273–296, 1986

Hauser ST, Jacobson AM, Lavori P, et al: Adherence among children and adolescents with insulin-dependent diabetes mellitus over a four-year longitudinal follow-up, II: immediate and longterm linkages with the family milieu. J Pediatr Psychol 15:527–542, 1990

Jacobson AM, Hauser ST, Lavori P, et al: Adherence among children and adolescents with insulin-dependent diabetes mellitus over a four-year longitudinal follow-up, I: the influence of patient coping and adjustment. J Pediatr Psychol 15:511–526, 1990

Johnson SB: Psychological factors in juvenile diabetes: a review. J Behav Med 3:95–116, 1980

Johnson SB: The family and child with chronic illness, in Health, Illness and Families: A Life Span Perspective. Edited by Turk EC, Kerns RD. New York, Wiley, 1985, pp 123–137

Kazak AE: Families of chronically ill children: a systems and social-ecological model of adaptation and change. J Consult Clin Psychol 57:25–30, 1989

Kemmer R, Bisping R, Steingruber H, et al: Psychological stress and metabolic control in patients with Type-I diabetes mellitus. New Engl J Med 314:1078–1084, 1986

Kohrman AF, Netzloff ML, Weil WB: Diabetes mellitus, in Pediatrics. Edited by Rudolph A. Philadelphia, PA, Appleton-Lange, 1987, pp 987–1002

Kovacs M, Brent D, Steinberg T, et al: Children's self-reports of psychological adjustment and coping strategies during the first year of insulin-dependent diabetes mellitus. Diabetes Care 9:472–479, 1986

Kuttner MJ, Delamater AM, Santiago JV: Learned helplessness in diabetic youths. J Pediatr Psychol 15:581–594, 1990

La Greca AM, Siegel LF, Wallander JL, et al (eds): Advances in Pediatric Psychology: Stress and Coping in Child Health. New York, Guilford, 1992

Mazze RS, Shamoon H, Pasmantier R: Reliability of blood glucose monitoring by patients with diabetes mellitus. Am J Med 77:211–217, 1984

Nathan DM, Singer DE, Hurtxthal K, et al: The clinical information value of the glycosylated hemoglobin assay. New Engl J Med 310:341–346, 1984

Rovet JF, Ehrlich RM: Effect of temperament on metabolic control in children with diabetes mellitus. Diabetes Care 11:77–82, 1988

Rovet JF, Ehrlich RM, Hoppe M: Specific intellectual deficits in children with early onset diabetes mellitus. Child Dev 59:226–234, 1988

Ruggiero L, Kairys S, Fritz G, et al: Accuracy of blood glucose estimates in adolescents with diabetes mellitus. J Adolesc Health
12:101–106, 1991

Ryan CM: Neurobehavioral complications of type-1 diabetes: examination of possible risk factors. Diabetes Care 11:86–93, 1988

Simonds S: Psychiatric status of diabetic youth matched with a control group. Diabetes 26:921–925, 1977

Stabler B, Surwit R, Lane J, et al: Type A behavior pattern and blood
glucose control in diabetic children. Psychosom Med 49:313–316,
1987

Stark LJ, Dahlquist LM, Collins FL: Improving children's compliance
with diabetes management. Clinical Psychology Review 7:223–242,
1987

Stein REK, Jessop KJ: General issues in the care of children with
chronic physical conditions. Pediatr Clin North Am 31:189–198,
1984

Weist MD, Ollendick TH, Finney JW: Toward the empirical validation
of treatment targets in children. Clinical Psychology Review
11:515–538, 1991

Wilson DP, Endres RK: Compliance with blood glucose monitoring in
children with Type-I diabetes mellitus. J Pediatr 108:1022–1024,
1986

Section IV

Suicide as Stressor and as Mediator of Stress

Chapter 12

Suicidal Behavior as a Response to Stress

Cynthia R. Pfeffer, M.D.

There is agreement among researchers and clinicians that youth suicidal behavior is a complex behavior involving important interactions among developmental, psychosocial, psychopathological, and biological factors that increase risk for this life-threatening behavior (Blumenthal and Kupfer 1988; Pfeffer 1986). In the United States, suicide is the third leading cause of death among 15- to 24-year-olds and the sixth leading cause of death in younger children, ages 5 to 14 years (National Center for Health Statistics 1992). It has been estimated that for every suicide among youth, ages 10 to 17 years, approximately 47 suicide attempts are reported (Andrus et al. 1991). Rates of suicidal acts have increased dramatically, especially among youth born after World War II (Klerman 1989). Such a cohort effect may be attributed to the stressful sequelae of living in a society with a rapid-paced lifestyle involving high degrees of family mobility, family disruptions caused by parental separation or divorce, and other factors including parental absence from the home because of work obligations or illness. A stress-diathesis model of vulnerability for suicidal acts may be proposed in which suicidal behavior is the outcome of interactions between personal adverse life experiences and psychopathological factors. In the present chapter I explicate recent research that highlights relationships between these factors and potential underlying determinants for the evolution of youth suicidal behavior.

Stress as Trigger for Suicidal Behavior

Multifaceted models have been described for processes leading to youth suicidal acts. Shaffer and colleagues (Shaffer 1988) proposed a linear additive model of risk for suicidal acts in which predisposing factors of an individual, such as depressive illness and personality disorders, are added to factors in the social milieu, such as suicide rates in the community, lack of social taboos against suicide, or media display of suicide, which are added to trigger factors, such as recent stressful events, altered states of mind, and availability of a suicide method, especially firearms. Such a model assumes that suicidal acts occur in vulnerable children and adolescents. It highlights stressful events as trigger factors that occur shortly before a suicidal act. Trigger factors have also been described especially in psychological autopsy studies of adolescents who committed suicide (Hoberman and Garfinkel 1988; Rich et al. 1990). Acute stressors noted retrospectively among youth suicide victims include school suspensions, rejections by parents or peers, family moves, loss of love relationships, arrests and jail terms, arguments, and work problems. Most of these studies did not report on other features of stress such as duration of stressful experiences, timing within specific developmental phases, and the physical and emotional condition of the child or adolescent at the time of stressful events.

A Stress-Diathesis Model for Youth Suicidal Behavior

Some investigators define stress as a transactional process involving a system of interdependent variables that mutually influence one another (Lazarus and Folkman 1984). Specifically, stress is a process involving bidirectional relationships between a person with unique characteristics and an environment with particular features. These relationships are stressful if they overwhelm a person's resources and endanger his or her well-being. This paradigm has received relatively sparse research attention with respect to risk for youth suicidal behavior.

Not all stressful encounters have the same significance for an individual's mental or physical health primarily because stress is a recursive process that is experienced over periods of time (Lazarus and

Folkman 1984). For example, a person's particular genetic, biological, and psychosocial characteristics and specific environmental variables, and the relationships between those characteristics and environmental variables at a particular point in time, may affect subsequent characteristics of that person and/or other environmental variables as well as their subsequent transactional relationships. As a result, new levels of vulnerability may occur subsequent to antecedent person–environment interactions. In this way, stress can be viewed as a profound mediator of suicidal behavior rather than a discrete trigger factor. Therefore, identification of key components of such a stress-diathesis model with respect to risk for youth suicidal behavior must be conducted within a framework of prospective multiple measurements of change over time and across stressful encounters (Lazarus and Folkman 1984). There has been little systematic research utilizing this approach for understanding the role of stressful events upon risk for suicidal behavior among youth.

Other important elements involve the significant impact of developmental processes within neurobiological, physiological, and psychosocial domains that may alter personal characteristics of children and adolescents. Developmental processes affect the quality of cognitive appraisal and styles of coping that researchers of stress postulate are essential for mediating the transactional relationships between a youth's personal characteristics and environmental factors (Brown and Harris 1978; Lazarus and Folkman 1984; Moos 1984; Spielberger and Sarason 1986). For example, a 3-year-old child, who according to Piagetian theory (Piaget 1952) would be in the stage of preoperations, can focus attention on one aspect of a situation but is not able to integrate this aspect with other aspects of the situation. If the child's mother suffers from a medical illness and feels too ill on a particular day to play actively with the child, the child may perceive that his mother is not able to play at other times too. In contrast, a 9-year-old child, who according to Piagetian theory would be in the stage of concrete operations, could appreciate that his mother, even though she is less energetic on one day, may be able to interact actively on another day. Children at the more advanced cognitive phase of concrete operations can classify experiences in such a manner that interrelated elements can be discerned and reorganized to fit new circumstances (Piaget 1952). In this stage of development, children can evaluate situations from various perspectives and can remember an initial experience after it has been altered by subsequent events.

Rutter (1989) suggested developmental principles that highlight the relationships between children's capacities to conceptualize events, the time of events, and the content of emotions when events occur. In the examples noted above, the younger child's affective experience of sadness associated with memories of his mother's illness probably is enduring and might lead to severe vulnerability to sadness. In contrast, the older child, who achieved a more advanced level of affect regulation, might be able to discriminate situations and modulate affect appropriately with regard to specific situations.

A stress-diathesis paradigm of risk for youth suicidal behavior proposes that suicidal acts of children or adolescents are outcomes of the transactional relationships between characteristics of the youngster and features of the environment. These relationships are mediated by cognitive appraisal and styles of coping, which may be modified by developmental, biological, and genetic processes. These multifaceted recursive processes influenced by the degree of stress at particular times can affect the incidence and prevalence of suicide and suicide attempts in children and adolescents.

Stressful Life Events

Characterization of stressful experiences has been an important aspect of investigations of suicidal behavior in adults. Such studies suggest significant positive relationships between suicidal behavior and an increased frequency and specific types of stressful life events. In the Lundby Study (Hagnell and Rorsman 1980), a 25-year prospective study of suicide in a general population sample in Sweden, suicide victims were compared with individuals who had died from natural causes and with a nonsuicidal control group. The investigators found that individuals who committed suicide had experienced more stressful life events in the week prior to and in the year before committing suicide. In the week of the suicidal deaths, high rates of humiliating experiences and loss of personal relationships or possessions had occurred. Changes in residence and major occupational problems had been more prevalent among the suicide victims.

Other research with adults suggests that stressful life events are significant risk factors for suicide attempts (Isherwood et al. 1982; Slater and Depue 1981). Stressful events are especially related to recurrent suicide attempts (Krarup et al. 1991; Kreitman and Casey

1988). Unhappy childhoods involving parental arguments, adverse home environments, and physical or sexual abuse have been reported retrospectively by adult suicide attempters (Krarup et al. 1991; van der Kolk et al. 1991).

In a methodologically elegant study conducted by Paykel and colleagues (1975), stressful life events in the 6 months preceding suicide attempts among adults admitted to an emergency service were compared with stressful life events in the 6 months preceding the onset of depression in adults admitted to the same emergency service, and with stressful life events of nondepressed and nonsuicidal adults recruited from the community. Suicide attempters experienced 4 times as many stressful life events as did the control subjects and 1.5 times as many stressful life events as did the depressed adults. Suicide attempters experienced an increasing frequency of life events in the 6 months before the suicide attempt and a *marked* elevation in stressful life events in the month preceding the suicide attempt. Compared with the control subjects, suicide attempters reported more serious arguments with a spouse, a new person's joining the household, serious illness of a relative, serious personal physical illness, and a court appearance for an offense. Compared with the depressed patients, suicide attempters reported more spousal altercations, serious illness of a relative, and engagement to be married. In fact, compared with the depressed patients and the control subjects, suicide attempters experienced a greater number of desirable life events such as engagement to be married, weddings, and promotion, as well as a greater number of undesirable life events such as death, separation, demotion, serious illness of a relative, jail, financial problems, unemployment for 1 month, court appearance, divorce, and business failure.

Studies of youth agree with the results highlighting the significant role of stressful life events on risk for suicidal acts in adults. Rosenthal and Rosenthal (1984) described high rates of physical abuse and neglect among preschool-age suicidal children. These children, compared with preschool-age children with behavior problems, were distressed by feelings of parental anger and of being unwanted by the parents. Pfeffer and colleagues (1993) noted that prepubertal suicidal psychiatric inpatients, who were compared with prepubertal nonsuicidal psychiatric inpatients and with children in the general community, had experienced a greater number of stressful life changes during school-age periods of development, especially related to problems in the family. Similarly, Myers and associates (1985) reported a greater number of stressful life events among prepubertal suicidal psychiatric inpatients then among prepubertal nonsuicidal psychiatric inpatients. Identification of timing and types of life events among prepubertal children was reported by Cohen-Sandler and colleagues (1982) for suicidal psychiatric inpatients, depressed nonsuicidal psychiatric inpatients, and nonsuicidal, nondepressed child psychiatric inpatients. The prepubertal suicidal children had had more cumulative stressful life events in their lifetimes that included more frequent sibling births; deaths of grandparents; parental hospitalization; parental separation, divorce, or remarriage; and introduction of another adult into the home. The suicidal children had experienced more stressful life events in the year preceding the hospitalization. These results are similar to those reported by Paykel and his collaborators (1975) suggesting that there are increased rates of stressful life events just before a suicide attempt and that suicidal children and adults experience a larger number of undesirable life events and high rates of entrance and exit life events.

Adolescence is a special developmental period, when rates of suicide are very high. Research methods using the psychological autopsy approach have made it possible to study relatively large numbers of youth suicide victims. Rich and colleagues (1991), reporting on 204 consecutive cases of suicide among people of all ages, suggested that interpersonal conflicts, separations, and rejections were the most prevalent life events. These distressing problems were most prevalent among adolescents and young adults. Conflict-separation-rejection occurred in 56% of individuals who were less than 19 years of age compared with 17% of individuals who were in their fifth decade. Brent and collaborators (1988) reported that the lifetime rate of environmental stress was similar among adolescents who had completed suicide and psychiatrically hospitalized adolescent suicide attempters. These lifetime rates of stressful events were higher than those reported in other studies (Robins et al. 1984) of community samples of 25- to 44-year-olds. Kosky and associates (1990) reported that adolescent suicide attempters, compared with adolescents who reported suicidal ideas, were more likely to have experienced persistent family discord characterized by hostility, quarreling, scapegoating, and verbal and physical abuse. However, there were no differences between these groups of adolescents in the quality of their relationships with their parents or their siblings and in the rates of family moves or disturbed relationships with other adults. An implication of this study is that the continuity between adolescents who report suicidal thinking and those who carry out suicidal acts requires further study.

Studies of community samples of adolescents suggest that parental arrest is more than twice as common and family dysfunction is almost twice as frequent among adolescents who report suicidal behavior as among those who do not (Joffe et al. 1988). When psychiatrically hospitalized adolescent suicide attempters were compared with adolescents in the general community, stressful life events were found to be significantly associated with suicidal behavior (Rubenstein et al. 1989). Adolescents who had attempted suicide had more problems with sexuality, achievement, family suicidal behavior, and loss of personal relationships. Another report (DeWilde et al. 1992) comparing adolescent suicide attempter patients, depressed adolescent patients, and psychiatrically healthy adolescents suggests that adolescent suicide attempters, compared with depressed patients or adolescent control subjects, experienced more separation from parents, more physical abuse, and a greater number of other stressful life events before the age of 12 years. After age 12 years, adolescent suicide attempters experienced more changes in living situations, parental divorce, and sexual abuse, and a higher number of total stressful life events. It was found that in the year preceding a suicide attempt, there had been a high frequency of changes in living circumstances, school problems, and total stressful life events. The importance of physical and sexual abuse, problems in peer relationships, problems in love relationships, family violence, and parental separation was noted in other studies of adolescent suicide attempters (see Adams-Tucker 1982; Brent et al. 1990; Deykin et al. 1985; Myers et al. 1991; Pfeffer et al. 1988).

Longitudinal studies of child and adolescent suicidal behavior are sparse but valuable in identifying predictors of suicidal acts. Salk and colleagues (1985) compared birth records of adolescents who committed suicide with birth records of those who did not report suicidal behavior. Predictors of suicide in adolescence were a greater number of prenatal, birth, and neonatal problems. The most significant stressful predictors for suicide were infant respiratory distress for more than 1 hour, no maternal antenatal care before 20 weeks of pregnancy, and chronic disease in the mother during pregnancy. The results of this study suggest that early adverse events related to birth may affect mechanisms leading to youth suicidal behavior at a much later time. Pfeffer and colleagues (1993) reported that early adverse life events, especially during the preschool- and school-age periods, predicted suicidal attempts in adolescents.

In summary, stressful life events experienced by children and adolescents are associated with suicidal behavior among youth. The timing and type of stressful life events are important features for predicting risk for suicidal acts among children and adolescents. Chronic accumulation of adverse life events, such as family violence, physical and sexual abuse, family discord, separations and other losses, and problematic interpersonal relationships, enhance risk for youth suicidal behavior.

Psychological Appraisal and Coping Mechanisms

Not all children or adolescents who experience adverse life events commit suicidal acts or think about wanting to kill themselves. This suggests that other factors may mediate between the occurrence of stressful life events and a suicidal outcome. As was noted earlier, stress involves processes that include cognitive appraisal of a potentially stressful situation as well as coping efforts. A number of researchers have suggested a cognitive-behavioral paradigm associated with risk for suicidal behavior in adults (Beck et al. 1985; Patsiokas et al. 1979; Schotte and Clum 1987). It may be inferred that certain intrapsychic processes associated with stressful events mediate behavioral responses such as suicidal behavior.

The concept of awareness is useful in connoting the psychological state of a child or adolescent that mediates the experience of adverse life events and an outcome, such as suicidal behavior. Awareness consists of components that are involved in the processing of information. These components include attention, perception, memory, intelligence, social understanding, and a capacity to integrate these complex domains. Relatively little research has been conducted to explicate these components with regard to suicidal behavior, especially among children and adolescents.

Shaffer (1974) found, in a study of 31 young adolescents, ages 12 to 14 years, who committed suicide, that their intelligence was unusually high. This finding has not been validated by other psychological autopsy studies. Furthermore, Weiner and Pfeffer (1986) did not find IQ differences between suicidal and nonsuicidal prepubertal psychiatric inpatients. They proposed that IQ tests may not be an optimal method to study cognitive processes distinguishing suicidal from non-suicidal youth but that specific domains of cognitive processes (e.g., memory and reasoning tasks) may be more fruitful areas of investigation.

A significant indicator of reasoning ability involves problem-solving skills. Compas and colleagues (1988) identified that children and adolescents, like adults, utilize a variety of coping strategies, among which are *problem-focused coping* that involves skills utilized to change the source of stress, and *emotion-focused coping* that involves efforts to regulate emotional states associated with stress. These specific coping skills have not been studied among suicidal children or adolescents. However, Asarnow and colleagues (1987) observed that prepubertal suicidal children, compared with disturbed nonsuicidal children, generated fewer active alternative methods to solve interpersonal problems and to regulate their affective and behavioral response to adverse life events.

The description of these coping deficits among suicidal children concurs with the research of Santostefano and colleagues (1984) indicating that prepubertal and adolescent suicidal psychiatric inpatients had difficulty imagining future action to solve problems. These investigators identified specific problem-solving skill deficits in that, for example, when a behavioral response required thought but not action, suicidal children and adolescents engaged in action and not imagination. This response suggested that fantasy was not invoked by suicidal children or adolescents to delay action or to decrease impulse expression. Santostefano and colleagues also found that, compared with the nonsuicidal child and adolescent psychiatric inpatients, the suicidal patients' images of active behavior were slower and less vigorous. This study highlighted the inability of suicidal children and adolescents to substitute thought for actions when a problem-solving task is necessary.

Other aspects of problem-solving deficits, especially regarding interpersonal conflicts, have been highlighted for adolescent suicide attempters (Rotheram-Borus et al. 1990). Compared with psychiatrically disturbed adolescents without a history of suicide attempts or psychiatrically healthy adolescents, female adolescent suicide attempters thought of fewer alternative approaches to solving problems. The lack of flexibility in conceptualizing various solutions to problems significantly characterized suicidal adolescents. Suicide attempters tended to dwell on problems significantly more than did adolescents who did not report suicidal acts. Compared with psychiatrically disturbed nonsuicidal adolescents, female adolescent suicide attempters characterized their lives as having positive life events that were unpredictable and not determined by their own acts but rather caused by external processes. The suicidal and depressed adolescents attributed negative life events to their own behavior. Other reports (e.g., Levinson and Neuringer 1971) pointed out that adolescent suicide attempters have few concepts about planning solutions to interpersonal problems.

Patterns of poor coping may lead to states of hopelessness and to perceptions of negative expectations of future events or poor sense of one's personal characteristics and capacities. States of hopeless perceptions elevate suicidal risk in adults (Beck et al. 1975, 1985). However, the relation between hopelessness and suicidal behavior in children and adolescents has not been consistently documented. This may be accounted for by varied methodological approaches of measuring hopelessness in youth (Kazdin et al. 1983), developmental aspects of cognition that may affect a youngster's understanding of time or causality (Carlson and Garber 1986), or the need to conduct more extensive research to identify whether other factors mediate associations between hopelessness and youth suicidal behavior (Spirito et al. 1991). Nevertheless, there is sufficient evidence that suicidal children and adolescents often have pessimistic expectations of future events, and when this happens such youngsters report an intense sense of hopelessness.

It may be presumed that states of hopelessness are, in part, an outcome of an individual's perceptions of not being able to solve sufficiently problems that arise from stressful life events. Kashani and colleagues (1989) provided a perspective on hopelessness in their developmental study of a general population in which they compared three groups of children, age 8 years, age 12 years, and age 17 years. This study found that there were no differences in severity of hopelessness in these age groups. One-third of the youngsters who reported high levels of hopelessness acknowledged recurrent suicidal ideation. However, only 0% to 4% of youngsters with absent to moderate degrees of hopelessness reported suicidal ideation. This study implied that children and adolescents are cognitively mature enough to experience hopelessness. These results have been validated by reports of positive associations between hopelessness and suicidal ideation or behavior in children (Asarnow et al. 1987; Carlson and Cantwell 1982;

Kazdin et al. 1983) and adolescents (Brent et al. 1988; Cole 1989; Spirito et al. 1988). In one report no relation between hopelessness and suicidal intent was found among minority female adolescent suicide attempters evaluated in an emergency and psychiatric outpatient setting (Rotheram-Borus and Trautman 1988).

Other constructs related to processing of information that encompass cognitive, emotional, and behavioral indices focus on components of ego functioning, a framework derived from psychoanalytic theory (S. Freud 1926/1959; A. Freud 1936/1946). In recent years, a focus has emerged on youth suicidal behavior and parameters of ego functioning involving impulse control, objective appraisal of situations connoted by the term reality testing, and use of ego mechanisms of defense that affect manifestations of self-reflection and emotional experience. For example, the maturity of ego functioning was compared among adolescent psychiatric inpatient suicide attempters and adolescent psychiatric inpatients who reported no history of suicidal ideation or suicide attempt (Borst et al. 1991) using the Loevinger's Washington University Sentence Completion Test (Loevinger et al. 1976). Suicide attempts were associated with higher levels of ego development among adolescent psychiatric inpatients who had a mood disorder and/or a conduct disorder. An important implication of this result is that adolescents with more mature ego functioning tend to regard sadness as part of themselves rather than to attribute sadness to external sources. These adolescents are more vulnerable to self-blame for environmental events and interpersonal problems. The findings from this study suggest that adolescents who attempted suicide but who had less mature ego functioning tended to externalize blame for adverse events. These adolescents held others responsible for their problems and attempted suicide as an act of impulsivity that was generated by angry feelings.

Pfeffer and colleagues (1986) reported on ego functioning associated with suicidal behavior in prepubertal psychiatric inpatients, outpatients, and nonpatients. In this study the authors found that suicidal behavior, especially among the psychiatric inpatients, was correlated with poor impulse control and with the use of multiple ego mechanisms of defense (A. Freud 1936/1946), especially introjection and displacement. These ego mechanisms of defense, according to psychoanalytic theory (Freud 1926/1959), operate as unconscious psychological processes that modulate subjective experiences related to painful ideas, affects, and emotions. That introjection was related to prepubertal suicidal behavior in psychiatric inpatients (Pfeffer et al. 1986) was supported by similar results of adolescent psychiatric inpatient suicide attempters (Recklitis et al. 1992).

In summary, there is strong evidence that styles of coping are associated with youth suicidal behavior. Because other factors, especially those involving psychopathology, elevate risk for youth suicidal behavior (Pfeffer et al. 1991a), additional research is necessary to discern whether coping styles that are observed among suicidal children are enduring traits that are independent of the presence of psychiatric disorders.

Biological Foundations of Suicidal Behavior

Technical advances in biological psychiatry have promoted the burgeoning of research on neuroendocrine components, neurotransmitter indices, and neurostructural aberrations associated with suicidal behavior in adults (Altshuler et al. 1990; Coccaro and Astell 1990; Mann and Stanley 1986; Mann et al. 1986, 1992; Ostroff et al. 1982; Roy et al. 1992; Träskman et al. 1981). Specifically, low cerebrospinal fluid levels of 5-hydroxyindoleacetic acid, low levels of homovanillic acid and dopamine in urine, and change in temporal lobe structures, specifically in the hippocampus and the parahippocampus, in suicidal adults were reported in these studies. Reports of high levels of serum cortisol in prepubertal suicidal children (Pfeffer et al. 1991b) and of low platelet imipramine binding in depressed suicidal children and adolescents (Ambrosini et al. 1992) complement research observations in adults of aberrations in the neurophysiology associated with suicidal behavior.

The etiological factors for these neurophysiological abnormalities associated with suicidal behavior are still to be clarified. Recent research suggests that adverse life events, especially early in life, may be implicated. There is evidence that gene expression regulates neuroendocrine and neurotransmitter functions and brain structure. Studies in nonprimates suggest that these processes are influenced by adrenal steroids whose activity may be enhanced by stressful environmental stimuli (McEwen et al. 1991). These genetic effects may be long-lasting. McEwen described the complex effects of gene expression, stressful stimuli, adrenal steroid factors, and brain function and structure in rats (McEwen et al. 1968). Specifically, he noted that in brains of rats there are receptors for corticosterone that are located in the hippocampus, a brain region important for cognition, memory, and affective states. McEwen suggested that damage to hippocampal structures can be induced by prolonged exposure to adrenal steroids that influence gene functioning to effect structural and functional changes in this brain region. Paradoxically, corticosteroids also are required for cell development in regions of the hippocampus in rat brain. The hippocampus functions to regulate hypothalamic-pituitary-adrenocortical axis responses to stress. Serotonin receptors in the hippocampus also respond to stress. In addition, the hippocampus responds to adrenal steroids by regulating calcium-almodulin–dependent adenylate cyclase activity, mechanisms that may be regulated also by gene expression. Thus, lesions in the hippocampus that are the result of excessive adrenal steroid levels that are induced by early stress may inhibit appropriate hippocampal responsivity to future stressful events. These lesions may lead to imbalances in regulation of hypothalamic-pituitary-adrenocortical axis functioning and to deficits in regulation of the serotonergic systems.

These research results emphasize the need to identify whether biological mechanisms in human brains become disorganized by the effects of intense early stress. Some indirect evidence to support this supposition is derived from research that suggests that human brain regulatory systems, which are disrupted by early stresses, are associated with risk for mood disorders. Post (1992) proposed that psychosocial stress early in life is associated with a first episode of mood disorder that, in turn, "kindles" a greater susceptibility for recurrent mood disorders. He further proposed that sensitivity to both early stressors and mood disorders becomes encoded at the level of gene expression. He suggested that these processes are related to the induction of the proto-oncogene c-fos and related transcription factors. This genetic dysregulation affects the more enduring functioning of certain neurotransmitters, neuroreceptors, and neuropeptides.

Because studies have documented the significant association of suicidal behavior with depression, Post's (1992) observations are important in hypothesizing relationships between early stressful life events and the biological underpinnings for suicidal behavior. For example, Post suggested that the quality of a stressor may have differential effects on oncogenes and transcription factors. This may result in variability in behavioral outcomes. In addition, because of the encoding of neurobiological factors, similar stressors that are experienced at a later point in life may not have to be as intense to induce recurrent behavioral responses. It may, therefore, be hypothesized that early severe stress induces a significant vulnerability to suicidal behavior and that recurrent suicidal acts in vulnerable persons may be precipitated by less intensive stress at a future time.

In summary, research has shown that neuroendocrine and neurotransmitter abnormalities have been identified in suicidal individuals. Studies using animal models and those with humans suggest that early stress induces gene responses that alter neurophysiological functioning. Such neuronal changes have long-lasting effects and are associated with heightened prevalence of mood disorders, a significant risk factor for suicidal behavior.

Conclusions

In this chapter I have reviewed theoretical concepts linking early adverse stressful events to the behavioral outcomes of suicidal behavior. Models defining stress incorporate the life event stimulus, an individual's perceptions of the stimulus, and coping responses. A stress-diathesis model of suicidal behavior in children and adolescents suggests that early stressful life events are risk factors for youth suicidal behavior and that this tragic behavioral outcome may be mediated by deficits in cognitive appraisal and coping mechanisms. Such deficits may be related to specific psychopathologies, such as mood disorders, which are significant risk factors for suicidal behavior. Additional research is necessary to explore the etiological mechanisms of youth suicidal behavior, especially those related to alterations in gene expression that influence neurobiological functioning.

Implications of these concepts are extensive, especially with regard to strategies for preventing youth suicidal behavior. Primary prevention involves identifying children at risk for early stress. Efforts to decrease potential stress may focus on parental social or psychological problems. Among children who have an early history of intense adverse life events, diagnostic assessments and treatment of psychiatric symptoms, especially those associated with mood disorders, may be helpful to avert a future suicidal act. Children and adolescents with a history of suicidal acts should be followed closely and interventions offered, especially at times of stressful events. Such interventions should not only focus on alleviating psychiatric symptoms but also enhance adequate coping mechanisms to deal with perceived stressful events.

References

Adams-Tucker C: Proximate effects of sexual abuse in childhood: a report of 28 children. Am J Psychiatry 139:1252–1256, 1982

Altshuler LL, Casanova MF, Goldberg TE, et al: The hippocampus and parahippocampus in schizophrenic, suicide, and control brains. Arch Gen Psychiatry 47:1029–1034, 1990

Ambrosini PJ, Metz C, Arora RC, et al: Platelet imipramine binding in depressed children and adolescents. J Am Acad Child Adolesc Psychiatry 31:298–305, 1992

Andrus JK, Fleming DW, Heumann MA, et al: Surveillance of attempted suicide among adolescents in Oregon, 1988. Am J Public Health 81:1067–1069, 1991

Asarnow JR, Carlson GA, Guthrie D: Coping strategies, self-perceptions, hopelessness, and perceived family environments in depressed and suicidal children. J Consult Clin Psychol 55:361–366, 1987

Beck AT, Kovacs M, Weissman A: Hopelessness and suicidal behavior: an overview. JAMA 254:1146–1149, 1975

Beck AT, Steer RA, Kovacs M, et al: Hopelessness and eventual suicide: a 10-year prospective study of patients hospitalized with suicidal ideation. Am J Psychiatry 142:559–563, 1985

Blumenthal SJ, Kupfer DJ: Overview of early detection and treatment strategies for suicidal behavior in young people. Journal of Youth and Adolescence 17:1–23, 1988

Borst SR, Noam GG, Bartok JA: Adolescent suicidality: a clinical developmental approach. J Am Acad Child Adolesc Psychiatry 30:796–803, 1991

Brent DA, Perper JA, Goldstein CE, et al: Risk factors for adolescent suicide: a comparison of adolescent suicide victims with suicidal inpatients. Arch Gen Psychiatry 45:581–588, 1988

Brent DA, Kolko DJ, Allan MJ, et al: Suicidality in affectively disordered adolescent inpatients. J Am Acad Child Adolesc Psychiatry 29:586–593, 1990

Brown GW, Harris T: Social Origins of Depression: A Study of Psychiatric Disorder in Women. New York, Free Press, 1978

Carlson GA, Cantwell DP: Suicidal behavior and depression in children and adolescents. Journal of the American Academy of Child Psychiatry 21:361–368, 1982

Carlson GA, Garber J: Developmental issues in the classification of depression in children, in Depression in Young People: Developmental and Clinical Perspectives. Edited by Rutter M, Izard CE, Read PB. New York, Guilford, 1986, pp 399–434

Coccaro EF, Astell JL: Central serotonergic function in parasuicide. Prog Neuropsychopharmacol Biol Psychiatry 14:663–674, 1990

Cohen-Sandler R, Berman AL, King RA: Life stress and symptomatology: determinants of suicidal behavior in children. Journal of the American Academy of Child Psychiatry 21:178–186, 1982

Cole DA: Psychopathology of adolescent suicide: hopelessness, coping beliefs, and depression. J Abnorm Psychol 98:248–255, 1989

Compas BE, Malcarne VL, Fondacaro KM: Coping with stressful events in older children and young adolescents. J Consult Clin Psychol 56:405–411, 1988

DeWilde EJ, Kienhorst ICWM, Diekstra RFW, et al: The relationship between adolescent suicidal behavior and life events in childhood and adolescence. Am J Psychiatry 149:45–51, 1992

Deykin EY, Alpert JJ, McNamara JJ: A pilot study of the effect of exposure to child abuse or neglect on adolescent suicidal behavior. Am J Psychiatry 142:1299–1303, 1985

Freud A: The Ego and the Mechanisms of Defence (1936). New York, International Universities Press, 1946

Freud S: Inhibitions, symptoms and anxiety (1926), in Standard Edition of the Complete Psychological Works of Sigmund Freud, Vol 20. Translated and edited by Strachey J. London, Hogarth Press, 1959, pp 75–175

Hagnell O, Rorsman B: Suicide in the Lundby Study: a controlled prospective investigation of stressful life events. Neuropsychobiology 6:319–332, 1980

Hoberman HH, Garfinkel BD: Completed suicide in children and adolescents. J Am Acad Child Adolesc Psychiatry 27:689–695, 1988

Isherwood J, Adam KS, Hornblow AR: Life event stress, psychosocial factors, suicide attempt and auto-accident proclivity. J Psychosom Res 26:371–383, 1982

Joffe RT, Offord DR, Boyle MH: Ontario Child Health Study: suicidal behavior in youth age 12–16 years. Am J Psychiatry 145:1420–1423, 1988

Kashani JH, Reid JC, Rosenberg TK: Levels of hopelessness in children and adolescents: a developmental perspective. J Consult Clin Psychol 57:496–499, 1989

Kazdin AE, French NH, Unis AS, et al: Hopelessness, depression, and suicidal intent among psychiatrically disturbed inpatient children. J Consult Clin Psychol 51:504–510, 1983

Klerman GL: Suicide, depression, and related problems among the baby boom cohort, in Suicide Among Youth: Perspectives on Risk and Prevention. Edited by Pfeffer CR. Washington, DC, American Psychiatric Press, 1989, pp 63–81

Kosky R, Silburn S, Zubrick SR: Are children and adolescents who have suicidal thoughts different from those who attempt suicide? J Nerv Ment Dis 178:38–43, 1990

Krarup G, Nielsen B, Rask P, et al: Childhood experiences and repeated suicidal behavior. Acta Psychiatr Scand 83:16–19, 1991

Kreitman N, Casey P: Repetition of parasuicide: an epidemiological and clinical study. Br J Psychiatry 153:792–800, 1988

Lazarus R, Folkman S: Stress, Appraisal and Coping. New York, Springer, 1984

Levinson M, Neuringer C: Problem-solving behavior in suicidal adolescents. J Consult Clin Psychol 37:433–436, 1971

Loevinger J, Wessler R, Redmore C: Measuring Ego Development, Vol 2: Scoring Manual for Women and Girls. San Francisco, CA, Jossey-Bass, 1976

Mann JJ, Stanley M (eds): The psychobiology of suicidal behavior. Ann N Y Acad Sci, Vol 487, 1986

Mann JJ, Stanley M, McBride A, et al: Increased serotonin and β-adrenergic receptor binding in the frontal cortices of suicide victims. Arch Gen Psychiatry 43:954–959, 1986

Mann JJ, McBridge PA, Brown RP, et al: Relationship between central and peripheral serotonin indexes in depressed and suicidal psychiatric inpatients. Arch Gen Psychiatry 49:442–446, 1992

McEwen BS, Weiss J, Schwartz L: Selective retention of corticosterone by limbic structures in rat brain. Nature 220:911–912, 1968

McEwen BS, Angelo J, Cameron H, et al: Paradoxical effects of adrenal steroids in the brain: protection versus degeneration. Biol Psychiatry 30:268–289, 1991

Moos R: Context and coping: toward a unifying conceptual framework. Am J Community Psychol 12:5–36, 1984

Myers KM, Burke P, McCauley E: Suicidal behavior by hospitalized pre-adolescent children on a psychiatric unit. Journal of the American Academy of Child Psychiatry 24:474–480, 1985

Myers KM, McCauley E, Calderon R, et al: Risks for suicidality in major depressive disorder. J Am Acad Child Adolesc Psychiatry 30:86–94, 1991

National Center for Health Statistics: Advance report of final mortality statistics 1989. Monthly Vital Statistics Report, Vol 40, No 8, Suppl 2. Hyattsville, MD, National Center for Health Statistics, Public Health Service, 1992

Ostroff R, Giller E, Bonese K, et al: Neuroendocrine risk factors of suicidal behavior. Am J Psychiatry 139:1323–1325, 1982

Patsiokas A, Clum G, Luscomb R: Cognitive characteristics of suicide attempters. J Consult Clin Psychol 47:478–484, 1979

Paykel ES, Prusoff BA, Myers JK: Suicide attempts and recent life events: a controlled comparison. Arch Gen Psychiatry 32:327–333, 1975

Pfeffer CR: The Suicidal Child. New York, Guilford, 1986

Pfeffer CR, Plutchik R, Mizruchi MS, et al: Suicidal behavior in child psychiatric inpatients and outpatients and in nonpatients. Am J Psychiatry 143:733–738, 1986

Pfeffer CR, Newcorn J, Kaplan G, et al: Suicidal behavior in adolescent psychiatric inpatients. J Am Acad Child Adolesc Psychiatry 27:357–361, 1988

Pfeffer CR, Klerman GL, Hurt SW, et al: Suicidal children grow up: demographic and clinical risk factors for adolescent suicide attempts. J Am Acad Child Adolesc Psychiatry 30:609–616, 1991a

Pfeffer CR, Stokes P, Shindledecker R: Suicidal behavior and hypothalamic-pituitary-adrenocortical axis indices in child psychiatric inpatients. Biol Psychiatry 29:909–917, 1991b

Pfeffer CR, Klerman GL, Hurt SW, et al: Suicidal children grow up: rates and psychosocial risk factors for suicide attempts during follow-up. J Am Acad Child Adolesc Psychiatry 32:106–113, 1993

Piaget J: The Origins of Intelligence in Children. New York, International Universities Press, 1952

Post RM: Transdirection of psychosocial stress into the neurobiology of recurrent affective disorder. Am J Psychiatry 149:999–1010, 1992

Recklitis CJ, Noam GG, Borst SR: Adolescent suicide and defensive styles. Suicide Life Threat Behav 22:374–387, 1992

Rich CL, Sherman J, Fowler RC: San Diego Suicide Study: the adolescents. Adolescence 25:855–865, 1990

Rich CL, Warsradt GM, Nemiroff RA, et al: Suicide, stressors, and the life cycle. Am J Psychiatry 148:524–527, 1991

Robins LN, Helzer JE, Weissman MM, et al: Lifetime prevalence of specific psychiatric disorders in three sites. Arch Gen Psychiatry 41:949–958, 1984

Rosenthal PA, Rosenthal S: Suicidal behavior by preschool children. Am J Psychiatry 141:520–525, 1984

Rotheram-Borus MJ, Trautman PD: Hopelessness, depression, and suicidal intent among adolescent suicide attempters. J Am Acad Child Adolesc Psychiatry 27:700–704, 1988

Rotheram-Borus MJ, Trautman PD, Dopkins SC, et al: Cognitive style and pleasant activities among female adolescent suicide attempters. J Consult Clin Psychol 38:554–561, 1990

Roy A, Karoum F, Pollack S: Marked reduction in indexes of dopamine metabolism among patients with depression who attempt suicide. Arch Gen Psychiatry 49:447–450, 1992

Rubenstein JL, Heeren T, Housman D, et al: Suicidal behavior in normal adolescents: risk and protective factors. Am J Orthopsychiatry 59:59–71, 1989

Rutter M: Pathways from childhood to adult life. J Child Psychol Psychiatry 30:23–51, 1989

Salk L, Lipsitt LP, Sturner WQ, et al: Relationship to maternal and perinatal conditions to eventual adolescent suicide. Lancet 1:624–627, 1985

Santostefano S, Rieder C, Beck SA: The structure of fantasied movement in suicidal children and adolescents. Suicide Life Threat Behav 14:3–16, 1984

Schotte D, Clum G: Problem-solving skills in suicidal psychiatric patients. J Consult Clin Psychol 55:50–54, 1987

Shaffer D: Suicide in childhood and early adolescence. J Child Psychol Psychiatry 15:275–291, 1974

Shaffer D: The epidemiology of teen suicide: an examination of risk factors. J Clin Psychiatry 49:36–41, 1988

Slater J, Depue RA: The contribution of environmental events and social support to serious suicide attempts in primary depressive disorder. J Abnorm Psychol 90:275–285, 1981

Spielberger CD, Sarason IG (eds): Stress and Anxiety, Vol 10: A Sourcebook of Theory and Research. New York, Hemisphere, 1986

Spirito A, Williams C, Stark LJ, et al: The Hopelessness Scale for Children: psychometric properties and clinical utility with normal and emotionally disturbed adolescents. J Abnorm Child Psychol 16:445–458, 1988

Spirito A, Overholser J, Hart K: Cognitive characteristics of adolescent suicide attempters. J Am Acad Child Adolesc Psychiatry 30:604–608, 1991

Träskman L, Åsberg M, Bertilsson L, et al: Monoamine metabolites in CSF and suicidal behavior. Arch Gen Psychiatry 38:631–636, 1981

van der Kolk BA, Perry JC, Herman JL: Childhood origins of self-destructive behavior. Am J Psychiatry 148:1665–1671, 1991

Weiner AS, Pfeffer CR: Suicidal status, depression, and intellectual functioning in preadolescent psychiatric inpatients. Compr Psychiatry 27:372–380, 1986

Chapter 13

A Test of the Diathesis-Stress Model of Adolescent Depression in Friends and Acquaintances of Adolescent Suicide Victims

David A. Brent, M.D.
Grace Moritz, A.C.S.W.
Laura Liotus, B.S.

T he diathesis-stress model of depression has gained wide acceptance (Hammen 1992). In brief, this model presupposes that certain factors render individuals vulnerable to depression, but that the expression of depressive symptomatology is most likely to emerge under stress. Lon-

This work was supported by both the Commonwealth of Pennsylvania's state appropriation to Services for Teens at Risk (STAR) of Western Psychiatric Institute and Clinic, and the National Institute of Mental Health (MH-44711) "Youth Exposed to Suicide." The authors gratefully acknowledge the contribution of Ms. Karen Rhinaman, who assisted in preparing this manuscript. In addition, a special note of thanks to the staff who worked on this project: Chris Allman, B.S.; Lisa Balach, B.S.; Amy Friend; Kelly Harrington, B.S.; Mary Remele; Claudia Roth, B.S.; and Joy Schweers, M.Ed.

Many of these results were first published in Brent DA, Perper JA, Moritz G, Allman C, Schweers J, Roth C, Balach L, Canobbio R, Liotus L: "Psychiatric Sequelae to the Loss of an Adolescent Peer to Suicide." *Journal of the American Academy of Child and Adolescent Psychiatry* 32:509–517, 1993. Copyright 1995, American Academy of Child and Adolescent Psychiatry. Reprinted with permission.

gitudinal studies of children at risk for depression by virtue of their attributional style or having a parent with an affective illness show that these vulnerable youth are more likely to evince depressive symptomatology in the face of undesirable life events (Hammen et al. 1990, 1991; Nolen-Hoeksema et al. 1986; Warner et al. 1992).

One particularly stressful event is the death of a relative or friend (Hammen and Goodman-Brown 1990; Holmes and Rahe 1967). Studies of the impact of the loss of a parent on surviving children suggest that depressive symptomatology is a frequent and enduring sequela (van Eerdewegh et al. 1982, 1985; Weller et al. 1991). Consistent with what the diathesis-stress model would predict, children who have lost a parent are most likely to become depressed if they have either a personal or family history of affective illness (van Eerdewegh et al. 1985; Weller et al. 1991).

Little is known about the impact of the loss of a friend due to sudden death. If the death is violent and witnessed, then posttraumatic stress symptomatology is likely to ensue (Pynoos et al. 1987). However, little is known about the course of grief and associated depressive symptomatology. It seems plausible that the death of a peer could be a particularly significant stressor among adolescents because peers take on increased importance during this stage of life (Hartup 1981).

Our own work on the impact of adolescent suicide on peers began as a test of the contagion hypothesis of suicide (Davidson and Gould 1986). In other words, we were interested in learning if the death of an adolescent to suicide put his or her social network at increased risk for suicidal behavior. We also examined, as secondary aims, psychiatric sequelae of exposure to suicide and the course of grief as a function of the nature of the exposure to the suicide ("stress") and vulnerability to depression ("diathesis").

As it turns out, we were unable to confirm the contagion hypothesis (Brent et al. 1992, 1993). Friends and acquaintances of adolescent suicide victims were no more likely to have attempted suicide up to 7 months after exposure to suicide than were unexposed, matched control subjects (Brent et al. 1992, 1993). However, we were able to demonstrate significant psychiatric sequelae associated with the loss, namely major depression and posttraumatic stress disorder (PTSD), in a substantial number of exposed peers of suicide victims.

In this chapter we describe the methods and results of this study and the implications of our findings for the diathesis-stress model of depression. We then use these results to make some observations on the boundary between bereavement and depression.

Methods

The Sample

The friends and acquaintances of 26 adolescent suicide victims were interviewed approximately 7 months after the death of the suicide victim. Parents and siblings nominated friends of the suicide victim with whom the victim had had a close and confiding relationship. Two friends whose names were nominated by both parent and sibling were picked at random and contacted. A third friend was obtained by asking the first two parent-nominated friends for names of other friends of the victim, and one was picked at random. Three acquaintances of the suicide victim were also chosen by having the friends nominate other same-age peers who knew the victim, but not as well as they themselves did. In most cases, three friends and three acquaintances were interviewed per network, for a total of 146 exposed peers. Of the exposed peers approached to participate in the study, 61% agreed.

Control Group

In order for the investigators to assess the impact of exposure, each exposed subject was matched to an unexposed community control. The community control subjects were obtained by geographic cluster sampling of communities that were matched to the communities of the suicide victims with respect to population density, median income, age, and ethnic distribution. The matching communities could not have had an adolescent suicide occur in the community, or in one contiguous to it, for at least 2 years. Ascertainment of targeted tracts was 98%. Unexposed control subjects were matched to the exposed peers on age (within 2 years), race, gender, and externalizing and internalizing scores (±10) on the Child Behavior Checklist (CBCL; Achenbach and Edelbrock 1983). Of those initially approached for a match, 71% consented to an interview.

Assessment

The exposed and unexposed subjects were assessed for past, current, and incident (onset within the past 7 months) disorder by use of the

Schedule of Affective Disorders and Schizophrenia for School-Age Children, Epidemiologic (K-SADS-E; Orvaschel et al. 1982) and Present Episode Versions (K-SADS-P; Chambers et al. 1985). Life events, psychosocial functioning, and family history of psychiatric disorder were obtained blind to proband diagnosis using standardized interviews, namely a structured life events interview (Brent et al. 1988), the Psychosocial Schedule (PSS; Lukens et al. 1983), and Family History–Research Diagnostic Criteria (RDC) (Andreasen et al. 1977), respectively.

The exposed probands' closeness to the suicide victim and their exposure to the suicide were assessed by using the Adolescent Relationship Inventory (ARI) and the Circumstances of Exposure to Death (CED), respectively. The ARI and the CED are semistructured interviews with acceptable psychometric properties (Brent et al. 1992, 1993). Additionally, symptoms of grief were assessed by administering a self-report instrument, the Texas Grief Inventory (TGI; Faschingbauer et al. 1977).

Psychiatric diagnoses were made using best-estimate procedures (Leckman et al. 1982) and DSM-III (American Psychiatric Association 1980) diagnoses, with the additional requirement that functional impairment in school, at work, with peers and family, or in the community needed to be present. Interrater reliability for proband diagnoses, family history, the ARI, CED, and life events was monitored throughout the study and was excellent (Brent et al. 1992, 1993). Because of the matched design, all data analyses are paired (Schlesselman 1982).

The two groups were very closely matched on gender, race, socioeconomic status, and proportion from Allegheny County (Table 13–1). Subjects in the exposed group were slightly older on average ($P <$ .0001), had CBCL scores that reflected more pathology ($P =$ .04), and were less likely to live with both biological parents ($P =$ .0008) (Table 13–1). Subjects in the exposed group were also more likely to have had a previous personal and family history of several psychiatric disorders (Table 13–2).

Results

Incident Disorders

The 7-month incidence of disorder in the exposed group subsequent to exposure to suicide was compared with the 7-month incidence of disorder in the unexposed control subjects (Table 13–3). The exposed group did in fact show higher rates of new-onset depression (29% vs. 5%, χ^2 = 25.0, P < .0001), suicidal ideation with a plan or an attempt (7% vs. 2%, χ^2 = 3.8, P = .05), and PTSD (P = .004), but not suicide attempts. The exposed subjects also showed worsening of substance abuse (9% vs. 0%, P = .0001) (data not shown in Table 13–3). However, there was no significant increase in the rate of suicide attempts in the exposed group. Moreover, almost all of the increase in suicidal ideation was explained by incident depression in the exposed

Table 13–1. Demographic characteristics of the peers exposed to suicide and of the matched control subjects

	Exposed (n = 146)	Control (n = 146)	χ^2 or t test	P
Sex (% male)	54.1	54.1		
Age				
Mean	18.4	17.5		
SD	2.0	1.7	6.43[a]	<.0001
Race (% white)	97.2	100.0		
SES (%)				
I	5.5	2.8		
II	27.6	21.4		
III	33.8	34.5		
IV	27.6	33.3		
V	5.5	8.3		
County of origin (% Allegheny)	45.2	43.8		
Lives with both biological parents (%)	47.6	66.2	11.2	.0008
CBCL [mean (SD)]				
Internalizing	53.5 (10.3)	51.5 (9.0)	1.9[a]	.06
Externalizing	53.1 (10.2)	51.9 (8.4)		
Total behavior	54.1 (12.4)	51.7 (9.9)	2.04[a]	.04

Note. SD = standard deviation; SES = socioeconomic status; CBCL = Child Behavior Checklist (Achenbach and Edelbrock 1983).
[a] t test.

group. These findings were consistent across males, females, friends, and acquaintances (Brent et al. 1992, 1993). The median time to onset of depression in the exposed group was within 1 month of exposure. The median duration of depression was at least 6 months, with the majority (64%) of incident cases of depression still ongoing at the time of the assessment.

When the entire sample was examined, three risk factors emerged as being associated with new-onset depression: previous major depression (16% vs. 6%, $\chi^2 = 5.4, P = .02$), family history of depression (64% vs. 37%, $\chi^2 = 11.2, P = .008$), and interpersonal conflict within the previous 12 months (71% vs. 35%, $\chi^2 = 21.4, P < .0001$). By use of paired logistic regression, it was determined that exposure to suicide conferred a 3.4-fold risk for incident depression (95% confidence interval [CI] = 2.1 to 5.1), after adjustment was made for previous ma-

Table 13–2. Baseline differences in prevalence of risk factors for new-onset psychopathology between the peers exposed to suicide and the control group

History of psychiatric disorder[a]	Exposed (*n* = 146) (%)	Control (*n* = 146) (%)	χ^2	*P*
Personal history of psychiatric disorder				
Any	62	35	22.2	<.0001
Major depression	20	10	5.5	.02
Conduct disorder	22	9	10.3	.001
Substance abuse	30	10	18.7	<.0001
Attention-deficit disorder	16	8	5.3	.02
Any psychiatric treatment	33	13	16.5	<.0001
Family history of psychiatric disorder in first-degree relatives				
Any	85	72	7.1	.008
Major depression	51	37	5.2	.02
Bipolar II disorder	7	2	7.0	.008

[a]Diagnoses based on DSM-III criteria (American Psychiatric Association 1980).

jor depression (relative risk [RR] = 1.8, 95% CI = 1.0–3.2), family history of major depression (RR = 1.5, 95% CI = 1.0–2.2), and interpersonal conflict (RR = 1.9, 95% CI = 1.3–2.8). In the absence of any risk factors, exposure conferred a 3.4-fold relative risk of depression (95% CI = 0.3–38.8), but in the presence of at least one risk factor, the relative risk of depression was 9.8 (95% CI = 3.4–24.5) (Figure 13–1).

Risk Factors for the Development of New-Onset Depression Among the Exposed Group

Those exposed subjects who developed new-onset depression differed from those who did not on a variety of domains (Table 13–4). Those with new-onset depression were more likely to have had a personal (P = .05) or family history of depression (P = .02), to have been exposed to interpersonal loss (P = .0006) or conflict (P = .0001) in the previous 12 months, and to have been closer to the suicide victim, as measured by the ARI (P = .0003). Subjects in the depressed group showed much greater manifestations of grief (P < .0001) and were much more likely to have known the victim's plans before the suicide (P = .04), to have felt that they could have prevented the suicide (P = .007), and to have had a conversation with the victim within

Table 13–3. Incident psychiatric disorder in peers exposed to suicide and in control (unexposed) subjects

Incident psychiatric disorder	Exposed (n = 146) (%)	Control (n = 146) (%)	χ^2	P^a
Any psychiatric disorder	37	8	29.4	<.0001
Major depression	29	5	25.0	<.0001
Substance abuse	1	0		NS
Conduct disorder	0	0		NS
PTSD	6	0	Binomial	.004
Suicidal ideation with a plan or suicide attempt	7	2	3.8	.05
Suicide attempt	3	1		NS

Note. PTSD = posttraumatic stress disorder.
[a]NS = not significant.

Table 13–4. Risk factors for new-onset depression among the peers exposed to suicide

Risk factor	New-onset depression (n = 42) (%)	No depression (n = 86)[a] (%)	χ^2	P
Previous psychiatric disorder				
Any affective disorder	24	11	4.0	.05
Major depressive disorder	17	6	3.9	.05
Family history of psychiatric disorder (rates in first-degree relatives)				
Any psychiatric disorder	57	41	9.5	.002
Affective disorder	30	20	5.4	.02
Major depression	25	16	5.4	.02
PTSD	4	1	4.3	.04
Life events in prior 12 months [mean (SD)]				
Interpersonal conflict	1.2 (1.1)	0.5 (0.9)	1094.5[b]	.0001
Interpersonal loss	1.1 (0.9)	0.6 (0.8)	1166.0[b]	.0006
Other stressors	3.6 (2.7)	2.1 (2.0)	1174.5[b]	.002
Exposure to suicide[c]	49	19	11.0	.0009
Knowledge of victim's plans before death	33	17	4.2	.04
Felt could have prevented suicide	31	11	7.35	.007
Conversation with suicide victim within 24 hours of death	73.8	33.3	18.4	<.0001
Adolescent Relationship Inventory [mean (SD)]	61.5 (29.8)	41.4 (22.8)	3.83[d]	.0003
Texas Grief Inventory [mean (SD)]	51.4 (12.9)	67.7 (16.0)	5.11[e]	<.0001

Note. PTSD = posttraumatic stress disorder; SD = standard deviation.
[a]Eighteen subjects excluded from analyses because they were depressed prior to exposure.
[b]Mann-Whitney U test.
[c]Includes having witnessed suicide, discovered victim, or seen victim at scene of death.
[d]*t* test; higher score indicates closer relationship.
[e]*t* test; lower score indicates more severe grief.

24 hours of the victim's death ($P < .0001$). Finally, depressed subjects were much more likely to have either witnessed the suicide, discovered the body of the victim, or seen the victim at the scene of death ($P = .0009$).

Discussion

In this study, we intended to look at the "contagion" effect of exposure to suicide in the social networks of suicide victims. To our surprise, we failed to find evidence of contagion, as there was no increase in the suicide attempt rate, despite sufficient power to detect an effect size consistent with that reported in the literature (e.g., relative risk ≥ 1.5) (Cohen 1977). It is possible that our negative finding could be attributed to our refusal rate at various stages of sampling, with the resultant effect that incident suicide attempters were more likely to have refused to participate. However, given the high frequency of risk factors for suicidal behavior in the sample accumulated, it seems reasonable to expect to have found contagion in this sample as well.

Somewhat serendipitously, this study turned out instead to be an investigation of the impact of the loss of a friend due to suicide. Our findings are consistent with a diathesis-stress model of depression. The two main stressors were exposure to suicide and loss of a friend. In both instances, the greater the stress, the greater the probability of depression. That is, those with a more intense exposure, and those who were closer to the victim, were more likely to become depressed. In terms of a depressive diathesis, we conceptualized that both personal and familial vulnerability to depression would contribute to risk for depression, and, in fact, both were risk factors for the development of depression. Moreover, in keeping with the diathesis-stress model, those youth who had both the stress (exposure and loss) and the diathesis (personal and family vulnerability to depression) were the most likely to become depressed, as depicted in Figure 13–1.

The mechanism for the development of depression seems clearly to be one of loss leading to acute grief and activating a depressive diathesis. However, one might question why a nonfamilial loss would have such a profound impact on the exposed group. The impact of the loss may have been especially pronounced, in part, because the exposed group was at particularly high risk for the development of psychopathology. Furthermore, given the degree of personal and familial psychopathology in both the suicide victims and their friends, it is possible that they sought one another out and provided support for one another that they could not get from their families. There is evidence to buttress the view that more depressed youngsters place greater emphasis on peer-derived support and less emphasis on familial support (Barrera and Garrison-Jones 1992). If this was the case, then the loss of a friend for youngsters with the predisposition to depression would be particularly devastating. Finally, it is unclear if the loss of a friend due to suicide is more stressful than the loss of a friend due to other means. This latter question should be the subject of future investigations.

One issue that should be addressed is whether the depressive reactions manifested by the exposed group should be considered "normal bereavement" or major depression. We feel that those youth who meet criteria for major depression should be diagnosed as such, cur-

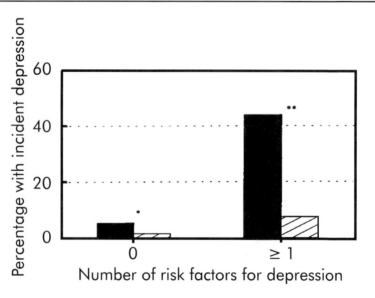

Figure 13–1. Risk for incident major depression in peers exposed to suicide (*solid bars*) and in control subjects (*hatched bars*) based on number of risk factors for depression. Asterisk indicates relative risk of 3.4 (95% confidence interval = 0.3–38.8). Double asterisk indicates relative risk of 9.8 (95% confidence interval = 3.4–24.5).

rent diagnostic conventions notwithstanding. First, the median duration of the depressive "reactions" (on average, at least 6 months) is most consistent with a depressive episode. Second, there was evidence of functional impairment, as required for the diagnosis of depression in this sample, thereby ruling out uncomplicated bereavement (American Psychiatric Association 1980, 1987). Third, the risk factors for the development of a depressive reaction subsequent to exposure—previous history of depression, family history of depression, and interpersonal discord—are all risk factors for depression per se (Hammen et al. 1990; Kovacs et al. 1984; Orvaschel et al. 1988; Puig-Antich et al. 1989; Weissman et al. 1986, 1987). Therefore, it is our view that these depressive reactions represent bona fide major depression and that the clinical practice of those evaluating bereaved individuals should be to diagnose depression when they see it.

These findings have implications for the treatment of depression. The loss of a friend is not currently considered to be a significant risk factor for depression, yet this study indicates that, under certain circumstances, it may be. Youth who present with major depression should be surveyed as to a history of interpersonal losses. Interpersonal therapy may be the most appropriate treatment for depressive episodes triggered by interpersonal losses (Moreau et al. 1991).

With respect to the proper response of a school to a student suicide, interventions have been recommended that are primarily oriented to prevention of contagion (American Association of Suicidology 1989; Centers for Disease Control 1988). Yet, the present findings suggest that imitative suicidality is rare and that a more common and enduring sequela of exposure to suicide may be major depression. If youth exposed to suicide are seen only once shortly after the suicide in a school setting, their responses might be attributed to "normal" bereavement. However, a depressive picture might emerge in some of this same exposed cohort when they are followed over time. Therefore, youth who meet the profile described in this study and who show significant dysphoria shortly after the death of a friend should be followed longitudinally and offered treatment if evidence of major depression becomes apparent.

This study does not address the specificity or generalization of these findings to other types of death besides suicide. Additional investigations are required to learn what the impact of a peer's death due to natural causes, accidental death, or homicide might be on that adolescent's social network. However, these results clearly indicate that the friends and acquaintances of suicide victims are likely to develop major depression as a sequela of such a loss.

References

Achenbach TM, Edelbrock CS: Manual for the Child Behavior Checklist and Revised Child Behavior Profile. Burlington, VT, University of Vermont, Department of Psychiatry, 1983

American Association of Suicidology, School Suicide Prevention Programs Committee: Postvention Guidelines. Denver, CO, American Association of Suicidology, 1989

American Psychiatric Association: Diagnostic and Statistical Manual of Psychiatric Disorders, 3rd Edition. Washington, DC, American Psychiatric Association, 1980

American Psychiatric Association: Diagnostic and Statistical Manual of Psychiatric Disorders, 3rd Edition, Revised. Washington, DC, American Psychiatric Association, 1987

Andreasen NC, Endicott J, Spitzer RL, et al: The family history method using Research Diagnostic Criteria: reliability and validity. Arch Gen Psychiatry 34:1229–1235, 1977

Barrera M, Garrison-Jones C: Family and peer social support as specific correlates of adolescent depressive symptoms. J Abnorm Child Psychol 20:1–16, 1992

Brent DA, Perper JA, Goldstein CE, et al: Risk factors for adolescent suicide: a comparison of adolescent suicide victims with suicidal inpatients. Arch Gen Psychiatry 45:581–588, 1988

Brent DA, Perper JA, Moritz GM, et al: Psychiatric effects of exposure to suicide among the friends and acquaintances of adolescent suicide victims. J Am Acad Child Adolesc Psychiatry 31:629–640, 1992

Brent DA, Perper JA, Moritz G, et al: Psychiatric sequelae to the loss of an adolescent peer to suicide. J Am Acad Child Adolesc Psychiatry 32:509–517, 1993

Centers for Disease Control: CDC recommendations for a community plan for the prevention and containment of suicide clusters. MMWR Morb Mortal Wkly Rep 37, No S-6, 1988

Chambers WJ, Puig-Antich J, Hirsch M, et al: The assessment of affective disorders in children and adolescents by semistructured interview: test-retest reliability of the Schedule for Affective Disorders and Schizophrenia for School-Age Children, Present Episode Version. Arch Gen Psychiatry 42:696–702, 1985

Cohen J: Statistical Power Analysis for the Behavioral Sciences. New York, Academic, 1977

Faschingbauer TR, Devaul RA, Zisook S: Development of the Texas Grief Inventory. Am J Psychiatry 134:696–698, 1977

Davidson L, Gould MS: Contagion as a risk factor for youth suicide, in Risk Factors for Youth Suicide: Report of the Secretary's Task Force on Youth Suicide, Vol 2 (DHHS Publ No [ADM] 89-1622). Rockville, MD, Department of Health and Human Services, 1986, pp 88–109

Hammen C: Life events and depression: the plot thickens. Am J Community Psychol 20:179–193, 1992

Hammen C, Goodman-Brown T: Self-schemas and vulnerability to specific life stress in children at risk for depression. Cognitive Therapy and Research 14:215–227, 1990

Hammen C, Burge D, Burney E, et al: Longitudinal study of diagnoses in children of women with unipolar and bipolar affective disorder. Arch Gen Psychiatry 47:1112–1117, 1990

Hammen C, Burge D, Adrian C: Timing of mother and child depression in a longitudinal study of children at risk. J Consult Clin Psychol 59:341–345, 1991

Hartup WW: Peer relations and family relations: two social worlds, in Scientific Foundations of Developmental Psychiatry. Edited by Rutter M. Baltimore, MD, University Park Press, 1981, pp 280–292

Holmes TH, Rahe RH: The social readjustment rating scale. J Psychosom Res 11:213–218, 1967

Kovacs M, Feinberg T, Crouse-Novak M, et al: Depressive disorders in childhood, II: a longitudinal study of the risk for a subsequent major depression. Arch Gen Psychiatry 41:643–649, 1984

Leckman JF, Sholomskas D, Thompson D, et al: Best estimate of lifetime diagnosis: a methodological study. Arch Gen Psychiatry 39:879–883, 1982

Lukens E, Puig-Antich J, Behn J, et al: Reliability of the Psychosocial Schedule for School Age Children. Journal of the American Academy of Child Psychiatry 22:29–39, 1983

Moreau D, Mufson L, Weissman MM, et al: Interpersonal psychotherapy for adolescent depression: description of modification and preliminary application. J Am Acad Child Adolesc Psychiatry 30:642–651, 1991

Nolen-Hoeksema S, Girus JS, Seligman MEP: Learned helplessness in children: a longitudinal study of depression, achievement, and explanatory style. J Pers Soc Psychol 51:435–442, 1986

Orvaschel H, Puig-Antich J, Chambers W, et al: Retrospective assessment of prepubertal major depression with the K-SADS-E. Journal of the American Academy of Child Psychiatry 21:392–397, 1982

Orvaschel H, Walsh-Allis G, Ye W: Psychopathology in children of parents with recurrent depression. J Abnorm Child Psychol 16:17–28, 1988

Puig-Antich J, Goetz D, Davies M, et al: A controlled family history study of prepubertal depressive disorder. Arch Gen Psychiatry 46:406–418, 1989

Pynoos RS, Frederick C, Nader K, et al: Life threat and posttraumatic stress in school-age children. Arch Gen Psychiatry 44:1057–1063, 1987

Schlesselman J: Case-Control Studies: Design, Conduct, Analysis. New York, Oxford University Press, 1982

van Eerdewegh MM, Biere MD, Parrilla RH, et al: The bereaved child. Br J Psychiatry 140:23–29, 1982

van Eerdewegh MM, Clayton PJ, van Eerdewegh P: The bereaved child: variables influencing early psychopathology. Br J Psychiatry 147:188–194, 1985

Warner V, Weissman MM, Fendrich M, et al: The course of major depression in the offspring of depressed parents. Arch Gen Psychiatry 49:795–801, 1992

Weller RA, Weller EB, Fristad MA, et al: Depression in recently bereaved prepubertal children. Am J Psychiatry 148:1536–1540, 1991

Weissman MM, John K, Merikangas KR, et al: Depressed parents and their children: general health, social, and psychiatric problems. Am J Dis Child 140:801–805, 1986

Weissman MM, Gammon D, John K, et al: Children of depressed parents: increased psychopathology and early onset of major depression. Arch Gen Psychiatry 44:847–853, 1987

Chapter 14

Siblings of Youth Suicide Victims

David C. Clark, Ph.D.
Ann E. Goebel, B.A.

The legacy of a deceased sibling can take any one of a number of different forms, including increased vulnerability to psychopathology, or increased resilience, increased maturity, and the strengthening of bonds between family members. According to some researchers and clinicians, these different types of outcomes are determined in part by the quality of the premorbid sibling relationship and/or by the circumstances of the death itself.

The Sibling Relationship

Only a modest amount of empirical research has been published describing the unique nature of the sibling relationship. Bank and Kahn (1982) hypothesize that sibling attachment forms in proportion to "sibling access" (i.e., access to similar experiences) so that those siblings who are the same sex and closer in age tend to become more emotionally close and more affectionate with each other. In the context of this definition, an identical twinship reared together would

From the Center for Suicide Research and Prevention, Department of Psychiatry, Rush-Presbyterian–St. Luke's Medical Center in Chicago, Illinois. This work was supported by a grant from the National Institute of Mental Health (MH-45501; "Affective Disorder, Substance Abuse, Teen Suicide, and Health Care Utilization").

represent siblings with highest access. Bank and Kahn point out that societal changes have encouraged greater interdependence between siblings in this century. For example, as families have decreased in size (the average family in the United States today has two children), sibling relationships have intensified. And as families have become more mobile, siblings remain one of the few constants in a fluid peer group. Bank and Kahn believe that the quality of sibling identification with each other exerts critical influence on the survivor's reactions to a sibling's death. If the relationship was conflicted before the death, "whatever conflicts the surviving children may have experienced while their sibling was alive must be sealed off" (Bank and Kahn 1982). Alternatively, if the relationship was characterized by overidentification, surviving siblings may end up living "two lives—their own and that of a dead brother or sister" (Bank and Kahn 1982).

Bereavement in Childhood and Adolescence

There is a common tendency to view bereavement as a brief or time-limited phenomenon, particularly in the case of children and adolescents. Because the young are perceived to be "sheltered" from the pressures of the adult world, because they are perceived to be more flexible and adaptable than their adult counterparts, and because they do not seem to dwell continuously on their grief after a death, many adults believe that young persons can digest the experience of losing a family member or friend by death in the space of a few months. Indeed, some grief investigators interpret evidence of adolescent grief persisting for more than 6 months as evidence of pathological processes and/or psychopathology (Brent et al. 1992).

We will argue, on the other hand, that the painful and dysphoric sequelae of youthful bereavement are likely to last *longer* than the 12 to 24 months usually estimated from profiles of adult widows and widowers. As Bank and Kahn (1982) have noted, "Death ends only a life: it does not end a relationship." The relationship interrupted in the case of child or adolescent bereavement is often one necessary for the surviving sibling to continue for reasons of maturation.

Bereavement, Grief, and
Mourning: Definitions

Mental health professionals, research scientists, and laypeople alike tend to use the terms grief, mourning, and bereavement interchangeably. Because consensual definitions facilitate clinical discussion and research communication, we advocate adoption of the definitions recommended by a National Academy of Sciences work group in their monograph summarizing current knowledge on the topic of bereavement (Osterweiss et al. 1984). In this schema, *grief* refers to the dysphoric feeling or affective response to the death of a loved one. *Mourning* describes the internal process of adaptation to death that culminates in an appropriate or maladaptive adjustment. Mourning also includes social rituals and other social expressions of grief. *Bereavement* is an umbrella term encompassing both the feelings of grief and the process of mourning; it represents the social process of coping along with various emotional responses to death.

The Quality of Childhood and Adolescent Grief: Descriptive Assessment of Grief Symptoms

The Adolescent Bereavement Consortium (David Balk, David Brent, David Clark, Barry Garfinkel, Madelyn Gould, Emily Harris, Gerald Koocher, Robert Pynoos, Elizabeth Weller, and Ronald Weller) sponsored by the W. T. Grant Foundation of New York City has reviewed the published literature and work in progress on the adolescent grief experience to develop a structured clinical interview, the Adolescent Grief Inventory (AGI), designed for use with children ages 10 to 19 years (Clark et al. 1994). The preliminary version included 142 questions representing eight conceptual domains:

- Reminiscences (i.e., attempts to actively remember or recapture, passive remembering, and the attendant feelings)
- Reunion fantasies in states of wakefulness or dream
- Experiences of disbelief (conscious and unconscious)
- Examples of identification with the deceased
- Participation in memorial activities or rituals
- Attempts to psychologically master the grief experience

- Behavioral changes not directly related to the experience of grief or sadness
- Personal conception of the grief process and recovery

Adolescent responses to the interview questions are probed, interpreted, and scored on a five-point scale by the interviewer based on the frequency and severity of reported grief symptoms.

In reliability exercises, AGI interviews with bereaved adolescents who had lost a family member by death in the last year were videotaped and circulated among eight clinicians for independent rating. This rating exercise allowed the consortium to establish good scoring reliability among raters. Items associated with low interrater reliability were dropped from the inventory.

A principal components analysis of the clinical ratings yielded a four-factor solution. Varimax rotation of the four-factor solution yielded four interpretable dimensions underlying the response scores that transected the eight hypothesized conceptual domains:

- Items related to active avoidance of remembering and the experience of painful, intrusive memories.
- Items associated with recalling of activities done together with the deceased, feelings of physical and emotional closeness with the deceased, behavioral imitation of the deceased, and identificatory behavior.
- Items related to heightened perceptual vigilance, vivid affective reactions other than sadness or euthymia, and some distancing of the self from the deceased.
- Items having to do with behavioral problems in school, experiencing of reminiscences as distressing, and pessimism about one's ability to transcend the grief experience.

These four dimensions characterize individual differences and so offer an empirical view of the experience of acute grief in adolescence. The first obtained factor, *painful intrusive memories/active avoidance,* may describe adolescents who have been overwhelmed or traumatized by the grief experience. Their responses indicate the presence of painful symptoms and an acute sense of vulnerability to disturbing, invasive, and often overpowering memories. The next two factors, *physical and emotional closeness/behavioral imitation* and *proactive affective compensation,* seem to relate to the different active coping styles associated with relief from distress and a sense of positive grief progress. The last factor, *misbehavior/distressful reminiscences/absence of grief progress*, may indicate that an unsuccessful coping style has been adopted. This particular study does not inform us about the typical time course of the symptoms and concerns illustrated by the four grief factors.

In one study of sibling bereavement, Balk (1983a) found that one-third of adolescents liked dreams about their dead sibling and found them comforting. In another study of sibling bereavement (Balk 1991), the same author found that adolescents were not necessarily capable of a consistent intellectual, logical, and rational understanding of death. Adolescents who understood the finality and universality of death in general terms often denied this reality when the death in question touched someone close to them. Similarly, adolescents often denied the fact that they themselves are vulnerable to death.

Sibling Suicide

The death of a sibling by suicide is a tragic event made more difficult by the relative immaturity of the surviving sibling. The surviving sibling's lack of experience with death and his or her relative immaturity render parental and other adult models of grief and bereavement particularly influential.

The literature on childhood and adolescent grief is vast but flawed by limitations in conceptualization and methodology. Despite long-standing clinical interest in the plight of adolescents who have lost a sibling, the professional and research literatures contain few empirical contributions that might guide our thinking and clinical intervention strategies. A number of theoretical papers, case studies, literature reviews, and dissertations have been published, but in aggregate they do little to define the experience, identify risk and protective factors, or clarify the long-term outcomes possible. A few of the more valuable studies are cited below.

Guilt

One of the most common reactions to the death of a sibling is guilt. In some cases, guilt is still present 5 or more years following the death of a sibling (Cain et al. 1964). Guilt may be manifested in physical reactions of crying, trembling, and sadness upon talking about the deceased sibling. Surviving siblings may mull over all the bad thoughts that they ever had about the deceased sibling. Many of the siblings feel at fault for the death or feel that they should have been the one who died instead (Cain et al. 1964; Hogan 1986). Their guilt is exacerbated at times when they find themselves laughing with friends and behaving like healthy teenagers—guilt can leave surviving siblings feeling that they should not be allowed to enjoy life.

Suicide rarely occurs in a vacuum. Often the surviving family members have suffered from the stress of caring for a mentally ill family member or the worry of suicidal threats for weeks, months, or years before the death (Hauser 1987). Some family members may feel a kind of relief at finally having this kind of chronic stress alleviated. Feelings of relief over the death of a loved one can themselves exacerbate guilt.

Adolescents who characteristically felt inordinate degrees of responsibility for their siblings are most vulnerable to exaggerated feelings of guilt and responsibility after the death. In one study of 10 sibling survivors of suicide, Todd (1980) found that 4 of the siblings fit this profile. Todd also found that siblings who felt pronounced guilt were sometimes motivated by guilt to relive the lost relationship—for example, allowing this to steer them into a career, such as one of the helping professions.

Anger and Denial

After a suicide, sibling survivors may feel abandoned and rejected by the deceased. Sibling survivors may be angry that the suicide victim did not let them know that he or she was considering suicide, or angry that the victim did not give them a chance to offer help. They may have offered help or tried their best to stop the suicide, and the victim may still have chosen to end his or her life. Surviving siblings may be angry at their brother or sister for leaving them behind or for leaving them with the emotional mess and pain of suicide aftermath. Because anger at the dead is socially unacceptable in most quarters, however, the surviving siblings may not feel permitted to express or acknowledge these feelings. Suppressed anger may be displaced onto other family members. Thus blame and scapegoating can come to block familial communication and add to the burden already experienced by surviving families (Hauser 1987; Ness and Pfeffer 1990).

Suicidal Ideation

Some studies have suggested that efforts to maintain a connection or to reconnect with a deceased family member (usually referred to as "reunion fantasies") are common in cases of youthful bereavement (Black 1984). Younger children's dreams may sometimes take the form of literal apparitions of ghosts. Adolescents, however, have a better appreciation for the difference between dreams and reality. As noted earlier, Balk (1983a) found that one-third of bereaved adolescents found dreams about their dead sibling comforting. Suicidal ideation and impulses are also common among surviving siblings and can be viewed in part as reunion attempts in fantasy. But such acts can also be motivated by surviving siblings' guilt or feelings that they should have been the one who died. Sometimes the surviving sibling becomes particularly accident-prone or engages in risk-taking behavior as an expression of these suicidal feelings. And, of course, it is important to remember that in cases of pathological bereavement or comorbid psychopathology, suicidal tendencies may represent the presence of major psychopathology and/or appreciable suicide risk.

Identification

Surviving relatives and family friends often see resemblances in the looks, habits, and personality of the surviving siblings that remind them of the deceased child. When the surviving sibling has a strong or excessive identification with the deceased, when family members and friends overaccentuate the identification, or when the similarities are simply great, the surviving sibling may become confused with the deceased and may be pushed to respond to or accept "replacement expectations" (Cain et al. 1964). Sometimes the identification with a deceased sibling can be so intense that the living sibling fears meeting the same fate as was met by their deceased brother or sister (Pollock 1986).

Questioning Why

The desire to find some plausible explanation for the death is an urgent, perhaps universal type of response to the tragic, abrupt, and ambiguous dimensions of a death by suicide. However, the search for these sorts of "conclusive reasons" can lead to overzealous "witch hunts" (i.e., finding an evil and powerful person to blame) and/or specious psychological theorizing. When a sibling is exposed to this kind of activity on the part of parents or other family members, the sibling generally has little recourse but to accept the adult theories of "what went wrong." The result may be that the surviving sibling blames himself or herself or fellow loved ones, or is unified with other family members against a nonfamilial agent (Todd 1980). This kind of premature closure generally hinders the sibling's ability to pose the unique questions that occur to him or her, to consider and explore the evidence independently, and to develop answers that seem personally meaningful.

Youthful Grief After the Suicide of a Friend: Findings From Controlled Studies

Controlled studies have the potential to identify symptoms that are unique to grief states, but few descriptive or controlled studies have considered anything other than parent loss in the case of children or adolescents. Two recent studies of adolescent grief after the suicide of a peer, though not a sibling, are particularly valuable to consider for this reason.

In one controlled study, Brent and colleagues (1992) interviewed 58 friends and acquaintances of 10 adolescent suicide victims 6 months after the deaths and compared incidence rates for psychiatric symptoms during the bereavement period with those for a matched group of 58 adolescents from similar communities. Almost two-thirds (62%) qualified for psychopathological diagnosis before exposure to the suicide, and more than one-third (36%) had received psychiatric treatment before. The incidence of a depressive syndrome was higher for the group exposed to the suicide of a friend, and risk for developing a depressive syndrome was higher for those with a personal or family history of major depression. Depressive syndromes tended to begin in the first month after the suicide, and most syndromes persisted beyond 6 months. Despite higher rates of depressive symptoms, the friends of suicide victims did not show a higher rate of *suicide attempts* during the 6 months following the death. The risk of developing symptoms of posttraumatic stress disorder (PTSD) was higher for those with a personal or family history of anxiety disorder, but the severity of PTSD symptoms was also correlated with the closeness of the preexisting relationship and with the experience of witnessing the suicide or finding the body. No subjects qualified for a diagnosis of PTSD, however.

In their discussion of these findings, Brent and colleagues hypothesized that exposure to the suicide of a friend precipitated a *pathological bereavement reaction* for many of the adolescents, manifested as a bona fide major depressive episode. They based their interpretation on observations that measures of grief and depression severity were intercorrelated, measures of grief and depression both were correlated with the closeness of the relationship to the suicide victim, the risk of developing major depression was higher for friends with a personal or family history of major depression, and the depressive syndromes were long-lasting—often 5 or 6 months in duration at the 6-month follow-up assessment.

Alternatively, one could hypothesize that the friends of suicide victims who evidenced a variety of depressive symptoms persistently over the 6-month period following the death were simply bereaved in a more severe or prolonged fashion than the investigators expected, but that the quality of grief was not patently pathological and the diagnosis of major depression is not justified.

In another controlled study, Hazell and colleagues (Hazell and Lewin 1993) interviewed 152 friends of two adolescent suicide victims 8 months after the deaths and compared prevalence rates for psychiatric symptoms in this sample with those in a group of 554 other adolescents attending the same two high schools. Friends of the suicide victims were divided into two subgroups: those who reported having a friend who had made a suicide attempt before ($n = 84$) and those who did not ($n = 68$). Bereaved students in the first subgroup showed more symptoms of suicidal ideation, suicidal behavior, depression, delinquency, somatizing, and drug use than did students who had not lost a friend by suicide. But bereaved students in the second subgroup failed to show more symptoms of any type than did students who had not lost a friend by suicide.

Students who had not lost a friend by suicide in the previous 8 months were also divided into two subgroups: those who reported having a friend who had made a suicide attempt before ($n = 92$) and those who did not ($n = 554$). Nonbereaved students in the first subgroup showed more symptoms of suicidal behavior and depression than did students in the second subgroup.

Hazell and colleagues interpreted the results to mean that friends of adolescent suicide victims are not particularly likely to be symptomatic 8 months later unless they had a preexisting vulnerability to suicidal behavior and other problems. These authors hypothesized that students who were friends with both an adolescent who died by suicide and one or more other adolescents who had attempted suicide were the most psychologically vulnerable group because emotionally vulnerable adolescents tend to congregate in social groups (Hazell and Lewin 1993).

Comorbidity Following Loss of a Sibling by Suicide

As discussed earlier, there is a paucity of studies defining the "average expectable" course of grief for children or adolescents, and consequently there is a tendency for investigators to invoke the label of "pathological grief reaction" or "comorbid depressive illness" in cases when the young person exhibits many depressive symptoms, or when his or her grief syndrome has lasted for a long time. In what follows we review some clinical studies that consider the boundaries between normal grief reactions and psychopatholgical states.

Depressive Illness

Studies of adult bereavement have demonstrated nearly equivocally that there is great overlap between symptoms of normal grief and symptoms of major depression (Clayton 1974; Clayton et al. 1971, 1972). Dysphoria in the initial period after a death is common, but in most cases such dysphoria decreases significantly over time. A mild depressive state is characteristic of most bereaved children and adolescents.

One of the most difficult questions confronting grief investigators is how to discriminate between those persons who are acutely bereaved and those who develop "pathological" bereavement or major depression superimposed on a "normal" grief state. Despite almost 75 years of theoretical formulation and debate, the problem remains far from solved. Even current-day psychiatric diagnostic criteria evade the problem. The official psychiatric nomenclature (DSM-III-R) discourages clinicians from making a diagnosis of major depression in cases of acute grief unless the grief reaction is abnormal or accompanied by "morbid preoccupation with worthlessness, prolonged and marked functional impairment, [or] marked psychomotor retardation" (American Psychiatric Association 1987, p. 361). Because many symptoms of acute depressive illness are also characteristic of grief states, and because "normal grief" has not yet been defined phenomenologically in any reliable fashion for any age group, it remains too easy for clinicians to label bereavement reactions as "pathological" and superimpose psychiatric diagnoses with minimal justification. The boundaries between grief and depressive phenomena need further clarification.

In one study of 201 close relatives or intimate friends of persons who died by sudden natural or violent causes, Vargas and colleagues (1980) found that features traditionally associated with pathological grief (e.g., depressive symptoms, anger, difficulty relinquishing the lost object) are characteristic of many or most bereaved persons, and that the concept of "pathological" grief may have less to do with phenomenology than with the frequency, intensity, and duration of these symptoms. Balk (1983a) interviewed 33 siblings to assess changes in their self-concept following the death of a sibling. He found that for many of these adolescents, the symptoms of grief (i.e., tears, shaking, and even shortness of breath) were still present when they spoke about their deceased siblings 2 or more years after the deaths.

Is comorbid depressive illness confined for the most part to those children and adolescents with a prior history of affective disorder? For example, in a study by Weller and colleagues (1991), children who had had an untreated psychiatric disorder prior to the death of a parent were more likely to develop a depressive illness during the early course of their grief. Likewise, Brent and colleagues (1992) showed that adolescents with a prior history of major depression were more likely to develop a depressive illness during the first 6 months following the death of a friend by suicide. Thus it is not yet clear whether the onset of depressive states in early months of acute grief represent 1) nothing more than severe, impairing, or long-lasting versions of normal grief reactions; 2) distinctly pathological forms of grief reactions; or 3) independent, comorbid psychopathology that has been triggered by an aversive life event (i.e., the death of a family member or close friend).

Implicit in these questions, of course, are profoundly different viewpoints about when children in mourning should be left to find their own ways of coping and when they should be offered treatment. Answers to these kinds of questions can be obtained only from well-wrought long-term follow-up studies. One strategy for discriminating among normal bereavement, pathological bereavement, and depressive illness lies in the development of age-sensitive criteria for assessing grief states without resorting to depression symptom inventories. A second strategy lies in longitudinal studies of preadolescents with and without a history of a major affective disorder. Studies like this would be valuable to compare the phenomenology, severity, and duration of bereavement reactions of children/adolescents with and without a prior history of affective disorder.

Posttraumatic Stress Reactions

The circumstances of a death by suicide can be more difficult for a child to understand than any other form of death. Parents usually have difficulty discussing the circumstances of suicides with their surviving children. The parents may give misleading explanations or may not discuss the death at all. This confusing situation is often compounded by neighborhood rumors and inaccurate media reports. Children tend to be aware of when portions of details about a familial death are being hidden from them. This results in the children's knowing and feeling things they are not *supposed* to know or feel. The incongruence between what children are told and what they actually know may contribute to chronic confusion, an inability to identify their own feelings, and a lack of understanding of the nature of the death. Understanding the cause of death is a part of the initial work of coping with loss.

Coping with death by suicide can be further complicated for children or adolescents who actually find or inadvertently view the injured body of a deceased sibling. Work by Pynoos (1992) provides strong evidence that children who have witnessed a violent injury or death often exhibit posttraumatic stress reactions that complicate the normal grieving process. Children who witness violent death, in contrast to death by natural causes, are confronted with two types of reminders: reminders of the loss itself and reminders of the violence. In cases in which the victim's sibling has witnessed the suicide or been among the first to discover the body, two distinct syndromes often emerge: one related to grief and the other to PTSD (Nader et al. 1990).

It is common for children who witness a suicide or find the body to develop persistent bad dreams and intrusive images, or to reexperience sounds from the scene of the suicide (Yule and Williams 1990).

For example, they will repeatedly visualize images of their sibling's wounded body. These disturbing and anxiety-provoking images may interfere with the sibling's ability to reminisce about the deceased brother or sister. Reactions that keep the child preoccupied with the traumatic details of the suicide may interfere with his or her ability to focus on and master the emotional aspect of loss.

Even in the absence of full-blown PTSD, suicide survivors often experience profound psychological numbing, emotional avoidance, and constriction in relation to the suicide. The bereaved may attempt to avoid thoughts of the event to protect himself or herself from reactions of intense horror and fear. Locations and situations that are reminders of the suicide may also be avoided. Helping the bereaved child to address and tolerate these reminders may initiate recovery from emotional constriction.

Behavior and Academic Problems

Sibling survivors sometimes report difficulty concentrating in school because of intrusive thoughts or disturbing associations (Dunne-Maxim et al. 1987; Gaffney et al. 1992). Balk (1983a) found that 25% of the 33 bereaved siblings he interviewed had developed academic difficulties since the time of the loss. Some sibling suicide survivors become preoccupied with the concept of death and suicide and cannot seem to focus on anything else.

Raphael (1983) hypothesized that some adolescents who suppress their grief, rather than express their grief or "work it through," may become aggressive, hostile, uncooperative, and destructive of property, with an associated increased risk of alcohol and drug use. When these behaviors are misunderstood as simply lawless or defiant, the child's problems are compounded by punishment (Wass 1984).

One long-term follow-up study of more than 11,000 9th-grade Minnesota public school students found that subjects who had lost a parent by death showed more delinquent behavior in 10th grade and committed more legal offenses in their early 20s, but that the trend toward more delinquency no longer pertained in their 30s (Bendickson and Fulton 1976; Gregory 1965; Markusen and Fulton 1971).

Somatic Symptoms

The most common somatic symptoms among bereaved children who experience such symptoms appear to be gastrointestinal problems, stomachaches, and headaches (Sood et al. 1992). Children may lose their appetite or suffer digestive problems like vomiting, diarrhea, or constipation. Younger children sometimes experience a regression to loss of bladder control. Others suffer from a feeling of emptiness in their stomachs, tightness in their throats, and disrupted sleep (Wass 1984).

Clinical Observations in the Course of a Psychological Autopsy Study

In April 1990 we began a 5-year National Institute of Mental Health–funded prospective community-based psychological autopsy study of adolescents who died by suicide in the Chicago metropolitan area. The study was designed to compare a series of adolescent suicide victims with a series of adolescents who died in a car accident and a group of matched living adolescents from the same neighborhoods as the suicide victims were from. To characterize the psychological state and behavior of subjects during the weeks preceding death (or preceding study admission, for the living group), we have been conducting lengthy individual structured clinical interviews with five "knowledgeable informants" per subject—ideally the subject's mother, father, closest-aged sibling, a close male friend, and a close female friend.

Thus one by-product of our investigation has been the opportunity to become acquainted with adolescents who recently lost a sibling by suicide and to listen to them describe their view of and knowledge about the tragic incident. Another by-product has been the opportunity to compare the siblings of adolescent suicide victims with the siblings of adolescents who died in car accidents. Although these observations about the grief experience of adolescent siblings are anecdotal and not the focus of our investigation, the robust sampling procedure (i.e., in about 75% of all consecutive adolescent suicides and car accident fatalities, families give their consent to and participate in interviews) and the structured nature of our contacts enhance the value of our observations.

We have noticed that parents who have lost an adolescent child by suicide often become acutely and intensely frightened about the prospect of losing another child in the same way—even in situations in which the child's distress or symptoms give little objective cause for concern. The anxiety about losing another child suddenly and unexpectedly by suicide is often unspoken and preconscious. In cases in which the adolescent who died by suicide was in some form of mental health care during the weeks preceding death, the parents may be too angry at the "failure" of a professional to access any further mental health services for the siblings, or they may despair about the ability of anyone to protect the family from further tragedy. Parents who have lost a child by suicide, if they have initiated contact with a support group for persons in their situation, may become exquisitely aware of the existence of other families who have lost two or three adolescent children by suicide (there are a number of examples of more than one sibling in a family dying by suicide in every large metropolitan area). The first instinct of many parents, in their protective concern for their surviving children, is to shield the siblings from participation in any research investigation, lest the experience prove too upsetting or destructive.

The parents, however, are typically willing to be interviewed. Reasons they give for participating include the opportunity to talk with a professional who listens intently and does not judge, to ask questions of a professional who has become acquainted with many other cases of suicide, and to share personal experiences with scientists in the altruistic hope that what can be learned will someday spare another family from experiencing the same tragedy. Once they have completed their own interview, and once they have had a chance to voice their fears about their surviving offspring, most parents who were initially reluctant decide that it would be a good thing to allow their children to talk with the clinicians who conduct our research study. Most of the grieving persons we interview, adults and adolescents alike, describe study participation as a positive and useful experience, which has generally been the experience of participants in many other studies using psychological autopsies reported in the literature (Shneidman and Farberow 1961; Litman et al. 1963, 1983; Shneidman 1981; Beskow et al. 1990).

Some of the adolescent siblings of suicide victims we have interviewed lack insight into the personality and condition of their deceased sibling. This is most often the case when the sister or brother who died had been afflicted with a major psychiatric disorder for a long period of time, and when the illness was characterized by pronounced irritability or volatility of mood at the time of death. Many of these surviving siblings were frightened by the erratic behavior of the

deceased and coped with their fear by avoiding the subject and forming a consciously distant sibling relationship.

Other grieving siblings continue to express anger and jealousy
about the attention the deceased received for a long period of time
prior to death and continues to receive after death. While the parents
were trying to access adequate care for the chronically or episodically
ill sibling, the needs of the other siblings may not have been met, or
may have been given a low priority. Many of the siblings in this situation engage in avoidance behaviors that are conscious and purpose-
ful. For example, one such sibling in our study busied himself with
a homework assignment during his sister's funeral service.

Still other siblings had developed a long-term caretaking relationship with the fragile or ill subject, which in many cases included
chronic, conscious feelings of responsibility to keep the brother or
sister alive. They motivated the family to access treatment in crisis
periods, tried to problem-solve for the ill sibling, and persistently worried about whether or not they were doing enough to make a difference. These surviving siblings often report feeling relief in the months
following the death, but also some guilt linked to this seemingly "inappropriate" reaction. After the death of a sister in whom he had invested an extraordinary amount of vigilance and counseling, for
example, one adolescent boy described feeling as though a physical
weight had been lifted from his shoulders and the emptiness in his
stomach had vanished. The same siblings, however, often report
a problematic void in their lives at a later point—perhaps because
their chosen life-and-death responsibility is no longer available. These
survivors often go through a long period of confusion and mild disorganization before achieving a new, firmer sense of identity and
purpose.

Apart from these patterns, we have not observed remarkable differences between the quality of grief in siblings bereaved by suicide
and siblings bereaved by car accident. This conclusion is consistent
with the limited empirical evidence available on the topic, but runs
counter to prevailing clinical theory (Ness and Pfeffer 1990). Those
who lost a brother or sister by suicide were certainly exposed to
a great deal more in the way of social stigma, curiosity, and sensation-
alism by other persons. The parents of adolescent suicide victims seem
to have a qualitatively different, though not necessarily more distressed, course of grief than do the parents of adolescents who died in
car accidents—and, of course, parents' grief exerts a strong influence

on the surviving offsprings' grief in numerous direct and indirect ways. But the death of an adolescent sibling by suicide does not seem to characteristically beg the same profound questions about personal worth, personal vulnerability, personal responsibility, fairness and evil, or the capacity to heal that we see in parents who have lost a child, or in children who have lost a parent by suicide.

The majority of the sibling survivors we have studied did not witness the act of suicide and did not encounter the corpse in the hours after suicide, so that here we are referring to cases in which traumatic exposure has not complicated the sibling's grief reaction. In our ongoing investigation of adolescent suicide, it is also important to note, we do not have provisions for studying the course of sibling grief reactions over time. Although many adolescents and their families have remained in touch with our research group for a variety of reasons, it is, of course, possible that we have enjoyed more consistent and long-lasting contact with those enjoying a more favorable course.

Secondary Impact of Sibling Death by Suicide

A death in the family is not simply an isolated, one-time stressor, but an event that initiates cascades of changes and secondary stressors that also have an impact on the survivors. All these resulting changes have a potential impact on the child's or adolescent's bereavement process.

Changes in Family Relationships

The quality and duration of the surviving parents' grief reaction directly influence the child's sense of safety and well-being, and the parents' reaction serves as one model of grief response for the child to consider. Correlations between the acute emotional distress of a child and his or her parent following the death of a sibling (Demi and Gilbert 1987) support the hypothesis that a child's ability to recognize and express his or her emotions is powerfully influenced by parental role modeling. One of the main issues facing sibling survivors is the degree to which parents are able to continue to participate in their remaining children's lives, or the degree to which they become demoralized and inoperative as parents.

If parents are so grief-stricken that they show less interest in their remaining children, become less involved in their children's daily lives, or neglect them, the offspring may effectively experience the loss of more than one person—that is, the deceased sibling and one or both of the bereaved parents. In cases in which acute bereavement impinges on a parent's prior history of psychopathology to yield frank psychopathology (e.g., depressive illness, alcohol abuse), the problems posed for the remaining offspring may be serious. In this situation, the surviving offspring may experience a need to suppress any feelings of sadness, grief, or depression of their own, because they may not want to worry or further burden a preoccupied or ill parent. In their parent's emotional absence, these children may grow up so fast and become so competent that they become premature caretakers—parents to their own parents (Dunne-Maxim et al. 1987).

When bereavement occurs during childhood or adolescence, the surviving sibling must integrate these changing family dynamics with his or her own changing developmental needs. For example, the adolescent may have been struggling for increased independence from the family when the death occurred. Gaffney and colleagues (1992) have shown how this struggle can be made more difficult or abandoned altogether in the face of parents whose guilt drives them to become overprotective. In this situation, some adolescents report feeling as though their every move is being monitored.

Families often feel so suddenly and unexpectedly diminished when they lose a child by suicide that parents continue to worry about the safety of the remaining children for a long time afterward. Contact with familial support groups sometimes acquaints family members with other families who have lost two or more children by suicide on different occasions, which of course fans their anxiety about losing another child by suicide. The need of surviving mothers and fathers to guard their remaining children is a common familial reaction in the first months following a youth suicide. However, if such a need persists, it can be stifling or suffocating for the children, particularly for adolescents who try to resume their quest for social independence as their bereavement progresses.

In a larger sense, parents create a family context for their surviving children's mourning work. Some grieving parents find it impossible to talk aloud about the deceased or about their grief with anyone else. This coping response inadvertently denies their offspring the opportunity to talk about their feelings, fantasies, or struggles. In the course of our adolescent psychological autopsy studies, many adolescents have volunteered that they are reluctant to talk about the death of their sibling in the presence of their parent because they fear the topic is too painful for the adult to tolerate. Ironically, many of those parents give the same reasons for not wanting to talk about the death in the presence of their adolescent children (Balk 1991).

By the same token, parents struggling with their own grief often report they do not have the energy, skill, or resources to attend to the psychological dilemma of their bereaved children. It is not always possible for bereaved parents, who are under acute strain, to consider the individual plights of all their grieving children. It is difficult for a surviving parent to address the facts that surviving siblings are at different stages of development, had different kinds of relationships with the deceased, grieve in characteristically different ways, and have different styles for handling the acute family crisis. When surviving parents do make a conscious effort to attend to their children, the effort is often guided by an assumption that the children are struggling with issues similar to those faced by the parent. The problem for the sibling survivor of suicide in this situation is one of generic expectations: parents may expect or "schedule" all family members to talk, grieve, and visit the cemetery in a lockstep fashion, without sufficiently considering individual differences. Although it is valuable to spend time together as a family, and valuable to spend time together discussing personal feelings about the child who died, it is also important to respect individual differences in the pace and rhythm of bereavement. As Wortman and Silver (1989) have pointed out, there is a great deal of untested "conventional wisdom" about optimal ways to grieve. Stereotypes about the grief process place an unfair burden on bereaved individuals and sometimes shape misguided treatment efforts by parents and professionals alike.

Hogan (1986) found that in the early stages of the grief process, many of the 40 surviving siblings who answered her self-report questionnaire felt that the other siblings were handling their grief better than they themselves were. It may be that the general reluctance to discuss individual grief and the imposition of generic expectations about the expression of familial grief lead the siblings to feel out of step and believe that everyone else is handling the loss better.

Parents' individual grieving styles not only affect the surviving children but also can have a significant impact on the marriage and thus on the family as a whole. In his review of the literature, Lieberman (1989) found increased divorce rates among spouses who had lost a child. He also found positive changes in the marriage relationship, such as increased spousal communication and support. However, in his own 7-year follow-up study of families who had lost a child, Lieberman found that most marital relationships were injured or destroyed. The marital stress attendant on the loss of a child, particularly when death is by suicide, is often severe.

Changes in Peer Relationships

After losing a sibling, many children experience a change in their peer relationships as well (Balk 1983b; Gaffney et al. 1992). Peer relationships may improve and be strengthened because peers may prove to be a strong source of support when other relationships flounder. Some peers, however, are uncomfortable about how to respond to a grieving friend. An example of youth suicide often becomes the focus of intense discussion and speculation in a community. The stigma and horror invoked by suicide in the minds of many families lead some people in the community to view the surviving family members as "undesirables." More sympathetic peers may avoid the topic to avoid unleashing painful memories. Bereaved adolescents who found opportunities to talk openly and honestly about their loss, expressing their needs to friends, fared the best according to Balk (1983b).

Bereaved children sometimes have problems initiating and maintaining close relationships after a familial death. The surviving siblings may themselves be reluctant to form new relationships for fear of exposing themselves to future losses. Others react in the opposite manner, actively seeking replacements for the lost brother or sister (Raphael 1983). Still others become clingier in those relationships they already have, placing strain on existing friendships.

Antecedent/Premorbid Risk Factors

Parkes's (1990) study of 54 psychiatric patients revealed a number of risk factors for developing psychopathology after bereavement:

- Experiencing of sudden and multiple deaths
- A history of major psychopathology after a previous bereavement experience
- Low trust of the self and others, anxious parents, and (in adolescents) compulsive independence

In the latter case, Parkes found that compulsively independent adolescents are likely to show delayed grief reactions.

Krupnick (1984) and Medalie (1990) identified a list of risk factors for pathological bereavement that they felt were specific to children following the death of a parent or sibling:

- Losses occurring before the age of 5 years or during early adolescence
- Loss of mother for girls younger than 11 years and loss of father for boys in adolescence
- Psychological problems predating the death
- Conflicted relationship with the deceased prior to the death
- Having an overly dependent surviving parent
- Lack of family or external support
- Unstable home environment
- Parental remarriage
- Lack of a prior understanding of death
- Unanticipated death
- Death by suicide or homicide in general

Coping, Protective Factors, and Resilience

Methods of Coping

Bereavement may be viewed as a challenge to the adaptive capacities of the person affected. Successful adaptation signifies not only the remission of dysphoric symptoms of grief but also a positive achievement with consequent skill growth representing an expanded repertoire of coping skills.

Wortman and Silver (1989) have argued persuasively that prevalent models of "better" ways to grieve and mourn are rarely based on systematic longitudinal research. They maintain that the following clinical truisms are no more than unsupported "myths": 1) depression after a loss is inevitable and must be experienced before healing can start; 2) failure to experience distress after a death is a sign of psychopathology; 3) the bereaved must "work through" their loss; 4) the person who has experienced a loss by death will eventually recover from his or her feelings of grief; and 5) the bereaved must learn to accept the loss intellectually before recovery can truly be reached.

According to Wortman and Silver, coping with loss is an idiosyncratic process.

It is important to note that after experiencing the death of a sibling early in life, many surviving siblings feel that they were made more mature and more sensitive and empathic as a direct outgrowth of their painful experience and grief process (Hogan 1986). Some researchers have theorized that certain characterological and environmental factors enable some children to handle the stress of a sibling death without debilitating results. These factors may be viewed as protective or having a "steeling effect," according to Garmezy (1983, 1991).

Protective Factors

Theoretically, the ability to anticipate a death allows the bereaved to start grieving prematurely, thereby accomplishing part of their grief work before the loved one dies. This is rarely a possibility, however, in the case of suicide. Similarly, having a clearly defined concept of death is also a protective factor in bereavement. Adolescents who have already experienced the death of a loved one seem to be better equipped to handle the experience again.

Garmezy (1983, 1991) found that children who were regarded as well liked and friendly seemed to be protected from the harmful effects of stressors. These children were neither defensive or aggressive, but were cooperative and emotionally stable; they were reflective, not impulsive, youths. They had a positive sense of self and felt that they had power over their own lives. Garmezy also views the social/family environment as a potentially protective factor. Parents' showing concern for their children's future and education and defining roles for their children within the family seemed to act as protective factors. When no strong parental figure existed, having a single significant adult relationship, perhaps with a teacher or neighbor, proved to have an equally "steeling effect." Garmezy's findings can be consolidated into three broad protective factors: dispositional attributes within the adolescent himself or herself, emotional support within the family, and the existence of an external support system.

The Concept of Resilience

Horowitz (1990) hypothesized that a healthy grieving pattern is one in which the bereaved person uses both avoidance and purposive reminiscence, and that heavy reliance on either one to the exclusion of the other is an unhealthy pattern. His notion is that individuals should not remain at the beck and call of all of their grief experiences without relief; hence, intermittent periods of avoidance are in the service of healthy bereavement. Likewise, excessive avoidance leads to a failure to develop the necessary ability to tolerate the sadness and anguish associated with the death, failure to confront the changed realities of one's life situation, and failure to reorganize one's life in acknowledgment of the loss.

When surviving parents and relatives remain psychologically able to attend to the psychological needs of bereaved youth, when the surviving adults recognize the need of family members to grieve in their own idiosyncratic ways and on their own idiosyncratic timetables, and when the surviving adults are willing to participate in intermittent discussions and reminiscences about the deceased sibling, the bereaved child who is capable of a balanced repertoire of avoidance and purposive reminiscence is most likely to fare well. Evidence shows that surviving mothers are more likely to facilitate this successfully than are surviving fathers (Silverman and Worden 1992).

Studies indicate that young persons allowed opportunities to talk about their dead family member and allowed to maintain a place for that family member in their lives fare better. But the evidence also shows that most surviving parents have great difficulty assisting bereaved children in maintaining this connection by means of conversations or reminiscing. Hence, the child's ability to utilize or create intimate relationships (with other relatives, with neighbors, or with peers) that permit conversations about the deceased sibling is another important quality of resilience.

In a similar vein, Black's (1984) studies suggest that adolescents who have the capacity and make the effort to maintain psychological connections with a deceased family member are more likely to make better long-term adjustments. These "psychological connections" may take the form of handling or wearing treasured possessions, maintaining informal schedules for ongoing discussions or reminiscences, or talking aloud to a ghostly presence in private moments. Clearly some children spontaneously generate meaningful psychological connections and others do not. Children's efforts in these directions can be actively encouraged or discouraged by parents and other adults, but the evidence is that some children persist in the activities of resilience despite discouragement and barriers.

Pynoos (1992) stresses the importance of the child's/adolescent's ability to renegotiate the relationship with deceased family members, particularly parents, as he or she progresses through the rest of the normal stages of early development. Pynoos has found those who are able to successfully maintain a changing mental relationship with their deceased family members—one that is not a static representation of their relationship at the time of the death—are more likely to be resilient.

Although the need to remain psychologically connected with the deceased sibling through the remainder of childhood and adolescence may be developmentally vital, it seems clear that another aspect of "remaining connected" lies in the value of such connection for the mourning process. By preserving the deceased in some symbolic way, the child can alternate between painful reality testing and denial in fantasy at a pace commensurate with his or her psychological capabilities. The child can combat the fear that memories of the deceased will fade and become unreliable with time. The child can dose himself or herself episodically with as much or as little deidealization as required to facilitate the mourning process. The child can reconstrue the relationship in response to changing understandings and current psychological needs. And perhaps most important, the child can combat acute feelings of loneliness and abandonment. In all these respects, it is useful for siblings of youth suicide victims to maintain "psychological connections" with their deceased siblings.

Clinical and Research Implications

Clinical

Individual counseling can provide the support that will lead the surviving sibling back to his or her original level of functioning. Children and adolescents generally need the opportunity to explore their reaction to the grief individually.

We advocate application of a pulsed intervention model (Pynoos 1992) that anticipates and changes with the developmental challenges facing the bereaved child or adolescent. This model of intervention relies on both patient and therapist to discern what may (in the near future) be particularly developmentally challenging about the loss of the sibling. This intervention model entails initial work with the acute grief close to the time of the sibling death as well as planned and unexpected interventions at specific points of difficulty in the future—an approach that requires open communication between the patient and therapist over a long period of time. The main goal of this strategy is to provide the child with the support needed to maintain normal development.

Young persons who are experiencing grief can also be assisted at the family, classroom, and community levels. At the family level, security within the home environment can be restored. The family must be a stable and supportive place to whom the adolescent can go for solace and support. Because each family member is affected differently by the loss, the nature of each family member's grieving must be addressed and understood. Bereaved young persons can be helped at school by being reintegrated into the classroom by a supportive and understanding teacher. Within the community, there may be other children or adolescents experiencing similar losses with whom to do group work.

We have developed a model for group work with children and adolescents who have lost a family member by suicide in close collaboration with a local survivors support group. We recommend separate groups for preadolescents (e.g., 5 to 12 years of age) and adolescents. Within each of these age groups, inclusion of a wide age span has proved valuable. Sibling cohorts are permitted to join the same therapy group. To become eligible for group therapy, each child must already be aware of why he or she will be attending group meetings (i.e., because a family member died by suicide), and each child must participate in a psychiatric evaluation so that those children with a prior history of psychopathology, or current psychopathology too severe to manage in a group setting (e.g., suicide attempts, delusions or hallucinations), can be identified. Either of the latter two conditions is grounds for exclusion and referral to individual therapy.

The goals of the weekly youth group are to permit discussion of the children's curiosity about suicide, to facilitate discussion about personal grief thoughts and feelings, and to create a setting where the children can exchange observations about the impact of the death on their respective families. These groups tend to develop considerable cohesion and have often reached a planned termination in the form of a group memorial rite of the children's design after a year or so of group participation.

We have scheduled parent group meetings to run concurrently

with the youth group meetings. In the parent group, the focus is an educational one. The parents take turns posing questions and citing difficulties they are experiencing with their children. The others—parents and the professional facilitators—help the questioning parent sort through and understand the mixture of mourning, normal development, and problem behaviors represented by the examples raised.

Research

Too few empirical studies have been undertaken to permit any firm conclusions about the nature of the sibling grief experience. Most studies in this area suffer from a relatively small sample size, uncertain reliability of their observations and ratings, overreliance on single case studies, overreliance on surveys and self-report questionnaires to the exclusion of direct clinical interviews, and the absence of comparisons between information gleaned from interviews with young subjects and that gleaned from interviews with their parents or peers.

In one of the few suicide survivor studies that examined different types of grief reactions as they related to different relationships with the deceased (i.e., siblings, spouses, parents, children), Wrobleski and McIntosh (1987) found that siblings and spouses exhibited the most severe grief reactions and the most difficulty coping with the loss. Yet parents and children of the deceased remain the most common focus in studies of bereaved populations. This discrepancy seems reason enough to call for more studies comparing grief responses in suicide survivors by their relationship to the deceased, and more studies of surviving siblings of youth suicide victims in particular.

References

American Psychiatric Association: Diagnostic and Statistical Manual of Mental Disorders, 3rd Edition, Revised. Washington, DC, American Psychiatric Association, 1987

Balk D: Adolescent's grief reactions and self-concept perceptions following sibling death: a study of 33 teenagers. Journal of Youth and Adolescence 12:137–161, 1983a

Balk D: Effects of sibling death on teenagers. Journal of School Health 53:14–18, 1983b

Balk D: Death and adolescent bereavement: current research and future directions. Journal of Adolescent Research 6:7–27, 1991

Bank SP, Kahn MD: The Sibling Bond. New York, Basic Books, 1982

Bendickson R, Fulton R: Death and the child: an anterospective test of the childhood bereavement and later behavior disorder hypotheses, in Death and Identity. Edited by Fulton R. Bowie, MD, Charles Press, 1976, pp 274–287

Beskow J, Runeson B, Asgard U: Psychological autopsies: methods and ethics. Suicide Life Threat Behav 20:307–323, 1990

Black D: Sundered families: the effect of loss of a parent. Adoption and Fostering 8:38–43, 1984

Brent DA, Perper JA, Moritz GM, et al: Psychiatric effects of exposure to suicide among the friends and acquaintances of adolescent suicide victims. J Am Acad Child Adolesc Psychiatry 31:629–640, 1992

Cain AC, Fast I, Erickson ME: Children's disturbed reactions to the death of sibling. Am J Orthopsychiatry 36:873–880, 1964

Clark DC, Pynoos RS, Goebel AE: Mechanisms and processes of adolescent bereavement, in Stress, Risk, and Resilience in Children and Adolescents: Processes, Mechanisms, and Interventions. Edited by Haggerty RJ, Sherrod LR, Garmezy N, et al. London, Cambridge University Press, 1994, pp 100–146

Clayton PJ: Mortality and morbidity in the first year of widowhood. Arch Gen Psychiatry 30:747–750, 1974

Clayton PJ, Halikas JA, Maurice WL: The depression of widowhood. Br J Psychiatry 120:71–78, 1971

Clayton PJ, Halikas JA, Maurice WL: The bereavement of widowhood. Diseases of the Nervous System 32:597–604, 1972

Demi AS, Gilbert CM: Relationship of parental grief to sibling grief. Arch Psychiatr Nurs 1:385–391, 1987

Dunne-Maxim K, Dunne EJ, Hauser MJ: When children are suicide survivors, in Suicide and Its Aftermath. Edited by Dunne EJ, McIntosh JL, Dunne-Maxim K. New York, WW Norton, 1987, pp 234–244

Gaffney DA, Jones ET, Dunne-Maxim K: Support groups for sibling suicide survivors. Crisis 13:76–81, 1992

Garmezy N: Stressors of childhood, in Stress, Coping, and Development in Children. Edited by Garmezy N, Rutter M. New York, McGraw-Hill, 1983, pp 43–82

Garmezy N: Resilience in children's adaptation to negative life events and stressed environments. Pediatr Ann 20:459–466, 1991

Gregory I: Anterospective data following childhood loss of a parent, I: delinquency and high school dropout. Arch Gen Psychiatry 13:99–109, 1965

Hauser M: Special aspects of grief after suicide, in Suicide and Its Aftermath. Edited by Dunne EJ, McIntosh JL, Dunne-Maxim K. New York, WW Norton, 1987, pp 57–70

Hazell P, Lewin T: Friends of adolescent suicide attempters and completers. J Am Acad Child Adolesc Psychiatry 32:76–81, 1993

Hogan NS: An investigation of the adolescent sibling bereavement process and adaptation. Unpublished doctoral dissertation, Loyola University of Chicago, 1986

Horowitz MJ: A model of mourning: change in schemas of self and others. J Am Psychoanal Assoc 38:297–324, 1990

Krupnick JL: Bereavement in childhood and adolescence, in Bereavement Reactions, Consequences, and Care. Edited by Osterweiss M, Solomon F, Greene M. Washington, DC, National Academy Press, 1984, pp 99–141

Lieberman MA: All family losses are not equal. Journal of Family Psychology 2:368–372, 1989

Litman RE, Curphey T, Shneidman ES, et al: Investigations of equivocal suicides. JAMA 184:924–929, 1963

Litman RE, Curphey T, Shneidman ES, et al: The psychological autopsy of equivocal deaths, in The Psychology of Suicide. Edited by Shneidman ES, Farberow NL, Litman RE. New York, Jason Aronson, 1983, pp 485–496

Markusen T, Fulton R: Childhood bereavement and behavioral disorders: a critical review. Omega 2:107–117, 1971

Medalie JH: Bereavement: health consequences and prevention strategies, in Preventing Disease: Beyond the Rhetoric. Edited by Goldbloom RB, Lawrence RS. New York, Springer-Verlag, 1990, pp 168–178

Nader K, Pynoos RS, Fairbanks L, et al: Children's PTSD reactions one year after a sniper attack at their school. Am J Psychiatry 147:1526–1530, 1990

Ness DE, Pfeffer CR: Sequelae of bereavement resulting from suicide. Am J Psychiatry 147:279–285, 1990

Osterweiss M, Solomon F, Greene M: Introduction, in Bereavement Reactions, Consequences, and Care. Edited by Osterweiss M, Solomon F, Greene M. Washington, DC, National Academy Press, 1984, pp 3–11

Parkes CM: Risk factors in bereavement: implications for the prevention and treatment of pathologic grief. Psychiatric Annals 20:308–313, 1990

Pollock GH: Childhood sibling loss: a family tragedy. Psychiatric Annals 16:309–314, 1986

Pynoos RS: Grief and trauma in children and adolescents. Bereavement Care 11:2–10, 1992

Raphael B: The Anatomy of Bereavement. New York, Basic Books, 1983

Shneidman ES: The psychological autopsy. Suicide Life Threat Behav 11:325–340, 1981

Shneidman ES, Farberow N: Sample investigation of equivocal suicidal deaths, in The Cry for Help. Edited by Farberow NL, Shneidman ES. New York, McGraw-Hill, 1961, pp 118–128

Silverman PR, Worden JW: Children's reactions in the early months after the death of a parent. Am J Orthopsychiatry 62:93–104, 1992

Sood B, Weller EB, Weller RA, et al: Somatic complaints in grieving children. Comprehensive Mental Health 2:17–25, 1992

Todd S: Sibling survivors of suicide: a qualitative study of the experience of adolescent siblings whose brother or sister completed suicide. Unpublished doctoral dissertation, Boston University, Boston, MA, 1980

Vargas LA, Loya F, Hodde-Vargas J: Exploring the multidimensional aspects of grief reactions. Am J Psychiatry 146:1484–1489, 1980

Wass H: Parents, teachers, and health professionals as helpers, in Helping Children Cope With Death: Guidelines and Resources. Edited by Wass H, Corr CA. New York, Hemisphere, 1984, pp 75–130

Weller EB, Weller RA, Fristad MA, et al: Depression in recently bereaved prepubertal children. Am J Psychiatry 148:1536–1540, 1991

Wortman CB, Silver RC: The myths of coping with loss. J Consult Clin Psychol 57:349–357, 1989

Wrobleski A, McIntosh JL: Problems of suicide survivors: a survey report. Isr J Psychiatry Relat Sci 24:137–142, 1987

Yule W, Williams RM: Posttraumatic stress reactions in children. Journal of Traumatic Stress 3:279–295, 1990

Section V

Abuse and Its Traumatic Impact

Chapter 15

Physical and Sexual Abuse and Mental Disturbances in Children

Sandra Kaplan, M.D.
Elizabeth T. Pinner, B.A.

In this chapter we address the associated mental health problems, assessment, and treatment needs of children who have experienced the stresses of childhood physical or sexual abuse. Symptoms related to both sexual and physical abuse, and the similarities of symptoms following abuse to the symptoms seen in children after experiencing or witnessing various other traumatic events (e.g., kidnapping, attacks, natural disasters, death) are discussed. Long-term effects of childhood physical and sexual abuse, including an increased risk for suicide, dissociative disorders, depression, and other psychopathology, as well as for the intergenerational transmission of violence, are also presented.

Physical Abuse of Children

Definition

The Child Abuse Prevention, Adoption, and Family Services Act of 1988 (Public Law 100-294) defines physical abuse as "the physical injury of a child under 18 years of age by a person who is responsible for the child's welfare, under circumstances which indicate that the child's health or welfare is harmed or threatened thereby, as determined in accordance with regulations prescribed by the Secretary of the Health and Human Services." Such responsible persons may be an employee of a residential facility, any staff member of a facility, or any

393

staff person providing out-of-home care. Physical abuse, as defined in The Family Court Act (1976) of New York State, is "the situation which results when a parent or other person legally responsible for a child less than 18 inflicts or allows to be inflicted upon such child physical injury by other than accidental means" (qtd. in Garbarino and Ebata 1983). Straus and Gelles (1986), the principal investigators of The National Incidence Studies of Violence in America, defined physical abuse on the basis of the Severe Violence Index of the Conflicts Scale, whereby any parental act that is identified on this scale (which includes kicking, biting, hitting with a fist, hitting or trying to hit with an object, beating, and threats with a gun or knife and actual use of a gun or knife) is thus considered physical abuse.

Prevalence

It was estimated that 36 per 1,000 children in 1975 between the ages of 3 and 17 years had a history of being abused (Straus and Gelles 1986). Straus and Gelles (1986), based on results from their study, estimated that in 1985, 19 per 1,000 children between the ages of 3 and 17 years were abused. This decrease in prevalence may be attributed to methodological differences between the two studies (in-person interviews in the 1975 study and telephone interviews in the 1985 study), increased public awareness, and/or legislation regarding child abuse. In addition, in the national incidence and prevalence study by the National Center on Child Abuse and Neglect, it was estimated that 25.2 per 1,000, or 1,500,000, children were maltreated during 1986 and 5.7 per 1,000 children were physically abused (National Center on Child Abuse and Neglect 1988).

Violence in the United States is considered a major childhood public health problem. It has been hypothesized that the stress of childhood physical abuse leads to violent behavior. The relationship may be a complicated one, with several mitigating factors. Nevertheless, the high rates of violence highlight the seriousness of the issue. There have been dramatic increases in homicide and suicide rates in this country. Between 1984 and 1988, homicide rates doubled for black males between 15 and 24 years of age (Webster and Champion 1992). Gunshot wounds are the leading cause of death in both black and white teenagers. Homicide is the 12th leading cause of death in the United States (U.S. Department of Health and Human Services 1991). Suicide rates of children and adolescents have doubled in the past three decades, and suicide has become the third leading cause of death for this population (National Safe Kids Campaign 1992).

Risk Factors for Abuse

The *ecological model of abuse* (Belsky 1980) is the commonly accepted paradigm of risk factors for abuse. In this paradigm, child abuse is viewed as the manifestation of parental vulnerabilities (e.g., mental illness, substance abuse) combined with child vulnerabilities (e.g., low birth weight, difficult temperament, a particular developmental stage) and social stressors (e.g., lack of social supports, poverty). Risk factors associated with child abuse that have been identified by the National Study of the Incidence and Prevalence of Child Abuse and Neglect include a) single parenthood, b) minority ethnicity, c) lack of acculturation, d) four or more children in the family, and e) young parental age (National Center on Child Abuse and Neglect 1988). Exposure to violence, either extrafamilial or intrafamilial, has also been identified as a risk factor for abuse (Kaufman and Zigler 1987).

Psychopathology in Abused Children

Information regarding psychopathology in abused children is generally obtained from studies of those abused children who have been referred for treatment. It has been reported that abused children tend to exhibit the following: depression (Green 1978a; Kaplan et al. 1986), impulsivity, hyperactivity (Martin and Beezley 1977), learning impairments (Kline and Christiansen 1975; Salzinger et al. 1984), conduct disorder (Kaplan et al. 1986; Kinard 1980), and substance abuse (Kaplan et al. 1986). Kaplan and colleagues (1986) and Salzinger and associates (1984), comparing physically abused children and adolescents referred to a child and adolescent psychiatric outpatient treatment program with nonabused pediatric outpatients, reported that the child abuse victims, compared with the nonabused pediatric outpatients, more often showed significantly more hyperactivity, conduct disturbance, anxiety, and tension. Furthermore, Kaplan and colleagues (1986) reported that abused children of psychiatrically disturbed parents were more often diagnosed as having a psychiatric disorder than were nonabused children of psychiatrically disturbed parents. Physical abuse histories have been reported in child psychiatric populations (Kashani et al. 1987) as well as in delinquent populations (Alfaro 1978). There have been to date no studies comparing psychopathology in abused children with that in abused adolescents.

Suicide and Abuse

The relationship between suicide and abuse is an important one to consider because suicide is the eighth leading cause of death (third among young people) in the United States. Approximately 20% of all injury-related deaths are suicides (Rice et al. 1989). That the stress of physical abuse on a child is intense can be inferred from the reported association between abuse and suicide. Green (1978b) reported self-mutilation in abused and neglected children. Pfeffer (1986) reported that child abuse was frequently found among families of children who attempted suicide. Farber and colleagues (1984), Kaplan (1986), and Rotheram and Bradley (1987) reported that adolescent runaways had high rates of suicide attempts and, in many cases, had a history of abuse. Deykin and colleagues (1985) reported that adolescents who attempt suicide are more likely to have been abuse victims than are adolescents who have not attempted suicide.

The psychiatric disorders reported in adolescent suicide completers, as identified by Shaffer (1987), are the same psychiatric disorders that have been reported in child and adolescent abuse victims (Kaplan et al. 1986)—namely, substance abuse, conduct disorders, and depression. Shaffer also reported discord in the family and that adolescent suicide attempters had a history of suicide of relatives.

The association between suicide and abuse may be related to several factors. First, the association between physical abuse and suicide may be secondary to the modeling of suicidal or aggressive behavior and impulsive behavior within the family. Second, the association may be secondary to increased biological risk for highly correlative disorders (e.g., substance abuse, mood disorders, impulsive conduct disorders) (Kaplan et al. 1983, 1986; Shaffer 1987). Third, the social isolation of abusive families may also increase risk for suicidal behavior (Shaffer and Fisher 1974; Salzinger et al. 1983; Spinetta and Rigler 1972).

Dissociation and Abuse

Dissociative disorders are believed to be a response to trauma and have been found in patients with posttraumatic stress disorder (PTSD). Although there have been few studies of the relationship between childhood stress and dissociative disorders, the relationship of dissociation and childhood abuse was addressed by Sanders and Giolas (1991), who reported significant correlations between dissociation and both physical and sexual abuse.

Psychopathology in Parents of Abused Children

Studies of psychopathology in abusive parents have reported depression (Bland and Orn 1986; Kaplan et al. 1983; Wolfe 1985), aggression (Kaplan et al. 1983; Wolfe 1985), more physical and verbal aggressive behaviors when interacting with the child, a tendency toward negativity, increased somatic concerns, aversive controlling behaviors when interacting with the child, and increased arousal to aversive child stimuli (Wolfe 1985). In particular, abusive fathers have been found to more often be diagnosed as having alcoholism, antisocial personality disorder, or labile personalities compared with nonabusive fathers (Kaplan et al. 1983).

Intergenerational Transmission of Child Abuse

It has been suggested that nearly one-third of severely neglected or abused children (physically or sexually) will maltreat their own children (Kaufman and Zigler 1987). However, with the presence of one supportive parent, a supportive spousal relationship, and relatively few stressful events, this risk is decreased (Kaufman and Zigler 1987).

Mothers of abusive children have been found to have little social interaction outside the home. It has been reported that they are less often employed outside the home and tend, in general, to be socially isolated from their peers as compared with nonabusive mothers (Salzinger et al. 1983). Such social isolation for the parent may in fact lead to a lack of childrearing acculturation (Salzinger et al. 1983).

The intergenerational transmission of violence may be viewed as a consequence of childhood coping with physical abuse. In this view, the child is thought to idealize his or her perpetrator and become acculturated to violence. The notion is that violent behavior itself is the response to the original stress, which itself was violent. Longitudinal research by the National Institute of Justice (NIJ) of over 1,500 cases comparing abused children with nonabused children found that physical abuse increased the likelihood of delinquency and criminality by over 40% (National Institute of Justice 1992).

Assessment and Treatment Planning for the Physically Abused Child and the Family

To adequately plan for treatment and to ensure protection, complete medical, developmental, and psychiatric evaluations are needed as screening procedures for all abused and neglected children. These assessments are necessary because, as already mentioned, physically abused children and adolescents are at risk for serious behavioral and emotional disorders, developmental disorders, and learning problems. When assessment is being undertaken, school records provide useful information about achievement, attendance, and behavior.

Physical examination findings of physical abuse, as outlined by the Council on Scientific Affairs of the American Medical Association (1985), include injuries such as bruises and welts, injuries resembling the object used to inflict the injury, fractures, internal injuries to organs, and head trauma. The Council on Scientific Affairs (American Medical Association 1985) reported that characteristically, the injuries are more severe than could be reasonable attributed to the claimed cause.

Hospital Child Protection Committees

In hospitals, interdisciplinary and interdepartmental child protection teams assess cases of child abuse and neglect. These teams typically cooperate with those state agencies that are responsible for receiving and investigating child abuse reports and provide consultation to and education of hospital staff, trainees, and attending physicians.

Treatment

Because parents of physically abused children have increased risk for mental health and substance abuse problems, assessment and treatment for parental mental illness and substance abuse are important in order to accurately plan for parental rehabilitation and protection of children. Treatment plans should be comprehensive and involve treating the abusive parent as well as the abused child, in those cases in which the focus is on the interactional aspect of the cycle of abuse (Daro 1988; Wolfe 1985). Such a multidimensional view emphasizes that child abuse is a function of the degree to which the parents' health and environment enhance good parenting. Multidisciplinary treatment teams that operate at various levels of intervention have been found to be helpful (Daro 1988). These teams address, for example, individual psychopathology, family dysfunction, and lack of social supports.

The issues addressed in individual psychotherapy are different for parent and child. For the child victim this therapy needs to address issues of low self-esteem, the development of extreme passivity as a conflict resolution strategy, identification with and imitation of aggressive behavior, a sense of being damaged, depression, suicidal ideation, self-blame for the abuse, and substance abuse. Individual therapy for the parents needs to address parental knowledge of child development and conflict resolution strategies to use in lieu of violence.

As there is an unusually high dropout rate of abusive parents when they are referred to community mental health facilities, outreach is often needed. For example, the staff needs to be available 24 hours a day, and evening treatment times need to be an option to involve all parents.

There are two components to psychotherapy for the parents: 1) to provide parents with, when indicated, emotional support and positive parenting models and 2) to foster insight and enhance conflict resolution skills. These aims require a trusting therapeutic relationship established initially in the context of individual psychotherapy. Later, in conjoint family sessions, interactive issues, such as the scapegoating of the abused child and marital conflict, need to be addressed (Kaplan 1981).

Prevention

Various child abuse prevention strategies are currently employed: parental education programs, media campaigns, crisis hotlines, community socialization programs, and family support (visiting nurses or home visiting parental aides). Although the effectiveness of these programs is unclear, there is some evidence that the presence of home nurses reduces the rates of abuse (Rosenberg and Repucci 1985).

Child abuse prevention strategies also include efforts to abolish corporal punishment. The American Academy of Child and Adolescent Psychiatry (1988) has defined corporal punishment as the discipline method, used by a supervising adult, that inflicts pain upon a misbehaving child (child displays unacceptable behavior and/or inappropriate language). The following organizations have called for an end to corporal punishment: American Academy of Child and Adolescent Psychiatry, National Congress of Parents and Teachers, American Bar Association, American Academy of Pediatrics, National Education Association, and National Association of School Psychologists. All of these groups shun the notion of teaching children that violence is a primary method of conflict resolution.

Sexual Abuse

Several studies have suggested a link between childhood sexual abuse and increased risk for PTSD, a disorder that, by definition, occurs in response to an unexpected severe stressor. For example, McLeer et al. (1988) found that 48% of their sample of sexually abused children experienced symptoms that met the criteria for PTSD. The same researchers reported the incidence of PTSD to be as high as 75% in cases of incest (as opposed to lower rates for extrafamilial abuse). Sexual abuse may, especially in light of this association with PTSD, be a profound stressor.

Definition

Sexual abuse is defined as the sexual assault (causing harm or injury) of a child under 18 years old (National Center on Child Abuse and Neglect 1988). The following are examples of sexual assault: penile penetration of the child's genitals, anus, or mouth; fondling or other genital contact; prostitution of one's child; taking and/or disseminating obscene or pornographic photographs (or other depiction) of children for profit.

Prevalence

Several studies, utilizing both present and retrospective methodologies, in the past decade have reported the prevalence of sexual abuse. In 1983, 38% of a random sample of women in San Francisco reported having been sexually abused during childhood (Russell 1983). Yet, only 2% of the intrafamilial and 6% of the extrafamilial abuse was ever reported to the police. In 1985, Wyatt reported that in a multiracial community sample of women in Los Angeles, 45% reported having had unwanted sexual contact as children. In 1986, 22% of the women sampled in Calgary, Canada (Bagley and Ramsay 1986) reported sexual abuse during their childhood. That same year, the national incidence study done by the National Center on Child Abuse and Neglect (1988) estimated that 2.5 per 1,000 children (155,900 children) were sexually abused in the United States during 1985. This figure represents a threefold increase since 1980 (National Center on Child Abuse and Neglect 1988).

Depression, Suicide, and Sexual Abuse

Depression and suicide in victims of childhood sexual abuse have been documented by a number of studies. Depressive symptoms have been frequently reported. MacVicar (1979) reported that of all adolescents examined, those most vulnerable to depression were victims of sexual abuse. Sansonnet-Hayden and colleagues (1987) found a 71% incidence of major depression in sexually abused psychiatric inpatients.

The studies linking suicide and sexual abuse have been less specific. Nonetheless, a higher incidence of suicide attempts has been found in a population of abuse victims who were compared with non–sexually and non–physically abused control subjects (Sansonnet-Hayden et al. 1987), and Anderson (1981) reported four cases of adolescents who had made a suicide attempt following disclosure of a sexual abuse.

Dissociation and Sexual Abuse

Briere and colleagues, in several studies, found that sexually abused children, in addition to being at increased risk for depression and suicide as a consequence of the sexual abuse, exhibit more dissociative symptoms than control subjects with no history of abuse (Briere and Runtz 1987, 1988a, 1988b, 1989). van der Kolk and co-workers (1991) found that dissociative experiences were highly correlated with childhood traumas or stressors.

Psychopathology in Parents in Sexually Abusive Families

In cases of sexual abuse perpetrated by a parent, it has been reported that the perpetrators reveal an array of emotional and social problems. These individuals have been reported to exhibit high rates of alcohol and drug abuse (Strand 1986), personality disorders (Langevin et al. 1978, 1985), paranoia, anxiety, and depression (Williams and Finkelhor 1990). It has also been reported (Coons et al. 1989) that some male incest perpetrators tend to be sexually aroused by young children but not by adult females. There is, however, a dearth of information regarding the psychopathology in the parent who is not perpetrating the sexual abuse.

Assessment of Child Sexual Abuse

The American Academy of Child and Adolescent Psychiatry (1988) has issued guidelines for the clinical evaluation of child sexual abuse. It has been suggested that, first, the purpose of the evaluation needs to be established. The evaluation is intended to determine whether or not abuse has occurred and the degree of medical certainty; the specific needs for the protection of the child; and what treatment is necessary for any physical and/or emotional problems that are found.

Assessment of sexual abuse, according to the American Academy of Child and Adolescent Psychiatry guidelines, has several components, one of which is the physical examination. This examination, which is necessary to determine if there is any physical evidence of sexual abuse (e.g., chafing, abrasions, and bruising on inner thighs and genitalia; scarring, tears, and distortion in hymen, fossa navicularis, posterior fourchette, and labia minora; decreased amount of tissue in hymen; and enlargement of hymenal opening [see American Academy of Pediatrics 1991]) and, if such evidence is found, to provide any needed physical treatment, should, whenever possible, be performed by a physician known to the child or a pediatric gynecologist. It is also beneficial, when this is not possible, to allow the child to choose the sex of the examining physician. Furthermore, a trusted, supportive adult (nonperpetrator) should remain with the child during the examination.

If the child has been raped, or there is the possibility of acute trauma or infection, the examination should take place as soon as possible, especially when forensic evidence needs to be obtained. In such a situation, a physician's office is a preferable location to an emergency room, and the genital exam should be part of an overall physical exam so that it can be deemphasized from the child's perspective. If the child is unwilling to undergo the physical exam, it might have to be postponed until the child receives counseling and is able to cooperate.

Physicians should be sensitive about asking questions that might interfere with the ongoing examination by a mental health professional (Policy Statement from the American Academy of Child and Adolescent Psychiatry 1988).

Important components of assessment often include a developmental history; cognitive assessment; history of prior abuse or other traumas; relevant medical history; history of behavior changes; history of the parents' abuse as children; family attitudes toward sex and modesty; prior psychiatric disorders in child and/or parents; allegiances to respective parents; assessment of child's credibility; review of medical records, school reports, police reports, and any previous psychiatric reports; and talking with significant others.

Particular play materials facilitate the child interviews, which should be conducted without the use of any leading questions (American Academy of Child and Adolescent Psychiatry 1988). Such materials include drawing materials, a doll house, dolls, and toy telephones. Children's drawings may reveal sexual immaturity or hypermaturity (Aiosa-Karpas et al. 1991). The doll house may reveal the family's sleeping arrangements and daily activities. Anatomically detailed dolls are helpful in eliciting the child's terminology for anatomical parts and may facilitate disclosure (American Academy of Child and Adolescent Psychiatry 1988). Toy telephones may also ease disclosure, especially for preadolescent children.

Considerations of False Allegations of Child Sexual Abuse

Guidelines exist that aid in the assessment of the credibility of the child's account. According to the American Academy of Child and Adolescent Psychiatry (1988), for example, it is necessary to allow the child to use his or her own language and point of view when making descriptions. It is important that the interviewer be cognizant of degree of spontaneity, appropriate degrees of anxiety, corroborating evidence, behavior changes (those consistent with abuse), inclusion of detail, and consistency of allegations over time. When children show signs of abuse (through the use of doll-playing, drawings, etc.), have described the situation using age-appropriate language, and demonstrate the ability to distinguish fact from fiction and truth from lie, credibility increases.

False allegations tend to center around marital disputes (Green

1986; Yates 1991; Yates and Musty 1987). Deliberately false allegations are rare. More often, they are a result of misinterpretation and ambiguity.

Prevention and Treatment

Of the three types of prevention (primary, secondary, and tertiary), primary prevention, which is concerned with preventing abuse before it occurs, is most effective in enhancing the psychosocial outcomes of children at risk for being abused (Cohn and Daro 1987).

Primary prevention programs, usually in elementary schools, educate children about sexual abuse in the hope of providing them with the skills necessary to deter the abuse. In such prevention programs, the education consists of learning to say "no," learning that there are "good" and "bad" touches, learning that they, the children, are the "boss" of their bodies, and learning that blame rests with the perpetrator and not the victim. The children are instructed to report unwanted sexual contact to another trusting adult.

Schools use techniques such as pamphlets, coloring books, role playing, lectures, and films (Trudell and Whatley 1988; Wurtele 1987). Because of the sensitive nature of the information, parental involvement is usually sought.

Mental Health Treatment

There are several different treatment foci needed for the mental health treatment of sexual abuse: interdisciplinary, outreach efforts to engage families; 24-hour on-call mental health and substance abuse treatment for parents and children; parenting technique and child development education for parents; social skills training for children and parents; and case management with all agencies. Specific treatments designed to enhance parenting and family functioning include behavioral parenting therapies, marital therapy, and family therapy. Treatment should entail individual, family, and group psychotherapy.

Crisis intervention involves protecting the child from future abuse and monitoring suicide potential. In addition, it is necessary both during crisis intervention and during later psychotherapeutic efforts to encourage the ventilation of feelings regarding the abuse as well as to explore the reasons for the child's vulnerability and use these insights to help guide treatment.

The themes in group therapy with sexual abuse victims are believability, guilt and responsibility, trust and anger, powerlessness, court attendance, sex education, and other life crises and tasks. Family therapy addresses the specifics of sexual abuse, explores the individual contributions of each family member to the abuse, strengthens the parental coalition, and helps in the development of child nurturing in nonsexual ways. In individual psychotherapy with the child, the goals are to decrease anxiety and depression, improve self-esteem, diminish the sense of helplessness and self-blame while enhancing empowerment and assertiveness, correct cognitive distortions and any resultant age-inappropriate sexual behavior, and consolidate gender identity.

Guidance to Mental Health Professional Practitioners: Reporting Responsibilities

It is important for clinicians to obtain a copy of the state child abuse reporting law for every state in which they practice, as well as the juvenile court law that defines child abuse (because the legal definition may differ from personal interpretation).

State law requires the reporting of abuse, and civil and even criminal procedures may result from a failure to do so. State laws generally protect reporters, when the report is based on reasonable suspicion, so they need not fear retribution from accused parents. Some states have created criminal offenses for intentional false reporting of abuse. The extent to which immunity laws protect mandatory reporters for actions beyond the initial making of the report is questionable, and individual legal consultation is advised. For example, a mental health professional may be asked to serve on a multidisciplinary team that discusses information relevant to a child's case, to provide information from psychiatric records, to aid the investigation of a child abuse allegation, and/or to testify in a court proceeding as a result of the initial report.

The failure of the professional to provide information regarding the possibility of continued danger that an adult child abuser poses could result in legal action if that adult later abuses other children. This also holds true for an abused child in a foster home who presents physical danger to other children.

The child abuse reporting laws of most states specifically eliminate most legally privileged communications (e.g., those between mental health professionals). It is important to stress that the law on abrogation for privileged communications is a different law from that requiring mandatory reports of suspected child mistreatment. Once again, it is essential for mental health professionals to obtain specific legal advice about the impact of the laws of the states in which they practice.

In New York State, for example, the reporting procedure is as follows. Oral reporting to the New York State Central Register of Child Abuse and Maltreatment (SCR) is immediate by phone followed by a written report within 48 hours to the local Child Protective Services (CPS), and to the SCR when the child is being cared for away from the home. Those acting in a professional capacity are required to report if there is reasonable cause to suspect that a child has been abused or maltreated. Certainty is not required for reporting. "Reasonable cause" is when injuries are possible and are considered to be a consequence of neglect or nonaccidental. Further reporting information can be gleaned from an examination of the New York State Syllabus for Identification and Reporting of Child Abuse and Maltreatment (1994, The University of the State of New York).

References

Aiosa-Karpas CJ, Pelcovitz D, Kaplan S: Gender identification and sex role attribution in sexually abused adolescent females. J Am Acad Child Adolesc Psychiatry 30:266–271, 1991

Alfara J: Summary Report on the Relationship Between Child Abuse and Neglect and Later Socially Deviant Behavior. New York, Select Committee on Child Abuse, 1978

American Academy of Child and Adolescent Psychiatry: Guidelines for the clinical assessment of child and adolescent sexual abuse. J Am Acad ChIld Adolesc Psychiatry 27:655–657, 1988

American Academy of Pediatrics: Guidelines for the evaluation of sexual abuse of children. Pediatrics 87:254–260, 1991

American Medical Association, Council on Scientific Affairs: AMA Diagnostic and Treatment Guidelines Concerning Child Abuse and Neglect. JAMA 254:796–800, 1985

Anderson L: Notes on the linkage between the sexually abused child and the suicidal adolescent. J Adolesc 4:157–162, 1981

Bagley C, Ramsay RL: Sexual abuse in childhood: psychological outcomes and implication for social work practice. Journal of Social Work and Human Sexuality 4:33–37, 1986

Belsky J: Child maltreatment: an ecological integration. Am Psychol 35:320–335, 1980

Bland R, Orn H: Psychiatric disorders, spouse abuse and child abuse. Acta Psychiatr Belg 86:444–449, 1986

Briere J, Runtz M: Post sexual abuse trauma. Journal of Interpersonal Violence 2:367–379, 1987

Briere J, Runtz M: Controlling for family variables in abuse effects research. Journal of Interpersonal Violence 3:80–89, 1988a

Briere J, Runtz M: Symptomatology associated with childhood sexual victimization in a nonclinical adult sample. Child Abuse Negl 12:51–59, 1988b

Briere J, Runtz M: The Trauma Symptom Checklist (TSC-33): early data on a new scale. Journal of Interpersonal Violence 4:151–165, 1989

Cohn AH, Daro D: Is treatment too late: what ten years of evaluative research tells us. Child Abuse Negl 11:433–442, 1987

Coons PM, Bowman ES, Pellow TA, et al: Posttraumatic aspects of the treatment of victims of sexual abuse and incest. Psychiatr Clin North Am 12:325–335, 1989

Daro D: Confronting Child Abuse: Research for Effective Program Design. New York, Free Press, 1988

Deykin EY, Alpert JJ, McNamarra JJ: A pilot study of the effect of exposure to child abuse or neglect on suicidal behavior. Am J Psychiatry 142:1299–1303, 1985

Family Court Act, McKinney's Consol. Laws Book 29A, Part 1. St Paul, MN, West Publishing, 1976

Farber E, Kinast C, McCord W: Violence in families of adolescent runaways. Child Abuse Negl 8:295–299, 1984

Garbarino J, Ebata A: The significance of ethnic and cultural differences in child maltreatment. Journal of Marriage and the Family 45:733–783, 1983

Green A: Psychopathology of abused children. Journal of the American Academy of Child Psychiatry 17:92–97, 1978a

Green A: Self-destructive behavior in battered children. Am J Psychiatry 135:579–582, 1978b

Green AH: True and false allegation of sexual abuse in child custody disputes. Journal of the American Academy of Child Psychiatry 25:449–456, 1986

Kaplan S: Child psychiatric consultation to attorneys representing abused and neglected children. Bull Am Acad Psychiatry Law 9:140–148, 1981

Kaplan S: Runaway youth: psychiatric aspects. Child Psychiatry Grand Rounds Presentation, North Shore University Hospital, Manhasset, NY, February 10, 1986

Kaplan S, Pelcovitz D, Salzinger S, et al: Psychopathology of parents of abused and neglected children. Journal of the American Academy of Child Psychiatry 22:238–244, 1983

Kaplan S, Montero G, Pelcovitz D, et al: Psychopathology of abused and neglected children. Paper presented at the International Congress of Child Psychiatry and Allied Professions, Paris, France, July 1986

Kashani J, Beck N, Hoeper E, et al: Psychiatric disorders in a community sample of adolescents. Am J Psychiatry 144:584–588, 1987

Kaufman J, Zigler E: Do abused children become abusive parents? Am J Orthopsychiatry 57:186–192, 1987

Kinard E: Emotional development in physically abused children. Am J Orthopsychiatry 50:689–696, 1980

Kline D, Christiansen J: Educational and psychological problems of abused children. Final report, 1975 [ERIC microfiche ED111041]

Langevin R, Paitich D, Freeman R, et al: Personality characteristics and sexual anomalies in males. Canadian Journal of Behavioral Science 19:222–238, 1978

Langevin R, Handy L, Day D, et al: Are incestuous fathers pedophilic, aggressive, and alcoholic? in Erotic Preference, Gender Identity and Aggression in Men. Edited by Langevin R. Hillsdale, NJ, Lawrence Erlbaum, 1985, pp 161–179

MacVicar K: Psychotherapy of sexually abused girls. Journal of the American Academy of Child Psychiatry 18:342–353, 1979

Martin H, Beezley P: Behavioral observations of abused children. Dev Med Child Neurol 13:373–387, 1977

McLeer SV, Deblinger E, Atkins MS, et al: Posttraumatic stress disorder in sexually abused children. J Am Acad Child Adolesc Psychiatry 27:650–654, 1988

National Center on Child Abuse and Neglect: National Study of the Incidence and Prevalence of Child Abuse and Neglect (DHHS Publ No [OHDS]-81-30325). Rockville, MD, U.S. Department of Health and Human Services, National Center on Child Abuse and Neglect, 1988

National Institute of Justice: The Cycle of Violence. Washington, DC, U.S. Department of Justice, Office of Justice Programs, 1992

National Safe Kids Campaign, Washington, DC (Dr Koop) and the Scientific Publications Group. JAMA 267:3075–3076, 1992

New York State Syllabus for Identification and Reporting of Child Abuse and Maltreatment. The University of the State of New York, 1994

Pfeffer CR: The Suicidal Child. New York, Guildford, 1986

Rice DP, MacKenzie EJ, and associates: Cost of Injury in the United States: Report to Congress. San Francisco, University of California, Institute for Health and Aging, and Baltimore, MD, The Johns Hopkins University, Injury Prevention Center, 1989

Rosenberg M, Repucci ND: Primary prevention of child abuse. J Consult Clin Psychol 53:576–585, 1985

Rotheram MJ, Bradley R: Evaluation of imminent danger for suicide among youth. Am J Orthopsychiatry 57:102–110, 1987

Russell DE: The incidence and prevalence of intrafamilial and extrafamilial sexual abuse of female children. Child Abuse Negl 7:133–146, 1983

Salzinger S, Kaplan S, Artemyeff C: Mothers' personal social networks and child maltreatment. J Abnorm Psychol 92:68–76, 1983

Salzinger S, Kaplan S, Pelcovitz D, et al: Parent teacher assessment of children's behavior in child maltreating families. Journal of the American Academy of Child Psychiatry 23:58–64, 1984

Sanders B, Giolas MH: Dissociation and childhood trauma in psychologically disturbed adolescents. Am J Psychiatry 148:50–54, 1991

Sansonnet-Hayden H, Haley G, Marriage K, et al: Sexual abuse and psychology in hospitalized adolescents. J Am Acad Child Adolesc Psychiatry 26:753–757, 1987

Shaffer D: A critical look at suicide prevention in adolescence. Address to the Society for Adolescent Psychiatry, New York, April 29, 1987

Shaffer D, Fisher P: The epidemiology of suicide in children and adolescents. J Child Psychol Psychiatry 15:275–291, 1974

Spinetta J, Rigler D: The child-abusing parent: a psychological review. Psychol Bull 77:296–304, 1972

Strand V: Parents in incest families: a study in differences. Unpublished doctoral dissertation, Columbia University, New York, 1986 [Dissertation Abstracts International 47(8) 3191A, 1986]

Straus M, Gelles R: Societal change and change in family violence from 1975 to 1985 as revealed by two national surveys. Journal of Marriage and the Family 48:465–479, 1986

Trudell B, Whatley MH: School sexual abuse prevention: unintended consequences and dilemmas. Child Abuse Negl 12:103–113, 1988

U.S. Department of Health and Human Services: Position Papers From the Third National Injury Control Conference, Denver, CO, April 22–25, 1991

van der Kolk BA, Perry C, Herman JL: Childhood origins of destructive behavior. Am J Psychiatry 148:1665–1671, 1991

Webster DW, Champion HR: Epidemiologic changes in gunshot wounds in Washington DC 1983–1990, in Violence: A Compendium. Edited by Koop CE, Lundberg G. Chicago, IL, American Medical Association, 1992, pp 201–205

Williams LM, Finkelhor D: The characteristics of incestuous fathers, in Handbook of Sexual Assault: Issues, Theories, and Treatment of the Offender. Edited by Marshall WL, Laws DR, Barbaree HE. New York, Plenum, 1990, pp 231–235

Wolfe D: Child abusive parents: an empirical review and analysis. Psychol Bull 97:462–482, 1985

Wurtele SK: School-based sexual abuse prevention programs: a review. Child Abuse Negl 9:507–519, 1987

Wyatt GE: The sexual abuse of Afro-American and white American women in childhood. Child Abuse Negl 9:507–519, 1985

Yates A: False and mistaken allegations of sexual abuse, in American Psychiatric Press Review of Psychiatry, Vol 10. Edited by Tasman A, Goldfinger SM. Washington, DC, American Psychiatric Press, 1991, pp 320–335

Yates A, Musty T: Young children's false allegations of molestation. Paper presented at the 140th annual meeting of the American Psychiatric Association, Chicago, IL, May 1987

Chapter 16

Multiple Personality Disorder: A Legacy of Trauma

Richard P. Kluft, M.D.

In 1943, Stengel declared *multiple personality disorder* (MPD) extinct. Fifty years later, contemporary clinical investigators have demonstrated that MPD is a commonplace disorder that may afflict 3% to 5% of psychiatric inpatients who are screened for this condition (Boon and Draijer 1993; Ross 1991; Saxe et al. 1993). Placed in historical perspective, the clinical phenomenology of MPD (organized under the rubrics of a number of diagnostic or descriptive classifications) has been familiar to European and North American clinicians for centuries, but only at certain moments in history have the prevailing paradigms of the mental health sciences allowed it to be acknowledged and perceived as such (Kluft 1991b, 1993; see also Ellenberger 1970; Greaves 1993; Rosenbaum 1980).

Multiple personality disorder is a chronic and complex dissociative psychopathology (Kluft 1987b) characterized by lesions of identity and memory (Nemiah 1980). In DSM-III-R (American Psychiatric Association 1987, p. 272), the diagnostic criteria for MPD are as follows:

A. The existence within the person of two or more distinct personalities or personality states (each with its own relatively enduring pattern of perceiving, relating to, and thinking about the environment and self).

B. At least two of these personalities or personality states recurrently take full control of the person's behavior.

411

In DSM-IV (American Psychiatric Association 1994, p. 487), MPD has been renamed *dissociative identity disorder* (DID) and the diagnostic criteria modified somewhat. The DSM-IV criteria for dissociative identity disorder are as follows:

A. The presence of two or more distinct identities or personality states (each with its own relatively enduring pattern of perceiving, relating to, and thinking about the environment and self).
B. At least two of these identities or personality states recurrently take control of the person's behavior.
C. Inability to recall important personal information that is too extensive to be explained by ordinary forgetfulness.
D. The disturbance is not due to the direct physiological effects of a substance (e.g., blackouts or chaotic behavior during Alcohol Intoxication) or a general medical condition (e.g., complex partial seizures). **Note:** In children, the symptoms are not attributable to imaginary playmates or other fantasy play.

The older literature on MPD emphasized the presence of a small number of overt, distinct, well-articulated and polarized personalities. More recent findings based on the sequential reassessment of large numbers of patients who had achieved this diagnosis has revealed a very different picture. Kluft (1985b) studied 210 MPD patients and found that the natural history of the disorder involves most afflicted individuals' making very different presentations over the course of their patient careers; the vast majority of patients who satisfy DSM-III or DSM-III-R criteria at some points in time do not satisfy these criteria at others and may appear to have dissociative disorder not otherwise specified, or even no diagnosable dissociative psychopathology. He concluded that what is essential to MPD across its pleomorphic and polysymptomatic presentations is the presence within the individual of more than one structured entity with a sense of its own existence.

Kluft found that "the irreducible core of MPD is a persistent form of intrapsychic structure rather than overt behavioral manifestations" (1991a, p. 609). He stated, "MPD develops when an overwhelmed child who cannot flee or fight adverse circumstances takes flight inwardly, and creates an alternative self-structure and psychological reality within which and/or by virtue of which emotional survival is facilitated. This involves the alters, which allows the enactment of alternative approaches to trying circumstances" (p. 610). In an earlier report, Kluft (1985a) stressed that

> multiple personality disorder appears to develop as a dissociative defense in the face of overwhelming childhood events. The raison d'être of multiple personality disorder is to provide a structured dissociative defense against overwhelming traumata and the possible repetition of the same or analogous traumata. The emitted observable manifestations of multiple personality disorder are epiphenomena and tools of the defensive purpose. In terms of the patient's needs, the personalities need only be as distinct, public, and elaborate as becomes necessary in the handling of stressful situations. In childhood cases, investment in separateness and distinctness is usually minimal. Anything further results from hypertrophy or secondary autonomy of these processes, and from whatever narcissistic investments and secondary gains become associated with them. (pp. 231–232)

Similarly, dramatically enacted polarized behaviors, often regarded as most characteristic, are also secondary. Putnam et al. (1986) demonstrated that the most frequently encountered alters are child personalities and ones with specialized memory functions. However, from the perspective of the natural history of the disorder, personalities that the person had as a child, although very different from the major adult alters, may not have differed from what the patient's presentation had been at the time of the initial traumatizations (Kluft 1991a). As Kluft noted, "Therefore, what appears to be dramatically different at a later point in time may be the persistence of phenomenology that at one time blended so well with the initial personality presentation that it was indistinguishable" (Kluft 1991a, p. 610). That is, when a traumatized child forms another version of himself or herself either to hold an intolerable experience that can be ablated from awareness or to be unaware of it, MPD has been created intrapsychically. Such "isomorphic MPD" is the true paradigmatic expression of the condition. Thus, in youngsters, the alters are often muted and unelaborated in comparison with those of adults. The major signs of dissociative disorders with an MPD structure in children are those not of the personalities per se, but of the dissociative processes at work (Branscomb and Fagan 1992; Evers-Szostak and Sanders 1992; Fagan and McMahon 1984; Hornstein and Putnam, Chapter 17, this volume; Hornstein and Tyson 1991; Kluft 1984a, 1985a, 1985b,

1991b; McMahon and Fagan 1993; Peterson 1990, 1991; Putnam 1991a, 1991c, 1993b; Reagor et al. 1992; Tyson 1992).

When alters are shorn of their occasional epiphenomenological dramatic manifestations, what is important about alter personalities in both children and adults is the adaptational functions and strategies that they subserve and enact. This mission is supported by certain aspects of experience and knowledge being segregated from one another in a relatively consistent rule-bound fashion, as per Spiegel's (1986) description of dissociative information processing. Furthermore, the "emergence and manifest separateness" of the alter personalities are "not an inevitable and ongoing concomitant of these purposes and processes" (Kluft 1991a, p. 611).

The Study of Multiple Personality Disorder in Children

Aspects of the history of the study of MPD in adults have been described by a number of authors (e.g., Bliss 1986; Ellenberger 1970; Greaves 1980, 1993; Kluft 1987b, 1991b; Putnam 1989; Rosenbaum 1980; Ross 1989). The history of the study of MPD in children, however, has not excited equivalent scholarly interest. Until 1984 the entire modern clinical literature consisted of Ellenberger's (1970) fascinating and instructive account of the treatment of 11-year-old "Estelle" by Antoine Despine, Sr. Kluft (1984a) credits Despine with inspiring many of his therapeutic strategies. Despine's publications (1840) are difficult to locate and have not been translated into English. Fortunately, Fine (1988) has reviewed and summarized the contributions of this brilliant but overlooked pioneer.

In 1982, Elliott summarized unpublished diagnostic checklists and observations by several authors (e.g., Caul, Kluft, Putnam) in arguing that 1) MPD could be identified in children and 2) MPD was associated with child abuse and therefore the presence of MPD phenomena suggested the need to intervene in such cases. In 1984, Fagan and McMahon described a syndrome of "incipient multiple personality" in four children, consisting of dissociative symptoms that did not fulfill the full criteria for MPD. These authors also published a useful checklist of behaviors associated with dissociation. Also in 1984, Kluft described five children who had developed a complete MPD picture, and presented his own checklist (Kluft 1984a, 1984b). Kluft subsequently expanded his observations (Kluft 1985a, 1985b, 1986) and, later, described an additional three cases (Kluft 1990). In addition, he described situations in which mothers with MPD were found to have children with MPD, a constellation that had also been described by Coons (1985) and Braun (1985).

Weiss and colleagues (1985) described full MPD in a 10-year-old girl. Malenbaum and Russell (1987) reported MPD in an 11-year-old boy and his mother. Vincent and Pickering (1988) reviewed the literature and offered an overview. In the same year, Riley and Mead reported the development and successful treatment of MPD in a 3-year-old child. This case is remarkable for its having been assessed over a year before the development of the symptoms, and for the authors' having videotaped the initial assessment of the patient, and every other session but one (not taped because of technical problems) upon her return with dissociative symptoms and throughout her treatment.

Albini and Pease (1989) described early precursors of MPD-like phenomena in a traumatized child. In 1990, Peterson studied 21 cases of childhood MPD from the literature and conference presentations. He applied existing checklists to this group and argued that it would be productive to establish a diagnostic category of "dissociation identity disorder" to encourage the recognition and treatment of those children whose symptomatology was clearly dissociative but that lacked evidence of clearly defined alter personalities. He elaborated this position in a subsequent publication (Peterson 1991). Also in 1989, Carlson and Putnam attempted to integrate research on hypnosis and dissociativity and offered the hypothesis that the pathways into hypnotizability in children who were traumatized may be different from those in children who were not. This paper initiated a reconsideration of children's hypnotic and dissociative capacities and the relationship of these two capacities with each other.

Putnam (1991a, 1991c) summarized research findings bearing on the etiology of childhood dissociation. He also attempted to classify and clarify potential substrates for dissociative structures (Putnam 1991a). Hornstein and Tyson (1991), in the first study of hospitalized children with dissociative disorders, described their experience with 11 MPD children and 6 children with severe dissociative symptoms but without the clear-cut demonstration of alternate personalities. Both Putnam and Hornstein and Tyson referred to Putnam's Child Dissociative Checklist as a useful diagnostic measure. Putnam continues to study this instrument, which, although widely distributed, remains unpublished.

The year 1992 witnessed the publication of three instruments related to childhood MPD: the Child/Adolescent Dissociative Checklist of Reagor, Kasten, and Morelli; the Children's Perceptual Alteration Checklist of Evers-Szostak and Sanders; and an intriguing instrument for the retrospective assessment of childhood dissociation, the Childhood Dissociative Predictor Scale of Branscomb and Fagan. Furthermore, Tyson (1992) reported the application of various diagnostic checklists and offered some additional items based on his clinical experience. Putnam (1993b) condensed the literature and his research findings to develop a behavioral profile of the child with MPD or allied dissociative disorders. Also, the first detailed description of the play therapy of a child with a dissociative disorder was published by Mc-Mahon and Fagan (1993). Hornstein's most recent description of childhood MPD phenomena is presented in the present volume (Hornstein and Putnam, Chapter 17); a closely related publication by the same author was published elsewhere (Hornstein 1993).

An energetic but unsuccessful effort was mounted to advocate the inclusion of a category for dissociative disorders of childhood in the draft versions of DSM-IV. As more data accumulate, it is likely that a reasonable acknowledgment of this class of disorders will ultimately find its way into the official nomenclature. For the moment, children with this type of clinical phenomenology will be classified under *dissociative identity disorder* (300.14) or *dissociative disorder not otherwise specified* (300.15) (American Psychiatric Association 1994).

Hence, after a near-total absence of childhood MPD from the literature prior to 1983, over two dozen relevant contributions have been published in the course of a single decade. It is clear that appreciation of childhood MPD and allied conditions will grow rapidly and generate an increasingly rich literature.

Traumatic Antecedents of Multiple Personality Disorder: The Literature

Trauma and Dissociation

It is difficult to escape the conclusion that dissociative symptoms are often among the sequelae of traumatic experiences. Space precludes more than a selective review of this intriguing area. I will cite the adult literature because the study of dissociative phenomena in children remains complicated by the unfamiliarity of many child psychiatrists and psychologists with dissociative manifestations, and because the development of the capacity to perceive the passage of time is a complex process (Gibbon and Allan 1984) not taken into account in many studies of childhood traumatization. The baseline difficulty experienced by children in estimating the passage of time and in placing the elements of a complex experience in the correct sequence complicates research in this area (Putnam 1991c, 1993b).

In an important review, Putnam (1985) studied the presence of traumatic antecedents in the histories of patients with DSM-III dissociative disorders and concluded that "in most patients the precipitation of a dissociative reaction is associated with substantial psychological distress or traumatic experiences" (p. 86). Spiegel (1991; see also Spiegel and Cardeña 1991) reviewed many subsequent studies indicating the prevalence of dissociative responses to natural disasters, accidents, war, being held hostage, automobile accidents, and physical assault. He observed that the extreme discontinuity in personal experience caused by trauma was often accompanied by psychological reactions that incorporate discontinuities of experience such as dissociation. Spiegel summarized a rationale for this correlation:

> Dissociative defenses, which allow individuals to compartmentalize perceptions and memories, seem to serve a dual function. They help victims separate themselves from the full impact of physical trauma while it is occurring, and, by the same token, they may delay the necessary working through and putting into perspective of these traumatic experiences after they have occurred. They help the trauma victim maintain a sense of control during an episode of physical helplessness, but then become a mechanism by which the individual feels psychologically helpless once he or she has regained physical control. (Spiegel 1991, p. 261)

Boon and Draijer (1993) offer a review of trauma and dissociation that includes the impressive contributions of modern Dutch authors. For example, Albach (1991) and Ensink (1992) demonstrated that 44% of incest victims had had doubts about the reliability of their memories of traumatization, even when there was outside corroboration that the abuse had taken place. This is intriguing in connection with the recent findings of Briere and Conte (1989), who found that 59% of 450 incest victims had at some time forgotten their experiences of childhood sexual abuse (see also unpublished research quoted by Williams 1992), and Williams's (1992) discovery that 38% of 100 women with documented childhood abuse interviewed 17 years later did not report their abuse histories and that qualitative analysis of their reports suggested that the majority did not remember those experiences.

Vietnam combat veterans with posttraumatic stress disorder (PTSD) have been found to have higher scores on measures of dissociative symptomatology than combat veterans without PTSD, leading Bremner and co-workers (1992) to conclude that "dissociative symptoms are an important element of the long-term psychopathological response to trauma" (p. 328). Using a well-researched structured clinical interview for the diagnosis of dissociative disorders, Bremner and co-workers (1993) documented that Vietnam combat veterans with PTSD had higher scores in each of the five dissociative symptom areas studied (amnesia, depersonalization, derealization, identity confusion, and identity alteration), especially for amnesia. The veterans with PTSD often achieved scores similar to those made by patients with formal dissociative disorders.

Lenore Terr (1991) has attempted to synthesize her research, clinical experience, and interpretation of the literature to propose that childhood trauma can be divided into two subtypes with different posttraumatic profiles. Here only the phenomena of memory will be addresssed. Type I trauma follows upon the child's having experienced a single discrete traumatic event. Memory of the event is full, detailed, and "etched in." Type II trauma occurs in the aftermath of long-standing exposure to repeated untoward events. Amnesia, self-anesthesia, and distancing with autohypnotic defenses are common, with freqent impairment of memory. In the present author's experience this heuristic is useful, but the distinctions drawn are not absolute. He has seen several children with amnesia after documented single traumatic experiences. He speculates that future research will demonstrate an interaction among type of trauma, hypnotizability, dissociativity, and the response of those in the child's environment to the childhood traumatization. He further hypothesizes, on the basis of cases he has already assessed, that dissociative responses will be found after single traumatic events in highly dissociation-prone children (high hypnotizable and/or high dissociative) who are in environ-ments in which attempts are made to avoid dealing directly with the traumatic event.

In summary of the findings of this selective review and many other studies as well, there is a robust association between the historical experience of traumatization and the acute and long-term develop-ment of dissociative symptoms. Although amnesia has been the most thoroughly studied of the dissociative symptoms, those studies that have systematically assessed lesions of identity have documented their occurrence as well. Parenthetically, this connection is sufficiently compelling to have prompted the proposal of "brief reactive dissocia-tive disorder" as a new classification for DSM-IV (Spiegel 1991).

Trauma and Multiple Personality Disorder

The association of MPD with reported traumatic antecedents is con-troversial but very strong. The controversy, which is discussed below, concerns not whether MPD patients give histories of severe mistreat-ment during childhood, but whether the allegations of MPD patients should be accorded credibility.

Among modern MPD cases described in the lay press, "Eve" (Sizemore and Pitillo 1977) describes becoming aware of the presence of an alter personality after witnessing an industrial accident during which a man was cut in half at a sawmill. "Sybil" (Schreiber 1973) developed dissociative phenomena, including alter personalities, in the context of severe child abuse at the hands of her psychotic mother. William Milligan (Keyes 1981) is also said to have been the victim of terrible mistreatment as a child.

The scientific literature on MPD indicates that MPD patients are universally the victims of overwhelming childhood experiences and, in western cultures, as a group, are the survivors of child abuse. In their classic survey of 100 MPD patients, Putnam and co-workers (1986) found that 97% reported having been abused as children. Interest-ingly, the 3% who did not were also the patients that had entered treatment most recently (F. W. Putnam, personal communication, 1986). Putnam and his colleagues found that 83% reported sexual abuse, generally in the form of incest (68%). Repeated physical abuse was reported by 75%. The authors also found that 68% reported both sexual and physical abuse, and 45% said they had witnessed a violent death. Over 60% reported severe neglect.

Ross and co-workers (1989) studied a series of 236 MPD patients. The authors stated that there was evidence that 88.5% had been either sexually or physically abused, with uncertainty about whether abuse had occurred in many additional patients. Overall, 74.9% of the patients stated that they had been physically abused, and 11.1% were unsure whether this had occurred. With regard to sexual abuse, 79.2% reported such experiences, and an additional 8.1% were uncertain.

Coons and co-workers (1988) studied 50 MPD patients and found that 96% gave histories of childhood abuse; 68% reported sexual abuse, 60% reported physical abuse, and 22% reported neglect. Schultz and colleagues (1989) surveyed the therapists of 355 MPD patients and found that 86% of these patients reported histories of sexual abuse and 82% reported histories of physical abuse; 98% reported histories of abuse of one or both kinds. In another survey, Ross and colleagues (1990) studied structured interview data on 102 MPD patients and found that 95.1% reported histories of either physical or sexual abuse (82.4% and 90.2%, respectively).

In their comprehensive study of 82 patients with dissociative disorders, Boon and Draijer (1993) found that 65.1% had been physically abused and 60.3% had been sexually abused, and that there was a high prevalence of history of other overwhelming experiences. These authors postulated that amnesia for childhood led to their figures being rather low. It is of interest that almost all of the other studies involved patients who were already in treatment for dissociative disorders, whereas this study included many patients referred for diagnostic assessment whose treatment for a dissociative disorder had not begun.

Although these studies are based, in the main, on unauthenticated allegations from MPD patients, it is of interest that Bliss (1984) documented some allegations for 12 of 13 MPD patients, Coons and co-workers (1988) could document some allegations from 85% of a series of 20 MPD patients, and Dell and Eisenhower (1990) were able to obtain independent corroboration of some of the traumas alleged by 73% of their MPD patients.

When the focus shifts to the smaller case series and case reports of childhood MPD cases in the literature cited above, however, documentation of some of the patients' allegations is the rule rather than the exception. Most of the case reports indicate corroboration by other sources or that the traumas were first revealed by a witness or a perpetrator. For example, seven of the eight childhood cases described by Kluft (1984a, 1990) had documentation of the alleged source of traumatization, as did most of the cases described by Fagan and McMahon (1984). In one situation Kluft encountered MPD in a mother and son:

> When I began to treat mother, I had assessed the boy (then 6) along with his siblings and saw no evidence of dissociative symptoms. Two years later, one of the mother's personalities revealed that another had beaten the eldest son several times. She said that he had developed auditory hallucinations, amnesias, rapid fluctuations in appearance and voice, and a separate "scared" personality." The boy (now 8), his sister (5), and a brother (4) were seen. Brother could not be assessed adequately. Sister clearly dissociated traumatic events and idealized mother, but displayed no evidence of another personality. The 8-year-old boy had formed a scared, child-like personality that recalled the traumata and cowered in fear. In the midst of a family therapy discussion of discipline, the mother abruptly switched into an abusive personality and attacked the boy. His eyes rolled upward, and the cowering fearful personality emerged. The author had to intercede physically to stop the assault. When mother resumed a kind personality, son eye-rolled again, and resumed his usual personality. On inquiry, both he and his mother were amnestic for this horrible episode. Child welfare agencies were involved. The mother did no harm for several months and the boy achieved integration. Then mother abused the boy again and she was removed to a hospital. He maintained the prior integration but was found to have a complex personality based on identification with the aggressor mother, and abused his siblings. Treatment restored unity. (Kluft 1984a, pp. 126–127)

The follow-up on this family is of interest. As of this writing, the boy noted above, after a difficult adolescence during which he abused his sister over a period of time, and during which he returned for further treatment but had no signs of MPD, gradually stabilized, matured, and has been able to complete high school and specialized training. He was able to separate himself from his chaotic mother and her illness and his uninvolved father to find more stable object relations and role models. He became able to manage social relationships, date, and develop appropriate friends. Now in his 20s, he is gainfully employed in a technical field and has been promoted to supervisory capacities. He has married an appropriate young woman and is an active member of his church and several community organizations.

The daughter who dissociated the mother's attack on this boy herself became the target of the mother's abuse, developed MPD, and is the subject of another report (Kluft 1990). She was treated successfully for her dissociation but developed many Cluster B personality disorder features. She ultimately became estranged from her mother and filed new (and false) charges of abuse against her, leading to an exquisitely painful set of circumstances for all concerned. The youngest son never showed dissociative features of the classic varieties. He found ways to block out the world by withdrawal and intermittent elective mutism. It was not until his mid-teens that he was able to be engaged in productive therapy. The ultimate outcome for these two children remains uncertain.

Thoughts on a Current Controversy

As of this writing, there is intense media attention focused on the controversy surrounding the issue of whether allegations of childhood abuses reported by adults are credible. Skepticism is intensified if the alleged childhood mistreatment had been apparently forgotten, repressed, dissociated, and so forth and the memory has emerged or been retrieved in connection with therapy, or with some consciousness-raising discussion or publication about the delayed impact of forgotten abuse. Arguments are raised to invalidate apparent childhood memories that are retroactively deemed antecedent to some cluster of adult discomforts and distresses. Groups have been founded that challenge the idea that traumatic events can be repressed/dissociated and then later recalled; they maintain that the "memories" of abuse allegedly recovered are confabulations or false memories. It is not uncommon for such groups to advise those who feel they have been harmed by the recovery of false memories in their own treatment or the treatment of their children to seek legal redress in order to discourage the health care professions from what they choose to define as "malpractice."

Space precludes an extensive discussion of this volatile debate, which has been characterized by polarized opinions and flagrantly overgeneralized inflations of the probative values of both certain varieties of clinical experiences and laboratory studies. Unfortunately, the impairment of the objectivity of the participants in this imbroglio has been so pervasive that the author cannot recommend a single impartial review article in this critical area of study. The affective level and the adversarial nature of the discussion, replete with ad hominem attacks, resemble a holy war more than a process of scientific inquiry. Those who are primarily sympathetic with the complaints of those who allege childhood abuse are accused of participating in a witch-hunt to indict innocent parents and others; those who are primarily sympathetic with accused parents and others are accused of turning a deaf ear to the cries of the abused.

To summarize, with admitted oversimplification in the interests of brevity, there is ample evidence that memory is a reconstructive process subject to the impact of postevent information. There is evidence that some apparent memories describe events that have never occurred. There is also evidence that many recovered memories can be documented as accurate. The evidence that subjects can be induced to believe and report as memories events or bits of data that have not occurred comes both from laboratory studies and from clinical experience in finding that on occasion a patient represents as accurate recall an event that cannot have occurred. The evidence that recovered memories can be accurate comes largely from clinical experience.

To illustrate the complexity of this situation, two vignettes are offered. In the first, a woman who was once in treatment with the author recalled under hypnosis that she had murdered her divorced husband, fearing he would never cease to harass her. She described her act in exquisite detail and abreacted the experience with profound emotion. She truly believed in the accuracy of her recall and was thunderstruck 2 years later when a relative passing through the town in which the patient had lived discovered that the man was in fact alive and well.

In contrast, a second woman who was once in treatment with the author shortly after the publication of *Sybil* (Schreiber 1973) recovered under hypnosis experiences of abuse by her mother virtually identical to those described as inflicted upon "Sybil" by her psychotic mother. She also described her father's knowing of these torments but his doing nothing to stop them. The author frankly disbelieved the patient and was apologetic for his inquiries when he interviewed the patient's parents. To his amazement, the patient's father confirmed his daughter's recollections, even down to some singular details. The father was embarrassed by his having done nothing and simply said that he had not intervened because he loved his wife and had been brought up to believe that "raising children is the women's work."

When interviewed, the mother, who admitted to a history of psychiatric treatment, also confirmed the patient's recovered memories. When asked why she had treated her daughter as she had, she said, "Well, I was crazy then." She went on to explain that she had abused her daughter prior to the availability of chlorpromazine, which, when prescribed, had controlled her mental problems.

The state of the art is such that although it can be demonstrated that children and adults can be induced to incorporate leading suggestions and postevent information into their memory of events or sets of data, and thereafter may not be able to distinguish the introduced from the original material and may report the confabulated material with degrees of conviction equal to those with which they report the original material, it is neither accurate nor ethical to assert on the basis of such research that this has occurred in a given clinical situation. Many of these studies demonstrated that although inaccuracies and distortions may be induced, what is possible and occurs in a percentage of research subjects is not inevitably induced in all subjects exposed to a given experimental intervention. There is also the question of ecological validity. The experimental situation is different from the clinical encounter in terms of its demand characteristics and task expectations. The affective circumstances of the trauma victim are different from those of the subject of a laboratory subject. These are a few of many crucial and often bypassed considerations.

Conversely, it must be acknowledged that many clinicians in the trauma field have often erred on the side of credulity and have not been sensitive to the implications of research findings for their daily work. The author has frequently been attacked during lectures to audiences of mental health professionals by colleagues who insist that good clinicians always believe their patients, that patients do not make false allegations, and so forth. It appears that circumspection is in short supply at both poles of this dispute.

At this time it seems prudent to regard both extreme skepticism and extreme credulity about allegations of childhood abuse, whether the memory of the purported events has always been recalled or whether the memory stems from materials that emerge while a patient is in therapy, as statements of opinion and belief despite their apparent credible trappings and the prestige of those who voice them. In the individual case, clinical judgment informed by research findings and tested against corroborative evidence (when this is possible without doing harm to the treatment) is the best available guide. Recommended readings that represent major issues and perspectives with reasonable dispassion include Doris (1991), Ganaway (1989), Goodwin (1985), Herman and Schatzow (1987), Loewenstein (1991), Loftus (1979), Loftus and Doyle (1987, 1990), Orne (1979), Pettinati (1988), Schafer (1992), Spence (1982), Williams (1992), and A. Yates (1991). More recent publications have been tainted by the acrimony noted above.

Although all trauma does not lead to dissociation and all dissociation is not a sign of prior trauma, the accounts given by both children and adults alleging mistreatment must be treated with respect, approached circumspectly, and regarded as valuable clinical data. The current controversies should teach the contemporary clinician that the allegation of abuse is the beginning rather than the end of the search for understanding, and the confused and contradictory findings of today's literature should be humbling evidence that all too often it will not be possible to arrive at an understanding that is definitive, conclusive, and convincing to all concerned.

Models of Multiple Personality Disorder

Efforts to conceptualize the developed MPD psychopathology have often been based on an explicit or an implicit model or paradigm. Combining classifications offered by Stern (1984) and Putnam (1991c), there are many models currently under exploration: 1) supernatural/transpersonal, 2) psychological, 3) sociological, 4) role-playing/malingering/iatrogenesis, 5) trance state/autohypnotic, 6) split brain/hemispheric laterality, 7) temporal lobe/complex partial seizure/kindling, and 8) behavioral states of consciousness. To these might be added 9) the neural network of memory/information processing model (see Ansdorfer 1985; Li and Spiegel 1992; Spiegel 1990, 1991; J. L. Yates and Nasby 1993), 10) the neodissociation/ego states model (drawn from the work of Hilgard [1977/1986] by authors such as Beahrs [1982] and Watkins and Watkins [1979]), and 11) a basic affects model (Nathanson, in press), which has much in common with the behavior states of consciousness and the neural network of memory/information processing models. None of these models essentially precludes the operation of others, and none explains MPD but rather illustrates one possible mechanism by which it arises.

Space precludes more than a perfunctory overview of these models. Here the author can do no more than offer summary observations with selected illustrations, referring the interested reader to the cited articles for further details.

Supernatural/Transpersonal Models

Supernatural/transpersonal theories and models, in which it is speculated that the alters are demons, lingering spirits, the souls of those who have died but not passed on, and so forth, have never been in short supply. They have a venerable history, especially because MPD in its current form is the secular expression of the form and structure of the Judeo-Christian possession syndrome (Ellenberger 1970; Kluft 1991b). Although discounted by mainstream professionals, these ideas were inherent in the theories of Allison (1974, 1978), a major pioneer in the recognition and treatment of MPD, and are discussed in a recent book (Freisen 1991). *Dissociation,* the official journal of the International Society for the Study of Multiple Personality & Dissociation, receives several manuscripts advocating this explanation every year. There is no scientific evidence to accord this model credibility, but many religiously oriented clinicians continue to value it and use it to inform their clinical interventions.

Psychological Models

Purely psychological models have been plentiful but often have been based on theoretical considerations or the intensive study of one or a few MPD patients. No single psychological model has been proposed that is consistent with all known cases of MPD (Kluft 1984b, 1985a). A review of psychoanalytic contributions was offered in 1992 by Loewenstein and Ross. Many authors have tried to link the splitting of borderline personality disorder (BPD) defenses with the dissociation in MPD patients, but clinical studies have demonstrated repeatedly that not all MPD patients are borderline and that the resemblances between dissociative phenomena and splitting are more apparent than essential (see, e.g., Young 1988). Armstrong's (1991) recent work seems to have retired this argument.

Nonetheless, there appears to be a persistent clinical impression that important separation concerns play a major role in MPD psychopathology. Marmer (1980, 1991) has marshaled psychoanalytic evidence that with the failure of maternal and transitional objects, the person who will go on to develop MPD may take an aspect of self as self-object and initiate the experience of taking and perceiving self as object. More recently, Barach (1991) and Liotti (1992) have offered clinical and research-based arguments that many of Bowlby's ideas are consistent with observed MPD phenomena.

It seems likely that over time the aggregate psychological litera- ture will yield more useful explanations of why certain subgroups of MPD patients behave as they do, but no psychological model to date has been comprehensive enough to depict and explain the full spec- trum of MPD phenomena and processes.

Sociological Models

Sociological models of many dissociative phenomena have been of- fered, essentially depicting them as an attempt to live, at different times, by different systems of values or in a manner that compensates for controls imposed in certain societies. This is an attractive model for some culture-bound possession states in which the individual in the possession state is allowed to manifest behavior normally pro- scribed for him or her in a rigid culture (e.g., a woman behaving in a stronger manner than is deemed appropriate). However, such mod- els do not explain the majority of MPD phenomena and therefore are not sufficiently comprehensive.

Role-Playing/Malingering/Iatrogenesis Models

Models of MPD that focus on role playing, malingering, and/or iatro- genesis are attractive to those skeptical about the genuineness of MPD as a clinical entity. Nonetheless, the most sophisticated and widely cited studies of this genre (e.g., Kampman 1976; Spanos 1986; Spanos et al. 1985, 1986) are sadly deficient and fail to duplicate genuine MPD phenomena (Kluft 1982, 1991b; Kluft [ed] 1989; Put- nam 1991a, 1991c). Iatrogenic MPD has yet to be demonstrated and remains a conviction and belief of skeptics and those involved in law- suits with MPD plaintiffs or defendants. This having been said, it is well appreciated that occasional MPD patients, like others of the hu- man race, are not above using their symptoms for witting or unwit- ting secondary gain. Furthermore, it is very clear that a therapist's ineptitude or fascination with MPD phenomena can lead to the exac- erbation and/or the dramatization of these manifestations (Kluft 1982; Kluft [ed] 1989).

Trance State/Autohypnotic Models

Trance state/autohypnotic models are quite attractive because there is much research demonstrating the high hypnotizability of MPD patients, and a wealth of data relating chronic posttraumatic symptoms to the presence of high hypnotizability. Any model must account for this phenomenon. Some of the physiological phenomena of differences across MPD alters have intriguing parallels with findings from recent psychophysiological studies of hypnotized subjects. However, hypnotizability and dissociativity have been demonstrated to be separate phenomena in traumatized children, and dissociativity is the more correlated with the traumatization (Putnam 1985). Furthermore, there are no data to date that indicate that either hypnotizability or dissociativity per se is associated with the full phenomenology or psychophysiology of MPD. Putnam and co-workers (1990), for example, found that the psychophysiological differences across the feigned alters of high-hypnotizable control subjects were different from those found across the alters of patients with clinical MPD. In sum, any accurate model must incorporate this model but cannot be based completely upon it.

Split Brain/Hemispheric Laterality Models

Split brain/hemispheric laterality models are intriguing intellectually, but few data support them.

Temporal Lobe/Complex Partial Seizure/Kindling Models

Temporal lobe/partial complex seizures/kindling models were given premature prominence in the early 1980s despite the weakness of the data from which these models were adduced. Thus far there has been no demonstration of a correlation between dissociative and epileptic symptoms, and studies of such correlations have failed to find either epilepsy among MPD patients or robust multiplicity phenomena in epileptic persons with partial complex or generalized seizures with a frequency that would suggest a strong connection (Coons et al. 1988; Devinsky et al. 1989; Loewenstein and Putnam 1988). Nonetheless, it remains a favorite area of speculation by those attempting to find a biological mechanism for MPD and will doubtless be studied further.

Behavioral States of Consciousness Models

Behavioral states of consciousness models are extremely powerful because they span well-known developmental models with regard to states of mind and self structures, depend upon researched behavioral state phenomena in infants, and are most congruent with the psychophysiological study of MPD to date. In these models, "the alter personalities represent discrete behavioral states of consciousness with personality state–specific encoding of certain types of memory, behavior, and psychophysiology" (Putnam 1991c, p. 499). Putnam has authored a masterful statement of this kind of model (Putnam 1988), and Braun (1984) has a novel theoretical paper in this area that unfortunately has been perceived by many as so recondite as to be puzzling.

Because behavioral states of consciousness models are such a useful heuristic and address so much of the phenomenology of MPD, they must be taken into account in any comprehensive model. Two possible difficulties are noted with regard to these models. First, often the exposition in these models combines findings from the developmental states and state-dependency researches, and several state-dependency researchers believe their model has been overextended in the service of the behavioral states of consciousness models. Second, if the substrate of MPD alters is indeed the discrete behavioral states that could not, because of trauma, achieve a seamless fluency with maturation, should not the switches across alters in childhood MPD patients be rather grossly discontinuous instead of subtle in their manifestations? As befits an excellent model, both of these difficulties are amenable to resolution by future research.

Neural Network Models

Neural network models, which are recent arrivals on the scene, stem both from information processing and from cognitive science models (e.g., Anderson 1983; Ansdorfer 1985; Rumelhart and McClelland 1987; Li and Spiegel 1992) and in some cases are beholden to the mood-dependent memory research of Gordon Bower (e.g., Bower 1981). These models offer paradigms by which alters could be understood as being based upon the creation and activation of the nodes in a particular network. The MPD patient's executive consciousness at a given time would consist of those nodes activated above threshold at a given moment in time. A combination of stimulation and inhibition phenomena could be used to model co-consciousness, amnesia, flashbacks, the return of the repressed, and so forth. Although in their infancy, such models have endeavored to explain many of the complex MPD phenomena that have been bypassed by authors embracing alternative paradigms. Therefore, they deserve careful consideration in future research and model building.

Neodissociation/Ego States Models

In neodissociation/ego states models, the assumption is that the mind may have several simultaneously ongoing and autonomous centers of cognitive activity and/or that the mind is at best a plurality of selves that when congruous leave humans with the subjective illusion of unity, but when incongruous or in conflict give rise to the experience of several alternative self structures at work with different characteristics and the capacity to influence ongoing behavior. In both cases, multiplicity is seen as a norm, and pathological multiplicity is thought to occur when the boundaries across these states or processes become sufficiently robust to impair the usual mental commerce so that the parts may achieve full or partial control rather than participating in a process congruent with subjective and behavioral unity (e.g., Beahrs 1982; Watkins and Watkins 1979). It is intriguing that Hilgard, whose seminal work on hidden observer phenomena (e.g., 1977/1986) is essential to many of these conceptualizations, has tried to dissociate himself (Hilgard 1984) from the use of his work in these models. Clearly, these models are consistent with many laboratory observation and clinical findings and must play some role in a definitive conceptualization.

Basic Affects Model

Most recently, Nathanson (in press) has attempted to employ his application of the affect theories of the late Sylvan Tomkins to the understanding of MPD. In his basic affects model, Nathanson considers whether the personalities might be organized around different basic affects and/or affect scripts. Nathanson's work on shame scripts demonstrates that this model could bridge both the psychological and the psychophysiological dimensions of MPD. Because this model has not yet had a reading by the majority of scientific and clinical thinkers in the dissociative disorders field, its goodness of fit with other conceptualizations remains to be determined.

Summary

Of the available models, although most deserve further study, an over-arching model would have to encompass those findings that are consistent with the trance state/autohypnosis, behavioral states of consciousness, neural network, neodissociation/ego states, and, possibly, basic affects models. In any given case, the inputs of the other models, especially the psychological model, and less compellingly the role-playing/malingering/iatrogenesis model, must be given attention.

Etiology of Multiple Personality Disorder: Some Recent Conceptualizations

The "3-P" Theory

As the modern study of MPD was getting under way, three attempts were made to conceptualize the etiology of MPD. Braun and Sachs (1985) offered the "3-P" theory, describing predisposing, precipitating, and perpetuating factors associated with the development of MPD. These authors stated that predisposing factors included both "1) a natural, inborn capacity to dissociate; and 2) exposure to severe, overwhelming traumata, such as frequent, unpredictable, and inconsistently alternating abuse and love (especially during childhood)" (p. 42). They noted that good memory, intelligence, and creativity were contributants. Precipitating factors, as defined by Braun and Sachs, are those "that can be identified as being antecedent to the initiation of a set of intrapsychic processes and structures that lead to the formation of a new personality" (p. 48). The authors appreciated the vagueness of these factors and further explained that "the formation of an alternate personality occurs when a series of fragmented but defensively related episodes, linked by a common affective state, take on an identity of their own" (p. 49). They noted that perpetuating factors were personal (e.g., the individual's repeated use of dissociative defenses), interpersonal (e.g., family dynamics), and situational (e.g., direct exposure to further traumatic events).

Stern's Etiological Paradigm

Stern (1984) derived certain etiological hypotheses from the study of the literature and tested them against the given histories of eight MPD patients. He then summarized an etiological paradigm. The person who develops MPD will have a history of child abuse or neglect, and there will have been severe psychopathology in at least one caretaker. A history of physical and emotional abuse will be evident, and usually sexual abuse as well. The first splitting occurs in childhood in response to a situation of sudden high stress associated with the behavior of at least one other person, but later splits and the overt emergence of an alter may occur at a later time. It is likely that the individual grew up in an atmosphere of strict religious and/or mystical beliefs, but these were often the vehicle for other factors (e.g., the use of religion to excuse abusive acts). The individual will believe that he or she has had parapsychological experiences and out-of-body experiences and is likely to believe in reincarnation. Physiological phenomena, substance abuse, and amnesia will be found as epiphenomena rather than as etiological factors. Ongoing stressors will lead to confusion about identity and a high level of anxiety. The person will have average or above average intelligence. In retrospect, many of Stern's hypotheses have been confirmed, but others are not universal and may be related to the small size of his sample.

The Four-Factor Theory of Multiple Personality Disorder

Kluft (1984b, 1986) developed the four-factor theory of MPD, a theory that is accepted widely because of its flexibility and because it encompasses most other credible models of etiology in a relatively simple and pragmatic frame that can be used to inform therapeutic strategy. This theory holds that the individual who develops MPD will have 1) the biological capacity to dissociate, which will be mobilized when 2) the nondissociative defenses are traumatically overwhelmed by unfortunate life experiences. If this occurs, the individual will 3) develop alters in a manner consistent with his or her unique shaping influences and substrates. These adaptations will become relatively fixed and stable if there is 4) the inadequate provision of stimulus barriers to further overwhelming experiences, and/or the absence of sufficient restorative experiences from significant others. All of the factors in this model contain elements that have been documented as relevant.

The first factor—the biological capacity to dissociate—is basically a statement of a biological diathesis or vulnerability. In its first articulation, it was understood to be the biological component of hypnotizability without the component of suggestibility. Over time it has become clear that what Kluft called "dissociation proneness" includes hypnotizability (Kluft 1984b, 1986), dissociativity (Carlson and Putnam 1989; Putnam 1991b), and perhaps some developmental components related to the individual's not having achieved seamless transitions across states of mind, early forms of self experience, the management of affective states, and certain levels of synthesis across cognitive and neurological processes (Nathanson, in press; Putnam 1988; J. L. Yates and Nasby 1993). Studies reviewed elsewhere (Frischholz et al. 1992; Kluft 1986) have indicated the high hypnotic potential of the cooperative MPD patient; dissociativity has been documented in a variety of studies, most recently a study by Carlson and co-workers (1993). The other potential components of this dimension have been postulated in the models noted in the previous section, and research findings support aspects of many of these models.

The second factor—the presence of overwhelming childhood experiences that overwhelm the adaptive capacities of the child's ego—has been a major area of study. With regard to child abuse, findings and relevant controversies have been reviewed earlier in this chapter. It is important to note that stressors other than intentionally inflicted abuse have been understudied, a concern expressed by Kluft (1984b). Object loss, exposure to the death of a significant other, witnessing of a deliberately caused or an accidental death, and exposure to dead bodies may constitute sufficient stressors. Serendipitous exposures to death or severe injury, witnessing of the events of war or terrorism, or growing up in a neighborhood in which violence is endemic (e.g., see Putnam 1993a)—all may constitute intolerable stressors. One post–World War II displaced person was the sole survivor of a bomb attack that demolished his family's home and left him orphaned. A post–Vietnam War Southeast Asian immigrant dissociated while being forced to witness the slaughter of the male members of his family and the rape of the women.

Exposure to a severe threat to survival or to one's sense of physical or psychological integrity (e.g., severe sustained illness, pain, or debilitation; experiences that nearly led to death) may lead to MPD.

Experiencing cultural dislocation, being subjected to brainwashing by embattled parents in a custody battle, and being treated by different caretakers as if one were different genders may be sufficent to overwhelm a child, and, rarely, family chaos (usually with an alcoholic or psychotic parent) or excessive primal scene experiences may have unsettled some who have gone on to develop MPD.

It is important to appreciate that some factors may lower a child's resistance to the impact of trauma to the point that a lesser than usual amount of trauma may be able to overwhelm the nondissociative defenses. These factors include illness, fatigue, and pain; difficulties with separation and individuation; congenital anomalies or difficulties; and severe narcissistic hurts.

The third factor—the shaping influences and substrates that determine the form taken by the dissociative defenses—comprises both the intrinsic mechanisms of the components of the first factor (see above), the inherent potentials for psychodynamic dividedness associated with developmental concerns that may be disturbed by childhood events, and extrinsic influences. The components of the first factor have been noted above. All of the developmental lines discussed in the psychoanalytic literature may play a role in determining the qualities of the alter formation in a given case. For example, premature sexualization may lead to alters that appear to embody oedipal libidinal and antilibidinal concerns; concerns of separation and loss may lead to alters that behave as if they were governed by Mahler's (Mahler et al. 1975) concepts of separation and individuation or by the reaction patterns described by Bowlby (1988); excessive experiences of empathic failure may lead to alters that seem to enact Kohut's (1977) polarized selfobject configurations; and severe humiliation may lead to alters that enact all poles of Nathanson's (1992) compass of shame. Furthermore, normative processes such as introjection, internalization, and identification (including identification with the aggressor), and benign normative dissociative identity phenomena such as imaginary companionship are available as substrates as well.

In addition, extrinsic influences bear upon alter formation. In the last year, the present author, following up the implications of an alter's being named Michaelangelo, found a child with protector alters named after the various *Teenage Mutant Ninja Turtle* characters. Clearly, such an alter formation would not have been likely before the inception of this cartoon series. In 1978, the author had been stunned to find that the female alters of his first case of childhood MPD were named "Betty" and "Wilma," a not very disguised indication that his young patient was devoted to the television series *The Flintstones*. Children develop in the context of a particular culture, and that will be reflected in the alter formations of those children who develop MPD. The author has already encountered alters based on several contemporary rock stars, and the difficult-to-classify Madonna, and is apprehensive about the future of the introjective process.

For the first time in history, the MPD patients of the future are growing up with media exposure to explicit lessons on how to behave like an MPD patient. The author has recently evaluated a patient who was quite aware of these presentations and was somewhat guided by them.

Children who are brought up being encouraged to role-play and act from an early age (either by parents who are preparing them for a career in the media or by caretakers who take some pleasure in manipulating the child in this manner), and those who are exposed to numerous caretakers and/or to caretakers who impose contradictory expectations, demands, and reward systems, are being encouraged to be different at different times, not in the interests of acquiring healthy socialization, but to gratify unreasonable adult wishes. Closely related are those situations in which a child is being reared by a parent with MPD, with whom identification is inevitable. Many patients with MPD seem incapable of appreciating the deleterious impact of their modeling dissociative behaviors to their children (Kluft 1987a).

It is important to appreciate that here-and-now influences may be impacting on a child who has begun to develop an MPD configuration. A child's previous treatment, a child's exposure to the media and literature, the vulnerability of children to be led to produce what an interviewer appears to want from them (e.g., Doris 1991), inadvertent interview errors—all may play a role in determining what appears to be the clinical picture. The author has seen several videotapes in which children were led to endorse a series of MPD phenomena that did not seem to be present initially, but were incorporated by the children in their later accounts of their circumstances. Here the author does not refer to iatrogenic MPD, but instead to alters' being accorded names and attributes that clearly came from the therapists' leading inquiries. It is crucial to appreciate that not infrequently the child with MPD may go into an autohypnotic state and be extremely suggestible; what is said lightly may assume the compelling power of a strong posthypnotic suggestion.

One of the most powerful validations of the fourth factor—the inadequate provision of stimulus barriers and restorative experiences—is a series of observations made by Kluft (1984a, 1984b, 1985a, 1985b, 1986), D. Caul (personal communication, 1987), and F. W. Putnam (personal communication, 1987) that when children with MPD are protected from further traumatization and offered treatment, a sizeable minority cease to have MPD symptoms. Kluft and Caul noted this in connection with experiences treating childhood MPD, and Putnam remarked upon it as a clinical finding as well as identified it as a factor in the difficulty encountered in trying to initiate research studies. Kluft tried to elicit the apparently spontaneously integrated alters with hypnosis over months of observation in two cases and could not find evidence of residual separateness. Another intriguing set of unpublished clinical findings have emerged in connection with Kluft's (1986) prediction that a child with MPD who could not be made to feel safe would not be able to be treated successfully—that he or she would either need to retain the MPD as an anodyne to the continued overwhelming experiences or try to create an even more drastic defense, become self-injurious or suicidal, or develop psychosis. Kluft has since consulted to over four dozen therapists working with childhood MPD cases, each of whom was complaining that he or she could not achieve significant improvement, let alone the rapid responses to treatment that had been reported in the clinical literature. In no case was the child safe. In each case the child was still in the proximity of the alleged abuser, over whom there were no meaningful controls, or the child had been placed into an institution or in a foster care setting in which there were difficulties.

In one case example, a 9-year-old boy referred for suspected childhood psychosis was being raised in a manner that led to his being perceived as a deviant by his peers and that allowed him no privacy, no opportunity to disagree with adults, and no door on his room (lest he masturbate). The boy had developed MPD. He clearly was becoming skilled in autohypnotic withdrawal to block out his family, retreating into a world of fantasy in which imaginary companions had graduated to becoming alters. He also alleged sexual abuse by an uncle who frequently supervised him. The therapist, the present author, took a supportive stance with the boy and used the therapy to discuss autonomy with courtesy, perceiving that the parents' misguided efforts had been to make the patient a perfectly behaved boy in accord with a grandmother's rather outfashioned standards, in the process of which the boy had been totally crushed. The therapist insisted on family therapy as well as individual work and rapidly persuaded the mother to allow her son to have a door with a lock for his room, to drop those activities that made him a deviant among his peer group, to spend time away from the family in developing and visiting friends, and never to be left alone with the alleged abuser. The therapist lavished praise and reinforcements on the family for their changes and was informed that the uncle had decided to relocate. Within 2 months the boy was asymptomatic and functioning well at home and at school. Neither then nor on sequential follow-up could residual dissociative symptomatology be observed or elicited.

Until more useful conceptualizations are developed, the four-factor theory or the almost identical "3-P" formulation represent adequate heuristics for clinical use and to inform research considerations. Although the various more abstract models have much to offer, no current one encompasses the full spectrum of MPD phenomenology.

Etiology of the Overt Phenomenology of Multiple Personality Disorder

The unique clinical picture of MPD in a given patient at a given moment in time has an etiology of its own, apart from the existence of the MPD per se (Kluft 1985). Patients with MPD vary widely in their intelligence, creativity, and narcissistic investment in sustaining and manifesting the separateness of their alters (Kluft 1985a, 1991a). Furthermore, Axis II is where Axis I lives. Fink (1991) has outlined how different character pathology may impact the signs of MPD. MPD patients' manifestations and the frequency with which and circumstances under which the manifestations achieve overtness may be related to aspects of ego strength, Axis I and Axis II comorbidity, intercurrent stressors, external reinforcers and/or suppressants of the MPD phenomenology, and the relative harmony or disharmony of the personality system itself.[1]

---

[1] The discussion that follows is derived from Kluft 1991a, pp. 611–616.

That is, an intelligent and creative woman with MPD who is in financial distress, who is invested in the separateness of her alters and is rather histrionic in her character structure and comes to believe that if she is a fascinating and deeply hurt patient she may be retained in treatment despite her running out of funds, and whose alters are in conflict, may be both vulnerable and motivated to display both her pain and a panoply of overt dissociative psychopathology with frequent dramatic shifts among alters articulated in great detail. The alters are quite open about their memories of traumas and are likely to identify themselves and take efforts to ensure that their uniqueness is appreciated by the observer. Such a patient has no motivation to be secretive, and every motivation to manifest her MPD psychopathology.

In contrast, a highly productive scientist with MPD of equal complexity, who is obsessional in character and gratified in her work, and without major external stressors, and who is wishing across all alters to pass for unified and hoping to integrate smoothly before anyone takes notice of the few dissociative manifestations that she has failed to control, might appear to be no more than an "absent-minded professor," which was in fact how her colleagues perceived her. Her personalities took great care to cover over or rationalize any manifestations of her psychopathology. Highly motivated to be secretive about her conditions, and with her alters agreed about how to approach their shared life and the work of therapy, she minimized the emission of MPD phenomena outside of the office, and in session her alters, although very different in many ways regarding their memories, attitudes, and preferences, were rather subdued in their self-presentations.

Overtness is also affected by the structure of the personality system and the manner in which the alters communicate with one another. The alters constitute a system of mind and may subjectively experience one another as separate people. Furthermore, they may have complex inner relationships with one another, involving both alliances and enmities of many sorts. For example, some systems are characterized by incessant civil wars and/or efforts to take over control, whereas others are an extended support system to an alter that is understood to be "the real person." The nature of this inner world will impact on emitted phenomena.

In addition, overtness is highly affected by the resilience of the host personality, the one "out" most of the time during a particular period of time. A robust host will rarely be replaced by other alters, whereas a weak or overwhelmed one will frequently be displaced or abdicate. The presence of intercurrent traumas will raise the likelihood that the most customary arrangements will be upset and be replaced by the overt emergence of other alters. Likewise, the length of alters' emergences influences overtness. If an alter can emerge and do what it does in a brief period of time, it may not interrupt consciousness or change behavior enough to be noticed by the patient or by others.

If the alters cooperate, they may share memories, pass for one another, and come out in tandem to address complex issues, and there may be no evident symptomatology. If there is conflict without resolution, the host personality may be dominated by intrusive phenomena and appear to be psychotic or borderline rather than have MPD. Should the alters in conflict be able to impose their control periodically, there may be an overt fluctuation of clearly defined alters.

If alters influence one another by inner dialogue (usually heard as hallucinations within the head), there may be no manifestations. If they do so by imposing themselves on one another covertly or by coming out completely to seize control, they may appear as noted in the previous paragraph. The absence or presence of amnesia among the alters that are alternating executive control will also affect the noticeability of the MPD. When evidence of amnesia is lacking, the patient usually will only be noted to be moody, volatile, or some other descriptor indicating a fluctuation of affective states. As noted above, the alters' degree of commonality of motivation, the power of their investments in separateness, the strength of their determination to preserve secrecy, the potential for secondary gain, and the alters' creativity will also influence the final picture that the clinician encounters.

External contingencies are also important in some cases. Having significant others (including therapists) who either encourage or respond suppressively to MPD phenomena can be a crucial variable.

Summary

The essence of MPD is the presence of structured dissociated self states utilized in the service of defensive and adaptational purposes. The dramatic epiphenomena of the condition have long distracted attention from its reason for being. MPD has been found and treated in children as well as adults. Dissociation is a frequent response to the experience and the anticipation of traumatization; MPD is only one of many conditions in which this can be observed. Although most accounts of childhood traumatization in MPD populations are unconfirmed retroactive accounts, sufficient numbers of cases with documented traumatization have occurred to accept MPD as a posttraumatic condition. However, the vicissitudes of memory are many, and a patient's given account may or may not be historically accurate. (That is, in MPD the patient has been traumatized, but, as in any other condition, without corroborative evidence one cannot be sure that the trauma that is described is the trauma that occurred.) Current polarized positions that are a priori credulous or skeptical about patients' accounts are without scientific foundation, and possibly without ethical foundation also.

Eleven basic models for MPD have been offered. Among these, the trance state/autohypnosis, behavioral states of consciousness, neural network, neodissociation/ego states, and, possibly, basic affects models appear to offer productive if incomplete hypotheses that point the way to future research and informed clinical interventions. The psychological model, and at times the role-playing/malingering/iatrogenesis model, can contribute to the understanding of individual cases, but not the condition as a whole. Among the overall theories of the etiology of MPD, the four-factor theory (along with the very similar but somewhat condensed "3-P" theory) embraces known data and has been a useful source for suggesting clinical interventions and research strategies. The etiology of overt manifestations of MPD in a given patient at a given moment in time is subject to many influences that stem from the nature of the disorder, the characteristics of the patient's system of alters, and external stressors and pressures.

References

Albach F: Tussen amnesie en herbeleving. Herkenning van posttraumatische stressklacheten bij incestslachtoffers. Maandblad Geestelijke Volksgezondheid 2:134–155, 1991

Albini TK, Pease TE: Normal and pathological dissociations of early childhood. Dissociation 2:144–150, 1989

Allison RB: A new treatment approach for multiple personalities. Am J Clin Hypn 17:15–32, 1974

Allison RB: A rational psychotherapy plan for multiplicity. Svensk Tidskrift för Hypnos 3–4:9–16, 1978

American Psychiatric Association: Diagnostic and Statistical Manual of Mental Disorders, 3rd Edition, Revised. Washington, DC, American Psychiatric Association, 1987

American Psychiatric Association: Diagnostic and Statistical Manual of Mental Disorders, 4th Edition. Washington, DC, American Psychiatric Association, 1994

Anderson JR: The Architecture of Cognition. Cambridge, MA, Harvard University Press, 1983

Ansdorfer JC: Multiple personality in the human information-processor: a case history and theoretical formulation. J Clin Psychol 41:309–324, 1985

Armstrong J: The psychological organization of multiple personality disordered patients as revealed in psychological testing. Psychiatr Clin North Am 14:533–546, 1991

Barach PMM: Multiple personality disorder as an attachment disorder. Dissociation 4:117–123, 1991

Beahrs JO: Unity and Multiplicity: Multilevel Consciousness of Self in Hypnosis, Psychiatric Disorder, and Mental Health. New York, Brunner/Mazel, 1982

Bliss EL: Spontaneous self-hypnosis in multiple personality disorder. Psychiatr Clin North Am 7:135–148, 1984

Bliss EL: Multiple Personality, Allied Disorders and Hypnosis. New York, Oxford University Press, 1986

Boon S, Draijer N: Multiple Personality Disorder in The Netherlands: A Study on Reliability and Validity of the Diagnosis. Amsterdam, Swerts & Zeitlinger, 1993

Bower GH: Mood and memory. Am Psychol 36:129–148, 1981

Bowlby J: A Secure Base: Parent-Child Attachment and Healthy Human Development. New York, Basic Books, 1988

Branscomb LP, Fagan J: Development and validation of a scale measuring childhood dissociation in adults: the Childhood Dissociative Predictor Scale. Dissociation 5:80–86, 1992

Braun BG: Towards a theory of multiple personality and other dissociative phenomena. Psychiatr Clin North Am 7:171–193, 1984

Braun BG: The transgenerational incidence of dissociation and dissociative disorder: a preliminary report, in Childhood Antecedents of Multiple Personality. Edited by Kluft RP. Washington, DC, American Psychiatric Press, 1985, pp 127–150

Braun BG, Sachs RG: The development of multiple personality disorder: predisposing, precipitating, and perpetuating factors, in Childhood Antecedents of Multiple Personality. Edited by Kluft RP. Washington, DC, American Psychiatric Press, 1985, pp 37–64

Bremner JD, Southwick SM, Brett E, et al: Dissociation and posttraumatic stress disorder in Vietnam combat veterans. Am J Psychiatry 149:328–332, 1992

Bremner JD, Steinberg M, Southwick SM, et al: Use of the Structured Clinical Interview for DSM-IV Dissociative Disorders for systematic assessment of dissociative symptoms in posttraumatic stress disorder. Am J Psychiatry 150:1011–1014, 1993

Briere J, Conte J: Amnesia in adults molested as children. Paper presented at the annual meeting of the American Psychological Association, New Orleans, LA, August 1989

Carlson EB, Putnam FW: Integrating research on dissociation and hypnotizability: are there two pathways to hypnotizability? Dissociation 2:32–38, 1989

Carlson EB, Putnam FW, Ross CA, et al: Validity of the Dissociative Experiences Scale in screening for multiple personality disorder: a multicenter study. Am J Psychiatry 150:1030–1036, 1993

Coons PM: Children of parents with multiple personality disorder, in Childhood Antecedents of Multiple Personality. Edited by Kluft RP. Washington, DC, American Psychiatric Press, 1985, pp 151–165

Coons PM, Bowman ES, Milstein V: Multiple personality disorder: a clinical investigation of 50 cases. J Nerv Ment Dis 176:519–527, 1988

Dell PF, Eisenhower JW: Adolescent multiple personality disorder: a preliminary study of eleven cases. J Am Acad Child Adolesc Psychiatry 29:359–366, 1990

Despine A: De l'emploi du magnétisme animal et des eaux minérales dans le traitment des maladies nerveuses, suivi d'une observation très curieuse de guerison de neuropathie. Paris, Germer, Bailliere, 1840

Devinsky O, Putnam FW, Grafman J, et al: Dissociative states and epilepsy. Neurology 39:835–840, 1989

Doris J (ed): The Suggestibility of Children's Recollections. Washington, DC, American Psychological Association, 1991

Ellenberger HF: The Discovery of the Unconscious. New York, Basic Books, 1970

Elliott D: State intervention and childhood multiple personality disorder. Journal of Psychiatry and the Law 10:441–446, 1982

Ensink B: Confusing Realities: A Study on Child Sexual Abuse and Psychiatric Symptoms. Amsterdam, VU (Free University) Press, 1992

Evers-Szostak M, Sanders S: The Children's Perceptual Alteration Scale (CPAS): a measure of dissociation. Dissociation 5:91–98, 1992

Fagan J, McMahon PP: Incipient multiple personality in children: four cases. J Nerv Ment Dis 172:26–36, 1984

Fine CG: The work of Antoine Despine: the first scientific report on the diagnosis of multiple personality disorder. Am J Clin Hypn 31:32–39, 1988

Fink D: The comorbidity of multiple personality disorder and DSM-III-R Axis II disorders. Psychiatr Clin North Am 14:547-566, 1991

Freisen JG: Uncovering the Mystery of MPD. San Bernadino, CA, Here's Life Publishers, 1991

Frischholz EJ, Lyman LS, Braun BG, et al: Psychopathology, hypnotizability, and dissociation. Am J Psychiatry 149:1521–1525, 1992

Ganaway GK: Historical truth versus narrative truth: clarifying the role of exogenous trauma in the etiology of multiple personality disorder and its variants. Dissociation 2:205–220, 1989

Gibbon J, Allan L: Timing and Perception. New York, New York Academy of Sciences, 1984

Goodwin J: Credibility problems in multiple personalities and abused children, in Childhood Antecedents of Multiple Personality. Edited by Kluft RP. Washington, DC, American Psychiatric Press, 1985, pp 1–20

Greaves GB: Multiple personality: 165 years after Mary Reynolds. J Nerv Ment Dis 168:577–596, 1980

Greaves GB: A history of multiple personality disorder, in Clinical Perspectives on Multiple Personality Disorder. Edited by Kluft RP, Fine CG. Washington, DC, American Psychiatric Press, 1993, pp 355–380

Herman JL, Schatzow E: Recovery and verification of memories of childhood sexual trauma. Psychoanalytic Psychology 4:1–14, 1987

Hilgard ER: Divided Consciousness: Multiple Controls in Human Thought and Action. New York, Wiley, 1977 [revised edition, 1986]

Hilgard ER: The hidden observer and multiple personality. Int J Clin Exp Hypn 32:248–253, 1984

Hornstein NL: Recognition and differential diagnosis of dissociative disorders in children and adolescents. Dissociation 6:136–144, 1993

Hornstein NL, Tyson S: Inpatient treatment of children with multiple personality/dissociative disorders and their families. Psychiatr Clin North Am 14:631–648, 1991

Kampman R: Hypnotically induced multiple personality: an experimental study. Int J Clin Exp Hypn 24:215–227, 1976

Keyes D: The Minds of Billy Milligan. New York, Random House, 1981

Kluft RP: Varieties of hypnotic interventions in the treatment of multiple personality. Am J Clin Hypn 24:230–240, 1982

Kluft RP: Multiple personality in childhood. Psychiatr Clin North Am 7:121–134, 1984a

Kluft RP: Treatment of multiple personality disorder. Psychiatr Clin North Am 7:9–29, 1984b

Kluft RP: Childhood multiple personality disorder: predictors, clinical findings, and treatment results, in Childhood Antecedents of Multiple Personality. Edited by Kluft RP. Washington, DC, American Psychiatric Press, 1985a, pp 167–196

Kluft RP: The natural history of multiple personality disorder, in Childhood Antecedents of Multiple Personality. Edited by Kluft RP. Washington, DC, American Psychiatric Press, 1985b, pp 197–238

Kluft RP: Treating children who have multiple personality disorder, in Treatment of Multiple Personality Disorder. Edited by Braun BG. Washington, DC, American Psychiatric Press, 1986, pp 79–105

Kluft RP: The parental fitness of mothers with multiple personality disorder: a preliminary study. Child Abuse Negl 11:273–280, 1987a

Kluft RP: An update on multiple personality disorder. Hosp Community Psychiatry 38:363–373, 1987b

Kluft RP (ed): The David Caul Memorial Symposium Papers: Iatrogenesis and MPD. Dissociation 2:66–104, 1989

Kluft RP: Multiple personality disorder in children: an update, in Hypnosis: Current Theory, Research and Practice. Edited by Van Dyck R, Spinhoven P, Van der Does AJW, et al. Amsterdam, VU (Free University) Press, 1990, pp 169–179

Kluft RP: Clinical presentations of multiple personality disorder. Psychiatr Clin North Am 14:605–629, 1991a

Kluft RP: Multiple personality disorder, in American Psychiatric Press Review of Psychiatry, Vol 10. Edited by Tasman A, Goldfinger SM. Washington, DC, American Psychiatric Press, 1991b, pp 161–188

Kluft RP: The treatment of dissociative disorder patients: an overview of discoveries, successes, and failures. Dissociation 6:87–101, 1993

Kohut H: The Restoration of the Self. New York, International Universities Press, 1977

Li D, Spiegel D: A neural network model of dissociative disorders. Psychiatric Annals 22:144–147, 1992

Liotti G: Disorganized/disoriented attachment in the etiology of multiple personality disorder. Dissociation 5:196–204, 1992

Loewenstein RJ: Psychogenic amnesia and psychogenic fugue: a comprehensive review, in American Psychiatric Press Review of Psychiatry, Vol 10. Edited by Tasman A, Goldfinger SM. Washington, DC, American Psychiatric Press, 1991, pp 189–222

Loewenstein RJ, Putnam FW: A comparison study of dissociative symptoms in patients with complex partial seizures, multiple personality disorder, and posttraumatic stress disorder. Dissociation 1(4):17–23, 1988

Loewenstein RJ, Ross DR: Multiple personality disorder and psychoanalysis: an introduction. Psychoanalytic Inquiry 12:3–48, 1992

Loftus EF: Eyewitness Testimony. Cambridge, MA, Harvard University Press, 1979

Loftus EF, Doyle JM: Eyewitness Testimony: Civil and Criminal. New York, Kluwer Law Book Publishers, 1987

Loftus EF, Doyle JM: Eyewitness Testimony: Civil and Criminal. 1990 Cumulative Supplement. New York, Kluwer Law Book Publishers, 1990

Mahler MS, Pine F, Bergman A: The Psychological Birth of the Human Infant. New York, Basic Books, 1975

Malenbaum R, Russell AT: Multiple personality disorder in an 11-year-old boy and his mother. J Am Acad Child Adolesc Psychiatry 26:436–439, 1987

Marmer SS: Psychoanalysis of multiple personality. Int J Psychoanal 61:439–459, 1980

Marmer SS: Multiple personality disorder: a psychoanalytic perspective. Psychiatr Clin North Am 14:677–693, 1991

McMahon PP, Fagan J: Play therapy with children with multiple personality disorder, in Clinical Perspectives on Multiple Personality Disorder. Edited by Kluft RP, Fine CG. Washington, DC, American Psychiatric Press, 1993, pp 253–276

Nathanson DL: Shame and Pride: Affect, Sex, and the Birth of the Self. New York, WW Norton, 1992

Nathanson DL: Contemporary affect theory and dissociation: clinical and theoretical perspectives. Dissociation (in press)

Nemiah JC: Dissociative disorders, in Comprehensive Textbook of Psychiatry/III, 3rd Edition. Edited by Kaplan HI, Freedman A, Sadock BJ. Baltimore, MD, Williams & Wilkins, 1980, pp 1544–1561

Orne MT: The use and misuse of hypnosis in court. Int J Clin Exp Hypn 27:311–341, 1979

Peterson G: Diagnosis of childhood multiple personality disorder. Dissociation 3:3–9, 1990

Peterson G: Children coping with trauma: diagnosis of "dissociation identity disorder." Dissociation 4:152–164, 1991

Pettinati HM (ed): Hypnosis and Memory. New York, Guilford, 1988

Putnam FW: Dissociation as a response to extreme trauma, in Childhood Antecedents of Multiple Personality. Edited by Kluft RP. Washington, DC, American Psychiatric Press, 1985, pp 65–97

Putnam FW: The switch process in multiple personality disorder and other state-change disorders. Dissociation 1(1):24–32, 1988

Putnam FW: Diagnosis and Treatment of Multiple Personality Disorder. New York, Guilford, 1989

Putnam FW: Dissociative disorders in children and adolescents: a developmental perspective. Psychiatr Clin North Am 14:519–532, 1991a

Putnam FW: Dissociative phenomena, in American Psychiatric Press Review of Psychiatry, Vol 10. Edited by Tasman A, Goldfinger SM. Washington, DC, American Psychiatric Press, 1991b, pp 145–160

Putnam FW: Recent research on multiple personality disorder. Psychiatr Clin North Am 14:489–502, 1991c

Putnam FW: Dissociation in the inner city, in Clinical Perspectives on Multiple Personality. Edited by Kluft RP, Fine CG. Washington, DC, American Psychiatric Press, 1993a, pp 179–200

Putnam FW: Dissociative disorders in children: behavioral profiles and problems. Child Abuse Negl 17:39–45, 1993b

Putnam FW, Guroff JJ, Silberman EK, et al: The clinical phenomenology of multiple personality disorder: 100 recent cases. J Clin Psychiatry 47:285–293, 1986

Putnam FW, Zahn T, Post R: Differential autonomic nervous system activity in multiple personality disorder. Psychiatry Res 31:251–260, 1990

Reagor PA, Kasten J, Morelli N: A checklist for screening dissociative disorders in children and adolescents. Dissociation 5:4–20, 1992

Riley RL, Mead J: The development of symptoms of multiple personality disorder in a child of three. Dissociation 1(3):41–46, 1988

Rosenbaum M: The role of the term schizophrenia in the decline of multiple personality. Arch Gen Psychiatry 37:1383–1385, 1980

Ross CA: Multiple Personality Disorder: Diagnosis, Clinical Features, and Treatment. New York, Wiley, 1989

Ross CA: Epidemiology of multiple personality disorder and dissociation. Psychiatr Clin North Am 14:503–518, 1991

Ross CA, Norton GR, Wozney K: Multiple personality disorder: an analysis of 236 cases. Can J Psychiatry 34:413–418, 1989

Ross CA, Miller SD, Reagor P, et al: Structured interview data on 102 cases of multiple personality disorder from four centers. Am J Psychiatry 147:596–601, 1990

Rumelhart DE, McClelland JL: Parallel Distributed Processing: Explorations in the Microstructure of Cognition, Vols I and II. Cambridge, MA, The MIT Press, 1987

Saxe GN, van der Kolk BA, Berkowitz R, et al: Dissociative disorders in psychiatric inpatients. Am J Psychiatry 150:1037–1042, 1993

Schafer R: Retelling a Life. New York, Basic Books, 1992

Schreiber FR: Sybil. Chicago, IL, Henry Regnery, 1973

Schultz R, Braun BG, Kluft RP: Multiple personality disorder: phenomenology of selected variables in comparison to major depression. Dissociation 2:45–51, 1989

Sizemore CC, Pitillo E: I'm Eve. Garden City, NY, Doubleday, 1977

Spanos NP: Hypnosis, nonvolitional responding, and multiple personality: a social psychological perspective. Progress in Experimental Personality Research 14:1–61, 1986

Spanos NP, Weekes JR, Bertrand LD: Multiple personality: a social psychological perspective. J Abnorm Psychol 94:362–376, 1985

Spanos NP, Weekes JR, Menary E, et al: Hypnotic interview and age regression in the elicitation of multiple personality symptoms: a simulation study. Psychiatry 49:298–311, 1986

Spence DP: Narrative Truth and Historical Truth: Meaning and Interpretation in Psychoanalysis. New York, WW Norton, 1982

Spiegel D: Dissociating damage. Am J Clin Hypn 29:123–131, 1986

Spiegel D: Hypnosis, dissociation, and trauma: hidden and covert observers, in Repression and Dissociation: Implications for Personality Theory, Psychopathology, and Health. Edited by Singer J. Chicago, IL, University of Chicago Press, 1990, pp 121–142

Spiegel D: Dissociation and trauma, in American Psychiatric Press Review of Psychiatry, Vol 10. Edited by Tasman A, Goldfinger SM. Washington, DC, American Psychiatric Press, 1991, pp 261–276

Spiegel D, Cardeña E: Disintegrated experience: the dissociative disorders revisited. J Abnorm Psychol 100:366–378, 1991

Stengel E: Further studies on pathological wandering (fugues with the impulse to wander). Journal of Mental Science 89:224–241, 1943

Stern CR: The etiology of multiple personalities. Psychiatr Clin North Am 7:149–159, 1984

Terr LC: Childhood traumas: an outline and overview. Am J Psychiatry 148:10–20, 1991

Tyson GM: Childhood MPD/dissociative identity disorder: applying and extending current diagnostic checklists. Dissociation 5:20–27, 1992

Vincent M, Pickering MR: Multiple personality disorder in childhood. Can J Psychiatry 33:524–529, 1988

Watkins JG, Watkins HH: Theory and practice of ego state therapy: a short-term therapeutic approach, in Short-Term Approaches to Psychotherapy. Edited by Grayson H. New York, Human Sciences Press, 1979, pp 176–220

Weiss M, Sutton PJ, Utecht AJ: Multiple personality in a 10-year-old girl. Journal of the American Academy of Child Psychiatry 24:495–501, 1985

Williams LM: Adult memories of childhood abuse: preliminary findings for a longitudinal study. The APSAC Advisor, Summer 1992, pp 19–21

Yates A: False and mistaken allegations of sexual abuse, in American Psychiatric Press Review of Psychiatry, Vol 10. Edited by Tasman A, Goldfinger SM. Washington, DC, American Psychiatric Press, 1991, pp 320–335

Yates JL, Nasby W: Dissociation, affect, and network models of memory: an integrative proposal. Journal of Traumatic Stress 6:305–326, 1993

Young WC: Psychodynamics and dissociation: all that switches is not split. Dissociation 1(1):33–38, 1988

Chapter 17

Abuse and the Development of Dissociative Symptoms and Dissociative Identity Disorder

Nancy L. Hornstein, M.D.
Frank W. Putnam, M.D.

In the past decade, growing clinical and theoretical understanding of psychiatric syndromes related to trauma, psychiatric sequelae of physical and sexual abuse in childhood, and the phenomenology of dissociative disorders in adults has contributed to an enhanced recognition of the role dissociative symptoms play in the psychiatric presentations of traumatized children.

A number of researchers and clinicians have observed that the psychiatric sequelae of childhood sexual abuse can include a variety of disturbances (Bliss 1984; Bowman et al. 1985; Braun 1990; Briere and Runtz 1988; Conte and Schuerman 1988; Coons et al. 1988, 1990; Dell and Eisenhower 1990; Ensink 1992; Fagan and McMahon 1984; Famularo et al. 1992; Goodwin 1990; Hornstein and Putnam 1992; Hornstein and Tyson 1991; Kluft 1991; Kramer 1990; Loewenstein 1990; McLeer et al. 1992; Putnam 1990; Putnam et al. 1986; Rao et al. 1992; Ross et al. 1990; Schetky 1990; Shengold 1989; Sherkow 1990; Spiegel 1990; Stein et al. 1988; Terr 1990). These disturbances include

- Disturbances in identity (splitting, fragmentation)
- Disturbances in affect regulation (depression, mood swings, feelings isolated/dissociated from experience)

- Autohypnotic phenomena (trances, misperceptions, time distortions, psychogenic numbing)
- Memory disturbances (psychogenic amnesia, fugue)
- Revivification of traumatic experiences (flashbacks, hallucinations)
- Behavioral disturbances (inattention, poor impulse control)
- Self-injury and suicidality

For some of these cases of childhood trauma, the literature supports a theoretical model emphasizing the patient's use of dissociation. This model is seen as contributing to a further understanding of the patient's symptomatic presentation—his or her subjective experience—and is helpful for developing effective therapeutic approaches toward both adults (Bliss 1984; Braun and Sachs 1985; Chu and Dill 1990; Coons et al. 1988; Ensink 1992; Fink and Golinkoff 1990; Greaves 1980; Kluft 1987a, 1987b, 1991; Lovinger 1983; Putnam 1985, 1989, 1991; Putnam et al. 1986; Ross et al. 1989, 1990; Schultz et al. 1989; Spiegel 1991; Steinberg 1991; van der Kolk and Kadish 1987; Venn 1984) and children (Bowman et al. 1985; Briere and Runtz 1988; Dell and Eisenhower 1990; Donovan and McIntyre 1990; Fagan and McMahon 1984; Hornstein and Putnam 1992; Hornstein and Tyson 1991; Kluft 1984, 1985a, 1985b, 1986; Malenbaum and Russell 1987; Peterson 1990; Riley and Mead 1988; Vincent and Pickering 1988; Weiss et al. 1985).

As contemporary clinicians and researchers gathered clinical experience with these patients, they began culling the literature for historical corollaries of their present-day observations. They found that although child and adolescent dissociative disorders were clearly described in 19th- and early-20th-century clinical reports (Bowman 1990; Fine 1988), these disorders, along with their adult counterparts, later disappeared from clinical focus for much of the 20th century. The sudden increase in reports of patients with dissociative disorders caused initial controversy in modern psychiatry, with questions about the validity of the observers' perceptions in light of a century's passing with few reports of these phenomena.

Reasons for this historical dearth of clinical interest in and, correspondingly, reports on these disorders have been postulated (Putnam 1989). Among the limiting factors described was theoretical adherence to a model emphasizing repression rather than dissociation as a means of excluding information from conscious awareness.

Social scientists and historians have eloquently ruptured the myth of "pure scientific truth," showing how we, too, are vulnerable to fashions and trends, and how "what we see" is profoundly influenced by our theoretical constructs. Our own impression is that the advent of powerful antipsychotic medications led researchers to focus eagerly on the biogenetics of psychiatric illness, temporarily stalling investigations into the role a number of environmental influences, such as trauma and child abuse, play in the development of psychiatric disorders (not to mention their impact on "bioendocrinologic" and immune functioning). Similarly, there has been a resurgence of interest in psychiatric sequelae related to stress and trauma as other areas of psychiatric investigation reach limitations in their explanatory power.

Perhaps we now realize that our search for understanding is better served by a recognition that we do not need to choose between our "theoretical truths," which seem to compete with and contradict one another; rather, we can recognize that each of these "truths" attempts to capture and cognitively organize some element of observable reality, facilitating our understanding, investigation, and clinical work. The challenge then becomes searching for ways to integrate conflictual observations and theoretical understandings that we would like to reject, repress, or even dissociate.

In this chapter we present current research on dissociative disorders in childhood and on the relationship between dissociative disorders and childhood experiences of trauma and abuse. We include clinical illustrations of the role dissociation plays in the complex symptomatic presentation in these young patients. One should take note of an important but too often underemphasized point that will enhance understanding of the material to follow: Dissociation used as a defense, although integral (by definition) to the symptomatic presentation of dissociative disorders, is but one aspect of these patients' complex developmental adjustment to their experiences. The real utility of identifying dissociative symptoms lies in the recognition that a variety of disturbances in identity, affect modulation, behavioral control, and attention are present in children with dissociative disorders and are integrally related to past traumatic experiences. Thus, correct identification of dissociative symptoms has a tremendous impact on later diagnostic and treatment formulations in these cases, as well as implications for psychosocial intervention to prevent further trauma.

Dissociation and the Dissociative Disorders

To discuss meaningfully any topic, in this case "dissociation," one should have a clear definition or description of the phenomenon. In DSM-IV (American Psychiatric Association 1994), the "essential feature" of the dissociative disorders is "a disruption in the usually integrated functions of consciousness, memory, identity, or perception of the environment" (p. 477). The dissociative disorders include dissociative amnesia, dissociative fugue, dissociative identity disorder (formerly multiple personality disorder [MPD]), depersonalization disorder, and dissociative disorder not otherwise specified (DDNOS). The most extreme form of these disorders, dissociative identity disorder, involves alterations in consciousness, memory, *and* identity. One immediately runs into problems defining such constructs as "consciousness" and "identity" and differentiating the alterations in memory that represent dissociation versus those present in repression. A truly cogent discussion of this topic would require at the very least an entire chapter, if not an entire book, so interested readers are referred to two excellent discussions of this topic (Ensink 1992; Putnam 1989).

An abbreviated discussion should clarify the nature of the phenomenon being described. One conceptualization of dissociation emphasizes a "disturbance in consciousness." In this conceptualization, persons vary in the frequency and intensity of disturbances in the continuity of conscious awareness. There is a continuum from minor dissociations of everyday life (e.g., driving past your exit on the freeway) to the major forms of psychopathology involving dissociation, such as MPD. All patients with a dissociative disorder suffer from a variety of dissociative experiences such as amnesia, daze states, depersonalization, derealization, and fugue states (Putnam 1989). Putnam (1989) found that experiences of amnesia or time loss (i.e., time gaps) were the single most commonly reported symptom in patients receiving the diagnosis of MPD. Ensink (1992) provided useful criteria for differentiating dissociative "time-gaps" from other disturbances in consciousness. She noted that

> reports can be considered time-gaps only if they meet these criteria:
>
> 1. The person reports to have had no consciousness of the environment or her/his behavior.

2. The person can not describe any focus of attention. This differentiates experience [sic] of time-gaps from daydreaming, being absorbed in thoughts, or events excluded from awareness because the focus of attention was on another event.

3. The person has no conscious or voluntary control of behavior (like speaking, reading, writing), normally guided by consciousness. This criterion differentiates extensive time-gaps from passive behavior such as staring or sitting down and from complex but skilled acts normally not selectively attended such as driving a car.

4. Other people tend not to notice any difference in functioning of the person: This criterion differentiates extensive time-gaps from immediate [sic] evident disturbances in consciousness, such as coma, fainting, pseudo-epileptical attacks or more subtle changes in consciousness, such as staring, daydreaming, sleepwalking, etc.

This "operational description" of the dissociative symptom of "time-gaps" is included because it helps elucidate the kind of dissociative experience that clearly differentiates patients with dissociative disorders from those with other disturbances.

Identification of Dissociative Symptoms in Children

The children whose cases will be described in this section were part of a previously published study delineating the clinical profile of dissociative disorders in childhood and adolescence (Hornstein and Putnam 1992). In that study, behavioral and symptomatic presentations of two independently collected case series of children with dissociative disorders (64 cases)—44 with MPD and 20 with DDNOS—were compared with each other to test the construct validity of these diagnoses in children and adolescents.

The first series, collected by Hornstein (NH), was largely composed of children seen for evaluation and treatment in an inpatient unit at the University of California at Los Angeles. The second series, collected by Putnam (FP), was largely composed of outpatients seen either as part of a longitudinal research project on the psychobiological effects of sexual abuse conducted by the Laboratory of Developmental Psychology, National Institute of Mental Health (NIMH), or in consultation either with other National Institutes of Health research projects or at Children's Hospital National Medical Center, Washington, D.C.

The diagnoses of MPD or DDNOS were made using DSM-III-R criteria (American Psychiatric Association 1987) augmented by NIMH criteria based on clinical interviews of the children and their guardians, protective service caseworkers, teachers, therapists, and, in the case of inpatients, extended observation on the ward. Standard psychological testing was obtained for the majority of children. Parents or guardians also completed the Child Dissociative Checklist (CDC), a 20-item observer report measure under development in the Laboratory of Developmental Psychology, NIMH. The mean ages in these two series (NH and FP) were 9.55 ± 3.36 years and 10.84 ± 3.63 years, respectively. The two series consisted of 14 females and 16 males (NH) and 28 females and 6 males (FP). Twenty-two patients in each series received the diagnosis of MPD, and 8 (NH) and 12 (FP) patients received the diagnosis of DDNOS.

These children reported and/or were observed to have a variety of dissociative symptoms (e.g., trance or daze states, depersonalization, involuntary movements, passive influence experiences) and identity problems (e.g., alter personalities, spontaneous age regression, rapid changes in personality). Also, all of the children with MPD, and many of the children who received diagnoses of DDNOS, had demonstrable time gaps that would have met the "operational criteria" described previously (i.e., DSM).

Gathering interview data on amnestic experiences, or time gaps, in children is more difficult than gathering similar data from adult patients. The reasons for this include that children's development of adult time perception does not occur until late childhood and that the child's report of "not remembering" behavior can represent a "motivated forgetting" of their behavior to escape consequences or uncomfortable feelings. Identifying time gaps often requires interviewing strategies that take into account the child's developmental level supplemented with observational data obtained in a variety of settings that suggest discontinuities in the child's conscious experience.

Anchoring inquiry in the events of the child's daily life is the best approach for obtaining information about dissociative experiences in preadolescents. The interviewer may ask about gaps in the child's memory for common everyday experiences, such as times he is told that he has already eaten lunch when he thinks it is still morning, or times she is confused in class because she last remembered the teacher going over math problems on the board and now the other kids are all working on social studies. The child is asked to recount in his or her own words experiences they have had that are similar to these. The interviewer may also ask about experiences when the child requests to do an activity, only to be told, "But, you already did that."

To differentiate between dissociative experiences and "lying," or "motivated forgetting," it is useful to inquire whether the child ever got thanked for doing a chore he or she did not recall doing. An 11-year-old girl brightened when asked this question, replying "Oh yes, all the time. Just last night my Mom said 'Thanks for doing the dishes.' I thought she was teasing me because I didn't do them, but when I looked in the kitchen they were all done and my Mom was happy. I know she didn't do them either, so I can't guess who did because we were the only people at home." This child was previously assumed to be a chronic liar because of her disavowals of negative behaviors that had been observed by others.

Observing the child for incongruous or unusual behaviors during the interview and inquiring about these, as well as inquiring "What just happened?" when a child stares blankly, seems to change the subject, or seems suddenly confused about a question the interviewer asked, can reveal dissociative time gaps that occur during the interview itself. The child is asked to describe his or her observed behaviors so that possible gaps in recall can be ascertained.

Emotionally laden experiences are often occasions in which time gaps occur for dissociative children. Inquiry into experiences such as explosive outbursts, schoolyard fights, or intense family sessions can lead to discovery of dissociative processes. When a child seems to remember superficially, pressing the child for whether he or she actually remembers the occurrence, or remembers only what he or she was later told happened and has "blank periods" during the experience, can help the child describe his or her subjective experience. Children who do not dissociate revel in this chance to give detailed descriptions of what they feel and experience. Children who dissociate may describe control/influence phenomena or other aspects of their subjective awareness of dissociative experiences. An 8-year-old boy responded to requests for the details of his actual experiences during the frequent fights he was having by saying, "You know, the bad me just takes over. [How?] It kind of comes out my nose, and mouth and ears. [And then what happens?] Well, that bad me, it's got a hold on my arm, and it's running my legs too. I'm saying inside, 'No! Stop!,' but my legs just keep going, and then my arm is striking the other boy and I can't stop it. I also get a voice in my mind telling me to 'mind my own business.'"

When an approach that asks for details of a patient's subjective experiences is adopted, numerous misleading assumptions are avoided, as well as the danger of supplying information about symptoms that the child assents to for the sake of simplicity, which in turn gives the interviewer a false sense of knowing what is going on with the patient. Adopting this approach enhances understanding of children and adults with a wide variety of psychiatric difficulties and proves helpful in therapy as well as diagnosis.

Initially, there is no short-cut for experience in gaining access to this information from children and in distinguishing developmentally typical responses from unusual responses that are deserving of more detailed follow-up. With children who have been abused, gaining this access can be difficult and time consuming, because often a level of trust must be built with them before they will talk openly. In some ways, dogged attempts to understand their unique experiences, rather than to impose preconceived notions on them, enhance the trust-building process.

Observational or historical data that lead the experienced clinician to consider a dissociative disorder in a child's differential diagnosis include behavioral manifestations of dissociative time gaps. These manifestations include disavowal of witnessed behavior; amnesia; fluctuations in apparent attentional ability, concentration, knowledge, or performance; entrance into spontaneous "trance-like" states in which the child is oblivious to external stimuli (often leading to evaluation for seizure activity); and learning or reading difficulties.

In children with MPD, there are "switches" between different "states of consciousness" experienced as alternate personalities ("alters"). As in adults with MPD, alters in children with MPD manifest relatively stable patterns of behavior, affect, gestures, speech patterns (e.g., tone, pitch, complexity of language), manner of relating, and aspects of identity (e.g., gender and role identifications, name, age) that differ from one another.

The first clue that a child in the inpatient series had MPD came when an ordinarily ultrafeminine girl, calling herself Joanne, suddenly became rough and tomboyish, exhibiting differences in mannerism and voice tone during a baseball game. She insisted upon being called "Jo" in this setting. By the time she returned to the unit, she again was feminine, calling herself Joanne. When asked about the boyish "uniform" she still wore, and why she asked to be called "Jo" earlier, she initially stared blankly, and then she said, "Oh, I'm never really there when I have to do that boy stuff." When asked what she meant, she shrugged, later elaborating, "Oh, I think that some boy Jo that talks to me takes my place." She was asked how this works. Her replying, "I don't know really; I don't remember it well," was followed by her entry into a state in which she appeared dazed and then had an abrupt change in manner, saying, "I don't want to talk about this sh_t, Doc; Joanne don't bother anybody; this ain't really none of your concern." Needless to say, this was the first dissociative "change in personality" that was witnessed in her.

In children, these "switches" between alternate personality states are frequently observable as rapid age regression, sudden shifts in demeanor or personality characteristics, or marked variations in ability and skill level. The younger the child, the less elaborated these alters are relative to the often extensive elaboration of separate "personality characteristics" seen in the alters of adult patients with MPD. Kluft (1984, 1985a) has pointed out that children have relatively fewer resources through which their alters can express their separateness. In fact, children may be very subtle and resourceful in the ways their "alters" attempt to assert their separate identities, requiring close attention to detail on the part of the clinician.

A 9-year-old boy reported having three separate selves: a good, a bad, and a regular Larry. In the process of trying to understand whether or not these "selves" represented dissociative phenomena, the therapist asked the patient if it would be possible for others to identify which self he was at a given moment. He smiled slyly and said, "Yes, but they'd have to know how to." When the therapist asked, "What would they have to know," the patient replied, "Well, the good Larry is all in white and is a good Larry fairy, and the bad Larry is in red like a devil; the regular Larry is just plain skin." When the therapist asked the patient which Larry was speaking, the patient, with a broad smile, replied, "Well, I'm the bad Larry, since you're asking about all the problems; I'm wearing a red shirt and you're wearing red too." Further interviewing made clear that this boy's clinical presentation met the criteria for MPD.

Children's alters similarly have less investment in the "separateness" of their identities, and there tend to be less rigid amnestic barriers between the different personality states. Despite these differences, all of the children who received a diagnosis of MPD had symptomatology that met the full DSM-III-R criteria for the diagnosis.

None of the children in the inpatient series came with open revelations about "having different personalities." At most they complained of "hearing voices" or of behaving in ways they "couldn't explain" or could not "remember." They were unanimous in their secretiveness and fear that talking about their subjective experiences of dissociative phenomena made them "weirdos." They were fearful of what other children and adults would think of them if they "knew" about the dissociative phenomena," and in all cases one basis of the treatment alliance was the patients' expectation that their therapist would help them have more control so that these phenomena could be even more "private" than they were initially. There was relatively no observable secondary gain through "dramatics" or attention seeking from the disorder. In several of the children, the dissociative symptomatology was observed for some time before a diagnosis of MPD could be made. For two of the children, the diagnosis became apparent only on subsequent hospitalizations.

There are ongoing questions about the role of development in the elaboration and organization of dissociative experience into alternate personalities during childhood. In these cases, retrospective accounts of the children argued in favor of increasing trust in the therapeutic relationship, rather than developmental variables, playing a role in the eventual diagnosis. It is important to maintain a high index of suspicion in children with extensive abuse histories and the presence of some dissociative symptoms before MPD is ruled out, especially when symptoms suggestive of other disorders do not respond to usual treatment approaches.

Clinical Presentation of Dissociative Disorders in Children

All of the children with dissociative disorders in our sample, whether those with MPD or those with DDNOS, had numerous affective, anxiety, and attention/concentration problems and behavioral and learning difficulties that were suggestive of other diagnoses and that frequently played a role in their presentation for psychiatric treatment (Hornstein and Putnam 1992). Suicidal ideation was also frequently present in both groups, as were auditory hallucinations. The average child had received close to three psychiatric diagnoses before the diagnosis of a dissociative disorder. The most common prior diagnoses were major depression or depressive psychosis (45.3%), posttraumatic stress disorder (29.6%), oppositional defiant disorder (17%), conduct disorder (14%), and attention-deficit hyperactivity disorder (12.5%).

The presenting symptoms of depression, suicidality, auditory hallucinations, and behavioral problems seen in patients in our samples parallel symptom presentations reported for adult dissociative disorder patients (Bliss 1984; Coons et al. 1988; Kluft 1991; Putnam et al. 1986; Ross et al. 1989, 1990; Schultz et al. 1989) and for previously reported individual child cases and small clinical series (Bowman et al. 1985; Dell and Eisenhower 1990; Fagan and McMahon 1984; Hornstein and Tyson 1991; Kluft 1984; Malenbaum and Russell 1987; Peterson 1990; Riley and Mead 1988; Venn 1984; Vincent and Pickering 1988; Weiss et al. 1985). This parallel in symptom presentations supports the hypothesis that there is a syndromal pattern of symptoms shared by children, adolescents, and adults with MPD.

The dissociative symptoms observed in the children in our sample were reviewed earlier in this chapter, so in what follows we concentrate on the manifestations of the most common of the other symptoms with which the children in our sample presented.

Affect

A majority of the children had symptoms such as irritability, affect lability, depression, hopeless feelings, low self-esteem, self-blame, and so forth. Many had suicidal ideation, and some had attempted suicide. The children with MPD who had attempted suicide had made more serious attempts than had the children with DDNOS. In observing all of the children in this sample over time, some had chronic dysphoria, typically unresponsive to antidepressant medication, but most had a very reactive mood. They were up when things were going well, but had an exquisite sensitivity to slights, frustrations, alterations in the mood/attentiveness of caregivers, and extreme rejection sensitivity. Following a perceived injury to their self-esteem, their mood would plummet, suicidal ideation might emerge, and they might remain dysphoric for days.

In some of the children, there were identifiable alternate personalities who were sad, hopeless, and full of self-blame for the abuse they had experienced. Environmental "triggers" that in some way reminded the children of their abuse frequently precipitated a "switch" into one of these alternate personalities.

It was typical of these children that they held themselves responsible for abusive, neglectful behavior of others toward them and for other difficulties they experienced in relationships. Their feelings of hopelessness and worthlessness, although transitory, could nevertheless lead to quite serious suicide attempts such as running out in front of cars or, in the case of one young girl, attempting self-electrocution by inserting a knife in a light socket.

Anxiety and Posttraumatic Symptoms

All of these children could be described as "sick with worry"; often this related to realistic or at worst understandable concerns about the stability of their relationships, the endurance of the regard in which others held them, the well-being of their caregivers, and their own adequacy. Most had all the classic posttraumatic stress disorder symptoms of hypervigilance, hyperstartle, fears, flashbacks, avoidant behaviors, intrusive thoughts related to traumatic experiences, and traumatic nightmares.

The hours before bedtime were associated for many of the children with the emergence of intrusive thoughts about abuse that frequently occurred at home during these hours, and in this time period, often, dissociative symptoms such as spontaneous age regressions, amnesias, and "switches" in personality occurred. For other children, use of the bathroom facilities brought on sudden reactions of terror, flashbacks, or dissociative phenomena as well. An 11-year-old boy with MPD first showed signs of dissociation when he was discovered huddled in a corner of the bathroom, disoriented to location and the identity of a familiar caregiver. Later, it was discovered that this child had been repeatedly and violently sodomized, continued to experience pain with bowel movements related to his injuries, and had severe flashbacks whenever he attempted to use the toilet.

Conduct and Behavioral Problems

Many of these children had explosive temper outbursts, oppositional or disruptive behavior, and problems with aggression and fighting.

Although often accused of lying, they frequently had at least partial amnesia for their explosive, aggressive, and disruptive behaviors. These behaviors were often sudden, unpredicted, and out of keeping with the child's usual demeanor. Absent from these cases was the triad of enuresis, cruelty to animals, and fire setting.

The children's frequent misperceptions of interactions and their perception of threat, as well as rejection hypersensitivity, played a role in producing these problems. Often these abrupt behavior changes were preceded by a "switch" in personality in those children with MPD. The children with DDNOS had similar alterations in perception and cognition during their explosions, although they retained conscious recall and some ability to integrate these behaviors.

These kinds of behavior problems were frequently the reason for referral to inpatient treatment. Usually, when the dissociative aspect of the child's explosions was recognized, the child could be assisted to gain better control of these behaviors. Caregivers who were made aware of the kinds of perceptual and cognitive distortions that occurred when these children entered a state of defensive upset were also more effective at providing appropriate reassurance to these children, preventing the familiar eruption into aggressive behavior.

Sexualized play, inappropriate sexual behavior, compulsive masturbation, and promiscuity are frequently found in children with MPD, and 15% of the children, including some very young children, had perpetrated sexual assaults or abuse on other children. Most of the children were troubled by a variety of issues related to sexuality and their sexual identity. For some, sexual acting out was a way of compulsively reenacting their own experiences; for others it served as a reassurance that "they were normal," allaying fears of homosexuality in boys who were molested by male perpetrators, or attempting to affirm their attractiveness and control over relationships. For a few, there was sexual excitement in the victimization of others. Many of the children were vulnerable to revictimization by adults or other children.

Attention/Concentration and Learning Problems

The high levels of anxiety and posttraumatic symptoms in these children, and their dissociative trance states, amnesias, and so forth, frequently resulted in difficulty attending to lessons and concentrating on schoolwork. In some children there were significant auditory processing difficulties, learning problems, or difficulty with reading. Again, among the children who have been followed through their course of treatment, it has been noted that there has been remarkable amelioration of these difficulties as the internal disruption experienced by these children has been decreased. This is all the more surprising given in some of these children the past history of intrauterine exposure to alcohol and drugs and the past head trauma to which some of these children were exposed. Comorbid diagnoses are of course possible, but even when they are assumed present and treated as such, the better part of clinical wisdom is served through reevaluation as treatment progresses.

Dissociative episodes in childhood may at times be evident as perplexing variations in the child's knowledge, skill level, and performance. Different alters may have differing abilities and knowledge, or may have no conscious recall of having learned something when another alter is present. Marked variations on psychological tests assessing similar abilities may be seen, or there can be enormous variations on the same test on different days as the child experiences "switches" in personality.

The most striking example of this was a young girl who had evidence of nerve deafness on two subsequent but different examinations, but in different ears. Neurologically, her hearing was perfectly intact in both ears, but when she dissociated she had two different alters, each experiencing deafness in opposite ears; the deafness was a conversion symptom related to two separate traumatic incidents.

Hallucinations and Disturbances in Thought Processes

Auditory hallucinations were present in most of the children. In the majority of cases the child heard a voice or voices experienced as arising internally and as having distinctive characteristics such as age, gender, and personal attributes (e.g., "the voice of my father telling me I'm no good"). These are similar to descriptions by adults with MPD of their auditory hallucinations. Other types of hallucinations were also experienced, such as seeing "ghosts," having visual hallucinations of alters, and, less commonly, experiencing a variety of somatic and tactile hallucinations, often representing hallucinated reexperiences of a somatic or sensory element of dissociated traumas.

Frequent dissociation often leads a child to appear confused or disorganized at times. This more commonly occurs in stressful or emotion-laden situations and becomes less noticeable as treatment progresses. Apparent tangentiality can be an attempt on the part of a patient who is experiencing time gaps to "cover up" his or her symptoms. Many of the children in our sample routinely confabulated in attempts to cover up memory gaps, keeping others, as well as themselves, from being aware of them. None of the children had a persistent thought disorder. Dissociative experiences of having thoughts "removed" or "put into" the mind were present in some of the children with MPD, with the presence of the dissociative symptoms representing a statistically nonsignificant trend. These experiences are commonly reported by adult MPD patients, in addition to those with schizophrenic and bipolar illnesses (Fink and Golinkoff 1990; Kluft 1987a; Ross et al. 1990). Passive influence experiences (e.g., thoughts and feelings, complex bodily movements not felt to be voluntarily initiated, automatic writing) are commonly reported in adult MPD patients (Fink and Golinkoff 1990; Kluft 1987a; Ross et al. 1990). The experience of involuntarily initiated body movements distinguished the children with MPD in our sample from the children with DDNOS.

A number of clinical variables assist the clinician to differentiate between childhood dissociation and childhood schizophrenia. Of note, much lower rates of control and influence experiences, as well as much higher rates of delusional phenomena, have been reported in children with schizophrenia compared with children with MPD (Russell et al. 1989).

Overall Clinical Picture

Children with dissociative disorders have a complicated symptomatic picture related to the interaction between their use of dissociative defenses, the symptoms arising from past traumatic experiences, and the problems these children experience in regulating their affect and behavior, as well as establishing an integrated experience of self and others. In the next section, in which the development of these disorders is linked to traumatic experiences in early childhood, we note the symptomatic picture of these children and review the many facets of development that could be affected by experiences of extreme abuse and neglect in early childhood. The syndromal pattern present in children and adults with dissociative disorders clearly reaches beyond the use of dissociation as a defense. A full understanding of these patients requires an ongoing effort to understand the impact of trauma and neglect on psychological development.

Childhood Trauma and Dissociation

In the contemporary literature, profound dissociation is generally regarded as serving a defensive function in instances of overwhelming psychological and/or physical trauma (Ludwig 1983; Putnam 1985; Spiegel 1991). An oversimplified conceptualization of dissociation's defensive function is that traumatic experiences and their attendant affects are, through dissociation, segregated from ordinary conscious awareness, allowing the individual to continue functioning relatively unaffected by a trauma that would ordinarily be overwhelming. It may be a successful adaptation for many years (Archibald and Tuddenham 1965; van der Kolk and Kadish 1987), before the memories and feelings related to the trauma return as intrusive recollections, feeling states, fugues, delusions, depersonalization, and behavioral reenactment (van der Kolk and Kadish 1987).

Theoretical models have been advanced that emphasize the increased vulnerability of young children to overwhelming trauma and their natural tendency to rely on dissociative defenses in traumatic circumstances (Albini and Pease 1989; Braun and Sachs 1985; Donovan and McIntyre 1990; Fink 1988; Kluft 1985a; Lovinger 1983; Putnam 1989; Stern 1984). These theories gain support in part from numerous clinical descriptions of the prevalence of dissociative symptoms in adults and children as an acute and chronic response to traumatic experiences ranging from natural disasters (Terr 1990), painful and invasive medical procedures (K. Rao, N. L. Hornstein, and M. Stuber, unpublished data, 1992), and severe single traumas (Terr 1990; van der Kolk and Kadish 1987) to chronic and extreme sexual abuse (Bliss 1984; Bowman et al. 1985; Braun 1990; Briere and Runtz 1988; Conte and Schuerman 1988; Coons et al. 1988, 1990; Dell and Eisenhower 1990; Ensink 1992; Fagan and McMahon 1984; Famularo et al. 1992; Goodwin 1990; Hornstein and Putnam 1992; Hornstein and Tyson 1991; Kluft 1991; Kramer 1990; Loewenstein 1990; McLeer et al. 1992; Putnam 1990; Putnam et al. 1986; Ross et al. 1990; Schetky 1990; Shengold 1989; Sherkow 1990; Spiegel 1990).

Additional support arises from the documentation that a majority of adult patients with MPD report having experienced severe trauma during early childhood (Bliss 1984; Putnam et al. 1986; Ross et al. 1989, 1991; Schultz et al. 1989). Recent single case and small case series reports of dissociative disorders occurring in childhood and adolescence concur in these high reported rates of trauma and abuse (Bowman et al. 1985; Dell and Eisenhower 1990; Fagan and McMahon 1984; Hornstein and Tyson 1991; Kluft 1984; Malenbaum and Russell 1987; Peterson 1990; Riley and Mead 1988; Venn 1984; Vincent and Pickering 1988; Weiss et al. 1985).

In our series (Hornstein and Putnam 1992), an overwhelming majority of the children had experienced some identifiable trauma. In those with MPD, over 80% had documented histories of sexual abuse, and in 60% of the cases this was combined with physical abuse as well. Documentation of neglect was available in 80% of the cases. The percentages were only slightly lower in those patients with DDNOS. Additionally, over 70% of the children witnessed family violence.

The high percentage of documented abuse, neglect, witnessed violence, and other trauma in this large clinical series of children with dissociative disorders provides validation for the already existing literature linking traumatic, and particularly abusive, experiences in early childhood with the development of dissociative disorders.

Treatment Considerations

Reporting the percentage of children with dissociative disorders who have had abusive experiences and adumbrating their presenting symptoms and difficulties further our diagnostic capabilities and theoretical understanding of these conditions but barely brush the surface of the complexity of these children's life experience or the experience of being their therapist. What the statistics do not capture is the early onset of neglect and abuse; the extent, severity, and chronicity of the trauma; and the chaotic nature of the relationships with caregivers that was a reality for many of these children.

These children's clinical presentations become clearer when grasped as these children's attempt to develop a way to survive in and relate to a world populated by unpredictable significant others. From an early age, these children could not rely on having basic needs for nurturance and protection met; many experienced overt abandonment in addition to combinations of physical, sexual, and emotional abuse, domestic violence, exploitation, and sadism. The extent of the abuse, the age at onset, the degree of neglect, and the presence or absence of some stable adult relationship—all figure prominently in the degree of psychological disturbance each individual child has, as do the child's strengths, intellect, creativity, and disposition.

The child may have initially used dissociative defenses to manage an overwhelming trauma. With repeated trauma and neglect in the early years it is not only the specific traumas that are psychologically overwhelming. Many aspects of relationships become highly conflictual, dependency needs are in and of themselves overwhelming in this milieu, and affects become sources of danger and conflict. The child's internalization of these highly conflictual experiences produces within the child conflicts with aspects of his or her own identity. To integrate these conflicting identifications, with their associated affects and traumatic memories, would cause overwhelming anxiety. As a result, the child develops dissociated selves.

An aspect of the usual MPD child's adaptation is the organization of the dissociated "selves" or alters around the extremes of response that must be readily available to allow continued development in the face of repeated traumas. Fantasy assists the child in coping with overwhelming realities. Often each "alter" comprises a different fantasied representation of the child and the characteristics of the caregiver. With an environment that demands constant vigilance and self-protective responses, there is little time to focus on the development of internal regulation of affect and behavior. An effective adaptation to a world of repeated trauma becomes a handicap when called upon to develop trusting, intimate relationships, to focus on learning in school, or to behave in a predictable, consistent manner. The longing to trust in the caring response of another, to develop true intimacy, is at odds with the terror that past trauma may be repeated at any moment.

The role of the therapist becomes one of assisting the child with MPD to develop an increasing capacity for trust and intimacy, to build new capabilities for managing affect and behavior internally, to develop new defenses that aid in resolution of internal conflicts and past traumatic experiences without being overwhelmed, and, finally, to integrate the dissociated aspects of his or her personality. The prognosis depends on the establishment, first and foremost, of a nontraumatic environment for the child and on the ability of the child and therapist to develop a working therapeutic relationship.

Ensuring a safe, nontraumatic, nurturant environment can be daunting in an age of decreasing social and mental health services. Without ensuring such an environment, however, treatment can be only palliative; an attempt to remove the child's dissociative defenses is destructive and likely to fail. A number of refractory treatments, on closer inspection, have been found to have failed to address this issue adequately. What about the child who has a loving and stable foster family who lives in the heart of gang warfare in the inner city? What about the child whose needs for food, clothing, and shelter are met in an institution that provides little nurturance? The therapist of the child with MPD must be willing to roll up his or her sleeves and attempt to address these issues realistically. Creative partial solutions can be beneficial.

The degree of overall psychiatric disturbance in the child and his or her age, past experiences, strengths, and support systems become factors that influence how able the child is to develop a working therapeutic alliance and how quickly the therapy proceeds. Reports of individual and small case series have been optimistic about the rapidity to which childhood MPD can respond to treatment (Kluft 1985b; Kluft 1986; Riley and Mead 1988; Vincent and Pickering 1988; Weiss et al. 1985). Making the correct diagnosis is helpful for designing interventions that bring about improvements in the child's functioning.

When there was a favorable, nurturant environment and the resources for intensive treatment were available, and the child had considerable resiliency and capacity for developing intimacy despite having a severe dissociative disorder, treatment was indeed rapid and successful. Many cases do not fit this picture, however. In such cases, there has been some success, but the success was measured in small increments over greater lengths of time.

There is a need for further research on treatment outcomes, prognostic indicators, which approaches work best with which children, and so forth. An effective therapeutic approach relies on the bedrock of dynamically oriented therapy, supplemented with an understanding of dissociative processes that allows for limited hypnotic interventions that help the child contain overwhelming affects and memories; occasional cognitive and behavioral interventions; family work; and intervention with the school when necessary. Extensive review of treatment approaches would require an entire chapter, but the skills of most experienced child therapists do nicely with some added supervision by someone familiar with childhood dissociative disorders. There is also a need for longitudinal follow-up of cases of childhood dissociative disorders to ascertain course and outcome, the stability of integration as the child enters adolescence and adulthood, and the child's vulnerability to new traumas.

Summary

In this chapter we have provided a clinical overview of the phenomenology of childhood dissociative disorders, reviewed some of the relevant literature, and introduced some important theoretical considerations. The complexity of these disorders in childhood mirrors the complexity of the impact of trauma, abuse, and neglect on psychological development and functioning.

An exciting aspect of the study of these conditions in childhood is the opportunity for convergence of many different areas of psychiatric research and theoretical inquiry. The importance of recognizing dissociative disorders in children and providing treatment when possible, and of pursuing research in this area on which future treatment will be based, lies in the possibility of significant recovery from a severe form of psychiatric illness in individual cases. There are few pursuits that can be as demanding at times as therapeutic involvement with these children and their families. There are few experiences as rewarding as seeing a dissociative child respond to treatment.

References

Albini TK, Pease TE: Normal and pathological dissociations of early childhood. Dissociation 2:140–150, 1989

American Psychiatric Association: Diagnostic and Statistical Manual of Mental Disorders, 3rd Edition, Revised. Washington, DC, American Psychiatric Association, 1987

American Psychiatric Association: Diagnostic and Statistical Manual of Mental Disorders, 4th Edition. Washington, DC, American Psychiatric Association, 1994

Archibald HC, Tuddenham RD: Persistent stress reaction after combat: a 20-year follow-up. Arch Gen Psychiatry 12:475–481, 1965

Bliss E: A symptom profile of patient with multiple personalities, including MMPI results. J Nerv Ment Dis 174:197–202, 1984

Bowman ES: Adolescent multiple personality disorder in the nineteenth and early twentieth century. Dissociation 3:179–187, 1990

Bowman ES, Blix S, Coons PM: Multiple personality in adolescence: relationship to incestual experiences. J Am Acad Child Adolesc Psychiatry 24:109–114, 1985

Braun BG: Dissociative disorders as sequelae to incest, in Incest-Related Syndromes of Adult Psychopathology. Edited by Kluft RP. Washington, DC, American Psychiatric Press, 1990, pp 227–246

Braun BG, Sachs RG: The development of multiple personality disorder: predisposing, precipitating, and perpetuating factors, in Childhood Antecedents of Multiple Personality. Edited by Kluft RP. Washington, DC, American Psychiatric Press, 1985, pp 37–64

Briere J, Runtz M: Postsexual abuse trauma, in Lasting Effects of Child Sexual Abuse. Edited by Wyatt GE, Powell GJ. Newbury Park, CA, Sage, 1988, pp 85–99

Chu JA, Dill DL: Dissociative symptoms in relation to childhood physical and sexual abuse. Am J Psychiatry 147:887–892, 1990

Conte JR, Schuerman JR: The effects of sexual abuse on children: a multidimensional view, in Lasting Effects of Child Sexual Abuse. Edited by Wyatt GE, Powell GJ. Newbury Park, CA, Sage, 1988, pp 135–154

Coons PM, Bowman ES, Milstein V: Multiple personality disorder: a clinical investigation of 50 cases. J Nerv Ment Dis 176:519–527, 1988

Coons PM, Cole C, Pellow TA, et al: Symptoms of posttraumatic stress and dissociation in women victims of abuse, in Incest-Related Syndromes of Adult Psychopathology. Edited by Kluft RP. Washington, DC, American Psychiatric Press, 1990, pp 205–226

Dell PF, Eisenhower JW: Adolescent multiple personality disorder. J Am Acad Child Adolesc Psychiatry 29:359–366, 1990

Donovan DM, McIntyre D: Healing the Hurt Child. New York, WW Norton, 1990

Ensink BJ: Confusing Realities: A Study on Child Sexual Abuse and Psychiatric Syndromes. Amsterdam, VU (Free University) Press, 1992

Fagan J, McMahon PP: Incipient multiple personality in children: four cases. J Nerv Ment Dis 172:26–36, 1984

Famularo R, Kinscherff R, Fenton T: Psychiatric diagnoses of maltreated children: preliminary findings. J Am Acad Child Adolesc Psychiatry 31:863–867, 1992

Fine CG: The work of Antoine Despine: the first scientific report on the diagnosis and treatment of a child with multiple personality disorder. Am J Clin Hypn 31:33–39, 1988

Fink D: The core self: a developmental perspective on the dissociative disorders. Dissociation 1:43–47, 1988

Fink D, Golinkoff M: Multiple personality disorder, borderline personality disorder and schizophrenia: a comparative study of clinical features. Dissociation 3:127–134, 1990

Goodwin JM: Applying to adult incest victims what we have learned from victimized children, in Incest-Related Syndromes of Adult Psychopathology. Edited by Kluft RP. Washington, DC, American Psychiatric Press, 1990, pp 55–74

Greaves GB: Multiple personality: 165 years after Mary Reynolds. J Nerv Ment Dis 168:557–596, 1980

Hornstein NL, Putnam FW: Clinical phenomenology of child and adolescent dissociative disorders. J Am Acad Child Adolesc Psychiatry 31:1077–1085, 1992

Hornstein NL, Tyson S: Inpatient treatment of children with multiple personality/dissociative disorders and their families. Psychiatr Clin North Am 14:631–638, 1991

Kluft RP: Multiple personality in childhood. Psychiatr Clin North Am 7:121–134, 1984

Kluft RP: Childhood multiple personality disorder: predictors, clinical findings, and treatment results, in Childhood Antecedents of Multiple Personality. Edited by Kluft RP. Washington, DC, American Psychiatric Press, 1985a, pp 167–196

Kluft RP: Hypnotherapy of childhood multiple personality disorder. Am J Clin Hypn 27:201–210, 1985b

Kluft RP: Treating children who have multiple personality disorder, in Treatment of Multiple Personality Disorder. Edited by Braun BG. Washington, DC, American Psychiatric Press, 1986, pp 81–105

Kluft RP: First-rank symptoms as a diagnostic clue to multiple personality disorder. Am J Psychiatry 144:293–298, 1987a

Kluft RP: An update on multiple personality disorder. Hosp Community Psychiatry 144:293–298, 1987b

Kluft RP: Clinical presentations of multiple personality disorder. Psychiatr Clin North Am 14:605–630, 1991

Kramer S: Residues of incest, in Adult Analysis and Childhood Sexual Abuse. Edited by Levine HB. Hillsdale, NJ, Analytic Press, 1990, pp 149–170

Loewenstein RJ: Somatoform disorders in victims of incest and child abuse, in Incest-Related Syndromes of Adult Psychopathology. Edited by Kluft RP. Washington, DC, American Psychiatric Press, 1990, pp 75–111

Lovinger SL: Multiple personality: a theoretical view. Psychotherapy: Theory, Research and Practice 20:425–434, 1983

Ludwig AM: The psychological functions of dissociation. Am J Clin Hypn 26:93–99, 1983

Malenbaum R, Russell AT: Multiple personality disorder in an 11-year-old boy and his mother. J Am Acad Child Adolesc Psychiatry 26:436–439, 1987

McLeer SV, Deblinger E, Henry D, et al: Sexually abused children at high risk for post-traumatic stress disorder. J Am Acad Child Adolesc Psychiatry 31:875–879, 1992

Peterson G: Diagnosis of childhood multiple personality. Dissociation 3:3–9, 1990

Putnam FW: Dissociation as a response to extreme trauma, in Childhood Antecedents of Multiple Personality. Edited by Kluft RP. Washington, DC, American Psychiatric Press, 1985, pp 66–97

Putnam FW: Diagnosis and Treatment of Multiple Personality Disorder. New York, Guilford, 1989

Putnam FW: Disturbances of "self" in victims of childhood sexual abuse, in Incest-Related Syndromes of Adult Psychopathology. Edited by Kluft RP. Washington, DC, American Psychiatric Press, 1990, pp 113–131

Putnam FW: Dissociative disorders in children and adolescents: a developmental perspective. Psychiatr Clin North Am 14:519–531, 1991

Putnam FW, Guroff J, Silberman E, et al: The clinical phenomenology of multiple personality disorder: review of 100 recent cases. J Clin Psychiatry 47:285–293, 1986

Rao K, DiClemente RJ, Ponton LE: Child sexual abuse of Asians compared with other populations. J Am Acad Child Adolesc Psychiatry 31:880–886, 1992

Riley RL, Mead J: The development of symptoms of multiple personality in a child of three. Dissociation 1:41–46, 1988

Ross CA, Norton GR, Wozney K: Multiple personality disorder: an analysis of 236 cases. Can J Psychiatry 34:413–418, 1989

Ross CA, Miller SD, Bjornson L, et al: Structured interview data on 102 cases of multiple personality disorder from four centers. Am J Psychiatry 147:596–601, 1990

Ross CA, Miller SD, Bjornson L, et al: Abuse histories in 102 cases of multiple personality disorder. Can J Psychiatry 36:97–101, 1991

Russell AT, Bott L, Sammons C: The phenomenology of schizophrenia occurring in childhood. J Am Acad Child Adolesc Psychiatry 28:399–407, 1989

Schetky DH: A review of the literature on long-term effects of childhood sexual abuse, in Incest-Related Syndromes of Adult Psychopathology. Edited by Kluft RP. Washington, DC, American Psychiatric Press, 1990, pp 35–54

Schultz R, Braun BG, Kluft RP: Multiple personality disorder: phenomenology of selected variables in comparison to major depression. Dissociation 2:45–51, 1989

Shengold L: Soul Murder. New Haven, CT, Yale University Press, 1989

Sherkow SP: Consequences of childhood sexual abuse on the development of ego structure: a comparison of child and adult cases, in Adult Analysis and Childhood Sexual Abuse. Edited by Levine HB. Hillsdale, NJ, Analytic Press, 1990, pp 93–115

Spiegel D: Trauma, dissociation, and hypnosis, in Incest-Related Syndromes of Adult Psychopathology. Edited by Kluft RP. Washington, DC, American Psychiatric Press, 1990, pp 247–261

Spiegel D: Dissociation and trauma, in American Psychiatric Press Review of Psychiatry, Vol 10. Edited by Tasman A, Goldfinger SM. Washington, DC, American Psychiatric Press, 1991, pp 261–275

Stein JA, Goldring JM, Siegel JM, et al: Long-term psychological sequelae of child sexual abuse: the Los Angeles Epidemiologic Catchment Area Study, in Lasting Effects of Child Sexual Abuse. Edited by Wyatt GE, Powell GJ. Newbury Park, CA, Sage, 1988, pp 135–154

Steinberg M: The spectrum of depersonalization: assessment and treatment, in American Psychiatric Press Review of Psychiatry, Vol 10. Edited by Tasman A, Goldfinger SM. Washington, DC, American Psychiatric Press, 1991, pp 223–247

Stern CR: The etiology of multiple personality. Psychiatr Clin North Am 7:149–160, 1984

Terr L: Too Scared to Cry. New York, Harper & Row, 1990

van der Kolk BA, Kadish W: Amnesia, dissociation, and the return of the repressed, in Psychological Trauma. Edited by van der Kolk BA. Washington, DC, American Psychiatric Press, 1987, pp 173–190

Venn J: Family etiology and remission in a case of psychogenic fugue. Family Proc 23:429–435, 1984

Vincent M, Pickering MR: Multiple personality disorder in childhood. Can J Psychiatry 33:524–529, 1988

Weiss M, Sutton PJ, Utecht AJ: Multiple personality in a 10-year-old girl. J Am Acad Child Adolesc Psychiatry 24:495–501, 1985

Chapter 18

A Developmental-Interactional Model of Child Abuse

Spencer Eth, M.D.

In this chapter I examine the problem of child abuse from a longitudinal perspective by focusing on the pathological interactions and developmental dynamics of parents and children throughout the life cycle. It will be shown that dysfunctional behavioral patterns established in childhood evolve over time to culminate in the transmission of violence from one generation to the next. However, physical abuse is by no means a contemporary issue. For the vast majority of our species' history, children have been considered expendable property; most were not expected to survive the harsh environmental conditions and the ravages of disease, and their births and deaths hardly distracted their elders from the daily struggle for survival.

From antiquity to the early Christian era, parents routinely solved the problem of unwanted offspring by the practice of infanticide. Slowly, Western society began to accept the radical concept that each child is endowed with a soul. Killing came to be replaced by abandonment as the means of dispatching offspring. As the economic and social conditions improved and life expectancy lengthened, adults were able to assume greater responsibility for child care. Unfortunately, by the 18th century parental authority was commonly exercised in the form of intrusive and punitive discipline. Adults routinely flogged and beat their children in an effort to eradicate the devil, civilize the savage, and control the child. With the advent of the Industrial Revolution, youths with small and nimble hands were sent to work in the mines and factories throughout Europe. Only within the last century has society recognized the child's independent needs for safety and kindness (DeMause 1974).

Despite overall progress in the care of children, maltreatment has remained a major social problem and may actually be increasing in frequency. Although many definitions have been proposed, the simplest meaning of *child abuse* is the nonaccidental injury of a minor. Alternatively, *physical abuse* can be defined as the willful infliction upon any child of a cruel and inhuman corporal punishment or injury, while *neglect* is the failure to provide adequate food, clothing, shelter, or medical care. In 1986 over 1.5 million official reports of abuse and neglect were filed with the authorities in the United States, with about 25% arising from abuse alone, about 40% from neglect alone, and the rest from combined abuse and neglect (Kessler and Hyden 1991). Surveys have shown that about 14% of all adults recall having been physically abused as minors, with about 2% having been the victim of severe violence. It has been estimated that between 1.5 and 2.5 million children have been beaten by a parent at some time during childhood (Widom 1989b). The injuries sustained range from minor bruises inflicted by parents as corporal punishment to life-threatening injuries that in as many as several thousand cases each year lead to death.

The Traditional "Ecological" Model of Abuse

In a traditional perspective on child abuse, the phenomenon is viewed as the product of the interaction between three basic factors (Heins 1984): the abuse-prone parent, the abused child, and a stressful situation or incident arising in a violence-accepting culture. Although abusing parents show no consistent psychiatric diagnoses or personality types, they are commonly described as immature, impulsive, and overwhelmed (Wolfe 1985). Abusive parents are more easily annoyed and upset, are more isolated and alone, and are more fearful of external threat and control. They tend to report lower sense of self-esteem and are less able to empathize with their infants. These abuse-prone parents are more likely to respond with anger to distress in their children (Zeanah and Zeanah 1989).

Children are at greatest risk in infancy, with another lesser peak in the early teens, and they may be of either sex (Janson et al. 1982). Young children may be especially susceptible to abuse because of their greater need for care and attention, because they are less able to defend themselves or evade punishment, and because of their relative physical fragility (Friedrich and Einbender 1983). In infancy, low birth weight, prematurity, and congenital defects, especially if these conditions result in neonatal hospitalization, are child-specific risk factors (White et al. 1987). The concept of "fetal abuse" may be applicable to those congenital conditions that are the product of intrauterine neglect of proper prenatal nutritional and medical care, exposure to alcohol and illicit drugs, and infection with sexually transmitted diseases (Landwirth 1987). Undoubtedly for some of these gestational casualties, a pattern of abuse may already have been established at birth. As the child grows older, the continued presence of a mental or physical handicap increases the likelihood of maltreatment (Augoustinos 1987).

It may be hypothesized that early separations during the immediate postpartum period can result in difficulties in establishing the normal mother–infant bond. This initial failure in appropriate attachment may then lead to disorders of mothering, which could include abuse and neglect (Egeland and Vaughn 1981). Within the first 6 months of life, clusters of temperamental characteristics become recognizable. The infant with a "difficult" temperament shows irregular sleep and feeding schedules; slow acceptance of new foods; prolonged adjustment periods to new routines, people, or situations; and relatively frequent periods of loud crying. This pattern presents a problem in management for most mothers, especially those who are inexperienced or impatient. Commonly, a parent will respond to the demands of such a child by becoming confused, hostile, and inconsistent, if not abusive. Unfortunately, this potential for a poor fit between parent and infant can increase the child's difficulty and the parent's frustration (Chess and Thomas 1984).

In this ecological model, parental unemployment, poverty, single status, and young age are predisposing psychosocial stressors (Zuravin 1989). The addition of alcohol or illicit drugs to a tense family environment may serve as the precipitant for aggression, especially in a parent with personality traits of impulsivity, anger, and suspiciousness. At least half of abused children are subject to repeated abuse, as physical force tends to reflect a general pattern of child raising, rather than represent an isolated incident (Friedrich and Einbender 1983).

The value of this traditional model is that it conveys a degree of complexity to the problem of abuse. Intrapsychic, interpersonal, and social forces are together seen as salient in the process of physical abuse. The limitation of this model is that it is not designed to explain the evolving impact of abuse on parent-child interactions or on the child's psychological development. Such longitudinal issues may not be seen as necessary for a cross-sectional analysis of the determinants of an episode of abuse. However, these issues are crucial for the child psychiatrist who seeks to understand and interrupt the cycle of intra-familial violence afflicting our civilization.

The Developmental–Interactional Model of Abuse

Infancy and Early Childhood

Parental maltreatment of an infant can assume one of two general forms: either the very young child can be neglected, or he or she can be directly harmed. In the prototypical case of neglect, the infant is ignored or even abandoned for long periods of time. The predicament of neglect creates for the child a situation of maternal deprivation. Prolonged deprivation can result in the physical syndrome of non-organic failure to thrive (or deprivational dwarfism), with all of its attendant risks of morbidity and mortality.

The psychological consequences of maternal deprivation are also legion, with prominent displays of passivity, withdrawal, and developmental delays. The progression of response to an acute loss of parental care in an infant or young child between the ages of 6 months and 4 years has been characterized as "protest, despair, and detachment." After separation the child will immediately become distressed and start crying in an effort to summon his or her mother. If unsuccessful in that endeavor, the child grows increasingly apathetic and dysphoric. Finally, the child seems to relinquish hope and to lose interest in his or her surroundings (Bowlby et al. 1952). An ongoing lack of stimulation contributes to developmental retardation in language and in social and motor function (Rutter 1979). A similar constellation of symptoms was termed "anaclitic depression," in recognition of the comparability of the detached state of sadness, loss of appetite, and sleep disturbance to adult depressive disorder (Spitz and Wolf 1946).

The psychological picture of the physically abused infant and young child differs from that of the infant or young child who experiences maternal deprivation. The challenge for the abused child is not to overcome a lack of stimulation, but to contend with an overload of intrusive, painful, and unpredictable sensations. The infant responds to physical punishment by becoming increasingly irritable, whiny, fussy, colicky, angry, and irregular in biological rhythms. If the child is temperamentally difficult, these traits will markedly intensify. In effect, the young child already predisposed to unsoothable emotionality becomes a further irritant to an already stressed and aggression-prone parent. The consequence of this poor fit between parent and child is a vicious cycle of symptomatic child behavior eliciting an aggravating behavioral response from the parent. This situation thus presents the interactional dilemma of victim-precipitated violence occurring in the nursery within the first few months of life.

Attachment may be defined as a biologically based bond with a caregiver that affords the infant and young child protection, especially during the periods of stress in early childhood (Alexander 1992). Only by using the parent as a secure base can the child begin to effectively explore the environment. Further, on the basis of early experiences with the parent, the child develops expectations about relationships and the receiving and giving of care and love. Children may seek to recreate experiences congruent with their own relationship history, such that children of mothers who are hostile and punitive are likely to become angry and noncompliant. This adaptation to a not-good-enough mother may transform an otherwise temperamentally easy child into one who appears quite difficult. In this instance the young child may internalize his or her mother's aggression and learn both the provocative and the punitive roles (Zeanah and Zeanah 1989).

Abused infants may also be expected to develop insecure attachment behavior, with its typical features of avoidance, resistance, and disorganization. This pattern is distinguished from secure attachment, which has been found to predict greater competence with peers, ego resiliency, resourcefulness, empathy, and popularity in later childhood (Alexander 1992). Tragically, the abused child, who is most in need of reparative abilities, is most likely to be deficient in those valuable coping skills because of the abuse. In infancy such children may show accentuated separation and stranger anxiety. It is indeed tragic that a maltreated toddler may cling steadfastly to his or her abusive mother while actively avoiding other, potentially nurturing adults. In later years the same child as an adolescent may become entrenched in violent gangs, to the exclusion of other available, supportive youth groups.

Thus it can been seen that physical abuse disrupts and distorts the crucial tasks of infancy and toddlerhood as they relate to social relations and self identity: the establishment of secure, consistent, and trusting relationships with parent figures; the development of a basic sense of self; and the maturation of autonomous ego functions.

Middle and Later Childhood

By midchildhood the chronically abused youngster can present with deficits in physical, neurological, intellectual, behavioral, and emotional development (Toro 1982). Physical maldevelopment may be related to the lingering presence of birth defects, to the deleterious effects of nonorganic failure to thrive, and to the bodily stigmata of physical abuse. The neurological impairment may be constitutional or may have arisen as a result of injury-associated brain damage. Cognitive deficits may then be attributable to the neurological impairment, or the intellectual delays may be evident even in the absence of neurological findings (Augoustinos 1987). As a consequence of these deficits, these children experience academic hardships in school and may have diagnosable learning disabilities.

Terr (1991) has conceptualized childhood trauma as falling into two basic types: type I trauma, which follows from unanticipated single events, and type II trauma, which arises from long-standing or repeated exposure to extreme external events. The traumatic syndrome associated with chronic child abuse epitomizes the type II category. Children who have endured multiple beatings may be expected to exhibit both the common features of childhood trauma and those features characteristic of type II syndromes. Abused children contend with recurrent, intrusive visual memories of their mistreatment, especially when stimulated by reminders of their ordeal. Play and behavioral reenactments are often seen, frequently occurring as aggressive outbursts. Abused children may complain of trauma-specific fears that relate to some aspect of the abusive situation. As with all traumatized youngsters, abused children develop a new set of pessimistic attitudes about their personal future.

Abused children may employ the defenses of denial and psychic numbing (Terr 1991). They may avoid talking about themselves or their mistreatment in an effort to look normal. In extreme cases these children may "forget" their many episodes of abuse or even significant portions of their childhood. It has been argued that dysfunctional coping with interpersonal problems is characterized by daydreaming, fantasizing, and attempting to avoid or escape the problem (Compas 1987). Some repeatedly brutalized children learn the benefits of spontaneous self-hypnosis, depersonalization, and dissociation as a method of escaping unbearable experiences. Rarely, these dissociation-prone children elaborate over time imaginary alter egos that become the forerunners of multiple personality disorder.

Emotional disturbances found in abused children include constricted affect akin to psychic numbing, unremitting sadness, and profound rage. When observed at free play, abused children exhibit an utter lack of enthusiasm, imagination, and initiative, which may be an expression of their flat, anxious affect (Goodwin 1988). The term "frozen watchfulness" has been applied to the child's characteristic appearance (Ounsted et al. 1974). Terr (1991) has observed that the rage of the repeatedly abused child cannot safely be underestimated. The expression of that anger as aggressive reenactment and self-injurious behavior can assume life-threatening proportions even in the school-age child. Perhaps as many as 40% of abused children engage in direct forms of self-destructive behavior, self-mutilation, and accidental self-harm (Green 1978).

Compared with their nonabused counterparts, physically abused children demonstrate a greater number and frequency of behavior problems, including defiant noncompliance, tantrums, dysfunctional social skills, and poor school adjustment (Lamphear 1985). The combination of academic difficulties and disciplinary problems greatly increases the probability of school failure and suspension or expulsion, which tends to confirm the child's poor self-concept and sense of personal ineffectiveness. In particular, the abused child displays an overabundance of aggression directed toward peers and adults. In one well-designed study, 36% of children defined as harmed by physical abuse in early childhood received markedly elevated teacher-rated aggression scores, compared with just 13% of other children in a sample controlled for demographic and biological variables (Dodge et al. 1990).

It is easy to imagine how such an angry, distrustful, and hopeless child could engage in behavior that perpetuates a cycle of violence. As a "problem child" in school, this youngster will be a popular target for teasing and scapegoating by his or her schoolmates. The abused child who then reacts with stubborn, hostile, and provocative behavior toward his or her peers unwittingly encourages further social scorn. If the child also has poor impulse control and an angry temper, fighting becomes inevitable. After several such encounters, the youngster will have, for all intents and purposes, assumed the "bad child role" of being unmanageable and incorrigible. At home the abused child enmeshed in the "bad child role" has come to feel truly expendable, validating the parents' wish to dispose of the unwanted burden.

So-called problem children, who are perceived as unappealing, stubborn troublemakers, find themselves facing corporal punishment at school and physical attacks by peers. Understanding this cycle of victim-precipitated violence is prerequisite to an effective intervention strategy. Many abused children respond to their years of deviant environmental experiences with chronic cognitive biases in processing stimuli, with deficits in attending to and encoding relevant social cues, and with errors in overattributing hostile intent to others, producing ever greater hypervigilance and paranoid distortions. Further, these children access predominantly aggressive, as opposed to competent, responses from behavioral repertoires stored in memory, and then perceive the outcome of aggression as interpersonally and instrumentally positive. These processing patterns become self-reinforcing, contributing to a conspicuous display of aggression in childhood (Dodge et al. 1990).

To many it seems that the abused child has "learned" to be a victim from years of abuse at home, that he or she has come to confuse love with aggression in a masochistic desire for attention and affection. However, informed teachers and school personnel make every effort to apply positive reinforcers to modify the child's behavior. Unfortunately, these techniques often defy the principles of learning theory by failing to reduce the undesirable activities or to encourage more appropriate behavior in the abused child. Perhaps, as a manifestation of a profound confusion of love with aggression, the abused child desperately seeks physical contact in any form and at any cost. By so doing, the child is exhibiting a repetition compulsion of being beaten and mistreated with the perverse gratification of a need for love at the expense of pain. Or, for some children, the process of identification with the aggressor operates to replace the child's own feelings of humiliation and self-loathing with the fantasy of power and omnipotence invested in the abusive parent. For other children their violent reenactments serve as a means of destroying their identity as victim.

In another sense the pattern of allowing oneself endlessly to suffer abuse suggests that the child is attempting to convert the helpless experience of being a victim into the powerful role of eliciting the mistreatment. Anna Freud (1936/1966), in another context, has described this as the defense mechanism of turning passive into active. By provoking attack, the child no longer feels defenseless in an unpredictable world where at any moment he or she may be subject to assault. The belief that one has the ability to influence aversive events in a predictable fashion, even at the expense of accepting responsibility for the event, may be associated with good coping (Thompson 1981). Other work has found that the vast majority of children described their usual response to stressful episodes as primarily involving attempts to modify or influence the external circumstances, rather than relinquishing control (Band and Weisz 1988).

The immediate price the abused child must pay for feeling in control, and thereby decreasing the intolerable level of psychological anxiety, is the physical discomfort of being repeatedly hurt. This maladaptive, unconscious coping strategy successfully relieves anxiety by placing the child in the position of bearing the brunt of victim-precipitated violence. Over time, this coping strategy lacks flexibility to the demands of new situations and becomes increasingly maladaptive. Its repercussions in the context of individual play psychotherapy will be explored at the end of this section.

The chronically abused child has, in fact, endured "soul murder" (Shengold 1989). As Shengold (1989) explains, "Soul, or psychic, murder involves trauma imposed from the world outside the mind that is so overwhelming that the mental apparatus is flooded with feeling. The terrifying too-muchness requires massive and mind distorting defensive operations for the child to continue to think and feel and live" (p. 24). By analogy the abused child lives the life of a hostage held by sadistic terrorists who may at any moment beat, torture, or destroy their helpless captive. Former hostage Brian Keenan (1992) has portrayed his existence at the mercy of an extremist faction in Lebanon. Although subjected to innumerable indignities, Keenan suffered his 4-year ordeal as an adult. How much worse it must be to endure the same mistreatment during one's childhood.

The intrapsychic response to chronic abuse constitutes an area of intensive investigation and speculation. Repeated assaults can function as a stressor, causing a posttraumatic stress disorder (PTSD). This affliction in turn can result in ego regression and disorganization, narcissistic injury, and dysphoria that activate primitive defense mechanisms and disrupt reality testing (Green 1985). Besides using the defense of turning passive into active, the abused child may resort to splitting, projection, and denial as ways to modulate traumatic overstimulation and accompanying painful affects. The child may also adopt a style of frozen watchfulness and suspiciousness as a means to guard against parental attack. Although such defensive operations can suppress the awareness of parental sadism and the fear of annihilation, they may become rigidly reproduced in the face of a variety of new challenges (Pine 1986). Over time these pathological defensive structures could become the forerunners of major forms of psychopathology, as the child resorts to desperate measures to preserve an illusion of object constancy (Vaillant 1992).

Although most of the scientific literature contains reports drawn from clinical samples of children in inpatient or outpatient psychiatric treatment, with or without matched controls, there is a strong suggestion that physically abused children present with certain constellations of psychiatric symptoms. For example, one recent study examined 96 children ages 5 to 10 years, 61 of whom had been maltreated. The investigators found an increased incidence of attention-deficit/hyperactivity disorder, oppositional disorder, and PTSD (Famularo et al. 1992). Approaching the issue of abuse from the end point of a specific diagnosis, another recent team noted that of all children receiving the clinical diagnosis of borderline personality disorder, 39.6% had a history of abuse compared with only 9% of child patients with other conditions (Goldman et al. 1992).

Abused children are commonly brought for psychotherapy in an effort to control behavioral and emotional symptoms. The behavioral difficulty may assume the form of an attention-deficit, conduct, or oppositional-defiant disorder, which are grouped together in DSM-IV (American Psychiatric Association 1994) under the rubric of attention-deficit and disruptive behavior disorders. In the emotional realm, such disturbances as affective instability, anxiety, fears, depression, and relationship impairments may be evident. Often these symptoms are described as "acting out," insofar as they represent the direct expression through action of an unconscious wish or conflict in order to avoid awareness of either the idea or the affect that accompanies it (Vaillant 1992).

The primary goal of therapy for any abused child is protection from further maltreatment. It is beyond the scope of this chapter to explore the myriad issues that arise in a comprehensive plan to provide a safe and nurturing environment for the victimized child. Unquestionably, the psychotherapist has a central role in what frequently becomes a complex, multiagency effort. Meanwhile, within the confines of the therapeutic relationship, important transference themes will be negotiated. Initially in the playroom the child may appear amazed and overjoyed by an abundance of toys and the undivided attention of the therapist. The child revels in a newly recognized ability to capture and incorporate a good parent, thereby addressing long unmet dependency and protection needs.

The evocation of the child's capacity for object hunger and idealization signals the inevitable crash of disappointment. No therapist can gratify a child who feels so desperately empty. The patient responds with mounting disillusionment and rage as the image of the therapist is transformed from savior into tormentor. The reality of the unstructured setting and benign therapist is now of little comfort. Rather, under these circumstances the child responds in characteristic ways. First, the child becomes filled with anxiety and exhibits increasingly disorganized behavior in an atmosphere of almost palpable tension. Soon the child resorts to provocation as a tried and tested method to counteract feelings of helplessness and the threat of attack by the "bad" therapist. The psychotherapist's reliance on nonpunitive measures to control the child's destructive impulses initially fails to contain the child's fear of retaliation. The challenge for the therapist will be to maintain the neutral frame and support the child in the face of the terror of uncontrolled fury. Eventually, the child must contend with his or her own profound sense of defective emptiness and be capable of integrating the positive essence of the therapeutic alliance.

The process of treatment is not a linear working through of these developmental conflicts. New problems arise continuously, and old difficulties must be revisited. The period of provocation and limit testing around the reenactment of abusive interactions may seem interminable. Yet, over time the child's traumatic fixation should begin to give way with mastery of the memories of overwhelming helplessness and abandonment. Then commences the slow, painstaking work of fortifying the child's frustration tolerance, impulse control, interpersonal relations, and self-esteem. With corresponding progress in school performance and reduction in scapegoating, the child's life will mirror the gains seen in the session. If the child's family can provide security and stability, these positive changes can be consolidated and expanded.

Adolescence

In the half century following the introduction of the concept of adolescence, the conventional wisdom held that puberty heralded
a highly stressful epoch in the human life span (Offer and Schonert-
Reichl 1992). Normal adolescence was widely perceived as a tumultuous time of increased emotionality and symptomatology. Two
corollaries to this belief were the propositions that adolescents who
appear well adjusted may actually be quite disturbed, and the converse, that teenagers manifesting psychopathology are suffering from
adolescence and not mental illness. In fact, studies of nonclinical
populations have shown that a tumultuous course of adolescence is
the least common of three growth patterns. For the majority of youth,
independence is gradually achieved with generally manageable areas
of conflict (Offer et al. 1989). Most adolescents report self-satisfac-
tion and are without evidence of significant psychopathology
(Kashani et al. 1987). This heartening picture contrasts strikingly
with the lives of abused adolescents, who are symptomatic and "don't
grow out of it" (Masterson 1967).

Because the potential consequences of having been abused are
different for each sex, males and females will here be considered separately. Teenage boys with a history of physical abuse are at increased
risk for a variety of negative outcomes. Having had both academic and
disciplinary problems at school, these youngsters are likely to have
been suspended or expelled during their high school careers. As their
peers approach graduation, many of those abused boys who have not
already been expelled from school choose to leave on their own. Without an educationally supportive home, the constant challenge of progressing through grade levels in the face of learning and behavioral
disabilities often proves overwhelming. Under these circumstances
the option of leaving school to search for employment seems reasonable. Sadly, good jobs for high school dropouts even in robust economic times are scarce, and in the current recession virtually
nonexistent. Now the abused adolescent is confronted with the humiliation of failure in school and failure in the job market.

It is easy to imagine the multiple reasons that maltreated teenagers are at risk for substance abuse (Van Hasselt et al. 1992). Alcohol
and marijuana are, in the short term, effective methods to dull the
reality of life's disappointments, while the opiates are potent analge-
sics for the relief of the physical pain of abuse. Other drugs, such as

amphetamines and cocaine, appear as desirable ways to escape into a euphoric state, albeit only temporarily. A minority of drug abuse in adolescents may represent an available means of self-medicating clinical depression. What may begin as experimentation and occasional use can escalate into a pattern of daily use with associated tolerance and dependence, and in some instances culminate in an intentional or accidental overdose.

What in earlier childhood could be dismissed as mischief escalates in adolescence into frank delinquency. Retrospective studies have found that from 9% to 29% of all delinquents questioned report having been maltreated by their parents, while prospective studies of abused or neglected children find that 10% to 17% become delinquent (Widom 1989a). Further, it appears that among delinquents, the variable of abuse and neglect is correlated with a younger age at first offense, with a larger mean number of offenses, and with more violent forms of criminal behavior (Widom 1989a). For example, juveniles who were convicted of murder are twice as likely to have a history of physical abuse as delinquents who did not commit violent offenses (Lewis et al. 1988). This most severe form of aggressive violence has been seen as reflecting an early loss of object relatedness with consequent dehumanization and loss of control over aggressive impulses (Nichtern 1982). Formerly abused and neglected children tend to persist in their illegal activities, as evidenced by higher rates of arrests as adults (Widom 1989a).

Abused and neglected teenagers may associate with a juvenile gang that seems to offer a substitute "family." That membership in a group of violent, drug-abusing truants appears so desirable is testimony to the disaffection and alienation that these adolescents experience in their own homes. Aggressive tendencies are actualized in the frequent intergang skirmishes and criminal exploits. The dangers of this deviant lifestyle are protean. Youth gang members are frequently killed or maimed in car accidents or in confrontations with rival gangs or the police. In either case, the abused child's life is terminated in a violent, unnecessary death.

Maltreated adolescent girls also find themselves in serious difficulty in school for the same reasons as do their male counterparts. They too are prone to academic failure, disruptive behavior in class, and truancy, leading to expulsion or voluntary abandonment of their educational career. Similarly, teenage girls engage in substance abuse in an effort to escape by getting "high." Although delinquency is an increasingly common problem in females, a pattern of aggressive criminality is relatively rare in this sex.

Adolescent girls seem at greater risk than boys for turning anger against the self (Freud 1936/1966). Overt self-destructive behavior is increasing in prevalence during the last decade, with the reported female-to-male ratio for suicide attempts by teenagers varying from between 3:1 and 9:1 (Hawton 1986). It should be noted that the far rarer act of completed suicide remains more common in males. The adolescent's acting out of parental hostility directed against the child may be an important dynamic in suicidal behavior (Green 1985). Eating disorders, a group of psychiatric conditions occurring predominantly in females, appears also to be increasing dramatically among all social classes and ethnic groups in the United States (Pate et al. 1992). Disturbed parent–child relations and maltreatment may serve as a predisposing factor in this form or self-destructive behavior.

Encountered in most large cities is the growing population of teenage runaways. Both male and female runaways propelled by a desire to escape from a physically abusive home are especially likely to report symptomatology consistent with PTSD (McCormack et al. 1988). A principal reaction of traumatized adolescents is a premature closure of identity formation and a desperate flight into adulthood (Eth and Pynoos 1985). Experiencing a false sense of readiness to function independently and motivated by intense feelings of rage, shame, and betrayal, the teenager will begin an anxious search for new horizons. Tragically, adolescents traumatized by abuse are not well equipped to survive on the streets, plagued as they are by feelings of helplessness, anxiety, and even dissociation (McCormack et al. 1988).

Promiscuity, with its attendant risk of contracting a sexually transmitted disease, is an issue for both male and female adolescent victims of physical abuse. The desire for love and comfort, coupled with the newly aroused sexual drive, leads to frequent, though ultimately unsatisfactory, liaisons. Because of the careless, frequently self-destructive lifestyle adopted by many of these individuals, these affairs present the likelihood of pregnancy. Some of the women in this situation will avail themselves of the opportunity for legal abortion. However, many will choose to carry their pregnancies to term.

Imagine the sentiments of an abused adolescent who has become pregnant. She could well be a single, drug-using high school dropout with a casual attitude about nutrition and personal care. The adolescent, after finding herself pregnant, revels in the fantasy that her baby will offer her all of the love and kindness that she has failed to receive from everyone else in her life. The expectation that her child can gratify her unmet dependency needs establishes a role reversal that dooms her to eventual disappointment. In fact, her infant may be born small for gestational age, premature, or may even be born with birth defects as a result of inadequate prenatal care and possible fetal abuse.

The new mother, herself still a child, experiences overwhelming frustration over her baby's inability to deliver to her the love and attention she expects. This is a young woman who, while feeling so deprived and empty herself, is incapable of deriving the passive pleasure of motherhood. Having at one time been fantasized as representing the wished-for savior, the child now is invested with the hatred and rage displaced from the woman's feelings for her parents, boyfriends, and other persons who have abused and exploited her. Utilizing the primitive defenses of projection, splitting, projective identification, and identification with the aggressor, the young mother rejects and mistreats her own child. Should her child respond with irritability, this abused adolescent will retaliate, setting into motion another intergenerational cycle of violence and victimization.

Discussion

In this chapter I have discussed the problem of child abuse in the context of a developmental-interactional schema. By following the path of physical abuse from infancy through adolescence, an emergent pattern is traced that culminates in the transmission of violence from an abused mother or father to her or his child. The best estimate of the rate of intergenerational transmission of abuse appears to be about 30%, such that about one-third of all individuals who were abused or neglected will subject their offspring to one of these forms of maltreatment (Kaufman and Zigler 1987). This ratio is approximately six times greater than the base rate of abuse in our population.

The phenomenon of victim-precipitated violence commences in infancy, as the young child responds to maltreatment in ways that elicit maltreatment from an abuse-prone parent. Later, during school age, the child engages in behavior that provokes outrage and attack in a maladaptive effort to overcome feelings of helplessness. In adolescence, accident-prone and aggressive behavior carries the risk of motor vehicle injuries and fatal encounters with peers or police. The cycle of violence, from innocent victim to induced victim to perpetrator, is frighteningly real and a pervasive threat to our survival as a functioning society. People will select and shape their environments by their own behavior to conform with their intrapsychic needs. However, there remains the possibility of therapeutic intervention designed to detoxify the acting out of these abusive dynamics.

An idiographic model is suggested when a wide range of individual factors must be considered in order to appreciate the significance of a disease entity (Hyman et al. 1988). In this chapter I have addressed a process of fairly continuous physical abuse. However, abuse may begin and end at any age, with corresponding impact on developmental phase–specific issues (Eth and Pynoos 1985). In a later developmental phase the child will reconstruct the trauma according to the vicissitudes of contemporaneous conflicts and relationships (Goodwin 1988). By adulthood, the individual can present in psychotherapy with a potentially bewildering array of intrusive, dysphoric memories of abuse, transformed recollections of childhood trauma from subsequent years, and a distorted and disturbed capacity for human relatedness mirrored in the transference.

Lewis (1992) reminds us that the psychophysiological concomitants of maltreatment are highly variable. Disadvantaged children may have confronted any or all of the following: noxious intrauterine factors, including viral, hormonal, and toxic agents; pathogenic environmental conditions, such as overheating, crowding, isolation, and exposure to aggressive adults; and organism-specific responses to stress, which can affect crucial hormonal and neurotransmitter regulation. Often siblings raised in the identical home by the same parents will be subjected to vastly different child-rearing practices. In such instances abuse will be a "nonshared" environmental influence with differential impact across the sibship.

The explication of one paradigmatic life path traversed by an abused child is not intended to imply that other life trajectories are not possible. Early abusive trauma and adult functioning have no straightforward relationship; there are a wide variety of outcomes arising from similar circumstances (Martin and Elmer 1992). Further, even the end product of abuse described herein is likely to be the result of a multiplicity of other influences as well.

There are genetic factors that contribute to channeling one's life potential. However, as Rutter (1991) reminds us, it is a misconception to believe that genes impose a strict limit on outcome. He notes that children born to disadvantaged parents had significantly higher IQs when adopted into a privileged home. These findings suggest that a favorable rearing environment exerts a substantial effect on the developing organism. By implication, however, we should also assume that unfavorable environmental conditions will have significant deleterious effects, as is the case with child abuse.

Beyond the scope of this chapter, but of great salience to overall life adjustment, are the role and significance of protective factors (Widom 1989b). These hereditary, constitutional, and environmental influences can operate to neutralize negative experiences, such as physical abuse. In favorable cases a child may be insulated from the psychopathological consequences of parental maltreatment through a subtle interplay of these protective factors. A hypothetical model of stress invulnerability is appealing in its power to explain why certain children endure brutal abuse without succumbing to its effects. Unfortunately, methodological obstacles have prevented extensive study of stress invulnerability, and its relevance to abuse and trauma is largely speculative (Eth 1990).

Conclusions

Historians have long overlooked the scourge of abuse that was so common throughout the ages. Physicians, as well, apparently did not recognize, study, or comment upon this widespread pattern of the intentional physical injury of children. It has been only within the last 30 years, since the publication of Kempe and colleagues' (1962) landmark article on the battered child syndrome, that this condition has been clearly described in the medical literature. No doubt several factors have contributed to the centuries-old denial by doctors of this major public health calamity. Our professional history suggests that we must be cautious to guard against the tendency to romanticize and idealize the history of childhood to the exclusion of the indignities and suffering of children. As psychotherapists we observe that individuals frequently repress painful memories of their personal past. Collectively we may be employing a similar defense in or neglect of this important area of concern. However, our psychiatric understanding of the phenomenon of child abuse has been advancing in concert with society's greater devotion to the economic and social needs of our children. With focused resolve by both the medical and child welfare communities, the intergenerational transmission of violence can be, at the very least, attenuated. The survival of our species demands no less.

References

Alexander PC: Application of attachment theory to the study of sexual abuse. J Consult Clin Psychol 60:185–195, 1992

American Psychiatric Association: Diagnostic and Statistical Manual of Mental Disorders, 4th Edition. Washington, DC, American Psychiatric Association, 1994

Augoustinos M: Developmental effects of child abuse: recent findings. Child Abuse Negl 11:15–27, 1987

Band EB, Weisz JR: How to feel better when it feels bad: children's perspectives on coping with everyday stress. Developmental Psychology 24:247–253, 1988

Bowlby J, Robertson J, Rosenbluth D: A two-year-old goes to hospital. Psychoanal Study Child 7:82–94, 1952

Chess S, Thomas A: Origins and Evolution of Behavior Disorders: From Infancy to Early Adult Life. New York, Brunner/Mazel, 1984

Compas BE: Coping with stress during childhood and adolescence. Psychol Bull 101:393–403, 1987

DeMause L (ed): The History of Childhood. New York, Harper & Row, 1974

Dodge KA, Bates JE, Pettit GS: Mechanisms in the cycle of violence. Science 250:1678–1683, 1990

Egeland B, Vaughn B: Failure of "bond formation" as a cause of abuse, neglect, and maltreatment. Am J Orthopsychiatry 51:78–84, 1981

Eth S: Post-traumatic stress disorder in childhood, in Handbook of Child and Adult Psychopathology. Edited by Hersen M, Last CG. New York, Pergamon, 1990, pp 263–274

Eth S, Pynoos RS: Developmental perspective on psychic trauma in childhood, in Trauma and Its Wake. Edited by Figley CR. New York, Brunner/Mazel, 1985, pp 36–53

Famularo R, Kinscherff R, Fenton T: Psychiatric diagnoses of maltreated children: preliminary findings. J Am Acad Child Adolesc Psychiatry 31:863–867, 1992

Freud A: The Ego and the Mechanisms of Defence (1936), Revised Edition. London, Hogarth Press, 1966

Friedrich WN, Einbender AJ: The abused child: a psychological review. Journal of Clinical and Child Psychology 12:244–256, 1983

Goldman SJ, D'Angelo EJ, DeMaso DR, et al: Physical and sexual abuse histories among children with borderline personality disorder. Am J Psychiatry 149:1723–1726, 1992

Goodwin J: Post-traumatic symptoms in abused children. Journal of Traumatic Stress 1:475–488, 1988

Green AH: Psychopathology of abused children. Journal of the American Academy of Child Psychiatry 17:92–103, 1978

Green AH: Children traumatized by physical abuse, in Post-Traumatic Stress Disorder in Children. Edited by Eth S, Pynoos RS. Washington, DC, American Psychiatric Press, 1985, pp 133–154

Hawton K: Suicide in adolescents, in Suicide. Edited by Roy A. Baltimore, MD, Williams & Wilkins, 1986, pp 97–112

Heins M: 'The battered child' revisited. JAMA 251:3295–3300, 1984

Hyman IA, Zelifoff W, Clarke J: Psychological and physical abuse in schools: a paradigm for understanding post-traumatic stress disorder in children and youth. Journal of Traumatic Stress 1:243–267, 1988

Janson J, Williams SL, Burton A, et al: Epidemiologic differences between sexual and physical child abuse. JAMA 247:3344–3348, 1982

Kashani JH, Beck NC, Hoeper EW, et al: Psychiatric disorders in a community sample of adolescents. Am J Psychiatry 144:584–589, 1987

Kaufman J, Zigler E: Do abused children become abusive parents? Am J Orthopsychiatry 57:186–192, 1987

Keenan B: An Evil Cradling. London, Curtis Brown, 1992

Kempe CH, Silverman F, Steele B, et al: The battered child syndrome. JAMA 181:17–24, 1962

Kessler DB, Hyden P: Physical, sexual, and emotional abuse of children. Clin Symp 43(1):1–31, 1991

Lamphear VA: The impact of maltreatment on children's psychosocial adjustment: a review of the research. Child Abuse Negl 9:251–263, 1985

Landwirth J: Fetal abuse and neglect: an emerging controversy. Pediatrics 79:508–514, 1987

Lewis DO: From abuse to violence: psychophysiological consequences of maltreatment. J Am Acad Child Adolesc Psychiatry 31:383–391, 1992

Lewis DO, Lovely R, Yeager C, et al: Intrinsic and environmental characteristics of juvenile murderers. J Am Acad Child Adolesc Psychiatry 27:582–587, 1988

Martin JA, Elmer E: Battered children grown up: a follow-up study of individuals severely maltreated as children. Child Abuse Negl 16:75–87, 1992

Masterson JF: The symptomatic adolescent five years later: he didn't grow out of it. Am J Psychiatry 123:1338–1345, 1967

McCormack A, Burgess AW, Hartman C: Familial abuse and post-traumatic stress disorder. Journal of Traumatic Stress 1:231–242, 1988

Nichtern S: The sociocultural and psychodynamic aspects of the acting-out and violent adolescent. Adolesc Psychiatry 10:140–146, 1982

Offer D, Schonert-Reichl KA: Debunking the myths of adolescence. J Am Acad Child Adolesc Psychiatry 31:1003–1014, 1992

Offer D, Ostrov E, Howard KI: Adolescence: what is normal? Am J Dis Child 143:731–736, 1989

Ounsted C, Oppenheimer R, Lindsay J: Aspects of bonding failure: the psychopathology and psychotherapeutic treatment of families of battered children. Dev Med Child Neurol 16:446–456, 1974

Pate JE, Pumariega AJ, Hester C, et al: Cross-cultural patterns in eating disorders: a review. J Am Acad Child Adolesc Psychiatry 31:802–809, 1992

Pine F: On the development of the borderline-child-to-be. Am J Orthopsychiatry 56:450–457, 1986

Rutter M: Maternal deprivation, 1972–1978: new findings, new concepts, new approaches. Child Dev 50:283–305, 1979

Rutter M: Nature, nurture and psychopathology. Development and Psychopathology 3:125–136, 1991

Shengold L: Soul Murder: The Effects of Childhood Abuse and Deprivation. New Haven, CT, Yale University Press, 1989

Spitz RA, Wolf KM: Anaclitic depression: an inquiry into the genesis of psychiatric conditions in early childhood, II. Psychoanal Study Child 2:313–342, 1946

Terr L: Childhood traumas: an outline and overview. Am J Psychiatry 148:10–20, 1991

Thompson SC: Will it hurt less if I can control it? Psychol Bull 90:89–101, 1981

Toro PA: Developmental effects of child abuse: a review. Child Abuse Negl 6:423–431, 1982

Vaillant GE: The beginning of wisdom is never calling a patient a borderline: the clinical management of immature defenses in the treatment of individuals with personality disorders. Journal of Psychotherapy Practice and Research 1:117–134, 1992

Van Hasselt VB, Ammerman RT, Glancy LJ, et al: Maltreatment in psychiatrically hospitalized dually diagnosed adolescent substance abusers. J Am Acad Child Adolesc Psychiatry 31:868–874, 1992

White R, Benedict MI, Wulff L, et al: Physical disabilities as risk factors for child maltreatment: a selected review. Am J Orthopsychiatry 57:93–101, 1987

Widom CS: The cycle of violence. Science 244:160–166, 1989a

Widom CS: Does violence beget violence? A critical examination of the literature. Psychol Bull 106:3–28, 1989b

Wolfe DA: Child-abusive parents: an empirical review and analysis. Psychol Bull 97:462–482, 1985

Zeanah CH, Zeanah PD: Intergenerational transmission of maltreatment: insights from attachment theory and research. Psychiatry 52:177–196, 1989

Zuravin SJ: The ecology of child abuse and neglect: review of the literature and presentation of data. Violence and Victims 4:101–120, 1989

Section VI

Effects of Extreme Stress Factors on Developmental Processes

Chapter 19

Traumatic Stress in Infancy and Early Childhood: Expression of Distress and Developmental Issues

Richard D. Bingham, M.D.
Robert J. Harmon, M.D.

In this chapter we discuss extreme stress (trauma) in infants and young children (ages birth through 5 years). Trauma-related emotional disturbances of this age period will be described along with connections between early-occurring trauma and later psychopathology. In addition, we provide a developmental framework from which to consider the perception and meaning of potentially traumatic events early in life. The effects of trauma on development are also considered briefly. We close the chapter with a consideration of future directions.

There are strong reasons to separately consider trauma experienced by infants and young children. The early years of life are a time of rapid development and span a tremendous range of developmental capacities. The perception, impact, and response to traumatic stress

Dr. Bingham was supported by a National Institute of Mental Health postdoctoral training grant (MH-15442) and the W. T. Grant Foundation Endowment Fund of the Developmental Psychobiology Research Group (DPRG). The authors are grateful to a number of colleagues for their involvement: Robert N. Emde for his support; Joy D. Osofsky and Julie Evans for their helpful comments made on an earlier version; Nancy Murrow for her assistance with the final editing and typing; and members of the DPRG for their suggestions during the writing of this chapter.

499

will vary with these developmental capacities, and thus it is critical to consider the developmental context. Furthermore, extreme stress is at least as common in this age group as in later childhood. For example, one of the most common forms of trauma is intrafamilial violence. One form of this violence is child abuse. For half of the children who are abused, the abuse started by the time the child was 5 years old (Daro 1988). The Colorado Central Registry record of confirmed cases of child abuse for 1990 listed 37% of the cases as occurring in children 0 to 5 years of age (Colorado Central Registry staff, personal communication, 1994), and the children identified at older ages may have had a history of abuse dating back to preschool years. The greatest number of fatalities from child abuse occur in the period from infancy through the preschool years. Other family violence (e.g., spousal violence) may also be common when children are young, perhaps related to the demands of caring for infants and toddlers that may be stressful for new families. Children staying in shelters for battered women are commonly in the younger age groups, whereas adolescents are much less commonly found in these shelters (R. Rossman, personal communication, 1994). Infants and young children spend more time in the home than do school-age children and adolescents and therefore may witness more intrafamilial violence. Clinicians working in infant mental health have long been aware of the distress and impairments in infants and young children overwhelmed by abuse and neglect (Fraiberg 1980; Greenspan et al. 1987). These effects of abuse, as well as the effects of single-event trauma, are being conceptualized, at least in part, as posttraumatic disturbances (Drell et al. 1993).

Few empirical data are available on extreme stress in this young age group. In the absence of conclusions from such data, we hope that an outline of the relevant issues and concepts will help the clinician in making developmentally sensitive formulations of clinical problems as well as encourage future research in this area.

Early psychological trauma is an emotionally charged subject. The absence of research results allows extreme views to flourish. At one extreme is the view that infants and young children are protected from the detrimental effects of horrifying experience because they do not have lasting memories of the events. At the other extreme is the view that most emotional problems later in childhood and adult life can be attributed to trauma experienced very early in life. Many find the latter speculations intriguing. But if claims of detrimental effects of early trauma are not well thought through in terms of the developmental issues, then there is a risk that valid concerns about early trauma will be dismissed when exaggerated claims prove implausible. Again this points to the need for a developmental framework within which to structure and focus clinical formulations and to think about clinical situations and research issues related to early psychological trauma.

A better understanding of the effects of early trauma will also add to our knowledge of developmental trajectories of psychopathology across the life span. There are many important unanswered questions about how psychiatric disorders in infancy and early childhood relate to later disorder. A better understanding of these early origins may prove useful in our treatment of disturbed adolescents and adults who have histories of early traumatic experience. There is a growing body of research that identifies childhood abuse and neglect as a potentially important antecedent to later adult psychopathology (Bremner et al. 1993; Herman et al. 1989; Terr 1991), and some of this research especially implicates early abuse (Kluft 1991).

Lessons From History: Unacknowledged Distress

History provides abundant evidence about how easily the hurt of young children can be ignored, avoided, or rationalized away (Radbill 1987). Startling as it may seem, only in the last half of this century have the sadness and distress expressed by young children during prolonged separations (e.g., during hospitalization of the child or parent) been recognized and taken seriously (Bowlby 1973; Robertson 1953). This history of inattention to the emotional pain of children is in part related to the view that infants and young children are not seriously harmed by such distress. The history of relative indifference toward physical pain experienced by infants and young children reflects the same blindness. Perhaps the inability of infants to communicate their experience verbally and the self-protective avoidance of children's pain by adults combine to perpetuate this view. One of our goals in this chapter is to make clear that infants and young children can experience real terror. As a reminder of the risk that young children's experience of terror could again be denied, we briefly review how as recently as 50 years ago a special effort was required to make it generally recognized that infants deprived of maternal care and young children separated from their parents experience deep sadness and distress.

Two psychoanalytic researchers—René Spitz and John Bowlby—stand out as leaders in opening the eyes of both professionals and the public to sadness in infants and young children. A combination of sensitivity to the expression of emotional experience in infants and a drive to scientifically study these phenomena was necessary to overcome the prevailing views of their period.

Spitz systematically observed infants who had been separated from their mothers during the first year of life and infants who grew up with adequate physical care but had little contact or interaction with their caregivers. He took the important and innovative step of filming these infants. The result, *Grief: A Peril in Infancy* (Spitz 1947), was hard to ignore. Spitz's ability to feel the sadness in these infants, and not to turn away, allowed him to draw others' attention to their plight (Emde 1983). His carefully recorded observations were reported in papers on "anaclitic depression" and "hospitalism" (Spitz 1945, 1946).

Bowlby was well into his study of the role of early family life in childhood disturbance when, on behalf of the World Health Organization, he wrote the report *Maternal Care and Mental Health* (Bowlby 1952). This project enabled him to gather information and opinions from a wide range of researchers and clinicians from around the world who were knowledgeable about the effects of maternal deprivation and separation (Bretherton 1992). This experience further fueled his interests, leading eventually to the elaboration of attachment theory (Bowlby 1969, 1973, 1980). Like Spitz, Bowlby and his collaborator Robertson made a powerful film, *A Two-Year-Old Goes to Hospital* (Robertson 1952), which again convincingly showed the anguish young children can experience when separated from their parents. Again, the film helped others see what they had before somehow been unable to see or acknowledge. Bowlby's emphasis on the importance of real events in the child's external world as central determinants of children's emotional problems is echoed today by mental health clinicians' current interest in the effects of extreme stress.

There has been interest for decades in the impact of early psychological trauma. The early writings, however, typically were based on psychoanalytic case studies, and the traumas often did not involve the kinds of extreme stress being considered today. The sensitivity to anxiety in young children that came with the psychoanalytic approach was extremely valuable. Nevertheless, the fact that despite this sensitivity there was a failure to help recognize the actual terrifying events that some children experience is sad and unfortunate. There is now no denying the horrors that some young children must endure. It has in fact been the relatively recent and growing awareness of intrafamilial violence, including child physical and sexual abuse and spousal violence, that has brought a sense of urgency to this issue and raised many important questions about the relation between exposure to violence and the development of psychopathology.

Before going further with our discussion it is necessary to define what we mean by "extreme stress." As pointed out by Rutter (1983), the term *stress* has many different and even contradictory meanings. Despite the confusion and imprecision of the term, it has remained an important concept because it draws attention to important phenomena to be studied. The same is true for the concepts of "extreme stress" or "trauma." In this chapter, the terms *extreme stress* and *trauma* are used interchangeably. In our use of these terms we refer specifically to those experiences that involve overwhelming fright.

With this in mind we now turn to the main issues of this chapter. We first consider general developmental factors that influence the perception of danger and the expression of trauma in infancy and early childhood. We then briefly consider the impact of early trauma on developmental processes. Finally, we discuss the effects of and the psychopathology associated with extreme stress.

Developmental Considerations

There are several overarching developmental issues that need to be considered in a discussion of extreme stress in young children. In the first 5 years of life, development proceeds at a dizzying rate and spans extraordinary changes and transformations in the young child's capacities in all domains of development. For instance, in the emotional sphere there is a great leap from near complete dependency to considerable autonomy. In cognitive development, the trajectory of language passes from undifferentiated communication of distress or pleasure to quite articulate verbal negotiation of needs and expression of interests. Given these great leaps in the child's capacities, developmental issues require a central focus as we try to understand the impact of terrifying experiences in the first 5 years of life.

The developmental issues may be divided into three areas. The first area concerns the perception of threat and is related to the normal development of fear and appraisal of danger. The second area concerns changes in memory and representational capacity. The lasting effects of trauma derive from what has been learned and what is remembered, and because representational capacity is still developing in the early years, the effects of trauma may be quite different at different ages. The third area concerns consideration, in the context of these developmental issues, of the relevance of definitions and theory about trauma that have been derived primarily from clinical work with adults.

Perception of Threat and the Development of Normal Fear

Trauma, as we are defining it for this chapter, is precipitated by the experience of an overwhelming fright. An understanding of the early ontogeny of normal fearfulness can help sharpen our appreciation of the developmental issues regarding perception of threat and responses to fright as they relate to early trauma. Therefore, we first review some of what is known about the development of normal fear. Our discussion relies heavily on a review by Marks (1987) and the still excellent discussion of these issues by Bowlby (1973).

One of the prominent characteristics in the development of normal fear is the predictable sequence in which fears appear and decline. For example, separation fear is ubiquitous; it is found across cultures and in all types of children. This fear is normatively first expressed around age 8 months and then peaks at age 9 to 13 months and decreases from 2 years of age onward (Kagan et al. 1978; Smith 1979). Fear of the dark develops somewhat later and increases in early childhood, before waning (Bowlby 1973). Another important characteristic of fear development is that some cues are prepotent stimuli for fear. These cues require little or no experience to elicit fear responses, but may require maturation before being expressed. Fear of separation, fear of strangers, and fear of animals (e.g., especially snakes and spiders) are all examples of fear that is elicited by a specific cue. A pattern in the development of fear that is common to species as diverse and varied as puppies, human babies, and chicks is that of an initial lack of fear in infancy. During this early period, lasting through the first days or months of life, there is an indiscriminate approach to novel objects that is later replaced by wariness and fearful avoidance. The initial period of indiscriminate approach allows for affiliation and the development of familiarity and preference, and the subsequent period of fearfulness allows for self-protection.

In addition to changes in what elicits fear, there are changes in the expression of fear in the course of early development. In fact, fear as a differentiated emotional expression is rarely expressed until the middle of the first year of life. In the first 6 months of infancy there is little expression of wariness of novel objects and people. Loud noises, pain, or looming objects that may later elicit fear, in early infancy simply elicit a generalized expression of distress. By late in the first year, however, unmistakable expressions of fear are seen in a variety of situations.

These developmental changes are based on multiple interacting processes, and the precise nature of this complex process is not well understood (Marks 1987), although some of the relevant elements can be identified. One element that contributes to this developmental progression is the increase in perceptual discrimination that occurs over the first year. Along with these changes in perceptual capacity there are progressive learning and increase in available memory that transform the world from a place of almost complete novelty (barring the learning in utero) to a world in which certain perceptions and experiences become familiar and can be distinguished from those that are novel.

The perception of threat of serious bodily harm is likely a necessary element that creates the potential for an experience to be traumatic. Threat of harm is, in fact, an essential criterion in the common definitions of trauma. As we have mentioned above, some perceptual cues inherently (i.e., prepotently) elicit fear, whereas other cues for fear must be learned. From a biological perspective, it makes sense that the perception of serious threat might uniquely be a key ingredient in trauma because threat activates a complex set of psychophysiological responses as part of the "fight–flight" system for self-preservation. Threat cues range from simple direct sensory experience (e.g., a loud noise) to the complex experience of learning that a nearby nuclear reactor has leaked radioactive waste. Some prepotent cues, especially those that are simple sensory perceptions (e.g., pain, sudden approach) and lead to expressions of distress in early infancy and 1 year of age, are followed by convincing expression of fright. Other fears (e.g., fear of animals) do not develop for several years, even though they seem almost certainly to be prepotent. This variation in onset suggests that other developmental changes may be required before responses to certain danger cues are expressed. In addition, certain levels of nervous system maturation are required for the associative learning of fear responses. For example, taste aversion learning in rats becomes possible only gradually after several weeks of life (Schweitzer and Green 1982). As another example, in one study of human infants watching a doctor prepare to give an injection, when a similar injection had been given some weeks before, infants younger than 11 months of age rarely expressed fearfulness and thus did not seem to recall the association (Levy 1951). When threat cues do not inherently convey danger, and require more complex understandings, then the level of cognitive development and the knowledge base clearly determine whether or not there is an appraisal of danger.

From this background we can draw two conclusions: 1) that the nature of what is frightening changes with development, and 2) that infants and young children can, beginning at around age 6 months, clearly become extremely frightened on the basis of their own direct experience, given the right stimulus. This second point is especially important to highlight, because in the past too much emphasis was placed on the role of the parent's expression of fear as the primary elicitor of fear for children, a view that placed too little emphasis on the fact that children become terrified based on their own appraisals of danger (see Benedek 1985; Freud and Burlingham 1943; John 1941; R. S. Pynoos, personal communication, 1992). This is not to say that the emotional expressions of others (especially parents) are not important.

Models of the emotional processing of events commonly include a step involving a cognitive appraisal (Arnold 1960; Lazarus 1991). In addition to the appraisal of an event by the child himself or herself, the emotional expressions of others may also be used by the child in appraising the emotional meaning of an event. For example, when a stranger comes into a child's home, children often look on with a mixture of interest and wariness, but when their parent smiles, then the child approaches the stranger. Hagman (1932; as cited in Bowlby 1973) commented on this phenomenon of early "social referencing" (Campos and Stenberg 1981; Klinnert et al. 1983). From the experimental perspective, social referencing refers to the sequence of events involving, first, exposure to a novel event that typically generates both interest and wariness, then the infant's active search for the emotional expression or signal from another person, and, finally, the infant's approach to or withdrawal from the novel situation determined by whether the signal has a positive or negative emotional valence. This process has been studied quite extensively in children at around age 12 months and is mentioned here because it is relevant to the appraisal of threat. By 12 months of age, social referencing is well established (Klinnert et al. 1983). From infancy to early childhood, children grow in their understanding of emotional expressions of others and therefore can increasingly understand events through others' emotional responses as well as their own (Saarni and Harris 1989). Toddlers begin to learn more precise meanings of a number of discrete emotions (e.g., sadness and anger) but may have at an earlier age a greater sensitivity to fear signals than to other emotions because of the survival value of recognizing danger (R. D. Bingham, R. N. Emde, R. Landau, et al., unpublished manuscript).

Memory Development and Early Extreme Stress

One way that extreme stress may have a persistent damaging effect is through intrusive memories of the stressful event. Reliving the trauma through intrusive thoughts, dreams, flashbacks, or emotional distress following reminders of the event is the hallmark of posttraumatic disturbances. This reliving is so persistent and damaging that these intrusive experiences have been referred to as "malignant memories" (Schwarz and Kowalski 1990). Psychogenic amnesia is also a posttraumatic disturbance of memory, but one in which, instead of intrusion of memory, there is no accessible memory for a traumatic life event. That disturbances in memory are centrally related to trauma is also indicated by the connection between trauma and dissociative disorders, which in large part are disturbances in the integrative function of memory.

Types of Memories

Certain distinctions among types of memory are relevant for understanding early trauma. Although precise differentiation among types of memory becomes quite complex, a basic understanding of the distinction between *implicit* and *explicit* memory is useful and has been widely discussed in recent years (Schacter 1987). A related distinction is made in referring to *procedural* and *declarative* memory. Procedural memory refers to perceptual-motor and some cognitive skills and has been speculatively extended to include interpersonal expectations and transference (Clyman 1991). For the purpose of this discussion the more precise distinctions will not be made, and the terminology of implicit and explicit memory will subsume the other terms.

The intrusive symptoms and psychogenic amnesia mentioned above involve *explicit memory,* which is synonymous with the common usage of the term "memory," referring to memory that can be declared or stated in words (Schacter 1987). Explicit memory refers to the intentional, conscious recall or recognition of learned information. *Implicit memory* is demonstrated by a change in behavior based on prior learning even though the learned information is inaccessible to conscious retrieval. The concept of implicit memory has evolved out of the cognitive sciences and is not synonymous with the psychoanalytic concept of the dynamic unconscious. An example of implicit memory is subliminal learning of word lists that can be demonstrated through tested word associations even though the subject cannot recollect having seen the words (Squire 1992). Another example comes from the study of amnesia secondary to damage to the hippocampus and surrounding structures. Individuals with this type of dense amnesia are unable to retain simple word lists but can acquire new perceptual-motor skills (e.g., mirror writing). Thus, implicit memory refers broadly to memory that is nonconscious for a number of reasons but that nevertheless can be demonstrated through means other than directly declaring the presence of the memory. In other words, explicit memory is *knowing that,* whereas implicit memory is *knowing how.*

Understanding this distinction between explicit and implicit memory helps one recognize that posttraumatic disturbances may be expressions of either explicit or implicit memory, each resulting in different kinds of clinical problems. The problems related to explicit memory have been mentioned. Clinical phenomena such as reenactments and distress with reminders that occur without any recognition of the connection between the behavior and the past traumatic event are examples of problems related to implicit memory. This distinction between types of memory is also helpful in clarifying issues regarding the nature of memory for traumatic events occurring in the first years of life—an issue we return to after first summarizing what is known about memory for early trauma.

Memory and Early Trauma

There are no systematic studies of memory for traumas occurring in the first years of life, but there are several case reports that provide a starting point. We will limit our summary to case studies that focused on children and not discuss the clinical reports for adult patients showing evidence of memories for trauma in infancy. Terr (1988) has provided the largest case study and attempted to specifically examine several questions related to memory for early trauma. Because a major focus of this study was the accuracy of memories in children under the age of 5, the cases were selected on the basis of having sufficient outside reports or documentation by which the traumatic event could be independently verified. The 20 children selected had a wide range of fright or loss experiences, and findings were derived from a review of the author's own clinical records. The clinical interviews had been done at varying lengths of time after the traumatic event, with an average interval between the event and the interview of 53 months. There were several interesting findings. Children who were younger than age 28 to 36 months when the traumatic event occurred did not have verbal memories, but did have "behavioral memories." The term "behavioral memory" was used broadly, and by including practically any evidence of a lasting impact, including personality changes, it goes beyond even the definition of implicit memory. But there were more specific behaviors that strongly suggested the presence of implicit memory, if not clear explicit memory. These behaviors included replaying of the event with toys (when provided) and avoidance and fears of reminders. Some of the individual cases illustrating these findings were quite striking. Of the reexperiencing symptoms, posttraumatic play was frequently present, but nightmares were rare and flashbacks were not described at all. Terr noted that these behavioral representations were formed at all ages and were typically accurate. Children who were older than 36 months at the time of the traumatic event were more likely to have verbal memories of the event. Terr judged these memories to be generally accurate, although there were some deletions and additions to what was remembered.

Two case studies involving traumatic events—those of a car accident and a dog attack, with the children involved ages 9 and 21 months, respectively—are described in a recent chapter on posttraumatic stress disorder (PTSD) in infancy (Drell et al. 1993). The infant in the accident was seen at 22 months of age (13 months after the event), and the child attacked by the dog was seen at about 24 months of age (3 months after the event). Symptoms or behaviors that might represent explicit memory for the traumatic event and associated posttraumatic symptoms were described in both cases and included nightmares (although the content is very limited), demonstration of the traumatic event with toys (when the appropriate toys were provided), and some evidence suggesting intrusive thoughts. Again, verbal recollections were not given by these toddlers (who, of course, at the time of the evaluations had limited verbal skills). Whether these children have explicit memory of the event (i.e., memories either that they can spontaneously recollect or that intrude upon their consciousness) is debatable. However, the evidence for implicit memory is again quite convincing. Evidence for implicit memory is provided by the marked distress with exposure to reminders, avoidance and fears of objects associated with the traumatic event, recrudescence of stress symptoms with reexposure to strong reminders, and some posttraumatic play (at least when the appropriate toys were provided).

Memory in Infancy and Early Childhood

Given that disturbances of memory are central to the damaging effects of trauma, how do the profound changes in representational capacity and explicit memory that occur in the first years of life modify the effects of early trauma? Developmental changes in memory may influence the degree and nature of the impact of a traumatic event in early life. The phenomenon of infantile amnesia, which refers to the observation that most people do not remember events from before age 3 or 4 years (Howe and Courage 1993), suggests that memory capacity may be very different in the early years of life. Does this mean that before age 3 years most children are protected from the lasting effects of trauma that involve explicit memory? Although professionals and many laypersons recognize that extensive learning that does not involve explicit memory occurs in the early years of life, the fact that explicit memories are not generally recovered from the first several years of life does raise the question of whether or not the explicit intrusive posttraumatic memories are in fact formed in infancy and early childhood.

The answer to this question is taking shape in fascinating current debates on the nature of infantile amnesia and basic issues related to the development of mental representation in infants (Howe and Courage 1993; Mandler 1988). Empirical study of memory in infancy and early childhood has also begun to help answer this question.

Infantile amnesia has fascinated many while remaining an enigma (Howe and Courage 1993). As Howe and Courage (1993) point out, recent research on memory ability in preschool-age children has introduced an apparent paradox, namely, that 2- to 4-year-olds' memory for events is quite good (Fivush and Hudson 1990) even though this is a period from which few memories are available later in life. We now briefly review the research on memory in infancy and early childhood.

Fundamental memory capacity develops early. Long-term recognition memory is functional before birth as demonstrated by recognition of sounds presented prenatally (DeCasper and Spence 1986). One of the primary means of testing memory in early infancy has been through a procedure in which infants learn a contingency between the movement of a mobile and the kicking of their leg to which the mobile is connected (Rovee-Collier and Shyi 1992). Testing of this memory was done either as a simple forgetting paradigm without reminders or as a reactivation paradigm in which cues from the earlier training were presented on the day before the testing and probably reactivated the earlier memory. The simple forgetting paradigm gives evidence for only limited retention. At 3 months of age there was complete forgetting by 13 days (Sullivan et al. 1979). However, the reactivation paradigm demonstrated that if cues are reencountered, then the memory can be extended for as long as it was retained after the original encoding, and, most intriguing, suggested that infants may therefore be able to remember events for months or even years with repeated reactivation (Rovee-Collier and Hayne 1987). Using a different paradigm, Meltzoff and colleagues have shown that from 9 months onward, infants can imitate a novel action that they had witnessed but not performed (Meltzoff 1990). From this it was argued that if there is a higher-order representational system that develops separately from earlier habit or "procedural" modes of memory, then this system is functioning quite early, by midinfancy, rather than becoming functional only at the end of infancy.

The research that is perhaps most directly relevant to the subject of trauma is the study of event memory. Two- and 3-year-old children can produce coherent recall of previous events, both routine, common events such as a trip to the store, and unique, one-time events. In one study, 4-year-old children were able to recall events (e.g., a plane trip) that had happened around the age of 2½ (Fivush and Hamond 1990).

The emerging picture of infants and young children as having a fairly well developed memory capacity raises many new questions regarding memory for early traumatic events. This research is consistent with the clinical observations that infants and young children show clear evidence of remembering a traumatic event when their memory is cued in some way. These findings regarding nontraumatic events are also consistent with the clinical experience that meaningful psychotherapeutic work can be done in working with preschool-age children on frightening memories they have of traumatic events. Memories of events that occurred months or even years before the period of therapy may be accessed during the preschool years, but may not be available as more time passes and the child moves into the middle childhood years.

These findings notwithstanding, the question of whether infants and the youngest preschool-age children specifically have intrusive memory symptoms and recall without concrete reminders remains an open question. Even theorists who are very familiar with the work on early memory and who argue for a reevaluation of the concept of infantile amnesia still identify important developmental changes in autobiographical memory (Howe and Courage 1993; Nelson 1990). Nelson (1990) suggests that the development of language provides a way in which events may be reinstated and thus facilitates the persistence of memories and the learning of the personal and social functions of autobiographical memory. Howe and Courage (1993) emphasize the development of the cognitive sense of self as important for the developmental changes in autobiographical memory. These latter authors emphasize their point by suggesting that the term *amnesia* may even, in fact, be a misnomer, because the absence of autobiographical memories from this period of life is related not to developments in memory per se, but rather to developments in other cognitive domains.

In summary, it is clear that preschool-age children and even infants, given the right reminders, can remember traumatic events and experience considerable distress. These memories may be available to consciousness and may be worked with therapeutically, at least within these early years, even if they are not accessible later on. Intrusive memories of the type that are hallmarks of posttraumatic disturbances later in life may not occur in the same way as do memories of trauma in infancy and early childhood.

Determination of What Constitutes Trauma in Early Life

What are the events and experiences that represent extreme stress in the lives of infants and young children? As we have discussed, because perception and understanding change over the course of development, children at younger ages will not always perceive real threats as threats per se. Some events that are potentially traumatic for older children will not be so for infants or young children. However, there also are events that are experienced as threatening at practically any age. The types of events that are traumatic can be derived from this understanding. As Bowlby (1973) points out, being alone, even in adulthood, may be associated with greater risk of danger than is generally appreciated. There is no question, however, that being alone as an infant or young child is associated with markedly increased risk of harm (Bowlby 1973). Separation and being alone, as we have mentioned, constitute a prepotent stimulus for fear. In reference to loss of protection from a caregiver, van der Kolk (1987) suggests that "the earliest and possibly most damaging psychological trauma is the loss of a secure base" (p. 32). If the young child is alone and is also feeling threatened, then the terror is compounded.

Theories developed to understand the phenomena associated with traumatic stress come primarily out of experience with adults and assume a certain level of cognitive and emotional development. Because these competencies develop in early life, questions must be raised concerning the application of such formulations to an understanding of trauma in young children. Moreover, the very definition of trauma is for some tied to these models and hence raises basic questions about whether trauma as defined in adults is relevant to young children.

In fact, the definition of a traumatic stressor in infancy requires some modification from the standard definitions, which focus on the subjective experience. One common feature is that the event is appraised as threatening bodily harm or death to oneself or others, especially to those close (e.g., family) (American Psychiatric Association 1987; Pynoos and Spencer 1986). For infants this definition is problematic in that the threat of harm may be perceived only through concrete sensory perceptions, but not as a potential (e.g., when someone points a gun at another), and infants lack the concept of death. On the other hand, another subjective experience–based definition focuses on the experience of traumatic helplessness. Because infants are very dependent on others, it seems likely that they are more vulnerable to the experience of helplessness and perhaps potentially more at risk for traumatic stress.

Impact of Early Trauma on Development

As we noted earlier in this chapter, infancy and early childhood are times of astounding developmental change and transformation. In all domains of emotional and cognitive development, new capacities are emerging for the first time. This context of formative development raises unique concerns about the impact of early traumatic experience on development. There are many aspects of development that could be profoundly influenced by psychological trauma. A number of aspects of development—including regulation of fearfulness, development of trust and positive expectations, and emotional self-awareness and understanding—have clear conceptual links to experiences of extreme fright. In addition, it has been hypothesized that the avoidance that may follow traumatic experience can lead to impairments in the domain of cognitive development, including the capacity to symbolize. There is no substantial research examining the effect of trauma on these areas of development in young children. We will limit our discussion to research that raises questions regarding the potential effect of traumatic experiences on the development of fearfulness.

Experience and Modification of the Development of Fearfulness

Especially relevant to a discussion of the impact of traumatic experience are the investigations that identify how experience can have potent effects on modifying the development of fearfulness. In our discussion we will consider observations from nonhuman primates as well as humans. Although the concept of "critical periods" has been called into question for many developmental processes, in the development of fear there are some striking examples of this phenomenon. An example of a critical period in the development of fearfulness is the ease with which animals exposed to humans at an early age (before the onset of fear of novelty) remain nonfearful of humans, whereas in the absence of this early exposure, tremendous time and effort are required to overcome fearfulness to humans (i.e., to later tame an animal).

At the same time, normal social experiences are required for the development of adaptive fear responses. Social isolation or rearing with peers as opposed to rearing by the mother results in excessive fear of novelty (Suomi 1983). The expression of distress following separation also seems affected by aspects of the caregiving experience. Less contact in infant-parent dyads at 10 months of age is associated with less expression of distress when the infant is left alone (Kagan et al. 1978). The effect of social experience on stranger distress has also been investigated. Infants who were exposed to only a few unfamiliar adults, most of whom were babysitters, were more likely to be extremely distressed by strangers (Harmon et al. 1977; Morgan et al. 1975). Innate responses also become modified by experience. Rhesus infants who were shown pictures of rhesus threat displays showed fear responses even when reared in isolation. But when later moved to social groups, these monkeys showed no affective withdrawal or escape when faced with threat or attack (Sackett 1966). Apparently the lack of real social feedback (e.g., an actual attack following these pictures of threat displays) resulted in atrophy of the fear response.

An interesting and contrasting example of how early experience may significantly alter responses to later threat is provided by the work on "stress immunization." Infant rats exposed to the stress of rough handling or mild shock showed fewer signs of fearfulness and more effective adaptive avoidance when placed in a novel environment (Newton and Levine 1968). Simple extrapolations from these observations to the human infant are not possible, and it seems unlikely that extreme early stress would have an "immunizing effect." Still, the impressive degree of early plasticity and the nature of this plasticity may hold some clues for understanding early trauma.

Vulnerability to Trauma

Questions concerning vulnerability to or protection from stress related to a child's age and development remain an important area of continuing debate. When factors influencing the outcome of stress are considered in general, age is commonly cited as one of the important variables (Rutter 1983; van der Kolk 1987). Although age can be considered an important factor in a general model of the impact of stress, recognition that stressful events are complex and have multiple effects suggests caution in making generalizations. As noted by Rutter (1983), the particular stress of separation (studied as hospitalization) leads to the most pronounced distress between the ages of about 6 months and 4 years. This developmental pattern is related to the changes in attachment that bracket this period of increased vulnerability. Selective attachment before the age of 6 months is not well developed, and once a strong attachment bond is formed, it is not until 3 or 4 years of age that children have the capacity to both mentally represent and adequately maintain attachment relationships when another is physically absent.

Some of the most prominent theory about the impact of early traumatic experience places an emphasis on increased vulnerability for developmental reasons. Arguing from a biological perspective, van der Kolk (1987) has suggested that the immature central nervous system of the young child is particularly vulnerable to the effects of psychological trauma. Although this is intriguing, the limited empirical findings on posttraumatic symptoms have sometimes suggested that young children may show the least detrimental effects (Green et al. 1991), at least in the context of natural disasters.

Trauma and the Parent-Child Relationship

Behavioral and emotional regulation in early childhood is not separable from the functioning of the parent-child relationship. For the young child the parent is the source of protection as well as of nurturing care. When the child and/or the parent experience a threat toward the child, then both are challenged to respond in order to restore a sense of safety for the child. In infancy and early childhood the source of the threat is as likely to be from within the family, from one of the child's own parents, as it is to be from the outside. Trauma from within the family presents a different set of issues regarding the parent-child relationship from those presented by violence external to the family.

Intrafamilial Violence

Violence within the family, and certainly child abuse, represent a failure by the parent to provide safety and protection for the child. A failure to empathically understand the terror that the child experiences with such violence is often part of the problem. This lack of empathy also impairs the parent's ability to be responsive to the child's increased need for comfort and security that follows such a frightening experience. Overall, there is a pattern of underresponsiveness of the parent in his or her interaction with the child.

Violence External to the Family

In contrast to intrafamilial threat, when a child's life has been threatened by some event outside the family, parents themselves experience terror. Parents feel helplessness and shame about failing at their central role as protector. The assessment of whether or not, as a parent, one did enough to protect one's child inevitably follows a threat to one's child from outside the family. This is fundamentally an adaptive process in which an appropriate increase in protection can follow. An appraisal of failed responsibility and self-blame by parents commonly occurs in the initial phase of response to a child trauma and may or may not have a rational basis. During this time the world may suddenly seem more threatening, and routine judgments involved in monitoring a child's safety can be agonizing. The extent to which the parent supports and encourages exploration and independence and autonomy will be affected. Both the child and the parent are responding to the threat, and because the appraisals of children and adults often differ, and because of differences in temperament and experience, the responses and needs of each may be quite different. An adjustment in the regulation of safety and protection must be negotiated over time. The variability in the course of recovery of the parent as compared with the child's course of recovery often makes this process more challenging. In the course of this adjustment there may be "overprotectiveness," and the child may be viewed as highly vulnerable, or the child may seem "overdependent" and insecure. The child's development can be deleteriously affected if the parent is unable to modify these views as further experiences help restore a sense of reasonable safety. Successful adaptation leads gradually to a return of confidence in one's ability as a parent to realistically appraise potential threats and therefore provide protection without limiting exploration and the development of autonomy.

Trauma and Attachment

The concept of attachment disorders has been developed from the application of Bowlby's attachment theory to clinical practice in infant mental health. The nature of the disturbance and the context of abuse in which attachment disorders are often found suggest that an important overlap with the phenomenology of trauma is worth considering in some detail. Attachment and trauma also have relevant *conceptual* overlaps as well as important differences.

Implications of Research on Attachment in Relation to Trauma

A central thesis that Bowlby articulated in his theory of attachment—the need for protection of the young by adults—is the fundamental evolutionary reason that an attachment system exists (Bowlby 1969). He also identified the separate but related fear/wariness system that monitors the level of safety and danger. These two systems work together to maintain the infant's safety and thus are closely related. Attachment research, by focusing on attachment behaviors, has focused on what one could call the "response side" of the two systems. Attachment research has primarily examined the *way* in which the infant seeks reassurance and safety as an indicator of how the parent has provided a sense of security. Questions concerning *when* and *to what extent* the infant responds with fearfulness relate more specifically to the fear/wariness system—the "detection side" of the two systems. The study of trauma, in contrast to attachment, focuses on the sensitivity and dysregulation in the fear/wariness system (to use Bowlby's terminology). The empirical study of attachment, of course, does utilize a method that activates the fear/wariness system. The infant is separated from the parent in the "strange situation" paradigm (Ainsworth et al. 1978), which commonly produces brief, mild fearfulness, and this is then the context in which attachment behavior is examined. Behavior in this paradigm is influenced by both the attachment and the fear/wariness systems. This is illustrated by the finding that Japanese infants showed different proportions in the secure/insecure patterns of response in this paradigm, a finding that has been interpreted as likely being due to the fact that Japanese infants experience fewer separations from their mother. This difference in the experience of these infants resulted in a higher level of threat to be experienced in the separation. This variation in response reflects a different sensitivity in the fear/wariness system that then leads to different frequencies of the specific attachment behaviors that are used in determining attachment classification. Regulation of fearfulness and attachment are interconnected.

Another way to gain some perspective on the connections between the study of trauma and the study of attachment is to consider two relevant experimental animal research paradigms. The first is the extensive research on the effects of separation in nonhuman primates. Theory concerning trauma has drawn extensively from this experimental research (van der Kolk 1987). Studies of separation in infancy are relevant for the study of early trauma because separation is the prototypical fear experience of this period of life. The problem in considering separation as completely synonymous with trauma is that there are many other regulatory aspects of the relationship that are also disturbed by separation. Thus, it is probably not "just" lack of security and associated fearfulness that relate to the negative outcomes that have been described in this area of research, but disruptions in other domains as well. Extended separation probably leads to a complex set of consequences, one aspect of which is related to trauma. The second extensively studied animal paradigm is that of "learned helplessness." In the learned helplessness paradigm, comparisons are made between two groups of animals that both receive an equal number of painful stimuli (e.g., mild–moderate tail shocks in rats) but that differ in the extent to which the animal has some effective response to or control over the aversive stimuli. The effects on the animals who have control are minimal compared with the profound effects on the animals who lack control. This research has also been viewed as highly relevant to understanding trauma (Kushner et al. 1992). This focus on threat and helplessness is more specifically relevant to the field of trauma. However, separation does secondarily lead to helplessness. A sense of helplessness is created when the vigorous and repeated cries or calls by the infant are ineffective in bringing the mother back. This helplessness in the face of fear creates the potential for psychological trauma. The fact that important theory concerning the long-term effects of trauma derives from the study of nonhuman infant primates points to the need to better study the effects of trauma in human infants.

Attachment Disorders

With the background presented above, we can now examine some specific features of attachment disorders that we view as indicators of trauma. As we discussed, dysregulation of the fear/wariness system is a central aspect of trauma, and it is both under- and over-regulation of fearfulness that are often prominent in attachment disorders. Furthermore, the origin of attachment disorders suggests that frightening experience plays an important etiological role. In DSM-III-R (American Psychiatric Association 1987), reactive attachment disorder and PTSD share a characteristic that is unique among all the disorders in this system, namely, that of having diagnostic criteria that are based on etiological factors. For PTSD the presence of an extreme stressor is necessary for diagnosis, and for reactive attachment disorder, a history of frank neglect or harsh treatment. Subsequently, both DSM-IV (American Psychiatric Association 1994) and ICD-10 (World Health Organization 1992) have included a disorder of attachment (as discussed in Zeanah et al. 1993).

Criteria for attachment disorders have been developed primarily from maltreatment syndromes. This approach has been criticized as being too narrowly focused on the context of severe abuse and missing the importance of the broader range of clinically important attachment disturbances. The value of broadening the diagnosis to include a range of relationship disturbances has been articulated by Zeanah and Emde (1994). Recently, Richters and Volkmar (1994) have questioned whether attachment disturbances are central to reactive attachment disorder and also have highlighted the need for research to confirm the value of the etiological requirement of a history of pathological care. Although these issues remain, the fact that infants with reactive attachment disorder often have experienced extreme stress, and moreover show disturbances in regulation of fearfulness, suggests that this disorder is very relevant to an understanding of the impact of trauma.

Two subtypes of disorder have been identified—inhibited and disinhibited—and each has features that suggest dysregulation in fearfulness, but at the opposite extreme from that associated with the other subtype. Although the organizing concept for this disorder is a disturbance in "social relatedness," many of the behavioral criteria relate to fearfulness. In the inhibited subtype there is excessive fearfulness that may be expressed as hypervigilance around a particular individual (e.g., a particular family member). In the disinhibited subtype there is a lack of appropriate wariness with unfamiliar persons that is evident as indiscriminant sociability.

Zeanah and colleagues (1993), in arguing that it is important to broaden the scope of attachment disorders, delineate four subtypes, with the organizing principles for the classification being derived from developmental research on attachment rather than from "abuse syndromes." Even with this suggested classification, in which a broader range of relationship disturbances are identified and the context of abuse is not a central criterion, still the relevance of trauma for attachment disorders remains evident. In fact, some other aspects of posttraumatic behavior are further highlighted in this system. These authors delineate disorders of attachment from the normal range of attachment patterns by emphasizing that the disorders "represent more profound and pervasive disturbances in the child's feelings of *safety and security*" (Zeanah et al. 1993). Additional disturbances in safety and security that are also associated with trauma and are not described in the DSM-IV and ICD-10 attachment disorders are described as part of two of the four subtypes as described by Zeanah and colleagues. The descriptions by these authors are based on extensive clinical experience in infant mental health. A characteristic of children with one of the four subtypes, referred to as the "indiscriminant" type of attachment disorder, is "recklessness, accident proneness, and risk-taking" that often places the child at risk for physical harm (e.g., running from the caregiver into the street) (Zeanah et al. 1993). This recklessness is a characteristic that has been associated with trauma in both adults and children, and perhaps reaches its greatest level of dangerousness in the context of the impulsive adolescent (van der Kolk 1987; R. S. Pynoos, personal communication, 1994). Children with another subtype of attachment disorder, the "role-reversed" type of attachment disorder, typically act in very bossy and controlling ways with the caregiver. This behavior also has been identified in children following trauma and linked to the core experience of loss of control and helplessness in the face of the trauma.

Posttraumatic Disturbances

We first review PTSD in later childhood because it has received much more study than that in early childhood. Next we consider special issues related to the expression of posttraumatic symptoms at younger ages. We end this section with a brief discussion of connections between early trauma and later psychopathology.

Posttraumatic Stress Disorder in Childhood

Although there is a range of disturbances that can emerge from traumatic experience, PTSD is the psychiatric disorder that is most specifically linked to extreme stress. PTSD has historically been associated with the experience of combat by men in war. Experience with veterans from the Vietnam War, increasing recognition of posttraumatic responses to civilian disasters and violent crimes, and further articulation of a clinical theory (Horowitz 1986) all contributed to the establishment of PTSD as a diagnostic category in DSM-III (American Psychiatric Association 1980). PTSD is characterized by severe distress and disruption in functioning when the disorder is acute, and has the potential to become a chronic debilitating disorder. The potential for children to develop a chronic disorder in response to a traumatic event, a disorder that may then become increasingly resistant to treatment over time, underlines the importance of early identification and intervention. Only more recently has there been an increase in attention given to posttraumatic problems in children (Eth and Pynoos 1985). As a background for discussing posttraumatic disturbances in the first 5 years of life, we provide an overview of the clinical picture in older children.

Levy (1945) was astute in raising the question as to whether children who have had a frightening surgery may have traumatic responses that are comparable to soldiers' "war neuroses." He identified many of the core clinical phenomena that had been noted in medical writings and literature for centuries. The organization of the diagnostic criteria was modified somewhat in DSM-III-R, and symptoms were added or modified to be more relevant to children (Brett et al. 1988), but there is unlikely to be much change in DSM-IV (Davidson and Foa 1993). Posttraumatic symptoms are a mixture of external behaviors and internal experience. It is critical that children themselves be asked directly about their experience and possible symptoms, and this often requires that they have the opportunity to express these through drawing, play, and dramatization (Nader and Pynoos 1991). At the same time, reports from parents and teachers are essential because they may better report outward behaviors and patterns over time. Making connections between reminders of the frightening event and posttraumatic symptoms is useful in therapeutic work, but often challenging, so that getting reports from both children and other observers is quite important.

In addition to the criteria of exposure to an extreme stressor, the symptom criteria for PTSD are organized into three areas: reexperiencing of the traumatic event, avoidance of reminders and/or psychological numbing, and hyperarousal.

The reexperiencing of symptoms in children is similar to that in adults. Children do show distress when reminded of the frightening event, may report unwanted (i.e., intrusive) thoughts and images, have nightmares, and exhibit forms of reenactment. Children's symptoms also may be somewhat different from those expressed by adults. Nightmares may increase in frequency, but the content of the nightmares may reflect general childhood fears rather than contain specific reference to the trauma. Intrusive recollections may not be reported by the child, but there may be compulsive reenactment of aspects of the trauma in posttraumatic play. Almost any aspect of the traumatic experience may become a cue, and exposure to such a reminder can then lead to renewed fear or intrusive thoughts and may be accompanied by behavioral problems that can represent some form of reenactment.

Children do avoid thoughts and places that remind them of a traumatic experience and also may show restriction in affect. Children do not typically describe the changes in emotional experience in the ways that adults do (Nader and Pynoos 1991). Rather than identifying their emotional state as "numb," children may say they do not want to know how they feel. Behavioral changes can be observed that reflect a decreased range of interests, activities, and emotional expression. There has been some debate about whether or not psychogenic amnesia for aspects of the trauma occurs as commonly in children as in adults. Terr (1979, 1983), in her study of a group of children who had been kidnapped, did not find evidence for amnesia, although misperceptions were found. Others have observed various forms of memory distortions in traumatized children (Pynoos and Spencer 1986). The study of childhood trauma has added to this cluster the symptom of a negative future orientation that can be a dramatic departure from the hopefulness often seen in children.

Symptoms clustered under the heading of "hyperarousal," although somewhat loosely related, serve an important function of emphasizing the physiological aspects of PTSD. As with adults, children may show sleep disturbance, irritability, difficulty concentrating, hypervigilance, increased startle response, and bodily symptoms of sympathetic arousal. Sleep disturbances can be severe in children. There is some suggestion that young children may be more likely to express disturbance in arousal in a variety of non–rapid eye movement (REM) phenomena, including night terrors. Children may exhibit increased startle responses. Ornitz and Pynoos (1989) have suggested that the development of the startle response is vulnerable to early traumatic experience because this response does not fully mature until about age 8 years. An example of recurring autonomic hyperarousal is provided by a 6-year-old girl who would alternately feel her heart beating wildly in her chest and then not feel her heart beating at all (the latter of course being normal). This led to daily fears that her heart would stop.

Posttraumatic Stress Disorder in Infancy and Early Childhood

Clinical experience suggests that young children and infants may be profoundly affected by extreme stress, but data from systematic studies are lacking. Young children and infants, given their developmental capacity for monitoring and communicating their experience, are simply not able to report many of the symptoms of PTSD. The fact that a report of the symptoms cannot be elicited does not rule out the possibility that some of the same symptoms are being experienced. However, it does mean that PTSD is not easily or commonly diagnosed in this age group if the strict criteria are applied. In young children and in infants as young as 1 year, the core posttraumatic phenomena of fearfulness with exposure to reminders and a general increase in fearfulness can clearly be present. Increased fearfulness is expressed in an age-typical fashion with increased need for contact and comfort from parents (e.g., more clinging to parents and not wanting to sleep alone). This appears as a regression from the child's previous progress toward separation and autonomy, which require feelings of security. These behaviors are fundamentally adaptive in origin in that they increase protection from the parent. Clinicians may make a diagnosis of PTSD in infants and young children in the absence of all the necessary criteria in order to emphasize the important impact of an extremely stressful event. DSM-IV has acknowledged some of these issues, both by emphasizing that it is how the trauma is experienced that is important and by adding certain special notations for children. These notations include the behavioral response of disorganized or agitated behavior as a general reaction, as well as the acknowledgment that frightening dreams may not have recognizable content and that repetitive play of the trauma may occur, rather than recollections. Without more longitudinal study of clinical cases, however, it is unclear how the outcome (e.g., risk for chronicity) is similar to and different from adolescent and adult PTSD.

Zero to Three (1993), of the National Center for Clinical Infant Programs (NCCIP), has developed a diagnostic classification system for mental health programs in children from birth to age 4 years. Two types of "traumatic stress disorders" are identified: one resulting from a single event, and a second, from chronic, enduring, or multiple traumatic situations. Most of the symptoms of PTSD are listed as possible criteria for preschoolers who have verbal and other representational capacities, while a special note indicates that "children younger than 18 months, who have limited representational capacities, will less likely exhibit symptoms indicating reexperiencing the traumatic event. Underlying distress would more likely be manifest as disorders of affect, disregulation of eating and sleep, and social disturbance without symbolic representation" (Zero to Three 1993, p. 15). The attempt in this system to identify the different kinds of problems experienced by infants and young children who have been in enduring traumatic circumstances (in the United States this usually involves family violence) is laudable in drawing particular attention to the needs of these children. It seems likely the effects of chronic exposure to abuse will not fit neatly into a particular diagnostic category for all children and that more research is required to clarify what are the various outcomes that are possible.

Psychopathology in Adulthood

Over the past decade, clinical research has provided evidence that early trauma in the form of abuse and neglect may be an important antecedent to some forms of adult psychopathology. Some of this work suggests that the type of disorder, the severity, and the type of symptoms may depend upon the age and developmental level at which the trauma occurred (van der Kolk et al. 1991). For example, a dissociative disorder, multiple personality disorder (dissociative identity disorder), is thought to have its origin in early childhood abuse that could disrupt the development of a cohesive sense of self and consciousness in a formative period of self development (Kluft 1985). Alternatively, because dissociative processes are normally present in very young children, these mechanisms may be readily used in adaptation to extreme stress occurring in this period of development (Putnam 1991).

Another etiologically relevant association that has been suggested is that between childhood trauma and borderline personality disorder (Herman et al. 1989). Earlier theories of the etiology of borderline personality disorder suggested constitutional vulnerabilities or, as psychoanalytically conceptualized, early developmental arrests. The trauma-based theory has led clinical investigators to examine the frequency of a history of childhood abuse and neglect in patients with borderline personality disorder. Although the strength of this association varies, studies using interview assessments of past abuse indicate as many as 71% of the patients as having a history of abuse (Gunderson and Sabo 1993; Herman et al. 1989). The identification of posttraumatic symptoms of PTSD in patients with borderline personality disorder adds conceptual support to this association (Gunderson and Sabo 1993). From a clinical perspective it is striking that the borderline patient's overwhelming anxiety in response to mild suggestion of loss is so evocative of the distress of a young child terrified about being left alone in a frightening place.

Future Directions

As important as these links are between early trauma and later psychopathology, clearly quite complex models will be required to describe the role of trauma in shaping possible developmental pathways that may lead to continued distress or a return to a sense of safety. Rutter (1989) has outlined the many diverse elements that need to be considered in a realistic model of developmental psychopathology. We must be cautious about becoming too simplistic.

At the same time there has been little written on the possible intermediate link from early childhood mental health problems or syndromes and later psychopathology. There is a need to make bridges both conceptually and empirically between the approaches used to study the impact of early childhood trauma. These approaches include the study of the effect of abuse and neglect on development, the study of early childhood disorders associated with abuse and neglect (e.g., reactive attachment disorder), and the retrospective studies of the history of early trauma in individuals with adolescent and adult borderline personality disorder and multiple personality disorder. Increased understanding in these areas should increase our ability to help young traumatized children.

References

Ainsworth MDS, Blehar MC, Waters E, et al: Patterns of Attachment: A Psychological Study of the Strange Situation. Hillsdale, NJ, Erlbaum, 1978

American Psychiatric Association: Diagnostic and Statistical Manual of Mental Disorders, 3rd Edition. Washington, DC, American Psychiatric Association, 1980

American Psychiatric Association: Diagnostic and Statistical Manual of Mental Disorders, 3rd Edition, Revised. Washington, DC, American Psychiatric Association, 1987

American Psychiatric Association: Diagnostic and Statistical Manual of Mental Disorders, 4th Edition. Washington, DC, American Psychiatric Association, 1994

Arnold MB: Emotion and Personality, Vols 1 and 2. New York, Columbia University Press, 1960

Benedek E: Children and psychic trauma: a brief review of contemporary thinking, in Post-Traumatic Stress Disorder in Children. Edited by Eth S, Pynoos RS. Washington, DC, American Psychiatric Press, 1985, pp 3–16

Bowlby J: Maternal Care and Mental Health. Geneva, World Health Organization, 1952 [Originally published in Bull World Health Organ 3:355–534, 1951]

Bowlby J: Attachment and Loss, Vol 1: Attachment. New York, Basic Books, 1969 [2nd Edition, 1983]

Bowlby J: Attachment and Loss, Vol 2: Separation. New York, Basic Books, 1973

Bowlby J: Attachment and Loss, Vol 3: Loss, Sadness and Depression. New York, Basic Books, 1980

Bremner JD, Southwick SM, Johnson DR, et al: Childhood physical abuse and combat-related posttraumatic stress disorder in Vietnam veterans. Am J Psychiatry 150:235–239, 1993

Bretherton I: The origins of attachment theory: John Bowlby and Mary Ainsworth. Developmental Psychology 28:759–775, 1992

Brett EA, Spitzer RL, Williams JBW: DSM-III-R criteria for post-traumatic stress disorder. Am J Psychiatry 145:1232–1236, 1988

Campos JJ, Stenberg CR: Perception, appraisal and emotion: the onset of social referencing, in Infant Social Cognition. Edited by Lamb M, Sherrod L. Hillsdale, NJ, Erlbaum, 1981, pp 273–314

Clyman RB: The procedural organization of emotions: a contribution from cognitive science to the psychoanalytic theory of therapeutic action. J Am Psychoanal Assoc 39(suppl):359–383, 1991

Daro D: Confronting Child Abuse: Research for Effective Program Design. New York, Free Press, 1988

Davidson JRT, Foa EB (eds): Posttraumatic Stress Disorder: DSM-IV and Beyond. Washington, DC, American Psychiatric Press, 1993

DeCasper AJ, Spence MJ: Prenatal maternal speech influences newborns' perception of speech sounds. Infant Behavior and Development 9:133–150, 1986

Drell MJ, Siegel CH, Gaensbauer TJ: Post-traumatic stress disorder, in Handbook of Infant Mental Health. Edited by Zeanah CH. New York, Guilford, 1993, pp 291–304

Emde RN (ed): René A Spitz: Dialogues From Infancy—Selected Papers. New York, International Universities Press, 1983

Eth S, Pynoos RS (eds): Post-Traumatic Stress Disorder in Children. Washington, DC, American Psychiatric Press, 1985

Fivush R, Hamond NR: Autobiographical memory across the preschool years: toward reconceptualizing childhood amnesia, in Knowing and Remembering in Young Children. Edited by Fivush R, Hudson JA. Cambridge, UK, Cambridge University Press, 1990, pp 223–248

Fivush R, Hudson JA (eds): Knowing and Remembering in Young Children. Cambridge, UK, Cambridge University Press, 1990

Fraiberg S: Clinical Studies in Infant Mental Health. New York, Basic Books, 1980

Freud A, Burlingham DT: War and Children. London, Medical War Books, 1943

Green BL, Korol M, Grace MC, et al: Children and disaster: age, gender, and parental effects on PTSD symptoms. J Am Acad Child Adolesc Psychiatry 30:945–951, 1991

Greenspan SI, Wieder S, Lieberman A, et al (eds): Infants in Multirisk Families—Case Studies in Preventive Intervention (Clinical Infant Reports. Series of the National Center for Clinical Infant Programs: Third, Vol No 3, 3 Vols). Madison, CT, International Universities Press, 1987

Gunderson JG, Sabo AN: The phenomenological and conceptual interface between borderline personality disorder and PTSD. Am J Psychiatry 150:19–27, 1993

Hagman E: A study of fears of children of pre-school age. Journal of Experimental Education 1:110–130, 1932

Harmon RJ, Morgan GA, Klein RP: Determinants of normal variation in infants' negative reactions to unfamiliar adults. Journal of the American Academy of Child Psychiatry 16:670–683, 1977

Herman JL, Perry JC, van der Kolk BA: Childhood trauma in borderline personality disorder. Am J Psychiatry 146:490–495, 1989

Horowitz MJ: Stress Response Syndromes, 2nd Edition. Northvale, NJ, Jason Aronson, 1986

Howe ML, Courage ML: On resolving the enigma of infantile amnesia. Psychol Bull 113:305–326, 1993

John E: A study of the effects of evacuation and air raids on preschool children. Br J Educ Psychol 11:173–182, 1941

Kagan J, Kearsley RB, Zelazo PR: Infancy: Its Place in Human Development. Cambridge, MA, Harvard University Press, 1978

Klinnert MD, Campos J, Sorce JF, et al: Social referencing: emotional expressions as behavior regulators, in Emotion: Theory, Research and Experience, Vol 2. Edited by Plutchik R, Kellerman H. Orlando, FL, Academic, 1983, pp 57–86

Kluft RP (ed): Childhood Antecedents of Multiple Personality Disorder. Washington, DC, American Psychiatric Press, 1985

Kluft RP: Multiple personality disorder, in American Psychiatric Press Review of Psychiatry, Vol 10. Edited by Tasman A, Goldfinger SM. Washington, DC, American Psychiatric Press, 1991, pp 161–275

Kushner MG, Riggs DS, Foa EB, et al: Perceived controllability and the development of posttraumatic stress disorder (PTSD) in crime victims. Behav Res Ther 31:105–110, 1992

Lazarus RS: Emotion and Adaptation. Oxford, UK, Oxford University Press, 1991

Levy DM: Psychic trauma of operations in children. Am J Dis Child 69:7–25, 1945

Levy DM: Observations of attitudes and behavior in the child health center. Am J Public Health 41:182–190, 1951

Mandler JM: How to build a baby: on the development of an accessible representational system. Cognitive Development 3:113–136, 1988

Marks I: The development of normal fear: a review. J Child Psychol Psychiatry 28:667–696, 1987

Meltzoff AN: Towards a developmental cognitive science: the implications of cross-modal matching and imitation for the development of representation and memory in infancy, in The Development and Neural Basis of Higher Cognitive Functions. Ann N Y Acad Sci 608:1–37, 1990

Morgan GA, Levin B, Harmon RJ: Determinants of individual differences in infants' reactions to unfamiliar adults. JSAS Catalog of Selected Documents in Psychology 5:277, 1975

Nader K, Pynoos RS: Drawing and play in the diagnosis and assessment of childhood post-traumatic stress syndromes, in Play, Diagnosis, and Assessment. Edited by Schaeffer C. New York, Wiley, 1991, pp 375–398

Nelson K: Remembering, forgetting, and childhood amnesia, in Knowing and Remembering in Young Children. Edited by Fivush R, Hudson JA. Cambridge, UK, Cambridge University Press, 1990, pp 301–316

Newton G, Levine S: Early experience and behavior, in The Psychobiology of Development. Edited by Newton G, Levine S. Springfield, IL, Charles C Thomas, 1968, pp 102–141

Ornitz EM, Pynoos RS: Startle modulation in children with post-traumatic stress disorder. Am J Psychiatry 147:866–870, 1989

Putnam FW: Dissociative phenomena, in American Psychiatric Press Review of Psychiatry, Vol 10. Edited by Tasman A, Goldfinger SM. Washington, DC, American Psychiatric Press, 1991, pp 145–160

Pynoos RS, Spencer E: Witness to violence: the child interview. Journal of the American Academy of Child Psychiatry 25:306–319, 1986

Radbill SX: Children in a world of violence: a history of child abuse, in The Battered Child, 4th Edition. Edited by Helfer RE, Kempe RS. Chicago, IL, University of Chicago Press, 1987, pp 3–22

Richters MM, Volkmar FR: Reactive attachment disorder of infancy or early childhood. J Am Acad Child Adolesc Psychiatry 33:328–332, 1994

Robertson J: A Two-Year-Old Goes to Hospital [Film]. New York University Film Library, 1952

Robertson J: Some responses of young children to the loss of maternal care. Nursing Times 49:382–386, 1953

Rovee-Collier C, Hayne H: Reactivation of infant memory: implications for cognitive development, in Advances in Child Development and Behavior. Edited by Lipsitt LP, Spiker CC. New York, Academic, 1987, pp 185–238

Rovee-Collier C, Shyi G: A functional and cognitive analysis of infant long-term retention, in Development of Long-Term Retention. Edited by Howe ML, Brainerd CJ, Reyna VF. New York, Springer-Verlag, 1992, pp 3–55

Rutter M: Stress, coping, and development: some issues and some questions, in Stress, Coping, and Development in Children. Edited by Garmezy N, Rutter M. New York, McGraw-Hill, 1983, pp 1–41

Rutter M: Pathways from childhood to adult life. J Child Psychol Psychiatry 30:23–51, 1989

Saarni C, Harris PL (eds): Children's Understanding of Emotion. Cambridge, UK, Cambridge University Press, 1989

Sackett GP: Monkeys reared in isolation with pictures as visual input: evidence for an innate relearning mechanism. Science 154:1468–1473, 1966

Schacter DL: Implicit memory: history and current status. J Exp Psychol Learn Mem Cogn 13:501–518, 1987

Schwarz ED, Kowalski JM: Malignant memories: PTSD in children and adolescents after a school shooting. J Am Acad Child Adolesc Psychiatry 30:936–944, 1990

Schweitzer L, Green L: Acquisition and extended retention of conditional taste aversion in preweanling rats. J Comp Psychol 96:791–806, 1982

Smith PK: The ontogeny of fear in children, in Fears in Animals and Man. Edited by Sluckin W. London, Van Nostrand Reinhold, 1979, pp 164–168

Spitz RA: Hospitalization: an inquiry into the origins of psychiatric conditions in early childhood. Psychoanal Study Child 1:53–74, 1945

Spitz RA: Anaclitic depression. Psychoanal Study Child 2:313–342, 1946

Spitz RA: Grief: A Peril in Infancy [Film]. New York University Film Library, 1947

Squire LR: Memory and the hippocampus: a synthesis from findings with rats, monkeys, and humans. Psychol Rev 99:195–231, 1992

Sullivan MW, Rovee-Collier C, Tynes DN: A conditioning analysis of infant long-term memory. Child Dev 50:152–162, 1979

Suomi SJ: Models of depression in primates. Psychol Med 13:465–468, 1983

Terr L: Children of Chowchilla. Psychoanal Study Child 34:547–623, 1979

Terr L: Chowchilla revisited: the effects of psychic trauma four years after a school-bus kidnapping. Am J Psychiatry 140:1543–1550, 1983

Terr L: What happens to the memories of early childhood trauma? J Am Acad Child Adolesc Psychiatry 27:96–104, 1988

Terr LC: Childhood traumas: an outline and overview. Am J Psychiatry 148:10–20, 1991

van der Kolk BA: The separation cry and the trauma response: developmental issues in the psychobiology of attachment and separation, in Psychological Trauma. Washington, DC, American Psychiatric Press, 1987, pp 31–62

van der Kolk BA, Perry JC, Herman JL: Childhood origins of self-destructive behavior. Am J Psychiatry 148:1665–1671, 1991

World Health Organization: International Classification of Diseases, 10th Revision. Geneva, World Health Organization, 1992

Zeanah CH, Emde RN: Attachment disorders in infancy and childhood, in Child and Adolescent Psychiatry, 3rd Edition. Edited by Rutter M, Taylor E, Hersov L. Oxford, UK, Blackwell Scientific, 1994, pp 490–504

Zeanah CH, Mammen OK, Lieberman AF: Disorders of attachment, in Handbook of Infant Mental Health. Edited by Zeanah CH. New York, Guilford, 1993, pp 332–349

Zero to Three/National Center for Clinical Infant Programs Diagnostic Classification Task Force: Manual for the Diagnostic Classification of Mental Health and Developmental Disorders of Infancy and Early Childhood. Unpublished manuscript, Washington, DC, Zero to Three/National Center for Clinical Infant Programs, 1993

Chapter 20

Adoption: Its Benefits and Problems

Fady Hajal, M.D.

Adoption has existed throughout human history as a way of taking care of abandoned infants and children. The stories of Moses and of Oedipus attest to the presence of adoption in the early histories of Mediterranean peoples. The Babylonian Code of Hammurabi (1775 B.C.) is the earliest attempt to regulate its practice (Cole and Donley 1990). In modern times (post–World War II), and in the United States in particular, adoption has taken on new scope and dimensions, assuming new and unprecedented quantitative and qualitative features. Up to the 20th century the primary objective of adoption was to provide an infertile couple with the opportunity to raise a child. In that context the needs of the adults were paramount. In the 20th century, a new primary goal was set: that of providing for the needs of abandoned, neglected, and/or abused children (Hersov 1990). Some of these new features, such as cross-racial and transnational adoptions and adoptions of special needs children, have made adoption an even more challenging task for adoptees and adoptive families than it had been already. For some of these individuals and families, these features constitute additional sources of stress.

The rate of adoption by nonrelatives has gone up dramatically in the U.S. since World War II. The United States leads other countries in the number of adoptions (extrafamilial ones in particular). Although census data on adoption are lacking, the number of adopted children under age 18 in the U.S. was estimated to be 1.3 million (Zill 1985). This estimate represents roughly 2% of the child population in the U.S. Extrafamilial adoptions are estimated to constitute one-third of all adoptions; the remaining two-thirds of adoptions are intrafamilial (Hersov 1990). In the past 10 to 15 years, there has been a shift toward increasing rates of adoption of foreign-born children, of older children, and of children with "special needs." (The latter comprise children with significant problems or disabilities of a developmental, physical, or psychiatric nature, often including early histories of physical or sexual abuse, neglect, and significant physical or emotional deprivation.)

Many older adopted children are not relinquished by their parents voluntarily, but are forcibly taken away from their families following intervention by social services and the legal court system. In a number of these cases, and even in cases where parents have voluntarily relinquished their child at infancy or soon afterward, parents are petitioning the courts to have the child returned to their custody. Such requests are usually the beginning of a long process of custody litigation that can dramatically affect the child's emotional or physical well-being. The National Council for Adoption estimates that about 1% of the 30,000 adoptions a year in the U.S. are contested (Wilkerson 1992).

Adoption and Pathogenesis: Is There a Connection?

In the 1950s, studies and articles began to emerge in the clinical literature that focused on the emotional problems of adoptees, especially as evidenced by the overrepresentation of these persons in psychiatric clinical populations during childhood and adolescence (Brinich and Brinich 1982; Fullerton et al. 1986; Jerome 1986; Kim et al. 1988; Kotsopoulos et al. 1988; Piersma 1987; Rogeness et al. 1988; Schecter 1960; Schecter et al. 1964; Weiss 1984). Since that time, the question of the pathogenicity of adoption has loomed large in the field of adoption. The controversy remains very much alive today, and the question is an important one. Adoptees, adoptive parents, birth parents, social work professionals, mental health professionals, public policy–makers, ethicists, legislators, politicians, and governments have all become involved, and at times embroiled, in this debate over the advantages and risks of adoption.

Almost everybody recognizes that there are tremendous advantages to adoption. Those who benefit from adoption include 1) children that are left without caregivers committed to their well-being, nurturance, and support over a life span; 2) birth parents who find themselves saddled with an awesome responsibility that they feel unprepared or unable to carry out adequately (i.e., in the best interests of the child); and 3) adoptive parents who wish to add a child or children to their family and yet are unable to do so through their own reproductive means. At the social and public levels, adoption helps in providing a solution to the problem of abandoned, orphaned, abused, and/or neglected children, a solution universally held to be better (i.e., more advantageous) than alternatives such as childhood spent in orphanages, in institutions, and/or in a series of foster homes (Bohman and Sigvardsson 1990; Triseliotis and Hill 1990).

Although adoption presents many benefits, there has been a slanted focus in the recent clinical literature on the casualties, the problem cases that present with a confluence of clinical problems and an adoptive family member (generally the latter is the indexed patient or the symptomatic family member). It is important to note that adoption status does not automatically or even frequently lead to pathology. The majority of adoptees actually seem to turn out well adjusted. Studies comparing nonclinical adopted and nonadopted populations show that the two groups do not significantly differ along the psychological health–sickness continuum, even though adoptees seem to have greater adjustment problems (Brodzinsky et al. 1984a; Hersov 1985; Norvell and Guy 1977; Offord et al. 1969). Yet, adoptees are over-represented in clinical populations. This over-representation, however, may be related to complex factors, including attitudes of the adoptive parents toward adoption and the adoptee, and their greater-than-average tendency to use health care systems for the adoptee, partly related to the child's adoptive status and partly to their higher socioeconomic status (Brinich and Brinich 1982; Kirk et al. 1966). It may also be related to the reaction of health care givers to crisis situations involving adoptees and their adoptive parents. Health care givers may be biased, perceiving adoption as intrinsically traumatic and capable by itself of inducing deviant behavior to such a degree as to suggest (or even compel) a therapeutic intervention in most, if not all, cases. This over-representation may then represent patterns of referrals rather than necessarily or solely an increased rate of disturbance.

A Developmental, Life-Cycle Approach

It is generally recognized that adoption is a lifelong process involving several individuals and at least two family systems. Some of the individuals and families involved are visible, whereas others remain hidden and mysterious to one another. Therefore, adoption out of one family and into another is a major developmental interference and has immediate and/or delayed repercussions. These repercussions are triggered at each stage of the life cycle by new cognitive and dynamic configurations in the adoptee as well as in the family system.

In this chapter I focus on the unique developmental tasks that confront adopted children and adolescents and their families, and on the normative stresses they are likely to meet along the way. A helpful way of focusing on those supplemental tasks is to present them in the format of the "family life cycle outline" originally developed by Carter and McGoldrick (1980). This schema is organized around discrete phases in which families face specific tasks and elaborate specific patterns of organization until they come to a transition point where new tasks emerge and new structures are developed to carry out these tasks. It is during the transition from one stage to another, from one level of organization to another, that the risk for dysfunction is greatest and that symptoms appear (Hajal and Rosenberg 1991). Carter and McGoldrick's schema has been adapted to the stages of adoptive families by Hajal and Rosenberg (Table 20–1).

A central question faced by adoptive families is whether they are like any other (biologically formed) family, or whether the special way their family was constituted makes them different from other families. Kirk differentiates between adoptive families that "acknowledge" the difference and those that "reject" the difference (Kirk 1964). Most investigators and clinicians agree today that adoptive families are different. This difference is reflected in the additional tasks and challenges they face over the course of development (Hajal and Rosenberg 1991).

Circumstances of Birth and Adoption

Each phase of the life cycle potentially presents stress for the adoptee. At the outset, the circumstances of the biological mother's pregnancy may constitute a stress for her child. The emotional state of

Table 20–1. Adoptive families: life cycle outline (for traditional closed adoptions)

Phase	Emotional process of transition/prerequisite attitude	Developmental issues
Decision for adoption to take place	1. Accepting inability to reproduce successfully 2. Making decision to parent children outside bloodline	1. Accepting one's or spouse's inability to conceive 2. Differentiating between reproduction, sexual adequacy, and competence to parent 3. Dealing with spouse and extended family regarding genealogical discontinuity
Adoption process	Opening up oneself to public scrutiny	1. Affirming competence/self-regard 2. Seeking social validation of competence and adequacy regarding family formation/parenting 3. Mourning loss of bloodline
Adoption	1. Accepting new member into the family (child plus "images" of biological parents' families) 2. Child's managing transition from one family system to another	1. Mourning loss of fantasized biological child 2. Adjusting to instant parenthood 3. Effecting constitution of a "metafamily" 4. Bonding, for child as well as parents (and siblings, if any) 5. Accepting psychological parenthood (vs. genetic parenthood) 6. Realigning relationship with extended family to accept nonbiological child 7. Dealing with community attitudes toward adoption

Table 20–1. Adoptive families: life cycle outline (for traditional closed adoptions) *(continued)*

Phase	Emotional process of transition/prerequisite attitude	Developmental issues
Adoptive family with preschool-age child	Acknowledging adoption as a fact of family life by both parents and children	1. Disclosure of adoption: to tell or not to tell?; who, when, what, and how to tell? 2. Testing permanency of relationship 3. Dealing with responses to news of adoption
Adoptive family with latency-age child	Same as for with preschool-age child, in relation to extra-familial environment	1. "Family romance" fantasy stage: dealing with having two family sets, child's wish/fear of biological parents' contact, and parents' concerns about being good enough 2. Struggling with ambivalence-splitting and anxiety about being "returned" 3. Dealing with community reactions to the adoptive status of child
Adoptive family with adolescent child	1. Increasing flexibility of family boundaries 2. Accepting a different model of family (psychological vs. genetic bonding) 3. Accepting identity as combination of genetic base and adoptive upbringing 4. Maintaining sexual boundaries in the absence of firm incest taboo	1. Separation-individuation issues: achieving independence, not eviction 2. Differentiating between nuclear family and meta-family 3. Accepting adolescent interest in biological family as a help in the development of a stable identity 4. Struggling with sexual identity issues—images of biological parents vs. adoptive parents 5. Recontracting: adolescent's and parents' accepting adoption on both parts

Table 20–1. Adoptive families: life cycle outline (for traditional closed adoptions) *(continued)*

Phase	Emotional process of transition/prerequisite attitude	Developmental issues
Adoptive family with young adult	1. Accepting a multitude of exits from and entries into the family system 2. Coming to terms with "genealogical bewilderment" 3. Dealing with young adult's ability to reproduce and attach to blood relative	1. Establishing genealogical continuity if search for biological parent(s) is successful 2. Reaffirming ties within adoptive family 3. Recontracting: accepting adoption on both parts 4. Ensuring that potential mates are not biological siblings
Adoptive family in later life	1. Accepting shifting of generational roles 2. Taking care of adoptive parents	1. Disclosing one's adoption to one's own children 2. Dealing with genealogical discontinuity in one's and adoptive parents' lives 3. Adoptive parents' mourning biological progeny

the mother during a pregnancy, particularly if she had not wanted to become pregnant, can affect the fetus directly or indirectly. In addition, the prospective mother who had not wanted to become pregnant is often struggling with the decision of whether to keep the baby or whether to put it up for adoption. The quality of the fetal environment is directly related to her effort to create and maintain an optimal nutritional and humoral environment for her baby. Abstinence from alcohol and other substances that might harm the fetus is crucial, as is a regimen of good prenatal care.

Another potential source of stress for the child is the manner of transfer from the birth family and environment to the adoptive family. Distress is minimal when there is a smooth and early transition from birth mother to adoptive family. There is an increasing, yet still limited, trend to accomplish this transfer in an atmosphere of openness instead of the secrecy that has shrouded these transactions tradition-ally. The open adoption paradigm encourages contact between the birth parent(s) and the adoptive parents. The extent of the contact varies greatly from case to case and may include extensive contacts before birth, the presence of the adoptive couple during birth, and/or repeated and lifelong contacts among various members of the two families. In the case of an agreed-upon open adoption, the adoptive parents can prepare for the child to join their family and are able to bond with the baby almost from the time he or she is in the delivery suite. In addition, they will have a better sense of the physical and psychosocial backgrounds of the baby whom they are adopting than is the case with closed-records adoptions, in which secretiveness and a sense of mystery prevail.

When the baby is not transferred to its adoptive home in the early weeks or months of life, the adoption has the potential to be associ-ated with more stress. Much has been written about the deleterious effects of late adoptions on the mental and emotional health of the child (Frankel 1991; Fullerton et al. 1986; Murray 1984; Offord et al. 1969; Piersma 1987; Sorosky et al. 1975). Clinicians and investigators traditionally have classified adoption as early (child adopted before age 1 year or even 6 months) or late (child adopted after age 1 year and up to age 10–11 years, or even, yet rarely, in adolescence). The child in these cases will have established one or more attachments within his or her birth family. The longer an adoptee has lived with birth parents, siblings, and/or other relatives, the harder it will be for him or her to relinquish these focused attachments and to experience a smooth integration into his or her adoptive environment. Many of these children do not want to be adopted and, as a result, will have a harder time settling in with their new family. Adopted parents will need much more preparation than is usually provided. Older adoptees will likely keep alive in their minds the memory of their birth relatives, setting the stage for a more intense splitting of the two families (one bad, one good, in a fixed way or alternately) than one usually finds in adoptive families. When this occurs, adoptive parenting will most likely be more arduous and challenging than it usually is (Frankel 1991; Hersov 1990).

Furthermore, the circumstances of the birth environment of the older adoptee often constitute major stress or even traumatizing fac-tors. Abuse and neglect constitute major sources of stress that may affect the adoptee in significant and sometimes irreversible ways.

Other major sources of stress are years spent in an orphanage (as is the case in most foreign adoptions) or in a series of foster homes. Difficulty in trusting others and in establishing close relationships may lead some adoptees into a life of loneliness, isolation, and despair. The hope of all parties involved is that these adoptees will find a good fit with their adoptive homes, and the kind of nurturant, supportive environment that may compensate for the deficiencies in their earlier life, to help repair the harm done by months or years of abuse or neglect.

As the baby (or the older child) settles into the new home, the challenge of fitting in and accomplishing a smooth integration can vary in difficulty. The transition may be easy if the baby (child) matches the parents temperamentally, intellectually, and socioculturally. The parents usually find it easier to accommodate to a child whom they can identify as being like them—one who matches their fantasied idea of the biological child they would have had, had they been able to conceive. The greater the number of or the extent of differences between the adoptee and the adoptive parents, the harder is the adjustment. Mismatches between adoptees and adoptive parents have often been cited as a major cause of difficulties in adoptive families in the periods of latency and adolescence of the adoptee. An incompatibility of temperaments between parents and child is associated with an increased risk of intrafamilial conflict (Weiss 1984). Parental discontent may arise not only from specific sources such as a child's learning disability, school failure, delinquent acting out, impulsive behavior, and so forth, but also from the parents' unstated disappointment resulting from the discrepancy between the adoptee and their idealized fantasy biological child.

Conflict About Adoption

Another source of stress for the adoptee relates to the degree of acceptance that he or she receives from his or her extended adoptive family. Many adoptees are made to feel unwelcome by the relatives of their adoptive parents, being reminded every so often of their "foreign" status in the family. As a result they perceive themselves as second-class citizens. This experience can be intensified by the presence of biological children of their adoptive parents in the sibship. Some adoptees react by feeling like intruders in the family and live a somewhat isolated, alienated life within the family. This situation may be compounded when the adoptee comes from a different ethnic or racial background, or even a different gender, from that of the rest of his or her siblings.

Another source of potential stress is the degree to which adoptive parents have worked through their feelings and conflicts about their inability to conceive and their decision to adopt. An adoptee (baby or older child) who enters a home that is smoldering with conflicts may eventually be resented when he or she presents the slightest hint of difficulty. Developmental conflicts are often misread and transformed into major long-term conflicts between parents and child, perpetuated by the underlying parental conflicts over the need to adopt (Austad and Simmons 1978). The adoptee becomes by then a pawn in the marital conflict, an easy target for scapegoating and blaming. When this occurs, an often irreversible wedge is created between the adoptee and the adoptive parents.

Disclosure of Adoptive Status

The next major challenge facing adoptive families is the question of disclosing the fact of adoption to the child (MacIntyre and Donovan 1990). Parents struggle with questions such as when to tell the child and what to tell him or her. They agonize over how the child will react. McWhinnie (1969) has described three periods when children bring up the question of their origins in discussions with their parents. Between ages 3 and 5, children engage their parents in spontaneous questioning looking for simple factual information about their origins, the birth process, and so forth. Another time when adoptees bring home questions about their earliest past occurs around ages 9 to 10, when children engage in discussions with their peers about parentage and families. This period, which McWhinnie calls the phase of "Family Romance," is a time of potential crisis in the family. Finally, during adolescence the adoptee's preoccupation with birth family and the facts of his or her adoption raise anew the risk of crisis in the adoptive relationship, as will be described below. Adoptive parents must be prepared to tackle these difficult questions with their children, which includes being prepared for the strong feelings of fear, anger, shame, sadness, and the like that such questions inevitably provoke in the parents.

The general practice has been to begin early—when the child is between the ages of 2 and 4—telling adoptees about their origins. Usually, the stories told adoptees emphasize the warm reception in their adoptive home. These accounts are variations on the theme of the child's being chosen by the adoptive parents, including some cursory remarks about a birth mother (or birth parents) who was (were) unable to care for the child and who did well by allowing the adoptive parents to take care of the baby. Children at this age generally react minimally or even positively to the several versions of the chosen-baby story that they are told (Schwartz 1975).

It is only around ages 7 to 8, when a child's concept of reciprocity develops, that he or she begins to understand that being chosen has as its reverse being given up, because, the child surmises, he or she was not valued enough to keep (Brodzinsky et al. 1984b). It is at this point that adoptive status begins to be associated with ideas of badness of the self, or badness of the parents (birth parents as well as adoptive parents), and of feeling oneself marginalized, not belonging anywhere and not truly connected to the people one is living with, or in fact to anybody. Issues of loss become paramount from that time on (Brodzinsky 1990). This may be the first time that the child will feel acutely the loss of the birth family. This feeling of loss may be experienced as the loss of that fantasy of the birth parents that the child had elaborated and cherished in earlier years. The child had perceived his birth parents positively, believing, for instance, that they cared so much about him and that they relinquished him only out of love. Now, the child perceives the birth parents in a negative light: they gave him up, the child surmises, because they did not care about him, or because he was bad and they did not love him enough. A related fear (fantasy) develops here in the adoptee: the fear that his biological parents will come to claim him back and thus disrupt his relationships within his adoptive family. This negative perception of birth parents may eventually contaminate adoptees' perceptions of their adoptive parents. Some adoptees develop fantasies that their adoptive parents stole them from their birth family, or adopted them for purely selfish reasons.

The impact of these losses, and of other losses related to adoption in general, is aggravated by the fact that they go unmourned, because they are suppressed by the adoptee for fear of hurting others in the adoptive family. Adoptees are afraid of expressing their feelings of loss of their birth parents out of loyalty to their adoptive parents lest it be felt by the adoptive parents as ungratefulness (Berman and Bufferd 1986).

The cognitive realization that she has been relinquished by her birth parents ("real parents," as adoptees at this age often think of them, as opposed to the "fake" parents they are living with) leads the child to question the solidity and permanency of all parental ties. She may feel like a disposable commodity: discarded once, she could be so again. Hence the testing behavior that adoptive parents often describe during the latency years of their adopted children, when the children's provocative behavior seems designed to defiantly check the limits of tolerance of their parents. "How far do I have to go before you break down and get rid of me the way my birth parents did," the child appears to be asking himself and his parents. The adoptee's anxiety over the revocability of parent-child ties and the fear of dissolution of the adoption is a major source of tension in some families during latency. Often, it continues unabated into adolescence, making the child's teenage years a very difficult time for many adoptive families.

Another source of stress during the latency phase follows the sense of status loss felt by adoptees when their adoptive status becomes known to people around them. They experience not only a sense of being different but also a sense of not being as good as other children. This sense of inferiority may lead them to identify with troubled, problem children in their school or neighborhood, or to gravitate toward peers of socioeconomic status lower than theirs, creating a wedge between them and their disconcerted or disapproving parents. If not handled well, these conflicts can mushroom into more serious splits between adoptees and their parents during adolescence. From this background may develop a negative identity in the adolescent in later years.

Adoption and Learning Problems

Yet another source of stress during the latency phase occurs in cases where the adoptee exhibits learning difficulties and/or problems with impulse control (often consistent with a diagnosis of attention-deficit/hyperactivity disorder). During latency, adoptees are more at risk than nonadoptees of developing learning problems (Elonen and Schwartz 1969). A number of hypotheses have been advanced to explain this development. One hypothesis is that the secrecy that prevails around the facts of the adoption, or around feelings about the adoption, may lead to an inhibition of curiosity and of the impulse to learn. Another suggestion is that either the adoptive parents' fantasy that the child comes from a family of lower standing, or their own feelings of inadequacy (related to infertility), are projected onto the child, resulting in a self-fulfilling expectation that the child will not amount to much. Finally, there is the real possibility that poor pre-natal care and higher perinatal risks may have led to a mild degree of cerebral insult, producing an organically based developmental learn-ing disability (Kernberg 1985). In the latter case, learning problems are often associated with attention-deficit/hyperactivity disorder. The combination can be highly stressful, because it creates complications and conflicts for the child in both home and school environments, leaving him or her no respite from pressures to act better. Stein and Hoopes (1985) point out that subtle learning and behavioral distur-bances caused by neurodevelopmental problems in the adoptee may lead to "tragic family dysfunction" in light of the additional stresses that adoptive status imposes on these families.

The Question of Origins

Two questions haunt adopted children from latency onward: Who were my parents? Why did they give me up? These issues affect adoptees in a number of areas: cognitive performance (giving rise to learning inhibitions), relations with other family members, and, ulti-mately, sense of identity and self-esteem (Kernberg 1985). These ef-fects are modified or shaped by the child's temperament, experience, development, and environment.

The child's image of the circumstances of his or her conception and birth may also affect his or her attitude. A child who perceives himself or herself as the product of a loving relationship may weather these issues better than one who believes that he or she is the out-come of a violent act or the victim of parents who were irresponsible or unable to care for him or her.

Children develop their own narratives and continue to revise them as they grow older and more knowledgeable. These narratives and re-visions will serve to give meaning to each adoptee's predicament. Much of the stress of adoption can be related to the confusion gener-ated by the secrecy surrounding their origins that produces feelings of isolation, low self-esteem, lack of trust, and a preoccupation with fantasy (Lifton 1988). The adoptee's beliefs about his or her origins need to be confronted and integrated by all members of the adoptive family throughout the life cycle.

Adoption Crisis and Adolescence

During adolescence, the life cycle tasks of the adoptee and of his or her parents clash head on in a pattern that tends to aggravate tensions, widen the parent-adolescent gap, and create areas of special risk. The confluence of the developmental crisis of adolescence and adoptive status (for an individual and a family) can generate a highly flammable, explosive mixture for some adopted adolescents, rendering them more vulnerable to the eruption of behavioral or psychological disturbances. The synergistic effects of adolescence and adoptive status that lead to spiraling, escalating reactions of the adoptee and his or her family when conflicts and issues typical of this developmental stage begin to arise can turn this stage of the life cycle into a particularly trying time for adoptees and their adoptive families.

Four major areas in which a circular pattern of interactions complicates the resolution of an adolescent crisis for adoptees and their parents are considered here. These areas are genealogical discontinuity, identity formation, separation–individuation (or emancipation), and sexual development.

Genealogical Discontinuity

The adoptee's awareness of genealogical discontinuity is made more acute by the emergence of genital and procreative capacities in the adolescent; by a better awareness of biological links between generations; by the emergence of a sense of historical continuity (intra- and intergenerational), otherwise described as family life cycling; and finally by the physical changes that give the adolescent his or her definitive "looks."

In adolescence, adoptees' curiosity about their ancestry crystallizes in a desire to obtain information about their biological background, the adoption process, their genealogical history, and their birth family history. This curiosity comes about naturally in many adoptees. It is most likely related to new cognitive awareness of biological-historical continuity (one's "life cycle"). It is important to differentiate curiosity from the initiation of actual search behavior that usually comes later. Rarely do adolescents set out to search for their biological parents, even though they may spend an inordinate amount of time thinking about birth parents (Lifton 1988).

At the same time as their curiosity crystallizes, these adolescents experience an intensification of the family romance; they invest increasing amounts of energy and time in thinking about birth parents (the birth mother in particular). Dissatisfaction with oneself and with one's current adoptive family situation translates into wishing to be with one's birth family and dreaming about what things would have been like if one had gone on living and growing up with them (appeal of the "road not taken"). A "splitting" of parental sets is part of the same process, with the adolescent investing his or her current family with all the dark, negative feelings and energy (Fullerton et al. 1986). When tensions increase between adolescents and their adoptive parents, the wish to search can be used as a threat.

Confronted with their adolescents' genealogical preoccupations, adoptive parents often react negatively, perceiving their child's preoccupation as disloyalty and a sign of ungratefulness. The parents fear these preoccupations, for they perceive that their child is questioning the permanency of their relationship. Will they be abandoned by their child, back to the loneliness and feeling of deprivation of their earlier marital years when, in their struggle to conceive, they may have acutely felt the absence of children in their lives (Sorosky et al. 1980)? Their reaction can be one of intense fear and also anger. This reaction further strains their relationship with the adolescent and darkens the prospects of a positive resolution of the adoptive-adolescent crisis. The reaction of fear and particularly anger has led some adoptive parents to consider or seek the dissolution of adoption. These requests, and the rates of dissolution (or disruption) of the adoption, have gone up since the increase in the rates of adoption of older children and of children with special needs. As many as 10% of such adoptions were found to have been disrupted (Barth 1988; Festinger 1990).

Generally, however, it is important to remember that, search behavior notwithstanding, there is a strengthening of parent-child relationship after adolescence. Even adolescents and young adults who have searched and reunited with birth parent(s) will report an improvement in their relationship with their adoptive family. It is as if, at this point in their life, adoptees can truly and voluntarily "adopt" their adoptive parents (to use an expression coined by P. Kernberg [1985]).

Identity Crisis

As adopted adolescents grapple with such questions as "who am I" and "what sort of person am I becoming," they begin to feel that an essential part of themselves, their ancestry, is cut off. They become more acutely aware of differences in physique between them and their adoptive relatives. These differences imply to them deeper-seated dif- ferences in "genetic" structure. A sense of differentness pervades their feeling of being in the family. Alienation from both their adop- tive family and their biological roots leaves them in a state described by some as "genealogical bewilderment"—feeling rootless and searching for clues, while surrounded by invisible "hereditary ghosts," with many hereditary "unknowns" (Sants 1964; Toussieng 1962). A dual identity may emerge out of this cauldron of secrecy, uncertainty, and doubts, including a false (adoptive) self and a true (hidden because forbidden) self linked in fantasy to one's birth family (Lifton 1988). Possible negative outcomes of this process of frus- trated or distorted identity formation include 1) the development of a negative identity; 2) persistent feelings of insecurity and worthless- ness, and a depressive core; or, in some, 3) a sense of entitlement (they feel that they are "owed" things because they have been victim- ized, cheated by nature and society) (Fullerton et al. 1986; Lifton 1988; Tooley 1978; Wellisch 1952). Some of these feeling states lead to acting-out behavior to which adopted adolescents in distress all too often resort. The typical clinical psychiatric picture of the adopted adolescent in trouble is that of the adolescent with an exter- nalizing type of symptomatology and psychopathology, as found in the various forms of disruptive disorders. The typical diagnoses applied to adoptees are oppositional defiant disorder, attention-deficit/hyperac- tivity disorder, conduct disorders (from mild to severe forms), and, later, personality disorders (with impulsive, borderline, and/or anti- social traits).

Many adoptive parents, when faced with their child's identity crisis and alienation from them, will resonate (respond) with their own cri- sis of self-doubt regarding their identity and adequacy as parents (McWhinnie 1969). We have to remember that a number of parents will continue to feel that their parenthood is a socially ascribed role that was conferred on them by sociolegal means, rather than "natu- rally" acquired and thus legitimately earned. The conflicts between adoptee and adoptive parents are exacerbated when the parents (and adoptees) are unable to accept the differences between adoptive and biological parenthood, ending up with a devaluation of "psychological" ties, and undue glorification of "blood" ties, thus delegitimizing their authority and their rights and responsibilities. Lifton (1988, p. 262), herself an adoptee, reminds us that the ties that bind us are those of the heart.

Parents will also respond with an intensification of "genetic" anxieties regarding their adopted children. "Hereditary ghosts" haunt them as well as their adopted children. Fear of transmitted "bad blood" and of inherited immorality are all too frequent occurrences in these parents and families (Sorosky et al. 1980). These fears and concerns about hereditary differences may constitute an obstruction to intimacy—an obstacle to the establishment of a close empathic relationship between adoptees and adoptive parents.

Adoptees are generally not directly expressive of their preoccupations in this area; they act out instead their negative identity, their sense of badness and worthlessness. Their parents, on the other hand, can be very open about their "genetic anxieties." One parent, for instance, requested chromosome analysis on his adopted son.

Separation–Individuation (Emancipation)

Autonomy, for some of these adolescents, means the opportunity to "choose" or "reject" their adoptive parents, and other authority figures as well (Fullerton et al. 1986). What they show, however, is an intensification of their dependency conflicts, sometimes leading to counterdependent and inappropriate pseudo-autonomous actions. Given their sense of alienation from their family, their pressing wish for biological rootedness, and the ongoing interpersonal difficulties with their parents, a heightened sense of insecurity seems to predominate, including fears of rejection. They may perceive their parents as elusive and unreliable and, as a result, may set off on a search for stable objects (Sorosky et al. 1980).

On the other side, adoptive parents often will experience difficulty accepting the adolescent's separation and autonomy strivings. These strivings stir up in them fears of rejection or abandonment by the adolescent, as well as a reawakening of preadoptive feelings of isolation and loneliness. They may react to the threat of the adolescent's walking out of the relationship by infantilizing the adolescent or by becoming overprotective and/or permissive toward their child, all out of fear of losing their child's love, and as an attempt (sometimes a desperate one) to hold on to the child, or, more accurately, to induce—or seduce—the child to hold on to them. This reaction leads to anxiety, as well as in some cases a sense of omnipotence, in adoptees (Elonen and Schwartz 1969). Parental splitting and detachment constitute another type of reaction that can have disastrous implications, possibly leading to a precipitated emotional or physical cut-off, freezing the child out of the family, and thus increasing the adoptee's sense of total isolation and nonconnectedness.

Sexual Development

The lack of automatic incest barrier in the adoptive family may lead to an inhibition of sexual impulses and a slowing down of sexual emancipation and growth (Easson 1970). Fears of incestuous union with unknown biological relatives may inhibit adoptive adolescents' sexual activities. Also, adoptees may have fears of being rejected by potential dates or mates because of their adoptive status (Sorosky et al. 1980). Adoptive parents often overreact to expressions of sexuality and aggression in their adopted children. These reactions are based on their anxiety about the adoptee's following on the footsteps of his or her birth parents. Fusion of the adolescent's sexuality with actual (or assumed) illegitimacy in the child's background clearly triggers these fears and complicates parents' adjustment to their child's developing sexuality. In addition, there may be competitiveness and envy of the adolescent's blossoming sexuality and generativity (reproductive power), with the adolescent's sexuality and generativity acting not only as a counterpoint to the parents' waning sexuality but also as a reminder of the parents' inability to conceive, whether from infertility or for other reasons. The lack of an automatic incest barrier may put additional strain in the parent-child relationship, for some tempting parent and adolescent into some sort of sexual activity and for others leading them to increase the physical and emotional distance between them in order to resist giving in to sexual impulses. All of these issues may result in the adoptive adolescent's experiencing difficulties in assuming a stable sexual identity. Finally, there may be a blurring of generational roles related to an increased age difference between parents and child that increases the generational gap between them, leading the parents to take on a more moralistic, inhibiting, grandparent-type role with their adopted children.

The following letter, written by an adoptee to her unknown birth mother about whom she knew very little, illustrates the kinds of issues and questions that adopted adolescents struggle with in relation to their definition of self and to their conflicted concerns about their adoptive family and their birth family:

Dear . . .

Hi, how are you? My name is Beth and I'm your daughter. For about 4 years now, I have been really thinking about you. I have many questions that I need to ask you. I will list them and hopefully you will be able to answer them. Why did you leave me? Did you try to keep me? Who's my father? Do you think of me? Will I ever see you? Was I planned? Am I a mistake? Do I have brothers/sisters? What do you look like? What are your hobbies? Those are just some of the questions. I don't want to lay them all on you in one letter.

I guess I better tell you some things about myself. Well, I'm 15 years now. I'm a junior in high school. I play the guitar, clarinet and a little of the piano. I play soccer, basketball, softball, and swim during the summer. I heard you used to swim also. I also like to read and write. I guess I should also tell you a major issue that is about me. I am in a hospital. The reasons that I am here are for family problems, depression, self-destructiveness, suicide. I hope you are not in any way disappointed in me. I don't want you to feel guilty or anything but I think the center reason why I'm here is because I'm adopted. I don't know what kind of situation you were in when you got pregnant with me but you probably had a hard time deciding what to do. I know your parents, my grandparents, were divorced and you probably had money problems but I just want you to know even though you put me up for adoption I love you. You might not believe me but you are and always will be my real mother. You're the one who brought me into this world and I'll always love you.

One thing that I am afraid of is that you may not love me or even care about me. You might think that sounds ridiculous but that's how I feel.

I don't really know what else to write. I guess I'll tell you a little more about myself, well I'm 5′ 10″; I wear glasses, hopefully contacts soon; I've modeled before for a magazine. It was fun, but it was hard work. When I get older I hope to work with deaf kids. I used to want to be a physical therapist but then I found out how much science I needed, and forgot that idea. I have a lot of friends. Some are good and some are bad. I plan to hang around the better crowd in the future. Well I'm going to end this letter. I don't want to but it had to end sometime. So I hope to see you soon and re-member I love you.

Love always,
Beth
A.K.A. Joan [her presumed preadoptive name]

Protective Aspect of Adoption

Before this chapter closes, it is important to address the question of the protective dimension of adoption. Are there specific protective aspects to adoption, particularly for the "children of antisocial, or otherwise socially handicapped parents" placed early in infancy? Does adoption protect these children from later "social maladjustment"? Bohman and Sigvardsson (1990) carried out prospective outcome studies comparing adopted children, children placed for adoption but later returned to their biological mother, children placed in long-term foster homes, and control subjects. These authors concluded that growing up in a stable adoptive family seems to protect children against the risk of social incompetence and maladjustment, particularly when the family is well prepared psychologically for the task of rearing a nonbiological child.

Triseliotis and Hill (1990) identified factors that helped children who were in substitute forms of care achieve a clear sense of identity and a sense of security. These factors included "the quality of caring and attachments experienced in childhood, the knowledge and aware-ness about their heritage, genealogy, and personal history, and finally their experience of how other people perceive them and behave toward them and how they see themselves in relation to the rest of society" (p. 111). Triseliotis and Hill, too, believe that children growing up in adoptive homes achieve by adulthood a stronger sense of self and ap-pear to function more adequately at the personal, social, and eco-nomic levels when compared with similar children who were in foster care or who grew up in institutions. They also believe that adoption has a greater potential to reverse or compensate for earlier adverse circumstances than does foster or residential care. The impact of these early negative experiences can fade away when adoption allows the establishment of new positive attachments. (Triseliotis and Hill 1990).

Sorosky et al. (1980) have described factors that were found by these authors to correlate with good adult adjustment of adoptees. These factors included adoption at an early age, early awareness of being adopted, open channels of communication with adoptive parents, ease in being able to discuss birth parents, and, finally, the presence of siblings within the adoptive home.

Conclusions

Adoptive families differ from biologically formed nuclear and extended families. Yet, the frequent denial of, confusion about, and lack of appreciation for the exact nature of these differences cause additional stress for the adoptive family and the adoptee.

Adoptive families have attracted little attention from family therapists. They are rarely referred to in the family therapy literature. Some recent work has begun to correct this situation (Berman and Bufferd 1986; Hartman and Laird 1990; Reitz and Watson 1992; Schaffer and Lindstrom 1990).

Perhaps the pervasive changes that have affected the family structure of the American family, such as the increased prevalence and acceptance of divorce, of stepfamilies, of single-parent families, and of the ethnic diversity among families, have led to a more attentive and sympathetic perspective on adoptive families. The paradigmatic change that we are witnessing in the adoption field, the slow yet steady shift from sealed records adoptions to open adoptions, may have been facilitated by the toleration of diverse forms of family structure in the U.S. If children, in their postdivorce and remarriage families, can relate in constructive ways to several households and many layers of relatives and nonrelatives in their often very complicated stepfamilies, why could adoptees not be able to relate simultaneously to birth parents and adoptive parents in constructive and development-enhancing ways? We may be at the threshold of such a revolutionary change in the field of adoption. Some may argue that we have actually crossed that threshold and are well into the new era, one in which some of the traditional stresses associated with adoption will no longer be operative, but in which a new set of stresses may arise.

References

Austad C, Simmons T: Symptoms of adopted children presenting to a large mental health clinic. Child Psychiatry Hum Dev 9(1):20–27, 1978

Barth RP: Disruption in older child adoptions. Public Welfare 6(1):23–29, 1988

Berman LC, Bufferd RK: Family treatment to address loss in adoptive families. Social Caseworker 67:3–11, 1986

Bohman M, Sigvardsson S: Outcome in adoption: lessons from longitudinal studies, in The Psychology of Adoption. Edited by Brodzinsky DM, Schecter MD. New York, Oxford University Press, 1990, pp 93–106

Brinich P, Brinich E: Adoption and adaptation. J Nerv Ment Dis 170:489–493, 1982

Brodzinsky DM: A stress and coping model of adoption adjustment, in The Psychology of Adoption. Edited by Brodzinsky DM, Schecter MD. New York, Oxford University Press, 1990, pp 3–24

Brodzinsky DM, Schecter DE, Braff AM, et al: Psychological and academic adjustment in adopted children. J Consult Clin Psychol 52:582–590, 1984a

Brodzinsky DM, Singer LM, Braff AM: Children's understanding of adoption. Child Dev 55:869–878, 1984b

Carter EA, McGoldrick M: The family life cycle and family therapy: an overview, in The Family Life Cycle: A Framework for Family Therapy. Edited by Carter EA, McGoldrick M. New York, Gardner Press, 1980, pp 3–20

Cole ES, Donley KS: History, values, and placement policy issues in adoption, in The Psychology of Adoption. Edited by Brodzinsky DM, Schecter MD. New York, Oxford University Press, 1990, pp 273–294

Easson WM: Special sexual problems of the adopted adolescent. Medical Aspects of Human Sexuality 7(7):92–105, 1970

Elonen A, Schwartz E: A longitudinal study of emotional, social, and academic functioning of adopted children. Child Welfare 68(2):72–78, 1969

Festinger T: Adoption disruption: rates and correlates, in The Psychology of Adoption. Edited by Brodzinsky DM, Schecter MD. New York, Oxford University Press, 1990, pp 201–218

Frankel SA: Pathogenic factors in the experience of early and late adopted children. Psychoanal Study Child 46:91–108, 1991

Fullerton C, Goodrich W, Berman LB: Adoption predicts psychiatric treatment resistances in hospitalized adolescents. Journal of the American Academy of Child Psychiatry 25:541–551, 1986

Hajal F, Rosenberg EB: The family life cycle in adoptive families. Am J Orthopsychiatry 61:78–85, 1991

Hartman A, Laird J: Family treatment after adoption: common themes, in The Psychology of Adoption. Edited by Brodzinsky DM, Schecter MD. New York, Oxford University Press, 1990, pp 221–239

Hersov L: Adoption and fostering, in Child and Adolescent Psychiatry: Modern Approaches, 2nd Edition. Edited by Rutter M, Hersov L. Oxford, UK, Blackwell Scientific, 1985, pp 101–117

Hersov L: The Seventh Jack Tizard Memorial Lecture: aspects of adoption. J Child Psychol Psychiatry 31:493–510, 1990

Jerome L: Overrepresentation of adopted children attending a children's mental health center. Can J Psychiatry 31:526–531, 1986

Kernberg P: Child analysis with a severely disturbed adopted child. International Journal of Psychoanalytic Psychotherapy 11:277–299, 1985

Kim WJ, Davenport C, Joseph L, et al: Psychiatric disorders and juvenile delinquency in adopted children and adolescents. J Am Acad Child Adolesc Psychiatry 27:111–115, 1988

Kirk HD: Shared Fate. New York, Free Press, 1964

Kirk HD, Jonassohn KJ, Fish AD: Are adopted children especially vulnerable to stress. Arch Gen Psychiatry 14:292–298, 1966

Kotsopoulos S, Cote A, Joseph L, et al: Psychiatric disorders in adopted children: a controlled study. Am J Orthopsychiatry 58:608–612, 1988

Lifton BJ: Lost and Found. New York, Harper & Row, 1988

MacIntyre JC, Donovan DM: Resolved: children should be told of their adoption before they ask (Debate Forum). J Am Acad Child Adolesc Psychiatry 29:828–833, 1990

McWhinnie AM: The adopted child in adolescence, in Adolescence: Psychosocial Perspectives. Edited by Caplan G, Lebovici S. New York, Basic Books, 1969, pp 133–142

Murray L: A review of selected foster care–adoption research from 1978 to mid-1982. Child Welfare 63(2):113–124, 1984

Norvell M, Guy RF: A comparison of self-concept in adopted and non-adopted adolescents. Adolescence 12:443–448, 1977

Offord DR, Aponte JF, Cross LA: Presenting symptomatology of adopted children. Arch Gen Psychiatry 20:110–116, 1969

Piersma H: Adopted children and inpatient psychiatric treatment: a retrospective study. Psychiatric Hospital 18(4):153–158, 1987

Reitz M, Watson KW: Adoption and the Family System. New York, Guilford, 1992

Rogeness G, Hoppe S, Macedo C, et al: Psychopathology in hospitalized, adopted children. J Am Acad Child Adolesc Psychiatry 27:628–631, 1988

Sants HJ: Genealogical bewilderment in children with substitute parents. Br J Med Psychol 37:133–141, 1964

Schaffer J, Lindstrom C: Brief solution-focused therapy with adoptive families, in The Psychology of Adoption. Edited by Brodzinsky DM, Schecter MD. New York, Oxford University Press, 1990, pp 240–252

Schecter MD: Observations of adopted children. Arch Gen Psychiatry 3:21–31, 1960

Schecter MD, Carlson PV, Simmons JQ: Emotional problems in the adopted. Arch Gen Psychiatry 10:109–118, 1964

Schwartz EM: Problems after adoption: some guidelines for pediatrician involvement. J Pediatr 87:991–994, 1975

Sorosky AD, Baran A, Pannor R: Identity conflicts in adoptees. Am J Orthopsychiatry 45:18–27, 1975

Sorosky AD, Baran A, Pannor R: Adoption, in Comprehensive Textbook of Psychiatry/IV, 4th Edition, Vol 3. Edited by Kaplan HI, Freedman AM, Sadock BJ. Baltimore, MD, Williams & Wilkins, 1980, pp 2754–2759

Stein L, Hoopes J: Identity Formation in the Adopted Adolescent. New York, Child Welfare League of America, 1985

Tooley KM: The remembrance of things past. Am J Orthopsychiatry 48:174–189, 1978

Toussieng P: Thoughts regarding the etiology of psychological difficulties in adopted children. Child Welfare 41(2):59–65, 1962

Triseliotis J, Hill M: Contrasting adoption, foster care, and residential rearing, in The Psychology of Adoption. Edited by Brodzinsky DM, Schecter MD. New York, Oxford University Press, 1990, pp 107–120

Weiss A: Parent-child relationships of adopted adolescents in a psychiatric hospital. Adolescence 19:77–88, 1984

Wellisch E: Children without genealogy: a problem of adoption. Mental Health 13(1):41–42, 1952

Wilkerson I: Custody battle: is conception parenthood? New York Times, December 27, 1992, p. 20

Zill N: Behavior and learning problems among adopted children: findings from a U.S. national survey of child health. Paper presented at the meeting for the Society for Research in Child Development, Toronto, April 1985

Chapter 21

Family Transitions as Stressors in Children and Adolescents

Gene H. Brody, Ph.D.
Eileen Neubaum, M.S.

Parental divorce and remarriage are common experiences among American children in the 1990s. According to U.S. Bureau of the Census figures from 1989 (cited in Amato and Keith 1991), over 1 million children experience parental divorce each year. Estimates project that more than one-third of the children born during the past two decades will see their parents divorce (Grych and Fincham 1992). Using data obtained from the National Survey of Children, Furstenberg (1988) found that one-third of those age 16 and younger who had been born to married parents no longer lived with both biological parents. Using the same data, he further estimated that almost one-half of all children will spend some portion of their childhood living in families that do not include both biological parents. Furthermore, Glick (1984) estimated that 35% of all children born in the United States in the early 1980s will live in stepfamilies for some portion of their childhood. It is therefore likely that mental health professionals will at some point encounter children who have gone through these transitions in the past or are currently negotiating them (Grych and Fincham 1992).

To provide optimal support for children who are adapting to their parents' marital transitions, professionals must understand the nature of such transitions and have some idea of the challenges children face in adapting to these transitions. It was formerly believed that children who experienced parental divorce would be deeply and permanently harmed by the experience, and even today some agree with that assessment. Many of the research studies on parental divorce, however, suggest that the effects are less pronounced than was previously expected and to some extent time limited. Accordingly, it should not be assumed that children who have experienced their parents' marital transitions will automatically suffer from permanent, serious damage as a consequence. It is true, though, that the experiences of parental divorce and remarriage require children and adolescents to make numerous adjustments that affect many areas of their lives. Any life change of this magnitude is almost certain to be stressful for the person who is undergoing it.

The Nature of Marital Transitions

Professionals who work with divorcing families have begun to realize that divorce is not an isolated event taking place at a particular point in time, but rather a *process* (Emery 1988; Forehand 1992; Forehand et al. 1988; Grych and Fincham 1992; Hetherington et al. 1982; Wallerstein et al. 1988). For a considerable time before the legal termination of the marriage, family relationships are influenced by conflict between the spouses (Forehand 1992), decreasing commitment to the marriage that may be expressed in one or more trial separations (Wallerstein et al. 1988), and altered personal functioning among family members in response to the marital stress. The impact of divorce on family functioning does not end with the final decree, either, as family members face the tasks of redefining and reconstructing family roles and relationships, a process that can go on for years (Wallerstein et al. 1988).

The fact that divorce is a multistage process has implications for our conception of the "effects of divorce" on children. Many of the difficulties that children experience associated with their parents' divorce may well have begun years before the legal divorce in response to the stressors described above (Forehand 1992; Forgatch et al. 1988; Hetherington et al. 1982; Wallerstein et al. 1988). Characteristics of divorced families such as interparental conflict (Forehand 1992) and parents' difficulty in effectively disciplining their children (Forgatch et al. 1988; Hetherington et al. 1982) are particularly likely to have begun when the parents were still together. Because of this, any consideration of the impact of divorce on children must take into account the functioning of the family before the legal action took place, as well as the continued adjustments that families make afterward (Barber and Eccles 1992; Brody and Forehand 1988; Hetherington 1991).

More family transitions are likely to follow the divorce. Although the rate of remarriage has slowed in recent years (Bumpass et al. 1990), most people who divorce eventually remarry (Bumpass et al. 1990; Hetherington et al. 1992). Although women with children are less likely to remarry than are those without children (Bumpass et al. 1990; Hetherington et al. 1992), more than one-half of divorced mothers do remarry (Hernandez 1988); therefore, a considerable number of children will spend part of their childhoods in stepfamilies (Coleman and Ganong 1990; Hernandez 1988). This transition brings its own set of challenges and stresses to which children must adapt. The transitions, however, may not stop even there. Redivorce may take place, and may be followed by further remarriage and redivorce. Second marriages are slightly less stable than first marriages (Castro-Martin and Bumpass 1989), implying that a significant number of children will experience redivorce after their parents remarry (Bray 1988; Bumpass 1984; Furstenberg 1988). The children in such repeatedly reconstituting families experience stresses that become more or less chronic, to which they must spend a considerable amount of their childhood adjusting.

In this chapter we focus on some of the ramifications that ongoing family transitions may have for children's and adolescents' development and adjustment. We provide an overview of the research concerning the impact of divorce and remarriage on children, the possible interactions of the effects of divorce and remarriage with young people's developmental needs, and the specific effects of living through repeated family disruptions and reconstitutions. We then end the chapter with a discussion of those influences that can help children and adolescents involved in family transitions to adjust to their home lives and develop optimally.

Impact of Family Transitions on Children and Adolescents

Emery (1988) has pointed out that the most typical long-term response of children and adolescents to parental divorce is positive adjustment to the new family situation. Although children who have experienced parental marital transitions are at higher risk for psychological problems, those with problems serious enough to require psychiatric treatment are in the minority (Emery 1988). Accordingly, the literature on divorce and remarriage provides little specific information on the psychiatric conditions of the children involved in the studies. In two multimethod longitudinal studies performed by Hetherington and her colleagues of children's and adolescents' respective adjustment to parental divorce and remarriage (Hetherington 1989, 1991; Hetherington et al. 1982, 1992), no mention is made of any subjects experiencing psychopathology at the outset of the studies, or of excluding any prospective subjects on the basis of existing psychopathology.

Although in the study of adolescents (Hetherington 1991), assessments included the somatic complaints, schizoid, aggressive, cruel behavior, delinquent, anxious-obsessive, obsessive-compulsive, hostile-withdrawn, depressed-withdrawn, hyperactive, immature-hyperactive, and uncommunicative subscales of the Child Behavior Checklist (CBCL; Achenbach and Edelbrock 1983), no exact scores, or percentages of adolescents scoring above the clinical cutoffs, were provided for these subscales. These data simply were used for comparison, to indicate that adolescents from remarried families were more poorly adjusted than were those from divorced families, who were more poorly adjusted than were those from nondivorced families. Percentages of adolescents scoring above clinical cutoffs were indicated only for the total behavior problems subscale of the CBCL. It was determined, based on parent reports, that 45% of the adolescents in remarried families, 30% of those in divorced families, and 10% of those in intact families were experiencing clinically significant psychopathology (Hetherington 1991).

More information is provided through the National Survey of Children, which included a nationally representative sample of 2,258 children who were 7 to 11 years old in 1976 (Emery 1988). Even in this sample, however, psychopathology was measured only in terms of the percentages of children who had ever received psychological treatment. Again, no information was provided on specific diagnoses or types of problems experienced; reference was made only to general "emotional problems" (Zill et al. 1993). At the outset of the study, 13% of the children of divorced parents had received psychological or psychiatric treatment during their lives, compared with 5.5% of those in nondivorced families (Emery 1988). Zill and associates (1993) reported that by the time of the study's third wave of data collection, during which the respondents were 18 to 22 years old, 40% of the divorced-family offspring had received treatment, whereas only approximately 20% of the offspring from nondivorced families had received treatment.

The following is a brief overview of the available information on the adjustments required of children and adolescents during their parents' marital transitions, and the responses they commonly make.

Divorce-Associated Adjustments of Families

Changes in the Quality of Parenting

Divorce brings about changes in the ways in which parents relate to their children (Hetherington 1991; Wallerstein et al. 1988), as the emotional and organizational aspects of family life are rearranged. Particularly during the first 2 years after divorce, parents are often absorbed in their own problems, emotions, and stresses and are therefore less able to respond to their children's needs (Brody and Forehand 1988; Emery 1988). Divorced mothers experience more major adjustments and everyday problems than do married mothers (Forgatch et al. 1988), and the resulting stress contributes to their preoccupation. During the first year following divorce, custodial mothers are often less affectionate, less effective in communication, more punitive, less consistent and effective in their discipline, and less demanding of mature behavior from their children than are nondivorced mothers (Emery 1988; Hetherington 1991). Such attitudes may lead these mothers to perceive their children negatively, which may in turn lead to further negative parenting and an actual worsening of child behavior as a "self-fulfilling prophecy" (Brody and Forehand 1988). Divorced mothers' ability to parent effectively increases during the second year following divorce, although they tend to monitor their children less closely than do mothers in intact families, and relationships with their sons may be difficult (Hetherington 1991).

Although changes in the quality of mother-child relationships following divorce have been documented extensively, less information is available concerning postdivorce father-child relationships. Even in the midst of cultural change mandating equality in gender roles, children are seldom placed in their fathers' custody following divorce

(Emery 1988; Hetherington et al. 1982; Laosa 1988). Father-custody families make up only about 10% of single-parent families (Emery 1988). Like custodial mothers, custodial fathers experience disorganization of the home (Hetherington et al. 1982) and often feel overwhelmed by the responsibilities of single parenthood, although they are more likely than single mothers to obtain household help and are not as economically stressed (Emery 1988; Hetherington et al. 1982; Santrock et al. 1982).

Immediately after divorce, some noncustodial fathers reduce the frequency of their contact with their children in an attempt to spare themselves some of the pain of separation from them (Hetherington et al. 1982). Others, however, have as much contact with their children as do married fathers, sometimes increasing the amount of contact with the children over that which they had had before the separation (Hetherington et al. 1982). Initially, noncustodial fathers may become very permissive with their children, in an effort to keep their time together as nonconflicted and pleasant as possible (Hetherington et al. 1982).

After negotiating the first phase of divorce adjustment, parents must deal with family dynamics that are different from those experienced in nondivorced families. Relationships between the custodial parent (usually the mother) and the children often become intense and ambivalent, simultaneously closer and more conflicted than are parent-child relationships in intact families; this occurs particularly often in families with adolescents (Hetherington 1991). In addition, parents in divorced families, compared with those in intact families, often give their children more freedom, more power, and more responsibility (Hetherington 1991). Relationships with noncustodial parents (usually fathers) change even more than do those with residential parents. Hetherington and associates (1982) found that, over time, noncustodial fathers become less nurturant and more detached, show less affection, and ignore their children more. They become less permissive, attentive, and communicative, and use more negative and fewer positive sanctions. Loss of contact and involvement with the noncustodial parent is common (Amato and Keith 1991; Emery 1988; Furstenberg 1988; Hetherington et al. 1982). Even when contact continues, noncustodial parents' involvement in child care is often low, and parents seldom cooperate with each other in child-rearing matters even when the custodial parent remains involved (Furstenberg 1988).

Changes in Living Circumstances

Following divorce, it is common for mothers and children to experience a decline in socioeconomic status (Amato and Keith 1991; Emery 1988; Wallerstein et al. 1988). Even well-educated single mothers and their children often live in poverty (Forgatch et al. 1988). These circumstances may necessitate changes for the child such as moving to a new residence, changing schools, and coping with the initiation of or increase in maternal employment (Emery 1988).

Divorce-Associated Responses of Children

The literature on children's responses to parental marital transitions does not provide specific information on exact rates of particular behaviors. Rather, the behavior of children who experience parental marital transitions is described in general terms in comparison with that of children who have not experienced such transitions.

Externalizing Problems

During the divorce process, children often engage in disruptive behavior such as aggression, antisociability, demandingness, impulsivity, destructiveness, noncompliance, and conduct disorders (Brody and Forehand 1988; Camara and Resnick 1988; Emery 1988; Grych and Fincham 1992; Hetherington 1991). This type of conduct may be the most pronounced response to divorce, especially during the first year after the parents' final separation (Hetherington 1991). Although such behavior decreases markedly after the first year following divorce (Hetherington 1991), it can persist to some extent for more than 5 years (Grych and Fincham 1992; Hetherington 1991). Such behavior may be more prevalent, more lasting, and less likely to decrease among boys than among girls (Emery 1988; Hetherington 1991; Wallerstein et al. 1988).

Internalizing Problems

The existence of internalizing problems in children of divorce has not been as well documented through research as has that of externalizing problems, because, by nature, internalizing problems are less readily observed and measured (Emery 1988). Nevertheless, both research findings and clinical impressions suggest that children experience depression, anxiety, and loneliness following parental divorce.

They may become withdrawn or inappropriately dependent, blame themselves for the divorce, and fantasize about parental reconciliation (Emery 1988; Grych and Fincham 1992; Hetherington 1991). Children from divorced families who were interviewed in the National Survey of Children reported themselves to experience more general distress than did those from intact families, and their mothers reported them to be more depressed and withdrawn (Emery 1988). Such problems may be more prevalent among girls than among boys (Emery 1988).

Social and Interpersonal Relationship Difficulties

Social and interpersonal relationship difficulties can arise from externalizing and internalizing problems, as peers and other social agents react to the child's disordered behavior. Hetherington and associates (1982) found that, among 4-year-old children, disruptions in play behavior occurred following divorce. These disruptions included difficulty in engaging in imaginative, associative, and cooperative play; less time spent in play interactions with other children; more negative affect, negative behavior, aggression, and opposition toward other children; and less helping and sharing. Among the boys in this study, disrupted play behavior often resulted in rejection by other boys their age; this rejection persisted even after 2 years, when the boys' behavior had improved. Hetherington and associates also found that nursery school teachers behaved more negatively toward the boys from divorced families than toward those from intact families.

Guidubaldi and associates (1984), in their study of school-age children, found that teachers rated children from divorced families as more dependent and more unpopular with their peers than children from nondivorced families. Among adolescents, sexual activity may be initiated earlier among children from divorced families than among those from nondivorced families, and deviant activities such as smoking and drug use may be more common (Emery 1988; Hetherington 1991).

Academic Problems

Children from divorced families have difficulties in academic performance as measured by grades, standardized tests, teacher ratings, and likelihood of grade repetition (Emery 1988; Grych and Fincham 1992; Hetherington et al. 1982). Particular difficulties arise in tasks that require sustained attention, such as mathematical and other quantitatively oriented tasks (Hetherington et al. 1982). The academic difficulties encountered by children from divorced families, although not significantly different in severity from those encountered by children from nondivorced families (Emery 1988), may have a significant impact on academic achievement. In the National Survey of Children, the majority of adolescents who dropped out of high school were from divorced homes (Zill et al. 1993).

The difficulties that children of divorce have in school appear to be more a matter of emotional and behavioral problems that interfere with the ability to engage effectively in academic pursuits than a deficiency in academic skills. Problems may result from behavioral difficulties such as distractibility, inattention, off-task talking, impulsiveness, anxiety about failure, and generally disruptive behavior (Emery 1988; Grych and Fincham 1992). Hetherington and associates (1982) have suggested that the family disorganization, inconsistency, and poor parental control characteristic of recently divorced households account for these difficulties. Also, Emery (1988) has suggested that the increased responsibility for household tasks and family maintenance that children experience following parental divorce may interfere with their ability to complete homework and concentrate on achieving academically.

Self-Perceptions

Research concerning differences in self-perceptions in children following divorce is inconsistent (see Emery 1988 for review). Some researchers (Camara and Resnick 1988) have found that children from divorced homes have lower self-esteem than do those from intact families, whereas others (Bray 1988; Pasley and Healow 1988) have not found this to be the case. Forehand and colleagues (1988) found that, during the first year after divorce, adolescents perceived themselves to be less socially and cognitively competent than did matched control subjects from intact families; these perceptions of oneself as less competent may over time lead to actual reductions in competence.

Mental Health Problems

In studies of the mental health status of children from divorced families, rates of referral for treatment usually are used as an index of mental health problems, rather than specific descriptions of particular disorders. Children from divorced families are referred for mental health treatment approximately three times more often than are children from intact families (Zill et al. 1993), and this includes referral for long-term adjustment problems in addition to divorce-related stressors (Grych and Fincham 1992). Rates of referral for treatment, however, can be influenced by more than the child's mental health. Parental perceptions may influence referral rates, in addition to actual child adjustment (Brody and Forehand 1988; Grych and Fincham 1992); parents' perceptions that lead to increased referral to mental health services may result from the negative affectivity that, for many parents, accompanies divorce (Brody and Forehand 1988).

Long-Term Adjustment Difficulties

Longitudinal research suggests a variety of long-term social and psychological consequences for children from divorced and remarried families. Emery (1988) reviewed studies indicating that adults from divorced families reported greater anxiety, unhappiness, negative perceptions of life, difficulty in handling negative life events, poorer health, and less satisfaction with relationships than did those from nondivorced families.

Data from follow-up interviews with National Survey of Children respondents in early adulthood (Zill et al. 1993) indicated that problems arising during childhood from parental divorce can persist, and that new problems can arise as young people confront adult issues such as the process of mate selection, identity formation, and educational and career goal formation. These reinterviews were conducted when the respondents were 18 to 22 years old, and parental divorce had occurred 12 to 22 years earlier. Those who had experienced parental divorce by the age of 16 were twice as likely as those who had not to report poor relationships with their fathers and mothers; to have received psychological counseling; to have dropped out of high school, either permanently or temporarily; to experience psychological distress; and to have behavior problems. These problems *more often* showed up in early adulthood than in adolescence; some subjects who had adjusted relatively well as children and adolescents nevertheless experienced problems in early adulthood (Zill et al. 1993). Deterioration of the maternal relationship, increase in behavior problems, and receipt of psychological treatment increased from adolescence to young adulthood for females, but not for males (Zill et al. 1993). Parental remarriage did not have any beneficial effect for these respondents, as those from remarried families were found to have as many problems as, and sometimes more problems than, those from non-remarried families.

Fine and associates (1983) surveyed college students who had experienced parental divorce prior to age 11; divorce had occurred an average of 10 years before the survey. Subjects from divorced families perceived greater distance, poorer communication, less affection, less warmth, and fewer generally positive feelings in their relationships with their parents than did those from intact families.

Haurin (1992) studied the effects of childhood residence in two-parent, single-parent, and stepfamilies on the adjustment of black, white, and Hispanic young adults interviewed as part of the National Longitudinal Study of Work Experience. For blacks, longer time spent in a two-parent family was associated with a decreased chance of participation in serious illegal activities as a teenager; for whites, it was associated with less likelihood of teenage marijuana use or pregnancy, and greater likelihood of high school completion. For all ethnic groups, residence in a stepfamily before the age of 15 was associated with a greater likelihood of teenage marijuana use. For whites, residence in a stepfamily was also associated with a lower likelihood of high school completion and a greater likelihood of teenage pregnancy; for Hispanics, it was associated with a greater likelihood of participation in serious illegal activity. By the time the subjects were in their 20s, only stepfamily effects remained. Having lived in a stepfamily was associated with greater use of hard drugs among whites and Hispanics, and a greater likelihood of second-generation divorce among whites.

Parental marital transitions can have educational and economic consequences for children as well. Krein (1986) found that the 28- to 38-year-old men whose responses were included in the National Longitudinal Survey of Labor Market Experience completed fewer years of schooling if they had lived in a single-parent family before the age of 6, and that the longer they lived in such a family, the fewer number of years of education they had. Mueller and Cooper (1986) found that 19- to 34-year-olds in Minnesota who were from single-parent families had lower incomes, were more likely to require public assistance, were more likely to lack money for necessities, and were less likely to own homes. They were also more likely to be separated or divorced, and had their first children at younger ages.

The magnitude of these problems, however, must be considered in order to obtain an accurate picture of long-term adjustment. Zill and associates (1993) found that although those persons whose parents had divorced had twice the incidence of adjustment problems as those whose parents had not divorced, the ratings in the former remained well within the normal range. Fine and associates (1983) found that there was wide variation in perceptions of parental relationships among persons whose parents had divorced. Relationships with parents in those families in which divorce had occurred were not perceived as pathological; persons from divorced families, on average, rated their relationship with their parents as "average," as compared with persons from nondivorced families, who rated their relationship with their parents as "above average." Finally, Krein (1986) found that the difference in years of education completed by adults from one- and two-parent families was, on average, only around 1 year. Even the small differences reported by Krein, however, may have significant effects. In Krein's study, the adults from two-parent families were twice as likely to have completed high school or college. Zill and associates (1993) believe that the fact that people from divorced and remarried families experience significantly more problems indicates a significant risk to these families' well-being and that this risk should be taken seriously.

Remarriage-Associated Adjustments in Families and Children

During the 1970s and 1980s, the number of divorced people who remarry declined. Nevertheless, in 1987 there were 4.3 million stepfamilies in the United States, in which lived 5.95 million children who were born before their parent's current marriage (Glick 1989). Nearly 13% of all American children under 18 who lived in families headed by a married couple were stepchildren (Glick 1989). Thus, the experience of parental remarriage is one that an appreciable number of families undergo, and numerous adjustments are required during this transition.

Learning to live with a previously unfamiliar person is always challenging. Research findings indicating that children in stepfamilies often experience more adjustment problems than do those in divorced, single-parent families (Haurin 1992; Hetherington 1991; Zill et al. 1993) suggest that learning to live with a stepparent is particularly demanding. Children may perceive the addition of a stepparent to be an intrusion into an established family system, particularly if they have spent much time in a divorced, single-parent family (Hetherington 1991; Montgomery et al. 1992). It may also end the children's hopes for their parents' reunion, when such hopes exist. Stepfathers (the residential stepparent is more likely to be the stepfather) initially respond to these reactions by behaving as "polite strangers" (Hetherington 1991) toward their stepchildren; with time they usually disengage from emotional and caregiving involvement. As a result, children in remarried families are supervised and controlled less than are those in intact families (Hetherington 1991), perhaps because of lower maternal monitoring levels than in intact families along with stepfathers' detachment.

The intense mother-child relationships that characterize single-mother families (Hetherington 1991; Montgomery et al. 1992) must be renegotiated to include the stepfather, who, as noted above, may be perceived as an intruder. The increased freedom and power in the family that children of divorced mothers often experience may be withdrawn, as the custodial mother turns to the stepfather for assistance and support and the stepfather attempts to exert authority over the children (Hetherington 1991).

Children may fear that a good relationship with the stepparent constitutes a rejection of the noncustodial parent, leading to loyalty conflicts. The noncustodial parent also may have standards that conflict with those of the residential stepparent, inviting negative comparisons in the children's minds. The noncustodial parent may actually criticize the stepparent and his or her attempts to manage the children.

Uncertainty regarding relationships with various new steprelatives and the roles they are to assume can require a major family adjustment (Bray 1988; Cherlin 1981; Hetherington 1991). This uncertainty can create stress that makes relationships in stepfamilies less cohesive and more problematic than those in intact families (Bray 1988).

As with divorce, children experience both externalizing and internalizing problems following their parent's remarriage (Bray 1988; Hetherington 1991). In their families they experience less warm and more coercive exchanges, and less effective communication, with their mothers than do children in intact families. Young adolescents are particularly likely to respond to these situations by withdrawing from their families (Hetherington 1991). There is, however, a great deal of variability in children's responses to these changes (Hetherington 1991; Wallerstein et al. 1988).

Factors Associated With Children's Adjustment to Divorce and Remarriage

Brody and Forehand (1988) have pointed out that little attention has been directed toward understanding the specific aspects of divorce or remarriage that influence children's adjustment, although a considerable amount of work has been done on divorce as a global concept. The factors described in the following subsections are often related to differences in children's responses to family transitions.

Gender

Gender differences exist in children's responses to both divorce and remarriage (Barber and Eccles 1992; Forehand 1992; Grych and Fincham 1992; Hetherington 1989). Boys often exhibit more adjustment problems associated with parental divorce, particularly externalizing problems, than do girls (Brody and Forehand 1988; Grych and Fincham 1992; Wallerstein et al. 1988), although this is not universally true (Hetherington 1991). This increased number of adjustment problems in boys in divorced families may be because boys are more reactive to interparental conflict than are girls (Forehand et al. 1988) or because children may adjust best in the custody of the same-sex parent (Camara and Resnick 1988; Emery 1988; Santrock et al. 1982) and boys are usually in their mothers' custody. In divorced families, sons often have conflicted relationships with their mothers, whereas daughters often become very close to their mothers (Bray 1988; Hetherington 1991). Because of this difference in the quality of mother-child relationships, girls often adjust to divorce more easily than do boys.

Following the mother's remarriage, however, the situation often reverses. Although both boys and girls initially respond to remarriage with an increase in disrupted behavior (Hetherington 1991), with time boys often adjust well to the new marriage, whereas girls often do not (Hetherington 1991). Boys are more likely to eventually accept their stepfathers than are girls, who remain antagonistic (Brand et al. 1988; Hetherington 1991). For boys, the stepfather's introduction provides an additional supportive role model and a buffer against the negativism of the mother-child relationship, whereas for girls it interrupts the very close relationship with the single mother (Bray 1988; Hetherington 1991).

Santrock and associates (1982) found the reverse for father–stepmother families. Boys adjusted better in father custody families than did girls; after their father's remarriage, boys' adjustment worsened and that of girls improved. Evidently children who are of the same sex as the custodial parent form a close relationship with that parent, one that is interrupted by remarriage.

Age

Age at the time of divorce has been mentioned as an important influence on children's adjustment (Barber and Eccles 1992; Bray 1988; Forehand et al. 1988; Wallerstein et al. 1988), but the exact nature of its influence is not clear (Grych and Fincham 1992). Some contend that children adjust better if they are young at the time of the divorce (Guidubaldi et al. 1984; Wallerstein et al. 1988) because younger children have fewer experiences and memories of the predivorce family. Others expect children to adjust better if they are older at the time of divorce (Brody and Forehand 1988; Furstenberg 1988) because they are more independent and able to seek support outside the home. Zill and associates (1993) and Krein (1986) found that adults who experienced parental divorce before age 6 were less well adjusted than those who experienced it when they were older, with adjustment being measured on the basis of dimensions such as academic achievement and psychological distress.

Age is important in adjustment to parental remarriage, and adolescence appears to be a particularly difficult time at which to experience a parent's remarriage (Hetherington 1991). Adolescents adjust better than do younger children, however, to immediate authoritative parenting from their stepfathers (Hetherington 1991); the reasons for this are not readily apparent.

Family Structure

Children in families with a residential stepfather adjust differently than do those in families with a residential stepmother (Bray 1988; Fine and Kurdek 1992; Furstenberg 1988; Pasley and Healow 1988). The incorporation of a residential stepmother is more problematic (Fine and Kurdek 1992; Furstenberg 1988). Stepchildren included in the National Survey of Children evaluated residential stepmothers more negatively than they did residential stepfathers, particularly when the children had regular contact with their biological mothers (Furstenberg 1988). Fine and Kurdek (1992) found that 12-year-olds who lived with stepmothers reported lower self-esteem and more social problems than did those who lived with stepfathers. Perhaps the socially prescribed closeness of the mother-child relationship makes sharing of the maternal role more difficult than the traditionally less involved paternal role (Furstenberg 1988). Conversely, Fine and Kurdek (1992) suggested that problems in adapting to the stepmother may spring from problematic relationships with the natural mother, which may have led to the relatively uncommon father custody arrangement in the first place. Social stereotypes that portray stepmothers as "evil" or, conversely, dictate that they should feel immediate love for their stepchildren upon remarriage also can make adjustment in stepmother families difficult (Dainton 1993).

Parental Conflict Level

Parental conflict may be the most significant influence on children's adjustment to family transitions (Amato and Keith 1991; Forehand et al. 1988). Children experience more adjustment problems when divorce-associated conflict is high than they do when it is low (Forehand et al. 1988). Some of the negative effects that are attributed to divorce may actually arise from the conflict that accompanies the actual process of divorce (Barber and Eccles 1992). Parental conflict does not necessarily end or decline after divorce, and the ways in which it is handled are important to child adjustment. When parents work to resolve conflicts productively rather than destructively (Camara and Resnick 1988), and avoid involving the children in their disputes (Buchanan et al. 1991), the children may not be negatively influenced by the conflict. Fighting in the children's presence is detrimental (Forehand et al. 1988).

Quality of Previous Family Relationships

The quality of previous family relationships will influence adjustment to current family relationships (Forehand 1992; Hetherington 1991) through the expectations and behaviors that members have developed from their past experiences. An example is the difference, according to gender, of children's adjustment in stepfamilies arising from the differences in the mother-child relationship in single-parent families. In addition, Kalmuss and Seltzer (1986) found that remarried couples were more likely to engage in spousal violence than were nondivorced couples, regardless of the extent to which they were exposed to such violence in childhood. These authors interpreted their findings as evidence of the transfer of negative behavior learned in one marriage to the next, despite the remarried spouses' intentions not to repeat their mistakes.

Length of Time Since Transition

Child behavior and overall adjustment are the most disrupted immediately after a family transition but tend to improve over time (Forehand et al. 1988; Hetherington 1991). The significance of any behavior, therefore, should be evaluated in the light of the child's position in the adaptation process. Intensely negative child behavior and disruptions in parenting skill, for example, are typical during the first 2 years following a divorce and often resolve with time. If, however, they continue unabated for several more years, the family members may require help to resolve their conflicts. At some points in time, a particular behavior may be maladaptive, but at other times, it may be a necessary and appropriate part of adjustment. Soon after divorce, intense longing for the noncustodial parent and a strong desire to reunite the parents form a normal part of the child's process of grieving the loss of the predivorce family. Persistence of these feelings past the immediate postdivorce years, however, could be counterproductive for the child.

Individual Adjustment

The personal characteristics of individual family members are important to the quality of the interactions among family members. In the child, qualities such as self-esteem, social competence, intelligence, and assertiveness may enhance adjustment, whereas externalizing behavior and lack of social competence may impede it (Hetherington 1989; Hetherington et al. 1992). Parents' personality traits, their coping and problem-solving skills, and social support resources influence their effectiveness in managing their children (Forgatch et al. 1988). Characteristics such as lack of social skills, antisocial behavior, irritability, or depression in single mothers can interfere with their ability to elicit social support, distort their perceptions of their children, and compromise their parenting practices (Brody and Forehand 1988; Forgatch et al. 1988; Patterson and Forgatch 1990).

Stepparent Role

Hetherington (1991) found that most children adjusted to stepfamilies best when the new residential stepfather did not attempt to assume parental roles immediately, but started as a supporter of the mother's parenting and only gradually assumed authority himself. As noted above, young adolescents were the exception to this rule, benefiting most from immediate authoritative stepparenting.

Parental Resources

Resources such as social support (Barber and Eccles 1992; Forehand 1992) and financial assets (Barber and Eccles 1992) influence child adjustment through their impact on family climate and parental well-being. Conger and associates (1992) have suggested that financial difficulties cause parents to become angry, frustrated, and demoralized, conditions that impede skilled and sensitive parenting. In their study of married-couple families, Conger et al. (1992) found that financial pressures led to parental depression, marital conflict, and unskilled parenting, which in turn resulted in adjustment problems in adolescent boys.

Normative Adolescent Developmental Stresses and Adjustment to Family Transitions

Wallerstein and colleagues (1988) have noted that adjustment to the changes brought about by divorce "impose[s] psychological tasks upon the child that represent notable additions to the usual tasks of growing up in our society" (p. 198). A specific instance in which a child's developmental stage interacts with the demands of family transitions to make the stress greater than it would have been had either been experienced alone concerns parental divorce or remarriage during adolescence (Forehand et al. 1988; Hetherington 1991).

Several normative developmental transitions occur during adolescence, with which the requirements of family transitions interact. Because of the extensive social, emotional, and physical changes that adolescents undergo, it is normal for them to experience stress at this time. When divorce and remarriage occur during adolescence, the disruptions in family and personal functioning that accompany these transitions occur at a time when children particularly need a stable and supportive home environment to help them cope with the normative developmental stress (Barber and Eccles 1992; Forehand et al. 1988). Adolescence is also a time when young people normally begin to become independent from their families, and in single-parent families a considerable degree of independence may already have been attained. Family transitions can influence in several ways the normative process of attaining autonomy. Adolescents may choose to cope with the stresses associated with family transitions by disengaging from their families more quickly than is usual in order to distance themselves from the disruption. This premature disengagement may lead to negative consequences, including excessive peer orientation (Brody et al. 1988) and negativity in sibling relationships (Hetherington 1991). During remarriage, conflict surrounding issues of independence and autonomy become particularly salient (Hetherington 1991). The issues of parental authority, parental control, and child power in the family that always accompany remarriage become more highly charged, because they are superimposed upon a developmental stage in which the young person is particularly sensitized to these issues (Hetherington 1991).

In addition to these social and psychological issues, adolescents' physical development also makes adjustment to family transitions particularly challenging. Young adolescents' emerging sexuality, with the self-consciousness and desire for privacy that accompany it, may make them uncomfortable living with a biologically unrelated adult (Hetherington 1991). This may be particularly true for girls who acquire a stepfather, and may be part of the reason that, as Hetherington (1991; Hetherington et al. 1992) found, adolescent girls have particular difficulty in adjusting to maternal remarriage. Adolescents whose divorced custodial parent is dating, as well as those whose parents have remarried, may be confronted with the knowledge that their parents are sexually active, an idea that often makes adolescents uncomfortable (Hetherington 1991). Issues concerning appropriate levels of intimacy and displays of affection in the reconstituting family are also complicated by adolescents' emerging sexuality (Hetherington 1991).

Research findings provide further evidence for the difficulty of adolescents' adjustment to remarriage. In the Hetherington (1989, 1991) longitudinal studies, adolescents showed no positive adaptation to their parents' remarriages over the 26 months during which the adolescents were observed, unlike those children who were preadolescents at the time of the remarriage. Hetherington (1991) also found that in divorced single-mother families, girls who previously had adjusted well to their parents' divorce began to show an increase in behavior problems and conflict with their mothers upon entering adolescence. This increase exceeded that which took place normatively in nondivorced families. Caspi and Moffitt's (1991) study of early-maturing girls yielded similar findings, revealing that prior behavior problems among the girls in the study were exacerbated by the developmental stress of maturation.

Cumulative Stresses and Adjustment

When families undergo several consecutive transitions, and the stressors associated with them are repeated, child adjustment and the quality of later adaptations may be affected. Hetherington (1991) pointed out that the quality of family relationships before divorce will influence relationships in the divorced family, which will in turn influence relationships in the remarried family. Previous circumstances influence responses in the present and, through these responses, will affect situations in the future.

When previous circumstances include negative or stressful events, the result can be adjustment difficulties. Brody and Forehand (1988) speculated that when mothers have undergone many negative life experiences such as marital conflict, divorce-associated stress, financial problems, and health problems, maternal functioning will directly impact child adjustment. In a study of adverse life events and their impact on 6- to 10-year-old children, Beardsall and Dunn (1992) found the number of adverse life events that the children had experienced over the previous 3 years to be negatively related to the children's perceptions of their own competence. In this study, negative events were not predicted by either child temperament or maternal depression, so the association cannot be attributed to personal incompetence causing the problems.

Hetherington's (1991) work supports the idea that repeated family transitions may lead to cumulative difficulty in functioning. When adjustment differences emerged among children from intact, single-mother, and remarried families, children in intact families had the fewest problems, those in divorced families had an intermediate number of problems, and those in stepfamilies had the most problems, including externalizing and internalizing behavior and problems with social competence. In light of the benefits that stepparents bring into remarriage, such as social and financial support, the relatively poorer adjustment of children despite these benefits suggests that the children's capacity to cope with family transitions may be strained.

Serial Marriage: When Transitions Become Chronic

The possibilities of cumulative effects arising from family transitions and the stressful circumstances they entail are important in the consideration of a particular pattern of chronic family reconstitution, which Brody and colleagues (1988) termed "serial marriage." They defined serial marriage as the experience of three or more marriages as a result of repeated divorce. Many children may well be required to adjust to this pattern of family life. Bray (1988) and Castro-Martin and Bumpass (1989) noted that second and higher-order marriages are more likely to end in divorce than are first marriages. Bray (1988) and Furstenberg (1988) specifically stated that a significant number of children are likely to be involved in parental redivorce as a consequence. Furstenberg (1988) found that one-third of the children interviewed in the National Survey of Children whose custodial parents had remarried experienced a second parental divorce, and speculated that the proportion would have been even higher had redivorces among noncustodial parents been counted. Furstenberg (1988) concluded, "The total number of children who will experience three or more transitions during their childhood years is considerable and growing rapidly. For our sample, we estimate that approximately 1 child in every 10 will see their parents divorce, their custodial parent remarry, and then divorce again before they reach the age of 16" (pp. 249–250). The use of a nationwide probability sample in the National Survey suggests that these findings may well apply to the nation as a whole.

Brody and associates (1988) advanced several hypotheses concerning the unique effects of serial marriage on children, directly or indirectly (through parent characteristics). The proposed *direct* effects included deleterious influences from repeated periods of interparental conflict, attachment disruption, exposure to multiple periods of diminished parenting capacity, the acquisition of a learned-helpless perspective as a result of repeated exposure to the uncontrollable stressors surrounding family transitions, and the likelihood of repetition of the serial marriage pattern in the children's own adult lives. Parents who marry serially may have unrealistic expectations of marriage, may have personality characteristics that interfere with their ability to make family relationships succeed, and may transfer negative expectations and behaviors among failed marriages. Some of these hypotheses have been tested in research studies, most of which concerned the adjustment of adults who have divorced and remarried repeatedly. Limited information is available on children's adjustment in serial marriage families, and that which is available is oriented more toward atypical rather than general populations.

Adults and Serial Marriage

Most of the information concerning serial marriage in the general population comes from a series of studies carried out by Kurdek (1989, 1990, 1991). Kurdek (1989) found that marital history did not predict marital satisfaction in a sample of newly married couples that included both those who had married for the first time and those who had remarried. He suggested that problems associated with serial marriage may show up later in the relationship rather than at the time at which the couples were assessed (they were contacted approximately 1 month after their weddings), or that problems in serial marriage may be more strongly related to psychological processes than to marital satisfaction. Accordingly, Kurdek (1990) subsequently assessed differences in psychological distress among never-divorced, once-divorced, and multiply divorced men and women. He found greater psychological distress among serially married women but not men. Women's divorce history was associated with their experience of anxiety, phobias, paranoid ideation, and psychoticism, and with the global severity of their psychological symptoms. Women who had experienced more divorces reported more symptoms; their symptoms, however, were not severe enough for them to require treatment. Furthermore, divorce history explained only 2% to 4% of the variance in their personal adjustment; the amount of explained variance dropped to 1% to 3% when demographic variables were controlled. Kurdek (1990) therefore concluded that divorce history was a significant but weak predictor of psychological adjustment. He explained the differences in the findings for men and women in terms of women's socialization to be relationship oriented, which results in their greater investment in, and sensitivity to, the marital relationship. He concluded that "individual difference variables—rather than . . . marital history . . . —are important concurrent predictors of relationship quality in . . . newlywed couples" (Kurdek 1989, p. 1063).

These findings could have been influenced by the volunteer status of the study participants; persons who were not satisfied with their marriages may not have participated (Kurdek 1989). An opportunity to consider that possibility was provided in Kurdek's third study (1991), in which he examined data from a subset of a national probability sample. Using data from over 6,000 participants, he examined the relationships of divorce history to global happiness, depression, and general health. Divorce history was associated with happiness: nondivorced persons were happier than any who had divorced, once or several times. Persons who had had serial divorces were slightly less happy than those who had divorced only once, but the difference was not statistically significant. Divorce history was also associated with levels of depression; those who had not divorced were less depressed than those who had divorced once, and those who had divorced once were less depressed than those who had divorced more than once. As Kurdek (1991) noted, "The effects of divorce history were linear and cumulative" (p. 77) in a sample that was large and heterogeneous. Again, however, divorce history accounted for only around 3% of the variance in overall well-being. Kurdek (1991) once more concluded that divorce history is a significant, but weak, predictor of adult well-being in the general population.

The national probability sample that Kurdek (1991) examined was much more representative than the sample in his two previous studies (Kurdek 1989, 1990); however, the measures he used in the previous studies were much more comprehensive than the survey questions that were asked of the members of the probability sample. In the 1991 study, happiness and health were each rated using a single item. The strongest association for divorce history emerged for depression, which was measured using a 12-item scale. Although cost and time constraints would make it difficult, it would be interesting to know what would happen if Kurdek's earlier assessments were used with the probability sample.

Children and Serial Marriage

The information that is available concerning children's adjustment in serial marriage families is limited to a few studies of atypical populations, for whom serial marriage was an expression of pervasive personality and adjustment difficulties in the parents. Rosenbaum (1989) studied the family backgrounds of 159 young women who had been committed to the California Youth Authority (CYA) as juveniles in the early 1960s. These women came from strikingly similar, severely disturbed families, in which serial marriage was prevalent. The girls' mothers had been married an average of four times by the time the girls were 16, and had lived with a number of different men and borne children by them. Conflict arose in these families on issues involving perceived inequities among children of differing parentage. Nurturance was unavailable from these parents; mother–daughter role reversal was common. Rosenbaum described the mothers' lives as "a series of crises" (p. 39). A majority (82%) of the CYA girls became adult offenders.

Capaldi and Patterson (1991a, 1991b) used interviews, observations, questionnaires, standardized tests, and sociometric measures with over 200 9-year-old boys, their parents, their teachers, and their peers, to evaluate adjustment among children from lower-socioeconomic- and working-class families who had experienced multiple transitions that included at least two divorces. The sample was drawn from a comparatively high crime area, and families experiencing disruption were overrepresented. Child adjustment and number of family transitions were consistently associated; boys whose families had gone through more transitions had more problems and were more likely to engage in delinquent behavior as adolescents. Capaldi and Patterson interpreted this finding as support for Brody and associates' (1988) "hypothesis of disengagement from the family and increased peer orientation after transitions" (qtd. in Capaldi and Patterson 1991b, p. 495). The risk to children was greater in multiple-transition families than in single-mother families, and the number of transitions that boys experienced by age 9 predicted their adjustment at both age 9 and age 11.

In Capaldi and Patterson's study, families who had experienced one or more transitions were more likely than those who had not experienced a transition to undergo an additional transition during the 2 years of the study. This finding, according to Capaldi and Patterson (1991b), indicated that "the intact parent group may continue to be stable . . . into the boys' adolescence, whereas the families who have experienced transitions are less stable and likely to experience more transitions" (p. 501). Considering the effects of the combination of normative developmental stress with family transitions, plus the difficulty adolescents in particular experience with family transitions (especially remarriage), this likelihood could impact significantly on adolescent well-being.

Capaldi and Patterson (1991b) also found that higher levels of maternal and paternal antisocial behavior were positively associated with both maternal family transitions and mothers' failure to supervise their sons and be involved with them. This lack of maternal involvement contributed significantly to the boys' maladjustment. These results suggest that adjustment difficulties among children from multiple-transition families are explained by chronic parental and family maladjustment, resulting only in part from the periodic stresses accompanying transitions. Both transitions and child maladjustment apparently arise from parental maladjustment in atypical populations.

Children's Positive Adjustment to Family Transitions

The experience of parental marital transitions does not automatically produce severe or long-term disturbance in children. Children vary in their responses to family transition demands (Forgatch et al. 1988; Hetherington 1991; Hetherington et al. 1982; Wallerstein et al. 1988). Negative child outcomes and divorce may both arise from parental problems (Barber and Eccles 1992), particularly in serial-marriage families. Even in those situations in which children who have experienced family transitions are less well adjusted than are children from intact families, the differences are usually small (Forehand 1992) and child adjustment usually remains within normal levels (Bray 1988; Forgatch et al. 1988). Despite various stressors and demands on adjustment, many children who experience parental marital transitions adjust successfully and experience positive outcomes (Barber and Eccles 1992; Hetherington 1991). Although the experiences associated with family transitions can increase children's risk of developing adjustment problems, transitions can also benefit children. Divorce may end family conflict, and remarriage may increase financial and social support for them (Hetherington 1991). In the case of remarriage, children often become close to their stepparents, and many reconstituted families function well (Furstenberg 1988). Although families in transition do experience more stresses than intact families, not all of the stresses are negative; some are positive and serve to "balance out" the negative ones (Bray 1988).

Child characteristics such as intelligence, positive temperament, and social skill can help children respond effectively to the demands of family transitions. In addition, Hetherington and colleagues (Hetherington 1989; Hetherington et al. 1982) identified several social influences that can assist children in their adaptation. A family system that is as supportive as possible under the circumstances of the transition, particularly one that allows a close relationship with at least one parent, helps children to adjust well. When such a relationship with a parent is not available, closeness to another adult, such as a neighbor, a teacher, or a member of the extended family, is beneficial. A school environment in which schedules are regular, discipline is warm and consistent, and appropriately mature behavior is required provides children with a secure structure on which to rely during times of family change. A close friendship with at least one peer, and the ability to achieve academically or athletically, also enhance child adjustment.

As we come to understand more about the needs and functioning of families in transition, effective ways of dealing with the family must be developed that acknowledge the diversity of responses and promote positive functioning (Bray 1988; Furstenberg 1988; Hetherington 1991). For example, children can be taught coping strategies to help them deal with the uncontrollable stressors associated with their parents' marital transitions, thus decreasing the likelihood that the children will experience overwhelming distress or acquire a learned-helpless view of life. Children undergoing family transitions can be encouraged to regard their families as unique rather than deviant, or to regard a new stepparent as a contributor to the family rather than an intruder. They can be taught to avoid dwelling on negative emotions by planning enjoyable activities for themselves when they are feeling bad. They can learn to give up unrealistic goals, such as reuniting their divorced parents, in favor of building new, positive relationships with each of their single parents or stepparents (Nolen-Hoeksema 1992).

Conclusions

In working with children and adolescents whose parents are undergoing marital transitions, mental health professionals must be aware of the nature of the processes involved and of children's and adolescents' responses to them. Professionals must realize that marital transitions are not one-time events, but are processes that begin before, and continue long after, the legal divorce or remarriage. During the transitions children can experience such difficulties as externalizing and internalizing behavior problems, social and interpersonal relationship difficulties, and academic problems, some of which may continue into adulthood. Children's gender, age, and personality traits influence their adjustment to marital transitions, as do family variables such as interparental conflict levels and parents' social and psychological resources.

When families undergo multiple transitions, children encounter repeated stresses. The loss of attachment figures, repeated periods of diminished parenting capacity, and family reconfigurations are some of the experiences with which children must deal. The initial stress is often intense, but over a period of about 2 years children adapt to the new family situation, and most adjust well. The repetition of stressors, however, may have cumulative effects, as suggested by studies in which children in remarried families experienced more problems than did those in single-parent families. Children whose parents divorce repeatedly may experience particularly high levels of stress, but research on such families is still limited. Future studies of the impact of divorce and remarriage on children should include consideration of the parents' full marital histories, to determine whether child adjustment differs between once-divorced and multiply divorced families.

Although children and adolescents in divorced and remarried families are at greater risk for social and emotional problems than are those in intact families, they do not necessarily experience serious maladjustment. Parents, other family members, and professionals can offer ongoing support to these children that can minimize their adjustment difficulties and enhance their development. Future research should be directed toward further identification of those factors that promote positive adjustment to family transitions, as well as the most effective means of supporting children during times of family change.

References

Achenbach TM, Edelbrock CS: Manual for the Child Behavior Checklist and Revised Child Behavior Profile. New York, Queen City Printers, 1983

Amato PR, Keith B: Parental divorce and the well-being of children: a meta analysis. Psychol Bull 110:26–46, 1991

Barber BL, Eccles JS: Long-term influence of divorce and single parenting on adolescent family- and work-related values, behaviors, and aspirations. Psychol Bull 111:108–126, 1992

Beardsall L, Dunn J: Adversities in childhood: siblings' experiences, and their relations to self-esteem. J Child Psychol Psychiatry 33:349–359, 1992

Brand E, Clingempeel WG, Bowen-Woodward K: Family relationships and children's psychological adjustment in stepmother and stepfather families, in Impact of Divorce, Single Parenting, and Stepparenting on Children. Edited by Hetherington EM, Arasteh JD. Hillsdale, NJ, Lawrence Erlbaum, 1988, pp 299–324

Bray JH: Children's development during early remarriage, in Impact of Divorce, Single Parenting, and Stepparenting on Children. Edited by Hetherington EM, Arasteh JD. Hillsdale, NJ, Lawrence Erlbaum, 1988, pp 279–288

Brody GH, Forehand R: Multiple determinants of parenting: research findings and implications for the divorce process, in Impact of Divorce, Single Parenting, and Stepparenting on Children. Edited by Hetherington EM, Arasteh JD. Hillsdale, NJ, Lawrence Erlbaum, 1988, pp 117–131

Brody GH, Neubaum E, Forehand R: Serial marriage: a heuristic analysis of an emerging family form. Psychol Bull 103:211–222, 1988

Buchanan CM, Maccoby EE, Dornbusch SM: Caught between parents: adolescents' experience in divorced homes. Child Dev 62:1008–1029, 1991

Bumpass LL: Children and marital disruption: a replication and update. Demography 21:71–82, 1984

Bumpass LL, Sweet J, Castro-Martin T: Changing patterns of remarriage. Journal of Marriage and the Family 52:747–756, 1990

Camara KA, Resnick G: Interparental conflict and cooperation: factors moderating children's post-divorce adjustment, in Impact of Divorce, Single Parenting, and Stepparenting on Children. Edited by Hetherington EM, Arasteh JD. Hillsdale, NJ, Lawrence Erlbaum, 1988, pp 169–195

Capaldi DM, Patterson GR: Relation of parental transitions to boys' adjustment problems, I: a linear hypothesis. Developmental Psychology 27:489–495, 1991a

Capaldi DM, Patterson GR: Relation of parental transitions to boys' adjustment problems, II: mothers at risk for transitions and unskilled parenting. Developmental Psychology 27:496–504, 1991b

Caspi A, Moffitt TE: Individual differences are accentuated during periods of social change: the sample case of girls at puberty. J Pers Soc Psychol 61:157–168, 1991

Castro-Martin T, Bumpass LL: Recent trends in marital disruption. Demography 26:37–51, 1989

Cherlin AJ: Marriage, Divorce, Remarriage. Cambridge, MA, Harvard University Press, 1981

Coleman M, Ganong LH: Remarriage and stepfamily research in the 1980s: increased interest in an old family form. Journal of Marriage and the Family 52:925–940, 1990

Conger RD, Conger KJ, Elder GH, et al: A family process model of economic hardship and adjustment of early adolescent boys. Child Dev 63:526–541, 1992

Dainton M: The myths and misconceptions of the stepmother role: descriptions and prescriptions for identity management. Family Relations 42:93–98, 1993

Emery RE: Marriage, Divorce, and Children's Adjustment. Newbury Park, CA, Sage, 1988

Fine MA, Kurdek LA: The adjustment of adolescents in stepfather and stepmother families. Journal of Marriage and the Family 54:725–736, 1992

Fine MA, Moreland JR, Schwebel AI: Long-term effects of divorce on parent-child relationships. Developmental Psychology 19:703–713, 1983

Forehand R: Parental divorce and adolescent maladjustment: scientific inquiry versus public information. Behav Res Ther 30:319–327, 1992

Forehand R, Long N, Brody G: Divorce and marital conflict: relationship to adolescent competence and adjustment in early adolescence, in Impact of Divorce, Single Parenting, and Stepparenting on Children. Edited by Hetherington EM, Arasteh JD. Hillsdale, NJ, Lawrence Erlbaum, 1988, pp 155–167

Forgatch MS, Patterson GR, Skinner ML: A mediational model for the effect of divorce on antisocial behavior in boys, in Impact of Divorce, Single Parenting, and Stepparenting on Children. Edited by Hetherington EM, Arasteh JD. Hillsdale, NJ, Lawrence Erlbaum, 1988, pp 135–154

Furstenberg FF: Child care after divorce and remarriage, in Impact of Divorce, Single Parenting, and Stepparenting on Children. Edited by Hetherington EM, Arasteh JD. Hillsdale, NJ, Lawrence Erlbaum, 1988, pp 245–261

Glick PC: Marriage, divorce, and living arrangements: prospective changes. Journal of Family Issues 5:7–26, 1984

Glick PC: Remarried families, stepfamilies, and stepchildren: a brief demographic profile. Family Relations 38:24–27, 1989

Grych JH, Fincham FD: Interventions for children of divorce: toward greater integration of research and action. Psychol Bull 111:434–454, 1992

Guidubaldi J, Perry JD, Cleminshaw HK: The legacy of parental divorce: a nationwide study of family status and selected mediating variables on children's academic and social competencies, in Advances in Clinical Child Psychology, Vol 7. Edited by Lahey BB, Kazdin AE. New York, Plenum, 1984, pp 109–151

Haurin RJ: Patterns of childhood residence and the relationship to young adult outcomes. Journal of Marriage and the Family 54:846–860, 1992

Hernandez DJ: Demographic trends and the living arrangements of children, in Impact of Divorce, Single Parenting, and Stepparenting on Children. Edited by Hetherington EM, Arasteh JD. Hillsdale, NJ, Lawrence Erlbaum, 1988, pp 3–22

Hetherington EM: Coping with family transitions: winners, losers, and survivors. Child Dev 60:1–14, 1989

Hetherington EM: Families, lies, and videotapes. Presidential address to the meeting of the Society for Research on Adolescence, Atlanta, GA, 1990. Journal of Research on Adolescence 1:323–348, 1991

Hetherington EM, Cox MJ, Cox R: Effects of divorce on parents and children, in Nontraditional Families: Parenting and Child Development. Edited by Lamb ME. Hillsdale, NJ, Lawrence Erlbaum, 1982, pp 233–288

Hetherington EM, Clingempeel WG, Anderson ER, et al: Coping with marital transitions: a family systems perspective. Monogr Soc Res Child Dev 57, 2–3, Ser No 227, 1992

Kalmuss D, Seltzer JA: Continuity of marital behavior in remarriage: the case of spouse abuse. Journal of Marriage and the Family 48:113–120, 1986

Krein SF: Growing up in a single parent family: the effects on education and earnings. Family Relations 35:161–168, 1986

Kurdek LA: Relationship quality for newly married husbands and wives: marital history, stepchildren, and individual-difference predictors. Journal of Marriage and the Family 51:1053–1064, 1989

Kurdek LA: Divorce history and self-reported psychological distress in husbands and wives. Journal of Marriage and the Family 52:701–708, 1990

Kurdek LA: The relations between reported well-being and divorce history, availability of a proximate adult, and gender. Journal of Marriage and the Family 53:71–78, 1991

Laosa LM: Ethnicity and single parenting in the United States, in Impact of Divorce, Single Parenting, and Stepparenting on Children. Edited by Hetherington EM, Arasteh JD. Hillsdale, NJ, Lawrence Erlbaum, 1988, pp 23–49

Montgomery MJ, Anderson ER, Hetherington EM, et al: Patterns of courtship for remarriage: implications for child adjustment and parent-child relationships. Journal of Marriage and the Family 54:686–698, 1992

Mueller DP, Cooper PW: Children of single parent families: how they fare as young adults. Family Relations 35:169–176, 1986

Nolen-Hoeksema S: Children coping with uncontrollable stressors. Applied and Preventive Psychology 1:183–189, 1992

Pasley K, Healow CL: Adolescent self-esteem: a focus on children in stepfamilies, in Impact of Divorce, Single Parenting, and Stepparenting on Children. Edited by Hetherington EM, Arasteh JD. Hillsdale, NJ, Lawrence Erlbaum, 1988, pp 263–277

Patterson GR, Forgatch MS: Initiation and maintenance of process disrupting single-mother families, in Depression and Aggression in Family Interaction. Edited by Patterson GR. Hillsdale, NJ, Lawrence Erlbaum, 1990, pp 209–245

Rosenbaum JL: Family dysfunction and female delinquency. Crime and Delinquency 35:31–44, 1989

Santrock JW, Warshak RA, Elliott GL: Social development and parent-child interaction in father-custody and stepmother families, in Nontraditional Families: Parenting and Child Development. Edited by Lamb ME. Hillsdale, NJ, Lawrence Erlbaum, 1982, 289–314

Wallerstein JS, Corbin SB, Lewis JM: Children of divorce: a 10-year study, in Impact of Divorce, Single Parenting, and Stepparenting on Children. Edited by Hetherington EM, Arasteh JD. Hillsdale, NJ, Lawrence Erlbaum, 1988, pp 197–214

Zill N, Morrison DR, Coiro MJ: Long-term effects of parental divorce on parent-child relationships, adjustment, and achievement in young adulthood. Journal of Family Psychology 7:91–103, 1993

Chapter 22

Bereavement as a Significant Stressor in Children

Mordecai Kaffman, M.D.
Esther Elizur, Ph.D.

"Resilient" Versus "Vulnerable" Children

Children and adolescents who have experienced a traumatic life event such as death of a parent are expected to develop discernible affective, behavioral, and functional responses (Krupnick and Solomon 1987; Osterweis et al. 1984; Weller and Weller 1991). Although very few prospective studies of bereaved children have been carried out, those that have been done appear to confirm the fact that bereavement constitutes a risk factor for subsequent child psychopathology. Weller and Weller (1991) found that about one-third of a sample of bereaved youth met the DSM-III-R criteria for depression (American Psychiatric Association 1987), including symptoms such as chronically depressed mood, loss of interest in surroundings, augmented suicidal ideation, and sleep, appetite, and psychomotor disturbance. Kranzler and colleagues (1990) have reported significantly increased symptomatic behavior in a sample of preschool-age bereaved children compared with nonbereaved control subjects. In our own experience, for about 40% of preadolescent children without special adjustment problems before the bereavement, death of a parent in childhood constitutes an extremely traumatic event with rather long-lasting emotional and behavioral symptoms requiring some type of psychological intervention (Elizur and Kaffman 1982).

The severity, quality, duration, and long-term outcome of the particular bereavement symptoms vary considerably between two polar groups—those children perceived as "resilient" or "stress-resistant," and those children who are perceived as "vulnerable," as evidenced by their troublesome posttraumatic reactions (Luthar and Zigler 1991). In contrast to the "vulnerable" child, the "resilient" child continues developing as a functionally well adjusted individual despite the seemingly similar quality and severity of the traumatic blow experienced by each child. These differing outcomes may explain the often dissenting professional literature on the subject of bereavement reactions in childhood, including the contradictory findings from studies supporting or denying the idea that the death of a parent contributes to psychopathology in adult life (Birtchnell 1980; Bowlby 1980; Gregory 1966; Kendler et al. 1992).

Some studies based on a selected group of children have suggested that mourning reactions in children can be condensed to fit a standard model of bereavement irrespective of the diverse nature of the children's individual, family, and cultural circumstances. A further inspection of the literature, however, reveals that these data are based mainly on investigations of children in psychological treatment either before or after the trauma of death, and on retrospective recollections of adults who developed emotional problems many years after the loss of a loved one (Lloyd 1980; Tennand et al. 1980), as well as on studies based on children's reactions to temporary separation from parents (Bowlby 1960, 1980). It is clear that these samples of children cannot serve as a basis for generalization. In all probability, the methodological limitations of these studies contribute to the differences and contradictions in the conclusions of the various investigators about central issues such as the child's developing conception and understanding of death, differences between the mourning process in children and adults, duration of grieving in childhood, the child's ability to tolerate and express painful feelings related to the loss, and what constitutes the normal course and outcome of childhood bereavement.

Bowlby (1973) described three phases in the bereavement process of the child: protest, despair, and detachment. During the *protest* phase, the child expresses primarily anger, fear, and frantic attempts of reattachment to the lost parent. In the *despair* phase the child experiences sadness and depression, culminating gradually in an acceptance of the reality of the separation. Finally, in the phase of *detachment,* the child becomes open to new relationships, particularly to a new attachment with a parental figure. This model, like all models, should be considered a theoretical construct rather than a tangible reality. In our experience, few bereaved children fit into a consistent pattern of fixed consecutive stages. Bereavement symptoms of "protest," "despair," and "detachment" usually appear simultaneously during the early months of bereavement. Thus readiness and willingness for a new attachment to a substitute parental figure may already appear a few weeks after the loss, whereas the symptoms of "protest" can appear or persist up to the third year of bereavement.

Symptomatic Reactions of Bereaved Children

In this chapter we refer to findings from a 4-year prospective study, conducted in the framework of the Kibbutz Clinic, on the immediate and intermediate reactions—affective, behavioral, cognitive, and somatic symptoms—in 25 psychiatrically healthy children under the age of 10, who constituted a representative sample of all the bereaved preadolescent children of the Israeli kibbutz communes whose fathers had died in the Yom Kippur War of 1973 (Elizur and Kaffman 1982, 1983; Kaffman and Elizur 1979, 1983). It is important to note several characteristics of the children selected for this sample. Only children within their community with no special emotional and behavioral problems before the loss were included in the study. Any bereaved child who had received or was receiving psychological treatment, or had discernible developmental or psychological problems before the father's death, was excluded from the sample. All of the children had lost their father in war under similar circumstances (in battle) and during the same period of time. All of the families can be seen as belonging to the middle socioeconomic class, and all of the mothers had at least a high school education.

It should be stressed that in the kibbutz, both mothers and fathers are equally important attachment figures for the child. In general, the kibbutz father has a greater opportunity to be with his children than does the father in an urban family. Because children in the kibbutz are not dependent on their fathers as main providers of material needs, fathers are expected to be as effectively and affectively involved with their children as are mothers.

It should be noted that because of the communal structure of the kibbutz, there exist conditions that appear to ease the child's encounter with the trauma of the parent's death. Because food, lodging, clothing, day care, health needs, and educational requirements are provided by the community, the family need not fear economic insecurity, material deprivation, or any abrupt change in their daily routine. Life in the children's house remains stable, and in most cases, a couple of days after receiving news of the father's death the child returns to almost all regular daily activities. As a result, the child's contact with the mother's acute grief and with possible anxiety-provoking scenes and mourning ceremonials is relatively limited compared with that experienced by nonkibbutz children. Moreover, during the mourning period, kibbutz children are, even more than nonkibbutz children, surrounded by comfort, help, and support from people in their immediate community.

All these propitious conditions, however, were not enough to protect the kibbutz child from the disruptive impact of the traumatic event. In each phase of our 4-year follow-up study (6, 18, and 42 months after the loss), about 40% of the bereaved kibbutz children were found to react with severe problems and maladaptive behavior. Thus it appears that the tremendous importance of the father as a central attachment figure in the kibbutz child's emotional life far offsets the moderating influences of environmental conditions that help the child cope with the other stress situations.

"Pathological Bereavement"

Data for our conclusions were drawn exclusively from interviews with the widowed mother and the child's teacher. A basic premise in our study was that the diagnosis based on semistructured interviews with the child's mother and teacher has a reasonable degree of reliability and validity. Graham and Rutter (1968), among other authors, have shown that interviews with parents provide a valid basis for the detection of psychopathology in children, whereas the actual psychiatric examination does not necessarily lead to an accurate diagnosis, particularly with regard to diverse types of conduct disorder. In general, a high degree of agreement was observed between mothers' and teachers' reports, although mothers tended to underreport some of the school and social problems, while teachers overlooked particular grief and symptomatic reactions that appear mostly within the family setting. Our findings, therefore, appear to confirm the recent conclusions of Sanford and colleagues (1992) on the possible pitfalls of child psychiatric studies based on isolated parent- or teacher-reported data.

Independent interviews were conducted with the mother and teacher of each bereaved child during the three phases of the 4-year research. The guide questionnaire for the structured interview was compiled from an analysis of the salient symptoms reported in the literature on childhood bereavement and from a pilot study in which all of the reactions of eight preadolescent kibbutz children who had lost a parent in a car accident were recorded. The interview included an open-ended question probing the current predicament of the child and a structured checklist of 50 behaviors and symptoms that might be used to describe and assess the severity, duration, and frequency of each item. During the first phase of the research (3–6 months after the father's death) the interviewee was also asked to note which symptoms existed prior to the bereavement. These retrospective reports formed the pretraumatic profile of each child. Both available sources of information, mother and teacher, for each child were queried on the same items.

To prevent ambiguity in listing and assessing the bereavement reactions of the children, we recorded only symptomatic responses expressed by manifest behavioral changes that appeared or became exacerbated following the parent's death. Thus two distinct groups could be identified: children whose exceptional difficulties impaired their daily functioning and children who succeeded, despite the trauma, in adjusting to the new reality. Specifically, the label of "pathological bereavement" was applied in each phase of the study only to those children who met the following criteria:

1. The presence of multiple and persistent clinical symptomatology of sufficient intensity to handicap the child in his or her everyday life within the family, school, and children's group (*at least* eight impairing behavior symptoms of marked intensity). Only abnormal behavior and the impairment in the child's social functions that had persisted for *at least* 2 months were considered toward fulfilling the criterion.

2. The independent and concordant estimate by the mother and the teacher, on the one hand, and by the investigators, on the other hand, that the child's deviant behavior called for psychological intervention. A reliability test indicated a high rate of correlation (95%) among the separate appraisals of the mother, teacher, and investigators as to the need for professional help.

There was a significant increase in the incidence of behavior symptoms and grief reactions reported by all of the mothers and teachers of the bereaved kibbutz children compared with the incidence among those same children in the prebereavement period and with the representative samples of nonbereaved children matched by age and sex (Kaffman and Elizur 1977) (Table 22–1). *Immediately following the loss* we found a remarkable and significant increase in the average number of behavior symptoms in most of the children, as compared with the prebereavement profile. About 40% of the kibbutz children were judged to be experiencing "pathological bereavement" in at least two of the three stages of the investigation. Nearly 70% of the children showed signs of severe emotional disturbance in at least one of the stages. Only a minority of bereaved children—about one-third—did not show any overt signs of emotional impairment and were able to achieve satisfactory family, school, and social adjustment throughout the entire 4 years of follow-up. We did not continue our observations and interviews beyond the fourth postbereavement year because by then almost one-third of the bereaved children had been referred to psychological treatment, which, based on the original assessment criteria, excluded them from further consideration in the study.

Regarding the influence of the child's sex on the type and severity of bereavement reactions, we did not find significant gender differences except for the augmented prevalence of aggressiveness and outbursts of rage in boys at all stages of the investigation. We were unable to corroborate the generally accepted assumption that the psychological disturbance is greater if the death involves the parent of the same sex.

Death of a Parent During Wartime

One of the questions raised by a study on child bereavement in wartime is to what extent the findings can be generalized to other samples of bereaved children. Our clinical experience with kibbutz and urban Israeli children who have lost one of their parents under a variety of circumstances (suicide, illness, road accidents, etc.) suggests that these bereaved children respond to the loss with similar manifestations of grief and that their reactions and symptoms clearly resemble those of the children whose fathers were killed in war.

In the 1970s we (unfortunately) had ample opportunity to observe

Table 22–1. Frequency of behavioral problems, grief reactions, and "pathological bereavement" among 25 bereaved kibbutz children compared with 25 nonbereaved children

Type of reaction or symptom	Nonbereaved children (%)	Before loss (%)	Bereaved children			Significance	
			After loss			χ^2	P
			6 months (%)	18 months (%)	42 months (%)		
Main grief reactions							
Crying spells	8	4	86	60	43	Highly significant	
Sadness, moodiness	8	4	77	56	39	Highly significant	
Search for "substitute father"	—		54	44	48	Highly significant	
Main behavioral symptoms							
Overdependence, clinging to mother	12	8	59	64	61	12.68	P<.001
Separation problems	8	4	50	48	35	10.39	P<.01
Aggressive behavior	8	4	54	28	43	8.88	P<.01
Temper tantrums	4	4	45	40	52	10.96	P<.001
Discipline problems	8	4	45	52	48	9.92	P<.01
Restlessness	8	4	50	36	39	8.82	P<.01
Phobic fears	8	8	27	56	52	8.88	P<.01
Sleep problems	4	4	32	16	13	10.96	P<.001
Withdrawal, social isolation	8	8	18	24	39	Too small sample	
Learning problems (school ages)	8	—	19	16	17	Too small sample	
Health complaints	4	4	18	24	26	Too small sample	
Eating problems	4	4	29	32	39	Too small sample	
Enuresis	8	4	18	12	13	Too small sample	
Soiling	—	—	14	8	4	Too small sample	
"Pathological bereavement"	—	—	45	48	39	11.65	P<.001

the effects of stress experienced by kibbutz children during wartime. The Yom Kippur War (1973) was a relatively short one, lasting only 3 weeks. Throughout this period, the kibbutz successfully adopted the necessary measures to reduce the severity of the stress of war on the civilian population, particularly with regard to children (Kaffman 1977). In the 4-year period following the 1973 war, we observed no increase in emotional disturbances in the overall kibbutz child population. According to our records at the Kibbutz Clinic, the quantity and quality of the postwar psychological problems appeared to be similar to those of the pre-war period. In almost no case of kibbutz children referred for psychological consultation during or following the war were we able to establish that the stress conditions of the war were significant in the creation of the child's problems. The only clear exceptions were those cases in which the war affected the child and the family directly through the severe impact of death of a close family member. It is clear, therefore, that because of their extreme psychological vulnerability, children who lost their father either in war or in other circumstances constitute an exceptional group in the kibbutz setting.

Kibbutz and Nonkibbutz Children

In the second year of the children's bereavement it was possible for us to compare our findings in the original sample of 25 bereaved kibbutz children with those of 21 Israeli city children, matched for gender and age, who had also lost a father in the Yom Kippur War during the same period and under similar circumstances (Kaffman and Elizur 1983). Thus, at the second year of bereavement, the total sample included 46 children (25 boys and 21 girls; 31 preschool-age children [ages 3½–6], and 15 school-age children [ages 6–11½]). All of them were considered "normal" children without noticeable difficulties before their father's death. The data for the urban children were obtained from semistructured interviews with the mother of each child that took place 18 months after notification of the father's death, whereas the data for the kibbutz children included separate interviews with the mother and the teacher of each child.

Our findings indicate a similar pattern and incidence of grief reactions and behavioral symptoms as reported by mothers of both kibbutz and urban children. In both samples, 1½ years following the father's death, many of the children still exhibited evident manifestations of grief. The child still looked sadder than before the loss, had recurrent periods of moodiness, cried easily in response to slight frustrations, expressed feelings of longing for the dead father, and spent much time reminiscing (e.g., looking at photo albums, talking to the father's picture, recalling joining experiences). In most cases, however, the manifestations of the grief appear less frequently and with less intensity than in the first 6 months after the father's death. Mothers often spoke of both their own and their children's mourning process as "a painful open wound which gradually heals always with ups and downs."

In general, urban and kibbutz mothers gave very similar answers regarding the incidence of behavioral difficulties and the overall severity of the emotional impact of the loss on their children in the first 2 years following the loss. The percentage of children judged to be experiencing "pathological bereavement," as characterized by the presence of multiple and persistent clinical symptoms, was very high and similar for both kibbutz and urban children (48% and 52%, respectively). All these findings appear to confirm previous conclusions that for all children the death of the father has a severe and long-lasting impact on the child's emotional life.

We did find several differences between kibbutz and urban children, but only regarding the expressive content of the symptoms. These differences can be seen as related to sociocultural conditions. We observed, for example, a higher frequency of overly dependent behavior and phobic and night fears among urban children (67% vs. 52%). Clearly, the higher frequency of stressful changes, such as moving to a new neighborhood, change of school, and changes in mother's job and economic status, increases the city child's level of anxiety and insecurity. The urban children also tended more easily to cling to adult male figures in their immediate environment (67% vs. 18%). Moreover, among the urban children there was a significantly higher prevalence of denial of death, some of the children being influenced by religious ideas about the coming of the Messiah and the eventual resurrection of the dead.

Grief Reactions

Under the label "grief reactions" we included all of the affective-feeling responses of the bereaved child as reported by the surviving parent and the teacher. Some of the most common expressions of grief listed in our sample included gloomy moods, overt sadness, sobbing and tearfulness, spells of crying, longing, excessive reminiscing activity, exaggerated imitation or identification with the deceased parent, and continued preoccupation with the subject of death.

For most of the bereaved kibbutz and urban children (86%), there were reports of recurrent outbursts of crying and moodiness during the first 6 months of bereavement. Only a minority of the sample (23%) reacted with a facade of indifference, and these children were all under the age of 4 years. In several cases, the child did not connect the sadness directly to the father's death.

In the early months of bereavement, 75% of the children above the age of 3 years spent much time recalling specific memories of the dead father. Activities associated with this recollection included recurrently talking about the deceased father, recalling shared experiences, looking at photograph albums, listening to recorded conversations, holding or using his personal effects, and the like. In preschool-age children these reminiscences seemed to be connected with concrete events—shared experiences, presents, places—whereas the older children tended to speak less about their loss but spent more time looking at photographs, reading their father's letters, and occasionally even expressing their desire to go to the cemetery.

Obviously the intensity of activities of recalling the past depends to a large extent on the mother's willingness or ability to share her own feelings with her children. In some cases, it was the mother who refrained from conversation about the father and restrained the child's questions and reminiscences. In these cases the mother tried in various ways to "defend" the child and to keep him or her away from pain and sorrow by distracting his or her attention from any subject connected with the father's death. The degree of the mother's openness seemed influenced by many factors, such as, among others, the open or closed pattern of communication that had existed before the death of the father among members of the family.

Longing for the lost father was often expressed paradoxically by frequent and insistent search for a substitute father. About half of the bereaved preschool-age children announced verbally that they wanted to get a new father, or they attached themselves to a familiar man and demanded attention and signs of affection from him. Usually the kibbutz children turned to a close relative, but occasionally they chose the father of one of their peers in the children's group. Sometimes the idea of seeking a substitute father was the child's immediate and spontaneous response to the announcement of his or her father's death. This yearning for a new father reflects the child's strong need to alleviate the acute suffering caused by the father's absence, although sometimes children expressed their desire to get a substitute father in order to comfort the mourning mother.

The prevalence of most of the grief reactions in our study group of 46 bereaved kibbutz and urban children—the reactions occurring during the early months of bereavement in over 80% of the children—steadily declined to 37% during the second year, and to 25% by the third year. The only exception was the phenomenon of search for a substitute father, which was present in almost half of the bereaved children throughout all the phases of the study.

Behavior Symptoms

Behavior problems are related to the child's "fight-flight" behavioral style of coping with situations of pain, frustration, and stress. In contrast to the gradual decrease in the incidence of grief reactions, we found a persistently high rate of behavior problems throughout the entire follow-up period, including almost all known categories of childhood behavior disorders (according to the DSM-III-R nomenclature [American Psychiatric Association 1987]).

The augmented proportion of bereaved children with marked emotional disturbance (over 40%) throughout the follow-up period is strikingly higher than the comparative epidemiological data in matched samples of nonbereaved children of the same age and sex (Table 22–1). Surveys in representative samples of nonbereaved kibbutz children (Kaffman 1972; Kaffman and Elizur 1977) show a significantly diminished number of children in need of psychological help (13%) and a significantly lower proportion of behavior problems such as separation difficulties, overdependent behavior, aggressiveness, temper tantrums, restlessness, fears, and concentration difficulties.

The two most common clusters of behavioral problems found in our sample of bereaved children were

1. *Overanxious–dependent type* of problems, which included "internalized" reactions such as a) overdependency, separation anxiety, and clinging to mother (60% of the bereaved children compared

with 8% of the children before the trauma and 12% of the children in the nonbereaved group); b) various fears (such as fear of being left alone, of strangers, of darkness, of animals, and of imaginary creatures), sleep disturbances, night fears, and concern that something could happen to the child or to the surviving parent (44% of the bereaved children compared with 8% of the children before the loss and 8% of the children in the nonbereaved group); and c) repeated complaints about health (20% of the bereaved children compared with 4% of the children before the trauma and 4% of the children in the nonbereaved group).

2. *Antisocial-aggressive type* of problems, which included "externalized" responses such as a) aggressiveness, temper tantrums, restlessness, negativism, and disciplinary problems (40% of the bereaved children compared with 4% of the children before the trauma and 8% of the nonbereaved group); and b) school and learning problems (18% of the bereaved children compared with none of the children before the trauma and 8% in the nonbereaved group).

Many children also exhibited considerable increase in "regressive" symptomatic behavior such as eating problems, enuresis, and encopresis, as compared with both the pretraumatic situation and the nonbereaved group (Table 22–1), although because of the small size of the sample these findings did not reach statistical significance.

Course of the Bereavement Reactions

Generally, our findings point to the fact that the bereavement process is not a set of symptoms that start after the loss and gradually fade away. Rather, bereavement involves a succession of clinical pictures that blend into and replace one another.

The First Months

The child's immediate reaction to the sudden trauma of the father's death is expressed by a manifest emotional expression of pain and grief. In contrast to those studies that underscore "the absence of grief" in childhood mourning (Deutsch 1937; Nagera 1970), in our study it was found that the majority of children ages 2 to 10 reacted by crying, sadness, and varied expressions of longing. Responses of anger and protest are also frequent immediate reactions of the child to the loss. These responses among the children in our study did not replace manifestations of grief and sorrow, as some authors suggest (Wolfenstein 1968), but appeared together with them.

In our study the children utilized various defensive measures that helped them to mitigate the acute pain of grieving and enabled them to "gain distance and time" so that they could assimilate the shock gradually. The most common means of effecting this was the child's maintaining the belief that the deceased father is nearby although he may not be seen or heard. This was achieved by intense revival of the image of the lost father from the past (recalling joint experiences), as well as by denying the finality of death and expecting the father's return in the future. In contrast to the younger children who denied the loss and tended to talk a lot about the father as still present, most of the older children (ages 7 to 10) tended to gain distance by withdrawal, restraint, and ignoring the subject of death directly.

At the same time, and to an increasing extent throughout the first year of bereavement, the child began to examine the meaning and the implications of what had happened. Attempts to understand the concept of death were expressed in various ways in the early months of bereavement, either by translating the concept of death to concrete and familiar situations or by asking many realistic questions to gain understanding of the difference between "dead" and "alive." During the first months the child oscillated between the two opposing tendencies: the inhibitory tendency that, by denial and avoidance, limited the perception of the traumatic loss; and the reality testing tendency that enhanced perception and gradual acceptance of the father's death. The delicate interplay between these two tendencies enabled the child to accept the fact of death and come to terms with the many areas of uncertainty that threatened his or her world.

The Second Year

Eighteen months after the father's death, most children usually had achieved acceptance of the loss. Together with the decrease of the primary defensive measures (especially denial) and the painful understanding of the finality of the loss, there was a significant increase in the child's level of anxiety. This increased anxiety was expressed by the appearance of various fears among more than half of the children studied. Usually, these were fears about being left alone, apprehension that the mother may suddenly disappear or be inaccessible, and fears of injury and danger to oneself. Other reported fears concerned darkness, medical treatment, terrorists, various external threats, and animals. The most common fear was, however, the fear of being left alone.

The notable increase in the child's level of anxiety at this phase appears to be connected with the greater realistic perception of the irreversibility and permanence of the loss. Only at that point does the child perceive the full implications of the traumatic event. Eighteen months after the loss, it was clear that many children in our study sensed the world as dangerous and threatening and had many fears of being abandoned or injured. Dreams, essays, and drawings about the subject of death were frequent and can be seen as one of the child's ways to master anxiety.

The most common coping reactions at this period of anxiety and uncertainty are augmented dependency and demandingness. About two-thirds of the children in our study showed increased dependence on the mother, including difficulties in parting from the mother, clinging to her, looking for her at irregular hours, and constant requests for assistance and attention. Some children also extended this overdependency to teachers or other significant adults.

During each phase of the study, a greater incidence of fears (especially night fears) was found among the preschool-age children. Obviously, the younger the child, the greater his or her dependence on the parent as the principal object for satisfying his or her physical, emotional, and developmental needs.

Increased aggressive behavior, discipline problems, and restlessness characterized about 40% of the children 2 to 3 years after the father's death—three times more than in the prebereavement period. In about one-half of these cases the aggressive reactions were rated in the medium to severe degree of intensity. During the entire postbereavement period, expressions of hyperaggressiveness were significantly more frequent among boys and among children over the age of 6.

The increased incidence of eating problems (vomiting, poor appetite, or overeating) and regressive symptomatic behavior (thumb sucking, enuresis, and/or encopresis) observed during the early months remained stable throughout the follow-up period. They appeared in 25% of the children, especially the younger ones, usually as combined symptoms.

The Third and Fourth Years

We found in the last stage of the study that for many of the children, there was some evidence of symptomatic improvement and adjustment to the changed life circumstances. In this last stage, in comparison with the earlier two stages, there was a drastic decline in the rate of grief reactions. Manifestations of overdependence still typified about two-thirds of the sample, but there was a clear reduction in the anxiety level, separation difficulties, and severity of fears. The augmented aggressiveness and the concentration difficulties were also reduced. A considerable number of the children were reported to have returned to normal integration in the school and social frameworks. For many, there was also further adjustment to the new family situation, either to a new set of roles in a single-parent family, or to the extended family or to a stepfather. The attachment to an adult male figure was now more permanent and stable, as opposed to the tendency of changing the object frequently that characterized the first two stages after the loss.

During the 4 years of the study, there was a gradual rise in the frequency of two additional phenomena: general emotional restraint (including restraint on the subject of the father's death) and "exemplary behavior." These two reactions had characterized the older age group in the sample. The pattern of "good behavior" was expressed by the child's beginning to undertake new responsibilities and functions in the family and outside (e.g., care for a younger sibling, helping mother in household chores, diligence in studies, and social obligations). In most cases this pattern did not become rigid or neurotic and was the child's way of coping with the new situation by "accelerated maturity," which ensured the mother's and other adults' approval and strengthened the child's self-esteem and independence. In some cases, this reaction also reflected a certain type of identification with the father by the child's taking on family roles that had been the father's.

It should be remembered that despite the general trend toward symptomatic improvement and adjustment during the third and fourth years after the father's death, still more than one-third of the children (39%) showed signs of marked emotional impairment ("pathological bereavement").

Uneven Development of the Bereavement Reactions

In addition to individual differences in the nature of bereavement symptoms, we found a wide range of variability among the children regarding the course and development of the reactions. No stable pattern was found regarding the timing of appearance or disappearance of pathological reactions. We could not predict the degree of pathology that might appear in the child only on the basis of his or her clinical condition at a previous stage. Yet those children with symptoms of marked emotional impairment during the early months of bereavement appeared to develop the most severe and prolonged type of pathological mourning. However, there were other children who did not reveal any special pathology during the early months and yet deteriorated during the second or fourth year. In other words, the time that elapsed since the loss was not the principal determinant of the course of pathology. Hence, pathological mourning reactions appear to be either brief (2 to 6 months) or enduring (2 years or longer), immediate or delayed.

Factors Influencing the Severity of Bereavement

Manifold variables were found to be associated with the appearance and severity of the emotional and behavioral disturbance following the parent's death. Our findings suggest that it is the combination of several factors that determines the intensity of the bereavement response, rather than the exclusive influence of any single factor. Any of the eventual pathogenic influences could be either present or absent in a particular child with "pathological bereavement," thus indicating the complexity and multiplicity of the factors involved in the bereavement process. In analyzing the correlational pre- or posttraumatic variables associated with "pathological bereavement," we distinguish between three main categories: child variables, family variables, and circumstantial variables. On the whole, we found in our sample that the child's emotional responses during the early months of bereavement were largely determined by pretraumatic antecedent variables (temperamental attributes; overall coping abilities in response to frustration and environmental changes; emotional responsivity before the loss; the presence or absence of family conflict; prolonged separation from one or both parents before the death, etc.). Posttraumatic factors, on the other hand (the surviving parent's ability to cope with the stress of loss; the quality of the parent-child relationship; the proximity of a "surrogate" parental figure; as well as diverse social, cultural, and situational posttraumatic stresses), appear to play a paramount role in the determination of the final outcome, particularly throughout the second and third years of bereavement.

Child and Family Variables

Age and sex.   On the whole, neither age nor sex was found to be significantly related to the rate of "pathological bereavement" in any postbereavement stage. Although bereaved boys exhibited more motoric reactions, restlessness, aggression, and learning problems than did the girls, such differences did not reach statistical significance. However, when the effect of the interaction of age and sex was analyzed with regard to the total sample of bereaved kibbutz and urban children, a significantly higher rate of behavioral symptoms was found among the young boys, ages 3 to 6, than among the girls of the same age. A number of differences in the quality of grief and behavior reactions were found between the preschool-age children (age 3½–6 years) and the school-age children (6–11½) in both the kibbutz and urban samples. The younger children tended to be more spontaneous and actively engaged in recalling activities and talking about the dead father, and to frequently use denial regarding the finality of death. They tended to urge their mother to get married and find a surrogate father. On the other hand, most of the older children appeared to be afraid to allow feelings of longing to emerge. They dealt with the subject of death more symbolically through play, drawing, composition of diaries, and reading of selected books. Emotional restraint in verbal expression and general social withdrawal were frequently observed among the older children. Other significant differences between the two groups were a higher frequency of night fears, separation difficulties, and manifestations of overdependence and demandingness among the preschool-age children. Among the older children a higher prevalence of restlessness, aggressiveness, or unexpected "exemplary behavior" was found.

Temperamental characteristics.   We found a clear association between "pathological bereavement" and the child's temperamental level of self-control. Thus children in the low self-control group—the so-called high intensity children in the Thomas and Chess (1977) nomenclature (i.e., children with poor control of impulses, emotional lability, and a tendency to react with explosive rage to frustrations)— showed marked emotional and behavioral difficulties throughout the first 3 years of bereavement. On the other hand, overdependent and inhibited-withdrawn children tended to react with significant emotional difficulties only after the first postbereavement year, as more external pressure is exerted upon the bereaved child to return to independent and age-appropriate activities. Predictably, a consistent relationship was found between a high temperamental level of motor activity and a pathological bereavement reaction during all three phases of our study.

In general, no differences were found between kibbutz and urban populations with regard to pretraumatic temperamental variables and quality of bereavement. For both populations "pathological bereavement" was found to be related to low self-control, hyperactivity, and high withdrawal-inhibition temperamental traits. One exception, however, is the relatively lower correlation among the kibbutz children, in contrast to the urban children, between the temperament attribute of low adaptability and a poor bereavement outcome. One possible explanation for this finding could be related to the special conditions of the kibbutz, where the bereaved child does not face dramatic changes in physical, social, and educational settings following the loss.

Pretraumatic emotional difficulties.   Bereaved children who in the past had exhibited more than average or transient behavioral symptoms but before the father's death were considered by their mother, the teacher, and the investigators as "normal" children, often showed manifest relapse of the surmounted symptomatic behavior and tended to develop subsequent new emotional problems.

In many cases the situation was aggravated by unfavorable family conditions before the father's death (e.g., divorce, experience of long separation, or an obviously disturbed parent-child relationship), so that it was hard to differentiate between the individual child problems and diverse family factors.

Past separation experiences.   We found a significant relationship between pretraumatic long-term separation of the child from one of the parents (following divorce or circumstantial events), or previous experience of death in the family, and "pathological bereavement," particularly during the first 6 months after the parent's death. In children who had experienced short-term parent-child separations before the loss, however, no significant relationship was found at any phase of the study between this type of separation and the development of pathological responses. For these children a gradual mastering process, with "desensitization" to the experience of separation, appears to have evolved. It seems that the graded exposure to brief separation experiences in the presence of emotional support, followed by happy reunion, constitutes a very effective instrument to foster both readiness for independence and better tolerance to the stress of further traumatic separations. Conversely, as Bowlby (1973) and many others have pointed out, we have found that early experiences of repeated or prolonged stressful separations might preclude the establishment of basic trust in the parent-child relationship, handicapping them from dealing with subsequent loss and enhancing the likelihood that they will experience pathological bereavement if such loss occurs. On the other extreme, we found another group of high-risk children—those belonging to disproportionately child-centered families—who, always surrounded by overinvolved, overprotective, and overcaring parents, did not have age-appropriate separation experiences before the death of the parent, These children lacked the opportunity to profit from experience that might have prepared them for future stressful life events (Meichenbaum 1985).

Family conflicts.   We have found a clear connection between a previously disturbed family environment and the development of a pathological reaction during the first 2 years of bereavement. In families with a long-standing history of conflict and marital discord, children reacted to the loss of a parent with intense and pervasive problems. Among these children, the father was often peripherically involved with his children, and the mother was reported to have had considerable trouble in her relationship with the children before the father's death. When the pretraumatic relationship between the child and the deceased parent was characterized by excessive conflict, the child's bereavement reactions tended to be particularly intense. Bereaved children of divorced parents also showed marked emotional impairment during the first 2 years of bereavement. Thus, as suggested also by Raphael (1983), a prebereavement pattern of family conflict, particularly in the presence of frequent quarrels between the parent who subsequently dies and the child, tends to aggravate the bereavement reaction, eliciting feelings of intense guilt and confusion in the child.

Circumstantial Variables

Parental loss is a traumatic event that usually occurs in association with fundamental changes in the child's life. As noted above, in the Israeli urban population, in contrast to the kibbutz, the daily setting is less stable, and thus following the father's death the child is faced with immediate consequences, frequently involving changes in daily routine, location, and socioeconomic status. The relatively greater amount of psychological disturbance among the nonkibbutz children, therefore, may be partly related to the higher frequency of intercurrent life events and stressful changes in the family state of affairs after the loss of the father. In addition, the urban child has closer and more intimate contact with the acute grief reactions of the mother. All these circumstances appear to increase the level of anxiety and the child's feelings of insecurity, thus fostering increased dependent behavior and clinging attachment to the mother, who represents the remaining major provider of the child's basic emotional and instrumental needs. As noted above, urban children in the sample had more sleeping problems, night fears, and clinging behavior and were also more active in seeking a "substitute father" compared with their kibbutz counterparts.

Posttraumatic Factors

Mother's bereavement reactions.   The quality of the mother's grief response was found to be related to the child's problems, particularly during the early bereavement phase. When the mother exhibited overrestraint, withholding of emotional expression, and inability to share with the child expressions of grief, the child showed signs of considerable emotional distress during the first postbereavement months. This finding confirms the observation that emotional restraint in the surviving parent makes it difficult for children to express feelings, intensifies their experience of loneliness, and increases their anxiety and confusion in grasping the meaning of the sudden death (Furman 1974).

During the bereavement period, the child needs strong parental support, and when the parenting is inconsistent and characterized by reactions of confusion and anxiety, the child's bereavement process is impaired. Children who sense their mother's uncertainty and frailty may feel especially vulnerable and helpless in confronting a world that has become threatening and unpredictable. In our study the mother's ego strength in coping with the new situation proved to be a highly significant factor in determining the severity of the child's bereavement throughout the 4-year follow-up period. Children of "weak" mothers—those who did not return to their daily routine of activities within the first 6 months of bereavement and continued to exhibit helplessness and despair—were found to have a significantly higher percentage of problems than were children of mothers who adjusted successfully to the new reality and were able to return fully to work and to social and recreational activities. The mother's assertiveness, competence in parenting, coping ability, and capacity to maintain a positive relationship with the child constitute paramount influential factors in determining the quality and severity of the child's bereavement reactions.

Siblings.   The analysis of the reactions of 10 pairs of bereaved kibbutz siblings included in the kibbutz sample pointed to the influence of the family on the "bereavement profile" of the sibling (Kaffman and Elizur 1979). We found strong intrafamily similarities in the amount and severity of the symptoms exhibited by both siblings. Nine out of these 10 pairs of siblings were concordant as to the extent and severity of postbereavement morbidity. In four pairs of siblings, the "family bereavement profile" as expressed in parallel reports for each of them could be labeled as "pathological bereavement," with corresponding serious symptoms and marked impairment in functioning in both siblings. In the remaining five pairs of siblings, bereavement responses were also similar, but in the direction of normalcy, with only mild reactive behaviors for each of the siblings. This finding concurs with conclusions of previous research pointing to the fact that the severity of the child's symptoms is determined to a large extent by factors connected to the family's general level of functioning and its coping resources in dealing with stress (Luthar and Zigler 1991).

Availability of support systems.   Positive bereavement outcomes tend to be associated with an effective use of adequate support systems by both the surviving parent and the bereaved child. The availability of models and sources of support such as grandparents, aunts, uncles, older siblings, close friends, or any other surrogate parental figure who is able and willing to establish a good and stable relationship with the child usually decreases the risk of psychological morbidity. Only in a minority of cases, when a preexisting overly dependent attachment between the surviving parent and the child has persisted, does the introduction of a stepparent in the child's life lead to an increased rate of psychological difficulties in the family. In these cases the stepparent is rejected as an unwelcome outsider who is trying to displace the child from his or her central position in the family. The majority of the remarried mothers in our study group, however, reported a considerable improvement in the child's behavior following the stepfather's entrance into the family life. Evidently, the presence of a stable male figure to whom children can develop a positive attachment usually strengthens their sense of personal security and their feelings of "normal" family functioning and stability.

"Pathological bereavement."   A consistent connection was found between posttraumatic stressful situations and the child's "pathological bereavement" during the last two phases of the follow-up. Circumstances such as mother-child separation, conflicts between the surviving parent and other caregivers (educators, grandparents, other family members), or prolonged hospitalization of a close relative seemed to hinder the child's readjustment process particularly throughout the second and third years of bereavement.

Cultural influences.   The existence of differences in cross-cultural norms of grieving among different ethnic or socioeconomic groups has been well documented. Our findings show clear differences in the style and content of the mourning process among kibbutz and urban children—differences that can be seen as connected to the specific cultural attributes of each of the child-rearing methods. Thus, for example, urban children showed an intensified prevalence of denial of death. About one-half of the urban children, compared with only 8% of the kibbutz children, still used this defense mechanism in the second year of bereavement. Undoubtedly, cultural factors have decisive influence in strengthening and preserving the use of denial. Most of the kibbutz children learned to look at death more realistically, whereas some of the urban children came from homes where the mothers explained that "father is in heaven; he sees us and protects us," not because they were religious, but because they found it difficult to destroy the child's illusions about his or her father's coming back sometime in the future, trusting that time and maturation would help the child come to terms with the irreversibility of death. Several urban mothers tried to avoid discussing the subject and refused to respond to the child's attempts to clarify facts and gain understanding about death. One mother did not even tell her child that the father's body was buried in a grave. These examples clearly demonstrate how religious belief, or the adult's difficulty in coping with the finality of death, can reinforce the child's tendency to denial and makes it difficult for him or her to understand the full meaning of death. It should be noted that although these differences in sociocultural beliefs, norms, and practices influenced the type and quality of the grieving reactions, they did not affect the overall severity of the bereavement outcome or the intensity of the behavior symptoms.

The Victim Career

Between 1986 and 1990 we studied with particular interest the appearance and evolution of a dysfunctional and rigid postbereavement syndrome among young adolescents who adhered to and demanded official recognition of a permanent "victim status" following the death of a parent. Throughout this 5-year period our research team from the Kibbutz Clinic identified and treated a group of 12 such adolescents (7 girls and 5 boys), all of whom had lost a parent when they were 12 to 16 years old. They were referred for treatment at an average of 4 years after the death of the parent because of pervasive and persistent symptoms, including marked behavioral disorders, depressed moods, impairment in day-to-day functioning, and disturbance in interpersonal relationships. The severe symptoms, emerging soon after the parental death, did not meet the criteria for the diagnosis of any specific psychiatric syndrome, although they closely resembled a chronic adjustment disorder, with mixed disturbance of emotions, conduct, and functioning.

The single most striking symptom characterizing all these adolescents was their perception of themselves as "victims of life." For these adolescents the parental loss was seen as an irreparable and irreversible injury that would last the remainder of their lives, or, as one adolescent labeled it, "a life sentence." This implacable judgment was determined not by some objective court of law, but rather by the "victims" themselves, in close cooperation with significant persons in their immediate environment, and with no possible chance for reprieve. These bereaved youngsters firmly adhered to their inner belief that there is no way to reverse the dictates of this merciless destiny that blocks their way to happiness. Wherever they went they bared to all their burden like an open wound, one that they were convinced would never heal. In the absence of effective therapy, these adolescents will evolve into adults who continue to pursue their full-time career as "victims of life." They invested most of their energies in obsessive preoccupation with a pessimistic "half-empty glass" philosophy of life and neglected to search for positive content to fill their day-to-day functioning. Instead, they were consumed with bitterness, sadness, rage, and an endless search for revenge against their unjust fate.

The adolescents who fall into this syndrome of "victim status" can be divided into two main groups: those who adopt a pattern of acting out and aggressive behavior, and those with covert, internalized symptoms that are characterized by depressive moods, anxiety, and diminished interest and pleasure in almost all daily activities.

Adolescents in the first group tend to constantly criticize and denounce the surviving parent, who is seen as an evil, ruthless, hostile, overcritical person who makes the victim's life intolerable. In contrast, the deceased parent is deified and is seen as full of compassion, warmth, love, and understanding. Over a period of time, the overt family conflict becomes aggravated, and the adolescent feels increasingly overwhelmed with frustration and self-pity at having lost an overidealized parent while remaining at the mercy of a terrible monster.

In attempting to isolate the preconditions that facilitate the development and perpetuation of the "victim status," we found that one of the prime prerequisites is the existence of a reciprocal, complementary conflictual relationship with the surviving parent, who frequently also is caught up in the throes of chronic mourning. In some cases, the adolescent is locked in a mutually destructive and antagonistic relationship with the parent. In others, the adolescent is caught up in an overdependent and suffocating relationship with the surviving parent, which stifles his or her active coping skills for dealing with the loss and prevents later adjustment and growth. In still other cases, the adolescent's "victim status" is generated and maintained by overzealous and sympathetic adults in his or her immediate environment (e.g., grandparents, educators, neighbors) who reinforce the tragic elements of the loss and undermine the need for positive adjustment.

The situation may become exacerbated in cases in which the "victim" and those in his or her immediate social environment become locked in a destructive closed circuit, each caught up in a belligerent power struggle characterized by disturbed interpersonal relationships, endless fighting, and the development of a consistent pattern of oppositional behavior in the adolescent. When such a state of open warfare develops between the adolescent and the surviving parent, there is a consolidation of the perception of the living parent as a villain as compared with the deceased idealized parent. This reinforces the adolescent's identification with the "victim" role, justifies its maintenance, and reduces motivation for change. The "victim" is usually very convincing and meets with much support and sympathy from the many "good Samaritans" in his or her community, moved by the double tragedy of the "victim": the untimely death of a loved/loving parent on the one hand, and the pain of living with an unloving, rejecting surviving parent on the other. In spite of, or perhaps because of, the obsessive nature of the "victimization" belief, "victim" and "victimizer" become caught up in a destructive dance, the two held together by a magnetic-like pull in an endless struggle, with vicious mutual accusations and attacks, frequently accompanied by unrestrained explosions of hostility and aggression on both sides. The bereaved adolescent, caught up in his or her own repetitive, mono-ideaistic, self-hypnotic–like message of being an irreproachable sacrificial lamb, an innocent victim of tragic circumstances, becomes more and more convinced of the irreversible nature of the situation, and as such cannot be expected to change.

The second, smaller group of "victims" is that of "inhibited and insecure bereaved adolescents," who in the face of the traumatic loss of a parent withdraw from all active coping with life's challenges. These bereaved adolescents, perceiving themselves as "tragic victims," find rational explanations for their chronic mourning status and legitimize their exemption from fulfilling normative roles and functions together with their peers. They exhibit symptoms of depression, listlessness, tearfulness, anxiety, panic attacks, helplessness, impairment in social and occupational functioning, and persistent physical symptoms in the absence of organic pathology. They tend to pay frequent visits to the family doctor, often receiving (unnecessarily) large doses of medication, including antidepressants and tranquilizers.

It should be noted that this clinical picture of the "victim career" is not restricted to the trauma following the death of a parent. Any traumatic event (such as divorce, sexual abuse, loss of a loved one, accident or some form of injury, etc.) can result in a flight from coping with life's challenges, thereby transforming the loss or injury into a "living memorial."

Naturally, in all these cases the therapist's main aim should be to help the patient to shift from an impairing *victim status* to a healthy *survivor status*. We fully identify with Ochberg's (1991) credo that the therapist should have the aptitude "to guide a search for meaning, to recognize existential despair, to confront self-pity, and (particularly) to reinforce recognition of one's responsibility for one's own life." The necessary switch of the patient from a fatalistic victim status to an assertive and constructive position, of course, presents tremendous challenges even to the most experienced therapist.

Therapeutic Implications

In the literature there are conflicting opinions regarding the efficacy of professional help extended to the bereaved child and his or her family. Some clinicians assert that the negative impact of the loss of a parent in childhood on the personality of the child is unavoidable and that crisis intervention immediately after the event in no way diminishes the danger to the psychological health of the bereaved family (Pollack et al. 1975). In contrast, other researchers have stressed the usefulness of psychological assistance to the bereaved. In the words of Furman (1974), "We learned that when a child's parent dies he faces an incomparable stress, which threatens the further development of his personality. This danger can be avoided if the child can be helped to mourn his parent as fully as possible, and children from toddler age can be assisted in this task" (p. 11).

The nearly exclusive emphasis in the literature is on working through the mourning process and encouraging an emotional expression of the grief as the primary strategy for preventing a negative outcome from the crisis. In the light of our findings, this method seems rather limited in its scope and results. Although there is no doubt that open communication and emotional expression regarding the parent's death are very important, it would not be wise to propose this as a standard prescription in all cases. In our view there are additional significant factors aside from the style in which mourning has been worked through, particularly in the first years following the loss. Appropriate and effective intervention begins with the identification of the child at risk and a recognition of the influences of the surviving parent, of the school, and of the immediate community during the postbereavement period.

Identification of and Psychological Help for the Child at Risk

In the first few months after bereavement, particular attention should be paid to children with pretraumatic problematic personal or family adjustment, particularly if they have experienced prolonged separations from one of the parents in the past. Most of these children exhibit clinical symptoms soon after the first weeks and months of bereavement. In our opinion, for these children the first year is the "critical period" for intensive therapeutic intervention with both the child and his or her family, and recognizable clinical problems of the child should be treated immediately rather than years later when a severe pathology has already crystallized. To our regret, many professionals are unaware of the problems and stresses facing the child in the years immediately following the loss. Very often, at-risk bereaved children are referred for treatment 5 or more years after the loss. Our follow-up study suggests that the accepted notion that problems will fade in time by themselves is fallacious.

It is important to stress that although we emphasize the special vulnerability of the bereaved child, it is necessary to refrain from considering all bereaved children as "ill," "disturbed," or "exceptional." Such a stigma is liable to hinder children in their efforts to cope and to build a new positive identity for themselves. Similarly, pity, overprotection, and exaggerated "compassion" on the part of persons in the child's environment are liable to intensify the negative behaviors of the child, such as overdependence or fear of accommodation to the new reality.

Our findings indicate that clinicians must help the bereaved families in a more balanced manner. In the professional literature most of the recommended interventions for children who have lost their fathers have focused on helping the mother to cope with her bereavement. Insufficient attention has been paid to the fact that a large proportion of bereaved children go through a serious and prolonged crisis. Because of the mutual relationship between the condition of the child and that of the mother, we suggest that greater attention be paid to the mother-child system, in addition to focusing on the separate problems of the widowed mother and the child.

Suggested Tasks and Interventions in the Stages of Bereavement

The main implications of our research and our ideas regarding potential avenues of intervention during the process of bereavement are presented in accordance with the three stages during which we examined the children in our study.

The Immediate Stage: The Critical Weeks and Months After the Loss

Awareness and tolerance of the great variety of bereavement reactions.   It is important that the surviving parent, the members of the extended family, and teachers be cognizant of the wide variety of possible emotional, defensive, and behavioral reactions that the child may demonstrate in the first few months of mourning. An understanding of the normal bereavement process may reduce the concern, anxiety, and great confusion that are characteristic of the parent's behavior in the immediate stage. One must remember that the child's reactions may be varied and that there is no standard normal or uniform reaction. It is of extreme importance to accept temporary expressions of grief, anger, hysterical identification with the deceased father, denial of death, and diverse healthy ways of coping with the crisis employed by the child. Krupnick (1984) aptly summarizes this position as follows:

> It is important that parents learn about the grieving process in children so they will know what to expect and will not become alarmed about the differences between childhood and adult grieving. Anticipating that the child may ask distressing questions, such as when will there be a new parent . . ., may eliminate surprise and hurt. Children may manifest a superficially milder reaction to the loss because of the strong defenses that protect them from becoming flooded with overwhelming emotions. Preparing for and understanding such behavior and coping responses can help avoid or modify reactions of shaked hurt or anger in parents

that could intensify the child's feelings of confusion and guilt. (p. 128)

Explaining the fact of death.   Every child requires an adequate explanation of the concept of death. The difficulty in talking to the child on this subject lies generally in the anxieties, defenses, and confusion of the adult, more than those of the child. Our work has shown that the degree of children's ability to internalize the meaning of the loss and to reach cognitive control over the mysterious and threatening phenomenon of death depends, to a large extent, on the reaction of the adults around them. It is important to tell the child about the circumstances of the father's death, to assist the child in reaching some understanding, appropriate to his or her age, of the concept of death, and to provide all the relevant information regarding the tragic event that the child is able to absorb. It is necessary to help the child grasp death as something universal, inevitable, and independent of the child and his or her wishes. Clarifying the facts in a straightforward and clear manner can help the child in the bereavement process. Ignoring the subject, or creating a secretive atmosphere around it, will only heighten the anxiety level and increase unrealistic fantasies on the subject of death.

The surviving parent and other significant figures should be encouraged to listen to and patiently answer the young child's repeated questions. Sometimes the parent, who is also in active mourning, may find it hard to deal with the child's repeated queries. In such cases we found it advisable to seek external help, particularly from the teacher or the school psychologist.

Encouraging emotional expression.   It is of great importance that the adult accept and encourage the expression of pain, longing, anger, and anxiety on the part of the child. The child should feel free to express feelings that do not necessarily fit into the stereotype of grief, such as anger toward the father who has departed, feelings connected with a search for a "new father," and an egocentric concern over his or her own well-being.

During the first weeks of bereavement, the child needs to have access to a person with empathic understanding to whom the child feels close. When the mother shares her grief and longing with the child, when she reminisces about the father and talks to the child about him, she is actually helping the child express his or her own feelings in an uncon-

cerned manner. At this point in time, open, sincere, empathic transactions with a loved one make better sense to the child than any other
form of nurturing. Hiding or denial of the feelings of pain and grief
confuses the child and creates a barrier between him or her and the
adult world, adding a further loss to the loss he or she has sustained.

Immediate community outreach.   It is essential that the surviving
parent, as well as other significant figures in the life of the child, be
offered a clear avenue for support and consultation. An "open-door" arrangement, which allows the family to turn freely and legitimately for
counseling regarding any problem that may arise with the child, is likely
to be most useful. Psychiatric labels should be avoided so as not to injure
the family's feelings of competence. We observed in the course of our
research that this type of "on-call" help, which is offered and delivered
beginning with the stage of acute crisis, is better received by the grieving
family than continued and prolonged therapy or help offered at later
stages. The more time that elapses after the event, the less likely the
parent and child are to seek out professional help. Such a primary access
to a consultative therapeutic agency serves to encourage the parent in
seeking further help and advice concerning questions that may arise during the first years of bereavement.

The Intermediate Stage: The First and Second Years of Bereavement

A stable and secure framework is of utmost value for the child during
the first years of bereavement. It is essential to reduce as much as
possible further environmental changes and stresses. This may be accomplished in several ways.

A "strong," consistent mother.   It is of great help to the child if the
widowed mother is able to return gradually to her normal course of
work and care for the child while coping actively and effectively with
her new role as a single parent. Particularly in the first 2 years of bereavement, the child is in need of a parent who can provide the child
with the support and warm companionship he or she requires. Clearly,
when the mother is distressed and confused regarding her new role,
acts inconsistently, and displays helplessness, excessive self-pity, and
exaggerated dependence on her environment, the child's anxiety and
dependence needs increase.

Particularly in the case of children considered to be at high risk after the father's death, it is necessary to determine whether the mother is dealing with her own mourning process in a manner that prevents healing and raises obstacles in the process of recovery for herself and her child. To this end, we suggest meeting alone with the grieving mother to evaluate her daily functioning and adaptation to the loss. The clinician should explore the presence of encumbering emotional problems such as depressive features, interminable yearning for the lost figure, persistent blame, anger, or remorse. It is also useful to help the mother deal with any guilt feelings she might have over the right to enjoy pleasures of life and to plan future life, including the possibility of remarriage.

Among the possible mourning responses of the mother that are likely to be associated with "pathological bereavement" in the child are the following patterns:

- The mother may display an avoidance pattern characterized by extreme withdrawal and reluctance to communicate with her children in regard to her husband's death and the meaning that the loss has for her.
- The mother may experience protracted mourning, including total helplessness and active resistance in coming to terms with the reality and the inevitable consequences of the loss. Such resistance may involve actively perpetuating grief and perceiving the deceased partner as an object for idealization and worship while struggling actively against the normal process of "decathexis."

Both styles of maladjusted response have negative implications for the entire family. Clearly, the therapist must try to encourage the mother's return as quickly as possible to a normal daily routine that will replace the constant brooding over her pain and distress.

In cases of protracted mourning, we generally make use of other widows who can serve as a positive model of successful coping with their own traumatic experiences. In some cases professional intervention with the whole family may be necessary in order to restore disturbed hierarchical relationships. Frequently some of the mother's central functions are transferred to some other family members, and we have often seen a "parental child" acting as a mother-substitute, with pathogenic consequences for the mother and the child himself or herself, as well as for the siblings. We have found that in some cases major depressive reactions, even when they occur in the context of bereavement, may respond well to antidepressant medication in the context of comprehensive therapy.

The existence of a "substitute parent" and extended support systems.   Our findings indicate that it is helpful to encourage the child's bonding with an adult figure who can serve as an object for positive identification. In this effort, we do not aim for a transfer of love and devotion, but instead aim for the satisfaction of a developmental need of the young child. The availability of an extended family that provides several figures with whom the child can develop a satisfying bond reinforces the child's feelings of belonging and security and reduces his or her anxieties regarding the continuation of the family framework. Equally important, bonds of this sort may act as a counterweight to the close and sometimes overdependent bond between the bereaved child and his or her mother. In this regard, it is worth noting the importance of cooperation and coordination between the various systems involved in caring for the child. We observed that friction, competition, and conflicts between the surviving parent, grandparents, and educational staff added to the child's stress and aggravated his or her general condition.

Avoidance of additional separations and secondary stress situations.   As was described earlier, a stable framework that provides for the child's essential physical and emotional needs is a prerequisite for his or her successful coping with the crisis. A prolonged separation from the surviving parent or other significant figure, or a change in the location of home or attendance at a different school, adds to the anxieties of the child and diminishes the chances of his or her successful adjustment to the new reality. Very often in the early stages of bereavement, the widow feels the need for a new start or a change in her life circumstances. In such a case it is necessary to reduce the stress by proper preparation and explanation of the intended change to the child.

The Later Stage: The Third and Fourth Years of Bereavement

The growing child has to learn new social roles that strengthen feelings of autonomy. The existence of extrafamilial frameworks, such as school, the social peer group, and youth movements, can help the child to reorganize his or her life within the context of a new reality. In many cases, such supportive frameworks may provide external "compensation" and balance to the problematic nature and instability of some bereaved families. Educators, counselors, and other members of the community can assume an active role in assisting the bereaved child. We found that, with guidance and encouragement, the teachers in our sample were willing to cooperate in the therapeutic program and were ready to plan out specific activities for the improvement of the child's social integration.

General Preventive Work

Bereavement reactions of children are very strongly influenced by the social attitudes relating to the subject of "death" and by the nature of their previous encounter with death. Imposing a taboo on the subject, as well as protecting the child from an encounter with death (e.g., when coming across a dead animal, approaching a cemetery, meeting a friend affected by a family member's death) is detrimental to the child.

The Israeli reality, in which sudden death in the family is unfortunately not an unusual event, demands the preparation of the child for the contingency that he or she may have to cope with this problem. In recent years efforts have been made to develop general preventive techniques that prepare children in the event that this crisis should strike in their homes. Educators and other professionals can contribute in this preventive effort by preparing activity programs that help the child understand the meaning of death, as well as other distressing events such as war, separation, illness, and bereavement, as part of the world in which we live (Ayalon 1983).

One must remember that the loss of a parent is at all times a traumatic situation for the child. Whenever a bereaved child exhibits throughout a period of several months emotional difficulties, such as symptoms of insecurity and anxiety, marked aggressiveness, or regressive and overdependent behavior, professional advice and help are required. Hence, it is clear that in our view, although not all bereaved children may need regular treatment, some type of short-term psychological counseling or family therapy may be recommended. In all cases, however, adequate preventive measures and assistance to the at-risk bereaved child and his or her family, as well as the judicious use of community resources and social support networks, have been found to be invaluable in preventing psychological disturbance of a prolonged and severe nature.

Conclusions

For the bereaved preadolescent child, the degree of vulnerability and the severity of the bereavement process appear to be related not only to the specific reactions to loss and trauma but, to a great extent, to the baseline pretraumatic conditions, the quality of the surviving parent's responses, and the availability of a supportive and stable family and environment.

In our clinical practice, as well as in our follow-up studies, we have found no evidence to support theoretical assumptions that children react to the death of a parent according to a fixed pattern of sequential stages. Our research studies indicate that there is no definite prototype of childhood bereavement, but rather a wide range of individual patterns regarding the timing, quality, duration, and intensity of the grief and behavioral responses. Thus psychological impairment may appear immediately following the loss, or it may be delayed, appearing even a year or two after the traumatic event. It may be brief or extended, and can find expression consistently or during intermittent symptomatic periods. For this reason, a single or a short-term assessment of behavioral adjustment is not sufficient to draw conclusions about the overall quality and severity of the child's responses to the death of the parent. The symptomatic bereaved child may display one clear cluster or combined clusters of symptoms, particularly externalized acting out, internalized anxiety with basic insecurity, and/or regressive age-inadequate behavior. Although about 40% of the bereaved children in our follow-up studies showed evidence of "pathological bereavement," it should be stressed that among the remaining bereaved children in the study sample, over one-third did not exhibit any significant emotional difficulties during a follow-up period of 4 years.

In conclusion, it can be assumed that for a large proportion of children, the death of a parent at an early age is a serious traumatic event, and even those children who before the loss did not show any signs of maladjustment can be seen as "at risk." This vulnerability is particularly acute throughout the first year of bereavement. During the subsequent 2 to 3 years, there is a considerable reduction in the extent and intensity of affective grief reactions, although for many bereaved children the behavioral and emotional symptoms endure through the fourth postbereavement year. The common assumption that "time heals all" does not always hold true, and in the case of bereavement in preadolescence, adopting such a view may result in one's refraining from seeking psychological intervention for children at critical stages of the first 3 years after death of a parent.

References

American Psychiatric Association: Diagnostic and Statistical Manual of Mental Disorders, 3rd Edition, Revised. Washington, DC, American Psychiatric Association, 1987

Ayalon O: Precarious balance: coping with stress in the family (Hebrew). Tel Aviv, Sifriat Poalim, 1983

Birtchnell J: Women whose mothers died in childhood. Psychol Med 10:699–713, 1980

Bowlby J: Grief and mourning in infancy and early childhood. Psychoanal Study Child 15:9–20, 1960

Bowlby J: Attachment and Loss, Vol 2: Separation. New York, Basic Books, 1973

Bowlby J: Attachment and Loss, Vol 3: Loss, Sadness and Depression. New York, Basic Books, 1980

Deutsch H: The absence of grief. Psychoanal Q 6:12–22, 1937

Elizur E, Kaffman M: Children's bereavement reactions following death of the father (II). Journal of the American Academy of Child Psychiatry 5:474–480, 1982

Elizur E, Kaffman M: Factors influencing the severity of childhood bereavement reactions. Am J Orthopsychiatry 53:668–676, 1983

Furman E: A Child's Parent Dies. New Haven, CT, Yale University Press, 1974

Graham P, Rutter M: The reliability and validity of the psychiatric assessment of the child. Br J Psychiatry 114:581–592, 1968

Gregory Y: Retrospective data following childhood loss of a parent. Arch Gen Psychiatry 15:354–368, 1966

Kaffman M: Characteristics of the emotional pathology of the kibbutz child. Am J Orthopsychiatry 42:692–709, 1972

Kaffman M: Kibbutz civilian population under war stress. Br J Psychiatry 130:489–494, 1977

Kaffman M, Elizur E: Infants who become enuretics: a longitudinal study of 161 kibbutz children. Monogr Soc Res Child Dev, Vol 42, Ser No 170, 1977

Kaffman M, Elizur E: Children's bereavement reactions following death of the father. International Journal of Family Therapy 1:203–229, 1979

Kaffman M, Elizur E: Bereavement responses of kibbutz and non-kibbutz children following the death of the father. J Child Psychol Psychiatry 24:435–442, 1983

Kendler K, Neals M, Kessler R, et al: Childhood parental loss and adult psychopathology in women: a twin study perspective. Arch Gen Psychiatry 49:109–116, 1992

Kranzler E, Shaffer D, Wasserman G, et al: Early childhood bereavement. J Am Acad Child Adolesc Psychiatry 29:513–520, 1990

Krupnick J: Bereavement during childhood and adolescence, in Bereavement: Reactions, Consequences and Care: A Report by the Institute of Medicine, National Academy of Sciences. Edited by Osterweis M, Solomon F, Green M. Washington, DC, National Academy Press, 1984, pp 99–141

Krupnick J, Solomon F: Death of a parent or sibling during childhood, in The Psychology of Separation and Loss. Edited by Bloom-Feshbach J, Bloom-Feshbach S, and Associates. San Francisco, CA, Jossey-Bass, 1987, pp 345–374

Lloyd C: Life events and depression disorders reviewed: events of predisposing factors. Arch Gen Psychiatry 37:529–535, 1980

Luthar S, Zigler E: Vulnerability and competence. Am J Orthopsychiatry 61:6–21, 1991

Meichenbaum D: Stress Inoculation Training. New York, Pergamon, 1985

Nagera G: Children's reactions to the death of important objects. Psychoanal Study Child 25:360–400, 1970

Ochberg F: Post-traumatic therapy. Psychotherapy: Research, Theory and Practice 28:5–15, 1991

Osterweis M, Solomon F, Green M (eds): Bereavement: Reactions, Consequences and Care: A Report by the Institute of Medicine, National Academy of Sciences. Washington, DC, National Academy Press, 1984

Pollack P, Egan D, Vandenbergh R, et al: Prevention in mental health: a study. Am J Psychiatry 132:146–149, 1975

Raphael B: The Anatomy of Bereavement. New York, Basic Books, 1983

Sanford M, Offord D, Boyle M, et al: Ontario Child Health Study: social and school impairments in children aged 6 to 16 years. J Am Acad Child Adolesc Psychiatry 31:60–67, 1992

Tennand C, Bebbington P, Hurry J: Parental death in childhood and risk of adult depressive disorders: a review. Psychol Med 10:289–299, 1980

Thomas A, Chess S: Temperament and Development. New York, Brunner/Mazel, 1977

Weller E, Weller R: Grief, in Child and Adolescent Psychiatry: A Comprehensive Textbook. Edited by Lewis M. Baltimore, MD, Williams & Wilkins, 1991, pp 389–393

Wolfenstein M: Rage and repetition. Psychoanal Study Child 23:433–456, 1968

Epilogue

Implications for Clinical Practice and Research

Peter E. Tanguay, M.D.

In her introduction to this volume, Pfeffer, as editor, set a goal of revealing the important studies of the past two decades on the subject of the effects of acute and chronic stress on children's mental and emotional development. She and the other authors of this work have succeeded in giving us a rich overview of this important subject. Most chapters are written by the individuals who are themselves immersed in the experimental work of which they speak. Because of this, their knowledge is both timely and, often, encyclopedic. My task in this epilogue is to look back on the endeavor and attempt to intuit what is needed in the next decade if the field is to advance with efficiency. Put another way: How might a young investigator begin to plan a career in the field of stress research? Where should he or she begin? What wise counsels should he or she follow in planning a career of research? What has already "taken off" in the field? What is ready to take off?

It should be noted that this book does not solely present research findings, hypotheses, and models. Several chapters in the book, notably Eth's chapter on a developmental–interactional model of child abuse (Chapter 18) and Bingham and Harmon's chapter on the putative effects of early stress on infant development (Chapter 19), are presentations that I expect will be appreciated by persons primarily engaged in clinical evaluation and treatment. Eth's developmental–interactional model draws on the ideas of investigators such as Bowlby, Mahler, Anna Freud, and Ainsworth, and on the more recent observations of Terr and a small number of other clinicians who have described individual cases or groups of cases in their publications. The observations are primarily clinical, initially without use of structured instruments or more rigorous methodology. Ainsworth, of course, did develop a very structured approach to studying children, which itself has led to exciting work on attachment theory, but the latter is less a focus of the chapter by Eth. What we have in these two chapters are good clinical insights and a theoretical vantage point from which to understand them.

What is very exciting in this book is the demonstration of how well some aspects of the field of stress research are progressing, or how some parts are ready to advance. To continue the example invoked above, a young investigator, if he or she has not come up through the doctoral and postdoctoral path, but has instead followed the medical degree and residency path, should seriously consider taking a research fellowship. And he or she should choose an expert, the world's best expert if possible, to serve as mentor during that fellowship. Many of the authors whose work appears in this book are such experts. Suomi's studies of the effects of stress on primates (summarized by Higley and Suomi in Chapter 1) qualify him and his colleagues as exemplary mentors to anyone wishing to approach the study of the effects of stress from this viewpoint. Teicher and colleagues' ingenious application of clinical neurophysiological technology to the study of possible CNS changes resulting from severe stress (Chapter 2) would indicate that the senior members of their group could serve as excellent mentors for such work. Pynoos (Chapter 6) has developed one of the most rigorous approaches to studying acute and chronic stress. Mrazek and Klinnert's approach to the study of the effects of stress on children at risk for asthma (Chapter 7) is another model to emulate. Pfeffer, in her work on suicide (Chapter 12), and Brent and colleagues, in their studies of the effect of suicide on siblings (Chapter 13), use methods that are important tools to others who wish to pursue studies of stress and depression. Stuber and Houskamp's studies of the ramifications of the traumatic effect of "heroic" medical treatments for cancer or organ failure (Chapter 9) are unique in the field of child psychiatry. Putnam (see Hornstein and Putnam, Chapter 17) is a pioneer in the field of multiple personality disorder (dissociative identity disorder). All of the above individuals, as well as many of the authors in this volume, could be excellent mentors for anyone wishing to develop his or her career as a research investigator.

At the Intersection of Two Fields

Another observation that should be noted by beginning investigators is that many of the most important advances come not from within a field of research, but at the intersection of separate fields. One example, of some personal interest to me, is the manner in which our understanding of autism, which had come to somewhat of a impasse in the early 1980s, was subsequently advanced by new information that flowed from the fields of developmental psychology and developmental linguistics. The latter gave rise to a new understanding of "social communication" and its several specific domains, while the former provided additional information about the development of social interactions in infancy. Both have led to an entirely new view of autism and to new projects designed to expand this understanding. Another example, drawn from this book, is the manner in which work on attachment theory by Bowlby, Ainsworth, and Sroufe has been itself informed by Harlow's work with primates who have suffered maternal deprivation.

Even more to the point for one of the major interests of this book, work on the effects of stress trauma must be informed from the considerable work that has been done in the past two decades in cognitive research and in memory research. This work is alluded to in the chapters on posttraumatic stress disorder (PTSD) and on trauma, with several references to key articles on the subject. Desimone (1992) has summarized some of the recent findings. There are numerous memory systems, which are defined behaviorally or psychologically. One class of memory system underlies *declarative memory,* or *explicit memory* (i.e., memories of facts and events). These memories can be retrieved as conscious entities, though they are subject to continual reworking with time. Even the very act of recalling and discussing them can change their content. Within the class of declarative memory one can distinguish short-term memory from long-term memory. There are numerous material-specific systems in declarative memory, such as memory for faces, words, objects, and so on. In contrast to declarative memory, *nondeclarative memory,* or *implicit memory,* includes stimulus-response memory, habits, perceptual learning, conditioning, cognitive and motor skills, various types of priming, and habituation. It is possible that when one is under conditions of extreme stress, memories may be encoded as perceptual memories that may be unaccessible to the retrieval processes of declarative memory. If this were so, then one would not need to invoke "repression" to understand the unavailability of some traumatic memories, but would see these memories as representing a different type of memory from the start.

Experimental studies of memory must be studied by anyone wishing to work in stress research in humans. Pynoos (Chapter 6) and Hornstein and Putnam (Chapter 17) are well aware of this necessity and have taken into account in their chapters the insights gained from this work. The field of memory research will continue to expand, and future investigators will likely find that this research will be vital to the interpretation of their results.

Sweetening the Pot

There is another very important lesson to be learned from the work described in this book: If one wishes to study a particular phenomenon, such as the effects of stress on mental and emotional symptoms, it is very important to study those persons who are most likely to show such effects in a clearly unequivocal manner. Fornari and colleagues' study of the victims of an air disaster (Chapter 5) is an obvious example of this approach, as is Pynoos' study of the victims of severe trauma and abuse (Chapter 6).

In a similar vein, Kaffman and Elizur (Chapter 22) chose to focus their work on children who had lost fathers during the Yom Kippur War. The trauma was acute, and the event was recent enough at the time of their studies that they were able to study the manner in which environmental factors played a role in mitigating or exacerbating the child's response. Their findings challenged the findings of previous studies of bereavement, many of which had been carried out retrospectively, one or more years after the child's loss. There can be no substitute for immediate observation of the effects of stress combined with the use of good instruments.

Mrazek and Klinnert's chapter (Chapter 7) on the effects of stress on asthma is another excellent example of a longitudinal, prospective approach to the study of stress. The authors had noted that when children with asthma became anxious, they would develop a sudden sensation of tightening in the chest. To study the effects of stress on asthma, the authors recruited children prenatally who were *at risk* for asthma because one or both of their parents were asthmatic. In addition, they developed a model in which stress was defined in specific terms: a situation in which the mother's ability to parent was impaired by her being in a chronically unhappy marriage that resulted in maternal depression. They also defined stress as a situation in which maternal disinterest, insensitivity, or lack of knowledge about appropriate infant care might be expected to lead to poor infant care. The authors developed a method for assessing the latter risk at three points: during pregnancy, at the time of birth, and at 3 months of age. The method was not developed de novo, but was based on a lifetime of research carried out by Yarrow and her colleagues at the National Institutes of Health.[1] The authors found a strong association between their hypothesized risk factor and the development of asthma. How to interpret this finding, they noted, is less clear. The line of study that they are pursuing appears to be a robust one, and I expect they (and perhaps others as well) will tackle this question next.

Development of Models and Hypotheses

The models that one uses in research are of singular importance: they not only help determine what we look for, but control what we are likely to find and what we make of it. Some of the best models may be derived from animal studies. The chapter by Meaney and colleagues on hypothalamic-pituitary-adrenal axis stress responses (Chapter 3) is a superb example of such model building and should be required reading for all investigators of stress in humans. Likewise, the chapter by Bartlett and colleagues (Chapter 8) serves a similar role in presenting an overview of the experimental studies of the effects of stress on the immune system in humans.

Several models used by the various authors of other chapters are more global in nature, to the extent that they allow a wide array of observations made from a number of viewpoints to be included in an understanding of stress and its effects. The *ecological model,* described by Kaplan and Pinner (Chapter 15), and the *developmental–interactional model,* used by Eth (Chapter 18), are examples of the

---

[1] A point on the subject of instrument development: Try to use instruments that build on others' work if possible. The development of a good instrument can take years or even a decade or more, and any short-cut will get one to the point of being able to start one's research study as quickly as possible.

more global variety of models. Kaplan and Pinner view child abuse as a manifestation of parental vulnerabilities (secondary to mental illness, substance abuse, etc.) and child vulnerabilities (low birth weight, difficult temperament, etc.) interacting with social stressors (poverty, lack of social supports, etc.) to bring about the abuse. Various additional risk factors are considered: single parenthood, minority status, lack of acculturation, four or more children in the family, and young parental age. As was noted earlier, Eth draws on the ideas of Bowlby, Mahler, Anna Freud, and Ainsworth, and on the more recent observations of Terr and a small number of other clinicians who have described individual cases or groups of cases in the literature. As was also noted earlier, use of such a model leads to development of rich clinical descriptive material that fits broad theoretical vistas.

The *stress diathesis* model used by Pfeffer (Chapter 12) and by Brent and colleagues (Chapter 13) is also a global one. In this model, stress is described as a transactional process involving a system of interdependent variables that mutually influence one another. It is a process involving bidirectional relationships between a person with unique characteristics and an environment with particular features. These relationships are stressful if they overwhelm a person's resources and endanger his or her well-being. This viewpoint may permit a more global understanding of the phenomenon of stress, but may make it more difficult to quantify stress in terms of specific events and outcomes. Brent and colleagues are quite precise in their use of the model: some individuals are vulnerable to depression because of biological and psychological factors, but depressive symptoms emerge only after the person has experienced stress. The model is used to generate a hypothesis—that suicide of a friend could lead to increase in either depression or suicidal behavior in an individual—that was rigorously tested by Brent and colleagues and that resulted in two findings: suicidal behavior did not increase, but the incidence of depression did.

A last example of a more global model is given in Hajal's chapter on adoption (Chapter 20). The model, organized around the family life cycle outline of McGoldrick and Carter, is the *developmental lifestyle model*, which focuses "the unique developmental tasks that confront adopted children and adolescents and their families." As with most of the more global models, there is considerable future opportunity for investigators to begin to test the theoretical constructs underlying the models. Such work will require more precise specification of the variables of interest, and measurement of how they interact.

The *PTSD model,* used by Pynoos (Chapter 6), Stuber and Houskamp (Chapter 9), and Kazak and Christakis (Chapter 10) in their respective chapters is more precise and lends itself more easily to study. The model postulates that various specific acute or chronic trauma or stress leads to the development of a specific set of symptoms that constitute PTSD, as defined in DSM-IV (American Psychiatric Association 1994). The manner in which these symptoms occur and change with treatment or with specific events (such as experiencing reminders of the trauma) has been well documented by these investigators. Pynoos's work is an exemplary account of good stress research; it takes into account a number of important rules already discussed. Pynoos studied victims of fairly severe trauma; he developed a special interview instrument, tallied symptoms, and developed models that described types of response to severe trauma, how these varied with level of development, and how intervention itself becomes part of the experience of dealing with trauma. He also developed specific models of treatment, doing so in a cost-efficient manner that reflected the observation that there appear to be stages in the development of responses to trauma. Pynoos's work is based on careful observation. He has even taken persons who have been traumatized and studied their specific neurobiological responses. The neurophysiological variables he studied in this work were chosen on the basis of previous evidence that they might be disturbed as a result of trauma. He studied the manner in which the circumstances of the trauma affect outcome. Based on his findings, he introduced the notions of *traumatic reminders* and *secondary stressors.* Pynoos's work illustrates the degree to which long-term, intensive study, in which methods derived from the best work of others are carried out in a careful, informed, and logical fashion, can lead to important advances in knowledge.

Stuber's overall work on the stress of certain invasive medical procedures on children adds the dimension of temperament to the PTSD model. Temperamental differences (in which genetic factors may play a role) seem to partly determine the individual child's response to the stressful medical treatments. Stuber's meticulous work raises the question of whether there needs to be a redefinition of the symptoms of PTSD for use with traumatized patients.

Although the study of the role of diabetes as a stressor in children may not be as advanced as the study of the role of asthma as a stressor,

Garrison's thoughtful review (Chapter 11) of current studies of diabetes as a stressor suggests that this field, much like the field of asthma research, in which advances have been made by Mrazek and other investigators, is ready to develop. Garrison points out that observations have been made on the manner in which various factors may mitigate stress responses of children and adolescents to the onset of diabetes. Children who are knowledgeable about diabetes may be better able to cope. Whether children use and emotion-focused or problem-focused approach to their illness may also affect outcome. Temperament may predict how a child will respond to diabetes. These and other hypotheses have been advanced; they seem plausible but require more study. Any one could be the jumping-off point for a focused project.

Development of Research Instruments

Additional caveats are important to the beginning investigator: you must develop precise methods to diagnose subjects (or to select them on the basis of some defining characteristic), and you must acquire the best instruments for measuring the phenomenon (phenomena) of interest. Several chapters in this book provide excellent examples of research instruments that have proved important. Some of these instruments have been developed and perfected over many years. Hetherington, Wallerstein, Emery, and others (whose work is summarized in Brody and Neubaum's chapter on the effects of divorce on children and adolescents [Chapter 21]) have perfected a set of interviews useful for the study of children whose parents have divorced. These instruments have permitted investigators to reach a number of clinically important conclusions, especially about the different effects of divorce on young children and adolescents, including how these effects differ between boys and girls.

Pfeffer's chapter is one of several in which life-event scales are employed as a means of estimating stress. Scales such as these are quantifiable and can be used to identify the times at which stress may have reached a peak. Many investigators have used these scales successfully with adult subjects, but there is less experience in the use of these scales with children. Such a situation should be seen as yet another opportunity for some enterprising young academic to get to work.

Clark and Goebel, in their chapter (Chapter 14), describe another instrument, the Adolescent Grief Inventory (AGI). The AGI was found to be useful in the measurement of an adolescent's responses to the suicide of a friend or sibling. The authors described the careful way in which they used multiple raters to increase the reliability of items and then employed a principal components analysis to identify the important factors that characterized grief reactions in adolescents. At least two of the four factors that Clark and Goebel identified had some resemblance to symptoms described as characteristic of PTSD. A secondary lesson to be learned from this is that good instruments are not usually developed using a casual approach.

Good instruments take long effort and time to develop, and a willingness to throw out what does not work and try again. Pynoos's work is an even more impressive example of how rigorous attention to details leads to quality work. Like several other authors in this book, Pynoos studied victims of severe trauma. As noted earlier, he developed a special interview instrument and tallied symptoms; he then developed models that described types of response to severe trauma and how these responses varied with level of development. He studied how intervention affected his patients and itself became part of the recovery experience. Based on his findings, Pynoos developed, in a cost-efficient manner, specific models of treatment that reflect the stages in the usual response to trauma. His work has always been based on careful observation combined with the use of good instruments. More recently, Pynoos and his colleagues have extended their initial observations about the signs and symptoms of trauma in children and adolescents. Taking into consideration the symptoms of PTSD, he chose to study two neurophysiological phenomena: the startle response and disturbances in the electroencephalographic architecture of sleep. His findings are ready to be even more fully taken forward by others, though I expect we will be seeing more excellent work from Pynoos himself.

Multiple Personality Disorder: Ripe for Systematic Research

Kluft (Chapter 16) and Hornstein and Putnam (Chapter 17), in their respective chapters, provide us with an in-depth overview of multiple personality disorder (MPD). In 1943, MPD was declared nonexistent, but in the 1980s it returned to clinical awareness. The subject is controversial, but the opportunities for advancing our knowledge of this disorder and developing effective treatments are great. What has happened in the field of PTSD must happen in the field of MPD. Several rating instruments for measurement of the clinical characteristics of MPD have been developed, but more are needed. Kluft lists numerous models, and some of the more plausible ones must be studied. The field is ripe for reinterpretation of its hypotheses through information from the fields of cognitive sciences and memory research. There is also the opportunity to begin to define treatment more precisely, especially in terms of stages in treatment and specific methods used, much as Pynoos and others have begun to do in the case of PTSD. The field may be chaotic and controversial, but from such beginnings much good may come.

Treatment

Whether cognitive behavioral, psychodynamic, psychopharmacological, or family oriented, treatment of stress-related disorders must be based on the specific nature of stress (whether it is associated with acute or chronic trauma, whether it is secondary to the suicide of one's sibling, whether it is secondary to one's having cancer) and on the signs and symptoms that result. Pynoos and his colleagues (Chapter 6) have outlined the nature of one approach, involving focused interventions at various points in time, including initial psychological first aid, brief therapy, and, later, pulsed interventions and long-term therapy. The ecological family systems perspective of Kazak (Chapter 10) suggests ways in which family therapy interventions could be built upon her model. Haizlip and Corder (Chapter 4) suggest some very practical ideas aimed at helping large numbers of children and adolescents who are affected by natural disasters such as tornados and floods. Extension of their ideas to earthquake preparedness would be a logical step. As more becomes known about stress and its effects, more specific approaches will be identified and tested.

Even as this is being done, however, future investigators will do well to consider a related issue, namely the observation that much of the public seems to hold the view that the effects of stress may not be serious, or that if the effects are serious, the stressor will soon "be forgotten" by children and the immediate effects do not require treatment. This view is implicit, for example, in the reluctance of some of the parent survivors of the Avianca crash to maintain their children in treatment, even for a short period of time (see Chapter 5). Many parents who were among the hurricane survivors described by Haizlip and Corder (see Chapter 4) denied that the disaster would have any lasting effects on the children and did not bring their children for evaluation or help. Even such fundamental issues as recognition of the symptoms of trauma may be largely outside of the knowledge of many people. I recall my own anecdotal experience around this issue: I was at a dinner party with friends whom I had known for years. One woman had 4 months earlier been trapped in a department store fire with her children, and they had all barely escaped. She told me, reluctantly at first, of some strange symptoms she was having, which she feared might mean she was going out of her mind. Her symptoms were those of acute PTSD. She had never heard of PTSD, and the thought that what she was experiencing might be treatable had never crossed her mind. Knowing that what she was experiencing had been described in others made a major difference to this woman and led to treatment and resolution of her acute symptoms.

Conclusions

That this book has even been written is an indication of the rising interest on the part of mental health specialists in the psychological manifestations of stress. Like many developing fields, stress research is in a state of uncertainty and, occasionally, overcertainty. Now is the time for scientific rigor and careful work. Investigators must attend to the need for more precise definitions and diagnostic terminology. Animal studies should be closely tied to human models. Models should be testable, and should be tested. Clinicians must become aware of the major advances made in the scientific understanding of human memory and how these findings can be used to develop better human models for the effects of stress. Public health planners must be less dismissive about the long-term effects of severe stress on human lives. The subject of treatment must be addressed with vigor and candor: what works in the various forms of psychotherapy, and are there useful adjunctive psychopharmacological treatments? Models should be made explicit and should be studied as to their usefulness. In some areas of research, especially in that on PTSD, the work is well on its way to meeting the above goals. In other areas, such as the traumatic effects of medical interventions, and in the more contro-versial field of multiple personality disorder, the time seems ripe to launch some very productive work. When the sequel to this book is written, in another decade or so, it will be exciting to hear what has developed.

References

American Psychiatric Association: Diagnostic and Statistical Manual of Mental Disorders, 4th Edition. Washington, DC, American Psychiatric Association, 1994

Desimone R: The physiology of memory: recordings of things past. Science 258:245–246, 1992

Index

*Page numbers printed in **boldface** type refer to tables or figures.*